Designed for the maintenance of good nutrition of practically

all healthy people in the United States

Water-Soluble Vitamins / **Minerals**

Vita-min C (mg)	Thia-min (mg)	Ribo-flavin (mg)	Niacin (mg NE)[f]	Vita-min B₆ (mg)	Fo-late (µg)	Vita-min B₁₂ (µg)	Cal-cium (mg)	Phos-phorus (mg)	Mag-nesium (mg)	Iron (mg)	Zinc (mg)	Iodine (µg)	Sele-nium (µg)
30	0.3	0.4	5	0.3	25	0.3	400	300	40	6	5	40	10
35	0.4	0.5	6	0.6	35	0.5	600	500	60	10	5	50	15
40	0.7	0.8	9	1.0	50	0.7	800	800	80	10	10	70	20
45	0.9	1.1	12	1.1	75	1.0	800	800	120	10	10	90	20
45	1.0	1.2	13	1.4	100	1.4	800	800	170	10	10	120	30
50	1.3	1.5	17	1.7	150	2.0	1,200	1,200	270	12	15	150	40
60	1.5	1.8	20	2.0	200	2.0	1,200	1,200	400	12	15	150	50
60	1.5	1.7	19	2.0	200	2.0	1,200	1,200	350	10	15	150	70
60	1.5	1.7	19	2.0	200	2.0	800	800	350	10	15	150	70
60	1.2	1.4	15	2.0	200	2.0	800	800	350	10	15	150	70
50	1.1	1.3	15	1.4	150	2.0	1,200	1,200	280	15	12	150	45
60	1.1	1.3	15	1.5	180	2.0	1,200	1,200	300	15	12	150	50
60	1.1	1.3	15	1.6	180	2.0	1,200	1,200	280	15	12	150	55
60	1.1	1.3	15	1.6	180	2.0	800	800	280	15	12	150	55
60	1.0	1.2	13	1.6	180	2.0	800	800	280	10	12	150	55
70	1.5	1.6	17	2.2	400	2.2	1,200	1,200	300	30	15	175	65
95	1.6	1.8	20	2.1	280	2.6	1,200	1,200	355	15	19	200	75
90	1.6	1.7	20	2.1	260	2.6	1,200	1,200	340	15	16	200	75

[c] Retinol equivalents. 1 retinol equivalent = 1 µg retinol or 6 µg β-carotene.

[d] As cholecalciferol. 10 µg cholecalciferol = 400 IU of vitamin D.

[e] α-Tocopherol equivalents. 1 mg d-α tocopherol = 1 α-TE.

[f] 1 NE (niacin equivalent) is equal to 1 mg of niacin or 60 mg of dietary tryptophan.

Estimated Safe and Adequate Daily Dietary Intakes of Selected Vitamins and Minerals[a]

		Vitamins	
Category	Age (years)	Biotin (µg)	Pantothenic Acid (mg)
Infants	0–0.5	10	2
	0.5–1	15	3
Children and adolescents	1–3	20	3
	4–6	25	3–4
	7–10	30	4–5
	11 +	30–100	4–7
Adults		30–100	4–7

		Trace Elements[b]				
Category	Age (years)	Copper (mg)	Man-ganese (mg)	Fluoride (mg)	Chromium (µg)	Molybdenum (µg)
Infants	0–0.5	0.4–0.6	0.3–0.6	0.1–0.5	10–40	15–30
	0.5–1	0.6–0.7	0.6–1.0	0.2–1.0	20–60	20–40
Children and adolescents	1–3	0.7–1.0	1.0–1.5	0.5–1.5	20–80	25–50
	4–6	1.0–1.5	1.5–2.0	1.0–2.5	30–120	30–75
	7–10	1.0–2.0	2.0–3.0	1.5–2.5	50–200	50–150
	11 +	1.5–2.5	2.0–5.0	1.5–2.5	50–200	75–250
Adults		1.5–3.0	2.0–5.0	1.5–4.0	50–200	75–250

[a] Because there is less information on which to base allowances, these figures are not given in the main table of RDA and are provided here in the form of ranges of recommended intakes.

[b] Since the toxic levels for many trace elements may be only several times usual intakes, the upper levels for the trace elements given in this table should not be habitually exceeded.

NUTRITION THROUGHOUT THE LIFE CYCLE

NUTRITION THROUGHOUT THE LIFE CYCLE

Edited by

BONNIE S. WORTHINGTON-ROBERTS, MS, PhD

Professor, Nutritional Sciences Program; Nutritionist, Child Development and Mental Retardation Center, University of Washington, Seattle, Washington

SUE RODWELL WILLIAMS, PhD, MPH, RD

President, SRW Productions, Inc.; Clinical Nutrition Consultant, Davis, California; Formerly Metabolic Nutritionist, Kaiser-Permanente Northern California Regional Medical Center, Oakland, California; Field Faculty, M.P.H.-Dietetic Internship Program and Coordinated Undergraduate Program in Dietetics, University of California, Berkeley, California

Coauthors

ELEANOR D. SCHLENKER, PhD, RD

Professor and Department Head, Human Nutrition and Foods, The College of Human Resources, Virginia Polytechnic Institute and State University, Blacksburg, Virginia

PEGGY PIPES, MS, RD

Assistant Chief, Nutrition Section, Clinical Training Unit, Child Development and Mental Retardation Center, University of Washington, Seattle, Washington

CRISTINE M. TRAHMS, MS, RD, FADA

Chief Nutritionist, Clinical Training Unit, Child Development and Mental Retardation Center; Lecturer, Department of Pediatrics and Nutritional Sciences Program, University of Washington, Seattle, Washington

THIRD EDITION
with 92 illustrations

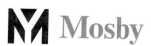
Mosby

St. Louis Baltimore Boston Carlsbad Chicago Naples New York Philadelphia Portland
London Madrid Mexico City Singapore Sydney Tokyo Toronto Wiesbaden

Vice President and Publisher: James M. Smith
Senior Acquisitions Editor: Vicki Malinee
Managing Editor: Janet R. Livingston
Assistant Editor: Jennifer L. Hartman
Project Manager: Carol Sullivan Weis
Production Editor: Karen Rehwinkel
Designer: Renée Duenow
Manufacturing Supervisor: Linda Ierardi
Cover Illustration: Jason Dowd

THIRD EDITION

Copyright © 1996 by The McGraw-Hill Companies, Inc.
Previous editions copyrighted 1988, 1992

Printed in the United States of America
Composition by Graphic World, Inc.
Printing/binding by Maple Vail Book Manufacturing Group

International Standard Book Number 0-8151-9427-7

95 96 97 98 99 / 9 8 7 6 5 4 3 2 1

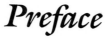

Preface

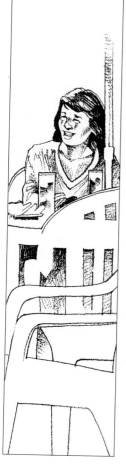

*T*he third edition of *Nutrition Throughout the Life Cycle* clearly and accurately presents the major special nutrition issues common at different periods of the life cycle. Our goal is to provide for students, teachers, and practitioners a unified view of the life cycle as a whole, with each life cycle stage supported by the nutrition foundations that are essential for positive development.

The perspective of interdependence in the life cycle has become increasingly significant in today's modern world as the lifespan has lengthened but, for many persons, not improved in quality. The quality of a lengthened life, genetically programmed from conception but dependent on a nourishing environment for fulfillment of this genetic potential, builds at each stage upon all past and present life experiences.

Our environment is rapidly changing and affecting individual lives in many ways, some of which are not always beneficial. In the midst of these changes is an increasing awareness that nutritional needs — so fundamental to human growth and development — do not exist in a vacuum. At each life stage nutritional needs are always interwoven with many other personal, socioeconomic, and cultural factors that make up the whole of life and influence positive growth and development and health in both subtle and obvious ways.

OBJECTIVES OF THE BOOK

This text is designed to meet the needs of a broad spectrum of students, with varying degrees of nutrition backgrounds, in courses in life cycle nutrition and for health professionals who work in both individual and community health programs. The text approaches nutrition from a basic developmental approach, maintaining a person-centered view of individual integrity. It presents nutrition needs on the basis of both physical growth and psychosocial development. It focuses throughout on positive health, for which nutrition provides a fundamental foundation.

SPECIAL FEATURES OF THIS TEXT

Throughout all its chapters, this text is distinctive in its breadth of topics discussed, comprehensive research base, and many practical and helpful applications to meet individual and group situations. References bring current scientific knowledge to a variety of modern situations and problems. Students can then further apply this knowledge to needs they discover for themselves. We provide a basis for students to weigh pros and cons and understand why the scientific method is important to decision making; often there are no "cookbook" answers to complex life problems and basic principles must be the guiding light. Such principles are highlighted here to help students see just how nutrition "works" in the lives of people at all ages.

The Core Life Cycle Chapters: The Developmental Concept

Chapters 3 through 9, the life cycle chapters, continue to provide the strong core of this text. We start where the life cycle naturally begins, with the young adult, especially the young woman, who conceives and nurtures new life to its birth. In-depth reviews of early fetal growth and development during pregnancy and breastfeeding of the newborn infant probe fundamental relationships of nutrition to maternal health and the outcome of pregnancy and to the following process of lactation. A clear foundation is laid for the varying nutritional needs of rapid infant growth and the slowed erratic growth of young children, revealing the lifetime importance of these early family and cultural food experiences and learned behaviors. The volatile nature of rapid adolescent growth and sexual maturation are discussed to display the increased nutrition and personal needs of teenagers coming of age in an increasingly complex society. The important theme of health promotion through the strengthening of a healthy lifestyle continues in chapters on the middle and older adult years. This information provides a basis for helping persons in the later years of adulthood to reduce their risks of health problems. These risks include those that affect food intake and use and thus nutritional status, as well as those that may lead to chronic disease.

Throughout the life cycle changes, we discuss responses to both physiologic and psychosocial needs that build positive health. Without these positive responses, nutrition and health problems develop and disease risks increase. Also, we have integrated material on body compositions and nutrition assessment with each life cycle stage to focus on changing status and needs during growth and development. In each life cycle stage, special attention is also given to addiction disorders that can ultimately compromise positive health.

NEW TO THE THIRD EDITION

Strategies for Nutrition Education boxes. To allow for greater specificity to each life cycle stage, we have included a *Strategies for Nutrition Education* box in each chapter, replacing the second edition's Chapter 10. Addressing contemporary topics such as *America's Changing Food Habits: Implications for Nutrition Education, Nutrition Counseling,* and *WIC: Providing Supplemental Food with Nutrition Education,* nutrition education issues are effectively integrated in the text's content.

Increased awareness of addiction disorders. New and enhanced discussion of addiction behaviors that can harm health, such as eating disorders, alcohol abuse, and tobacco use, have been added to many chapters.

Physical Fitness. Greater emphasis is given to physical fitness in each life cycle stage by presenting various ideas for health promotion.

Case studies. New case studies have been added to most chapters, allowing students to apply the content of the chapter to real-life situations.

LEARNING AIDS THROUGHOUT THE TEXT

Basic concepts. To immediately draw students into the topic for study, each chapter opens with a concise list of the basic concepts involved and a brief overview that sets the stage for the discussion to come.

Chapter headings. Throughout each chapter, the major headings and subheadings in special type indicate the organization of the chapter material. This makes for easy reading and understanding of the key ideas. Main concepts and terms are also emphasized with bold type and italics.

Definitions of terms. Key terms important to the student's understanding and application of the material in nutrition care are presented in three ways. First, when they are discussed in the text, they are identified in bold type. Second, they are brought out of the text into the margins for emphasis, often with interesting derivations along with the definition of the words. Finally, all of the key terms are listed alphabetically in a glossary at the back of the book for quick reference.

One Step Further boxes. At different places in the text, related material is placed in boxes to provide further explanation or application. These boxes contain expanded material that takes students a step further to increase their understanding of a key concept.

Case Study boxes. Case studies are highlighted in separate boxes throughout the text to focus the student's attention on related health needs or problems. Each case is accompanied by challenging questions for case analysis. Students can apply these examples to similar situations in their individual or community learning experiences.

Strategies for Nutrition Education boxes. In each chapter, nutrition education issues applicable to a particular life cycle stage are highlighted in a *Strategies for Nutrition Education* box. These boxes address contemporary themes of nutrition education, applicable to both the student and the professional.

Chapter summaries. Brief summary paragraphs review chapter highlights and help students see the *big picture*. Then they can return to any part of the material for repeated study and clarification of details as needed.

Review questions. To help the student understand and think through key parts of the chapter or apply it to health care problems, questions are given after each chapter summary for review and analysis.

Cited references. Carefully researched and updated background references throughout the text strengthen the material presented and provide resources for students who may want to dig further into a particular topic of interest.

Further annotated readings. To encourage further reading of useful materials to expand understanding of key concepts or apply the material in practical ways for nutrition care and education, a brief list of annotated resources is provided at the end of each chapter.

Appendixes. A set of appendixes supplies key reference tools for individual study or group projects. For example, nutritional assessment reference standards include anthropometric age-gender norms for body measures and weight-height tables for all ages, including older adults, as well as developmental growth charts from infancy through childhood.

Along with our publisher, we are especially grateful to the following reviewers, who gave their valuable time and skills to help us strengthen the third edition:

Mary E. Mohs, PhD, RD, LD
University of Houston

Alice C. Williams, PhD
Andrews University

Mary Etta Reeves, PhD
Appalachian State University

Kathleen Yadrick, PhD, RD
University of Southern Mississippi

Bonnie S. Worthington-Roberts
Sue Rodwell Williams

Contents

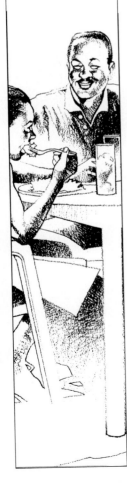

3 NUTRITION AND THE ADULT: THE YOUNG AND MIDDLE YEARS, 48

Sue Rodwell Williams
Eleanor D. Schlenker

5 LACTATION AND HUMAN MILK, 164

Bonnie S. Worthington-Roberts

8 NUTRITION IN ADOLESCENCE, 316

Bonnie S. Worthington-Roberts
Jane M. Rees

9   NUTRITION AND THE AGING ADULT, 380

Eleanor D. Schlenker

APPENDIXES

Nutrition Throughout the Life Cycle

1

Introduction to the Life Cycle: The Role of Nutrition

Bonnie S. Worthington-Roberts

Basic Concepts

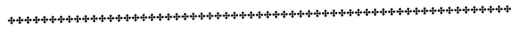

- ✔ *Each stage of the life cycle is associated with a distinct set of nutritional priorities.*
- ✔ *All persons throughout life need the same nutrients but in varying amounts.*
- ✔ *Health promotion and disease prevention are underlying lifetime goals.*
- ✔ *At times, especially in the later years, disease management may impact significantly on dietary planning.*

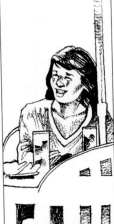

From beginning to end, the human life cycle is a fascinating sequence of events. From the moment of fertilization through the stages of growth, development, maturation, and aging, the interaction between genes and environment determines the details of the process. The importance of the genetic base cannot be ignored but it is clear that an assortment of environmental factors have the potential of significantly modifying the course of events. Nutrition is one of those influential factors demanding special attention.

This text considers in some depth the contributions that diet and nutrition make to support the growth and developmental process throughout the life cycle. Each chapter illustrates that in this health promotion process our food and its nutrients are essential to preventing deviations from the normal state or the establishment of acute or chronic disease.

THE NUTRIENTS: A BRIEF REMINDER

Survival requires not only oxygen and water but food as well. Food provides the energy required to support the body's life-sustaining processes; it also contains the materials needed to build and maintain all body cells. These materials are referred to as *nutrients;* each plays a role in assuring that the biochemical machinery of the human body runs smoothly.

Nutrients are classified in six categories (Table 1-1), including the energy-yielding **macronutrients** (carbohydrates, fats, and proteins), the **micronutrients** (vitamins and minerals), and water. Their basic features include the following:

1. *Carbohydrates* contain carbon, hydrogen, and oxygen combined in small molecules called sugars and large molecules represented mainly by starch.
2. **Lipids** (fats and oils) contain carbon, hydrogen, and oxygen as do carbohydrates, but the amount of oxygen is much less. **Triglyceride** is the main form of food fat.
3. *Proteins* contain carbon, hydrogen, and oxygen, plus nitrogen and sometimes sulfur atoms arranged in small compounds called **amino acids.** Chains of amino acids make up dietary proteins.
4. *Vitamins* are organic compounds that serve to catalyze or support a number of biochemical reactions in the body.
5. *Minerals* are inorganic elements or compounds that play important roles in metabolic reactions and serve as structural components in body tissues such as bone.
6. *Water* is vital to the body as a solvent and lubricant and as a medium for transporting nutrients and waste.

Triglyceride
(Gr *treis,* three; L *glycerinum,* glycerol) Chemical name for fat; a compound of three fatty acids esterified to glycerol base. A neutral fat, synthesized from carbohydrate, stored in adipose tissue. It releases free fatty acids into the blood when hydrolyzed by enzymes.

Amino acids
(*amino,* the monovalent chemical group NH₂) Carriers of essential element nitrogen; structural units of protein; specific amino acids being linked in specific sequence by peptide chains to form specific proteins.

TABLE 1-1 *Essential Nutrients in the Human Diet*

| | Energy Nutrients | | | | |
Carbohydrate	Fat (Lipid)	Protein (Amino Acid)	Vitamins	Minerals	Water
Glucose (or a carbohydrate that yields glucose)	Linoleic acid (omega-6) α-Linolenic acid (omega-3)	Histidine Isoleucine Leucine Lysine Methionine Phenylalanine Threonine Tryptophan Valine	A D E K Thiamin Riboflavin Niacin Pantothenic acid Biotin B-6 B-12 Folate C	Arsenic Boron Calcium Chloride Chromium Cobalt Copper Fluoride Iodide Iron Magnesium Manganese Molybdenum Nickel Phosphorus Potassium Selenium Silicon Sodium Sulfur Zinc	Water

From Wardlaw GM, Insel PM: *Perspectives in nutrition,* St Louis, 1990, Mosby.

DIET: INFLUENCES DURING THE LIFE CYCLE

Although food likes and dislikes probably determine largely what people eat, food choices also reflect socioeconomic status and budget, cultural experiences, religious beliefs, time constraints, health-related concerns, susceptibility to advertising, and other such factors. As one expert stated, "Food symbolizes much of what we think about ourselves."

Childhood Experiences

The food environment in which we are raised has a significant effect on food choices later in life. Environment reflects social and cultural preferences, which in turn are influenced by monetary constraints, limitations in the food supply, parental decisions about introduction of new foods to children, and an array of other variables. Innate food

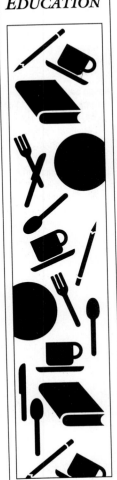

STRATEGIES FOR NUTRITION EDUCATION

America's Changing Food Habits: Implications for Nutrition Education

The American public has been receiving increasing numbers of messages from public health agencies and private health organizations regarding the relationship between diet and health. Food companies are also directing their attention to health concerns in the development and marketing of new food products. Of the nearly 13,000 new food products introduced to the marketplace in 1993, about 2500 made a health claim. Over two thirds of the products making a health claim were low or reduced in fat, cholesterol, or kilocalories, and about one third were low or reduced in sugar or sodium. Relatively few of the new products contained high levels or added amounts of fiber or calcium. Over the past 35 years the typical American diet has undergone many changes that are consistent with the Dietary Guidelines for Americans issued by the U.S. Departments of Health and Human Services and Agriculture. Food consumption data indicate that since 1960 intakes per person of cholesterol, sugar, and eggs have declined by 18 to 36 percent, while intakes of fresh vegetables, fish, pasta, and chicken have increased by 45 to 70 percent. Use of low-fat milk has increased by 4000 percent. Recent surveys suggest that over half of today's consumers are concerned about the level of fat in the foods they eat and the demand for reduced and low-fat food products continues to grow. Increasing their intakes of fruits and vegetables is a major concern of those consumers who are seeking more healthful diets. Other trends, however, are less encouraging. Americans are increasing their total energy intakes—up by 12 percent since 1980—despite their reduction in dietary fat, and all age groups are gradually gaining weight. Many new foods that are low or reduced in fat, or even fat free, are still high in kilocalories and can contribute to weight gain. Moreover, other important dietary goals are receiving little attention. Only 3% of consumers interviewed in 1994 were making an effort to lower their intake of cholesterol, and only 7% to 8% were attempting to increase their use of fish or high fiber foods or decrease their intake of salt. Yet these patterns are also critical to the development of healthy food behavior. It would appear that nutrition education messages have emphasized the reduction of dietary fat at the expense of other food issues. A more effective approach might be to encourage:

- A balanced diet to include a wide variety of foods
- The use of all foods in moderation
- Limiting intakes of fat, cholesterol, added sugar, and added salt
- Increasing intakes of complex carbohydrates, fiber, and calcium
- Monitoring total energy intake and expenditure to maintain a healthy body weight

Stillings, BR: Trends in foods, *Nutr Today* 29:6, 1994.
American Institute for Cancer Research Newsletter, Issue 47, Spring, 1995.

preferences do exist, such as the universal enjoyment of sweet foods and the dislike of sour or bitter substances. It is possible, however, to modify these preferences through the process of conditioning or learning. Some people learn, for example, to like very hot and spicy foods or foods that are very salty.

Social Situations

Special occasions are associated with the serving of specific foods. Foods often represent long established traditions within a family or cultural group. Also, family schedules dictate the family mealtime group. The traditional family meal occurs less frequently now than in times past and busy schedules often lead to eating outside the home. Some Americans have developed a pattern of **"grazing"** as opposed to "meal-eating." Negative nutritional effects may follow.

Grazing
Informal descriptive label for food pattern of frequent small snacks throughout the day rather than more formal regular meals. Term taken from animal pattern of constant eating in a pastureland.

Financial Resources

Family income certainly determines the kinds of foods selected. More affluent people tend to purchase more fresh vegetables and fruits and more meat, poultry, and fish. Income also dictates in most families the pattern of eating away from home. However, since cost of food in the United States is *relatively* inexpensive, differences in food choices of Americans are less than one might suspect.

Advertising

Billions of dollars are spent annually to entice the public to choose certain foods. Although the impact of such efforts was minimal at one time, the sophistication of modern advertising has markedly affected our pattern of product selection today. Whereas some of the advertising may promote important nutrition considerations, emphasis is often placed on sweets and other "goodies." Whatever the case, the force of advertising is now recognized to be substantial. This is true not only in the supermarket but also in the fast-food restaurant industry.

Daily Routine

Although we think of America as a society with much variation, a close look at any individual often discloses that the patterns of daily living include a rather limited food menu. People become locked into food choices that they enjoy, are readily available and affordable, and don't test their limited wishes to stray from "what is familiar." Children raised in an environment in which trying new foods is encouraged may very well accept the challenges of new food experiences better than children exposed to limited options.

Health Concerns

A growing number of Americans are concerned enough about health that they select foods in part based upon this factor. Some surveys indicate that half of the U.S. population considers health maintenance important when shopping for or ordering food. Real attention to proper food choices for promotion of health was sparked in the late 1960s by the "back to nature" movement, along with the recommendations of the American Heart Association that fat and cholesterol may contribute to coronary heart disease. Recent years have seen the publication of evidence that some cancers may also be "preventable" with choice of a good diet. These findings have not gone unnoticed by the general public. The food industry recognizes this and is now providing an array of products that are specifically of low-calorie, low-fat composition. Also, government regulatory agencies are in the process of reforming food labeling to present sound nutrition information for the consumer. These directions are very likely to continue to the year 2000 and beyond.

LIFE CYCLE NUTRITIONAL NEEDS

From the moment of conception, the human organism depends on nutrition for growth, development, and long-term survival. Prior to birth, the fetus must draw from maternal nutrient supplies and this process may continue after birth if the mother chooses to breastfeed her baby. Ultimately, an outside food supply provides the ongoing nutritional support for life. This nutritional support may come from both animal and plant food sources. An unlimited number of food combinations are known to satisfy nutrient needs. Consequently, people worldwide, consuming vastly different foods and food mixtures, demonstrate satisfactory growth and health.

Stages of the Life Cycle

Fetal and maternal needs. The **mammalian** fetus is completely dependent on nutritional support from the mother. The quantitative requirements are very small in the beginning but increase gradually until birth. During this time it is absolutely essential that a correct equilibrium be maintained among the various nutrients circulating in the maternal blood. This required biochemical **milieu** depends entirely on the mother's diet, her nutritional stores, and her metabolic idiosyncrasies. The adverse effects of nutritional-biochemical imbalance during **gestation** have been examined most frequently in animal models. Fortuitous observations of human experience, however, have contributed to our slowly growing knowledge base in this field. In general, the repercussions of abnormal nutrition depend on the stage at which a given nutrient factor acts, the nature of the nutrient considered, the intensity of the disequilibrium, and the species or strain of the animal studied. The types of repercussion are very different. They include death, tissue alterations, delayed growth, alterations of cellular differentiation, and malformations. Improvement in pregnancy outcome depends in part on motivating the pregnant woman to establish satisfactory diet and supplementation practices.[1]

Lactation. Establishment of **lactation** and continued production of sufficient high-quality milk also demands that the mother consume an adequate diet. While lactation is a high-priority physiologic process maintained even in the face of serious nutritional deprivation, without continuing nutritional support the quantity of milk production is generally hampered and milk quality eventually deteriorates. In either case, the nutritional well-being of the mother will be compromised as will eventually her health and preparedness for "mothering."[1,2]

Infancy. The first year after birth is a time in the life cycle when many changes occur in relation to food and nutrient intake. A number of factors influence these dramatic changes: (1) a rapid then gradually declining rate of physical growth, (2) maturation of oral structures and functions, (3) development of fine and gross motor skills, and (4) establishment of relationships with parents and family. As a result of these tremendous changes, infants prepared at birth to suck liquids from a nipple are at 1 year of age making attempts to feed themselves table foods with culturally defined utensils. The need for nutrients and energy depends on the infant's requirement for physical growth, mainte-nance, and energy expenditure. The foods offered to infants reflect culturally accepted practices. Infants' acceptance of food is influenced by **neuromotor** maturation and by their interactions with their parents. Well-nourished children at any month during infancy will consume a variety of food combinations.[3]

Preschool years. During the preschool years, the decreased rates of growth bring decreased appetites. Children learn to understand language and to talk and ask for food. Development of gross motor skills permits them to learn to feed themselves and to prepare simple foods such as cereal and milk and sandwiches. They learn about food and the way it feels, tastes, and smells. Preschool children learn to eat a wider variety of textures and

Milieu
(Fr *milieu*, surround-ings) Environment, social or physical. An important concept in nutrition, referring to both external socio-physical setting and internal biochemical environments, and the interacting balances between them.

Gestation
(L *gestare*, to bear) In-trauterine fetal growth period from conception to birth.

Neuromotor
(Gr *neuron*, nerve; L *motorium*, movement center) Movement involving nerve impulses to muscles.

kinds of food, give up the bottle, and drink from a cup. They demand independence and refuse help in many tasks, such as self-feeding, in which they are not yet skillful. As they grow older, they become less interested in food and more interested in their environment. They test and learn the limits of acceptable behavior.[3]

School age children. Between preschool and adolescence, children continue to grow slowly and demonstrate maturation of fine and gross motor skills. Individual personality develops and degree of independence increases. All of these changes influence the amounts of food consumed, the manner in which it is eaten, and the acceptability of specific foods. Food habits, likes, and dislikes are established, some of which are transient, but many of which form the base for a lifetime of food experiences. Environmental influences and parental behaviors reinforce or extinguish food-related behaviors. Parents need to provide appropriate foods and supportive guidance so that appropriate food patterns develop. The nutrition knowledge of the parents and other care providers positively influences children's requests for and acceptance of various foods. School feeding programs provide an opportunity for nutrition education.[3]

Adolescence. The adolescent period is a unique stage in the process of growth and development. It is characterized by a wide variability in norms of growth, increasingly independent behavior, and the testing of adult roles. This critical period of human development occurs at physiologic, psychologic, and social levels. These tumultuous changes do not occur simultaneously but at varying rates. Although adolescence may be defined as the teenage years between 12 and 20, physical maturation and changes in nutrient requirements actually begin at younger years and sometimes extend into the third decade.[3,4]

Teenagers assume greater responsibility for decision making in their own lives. In

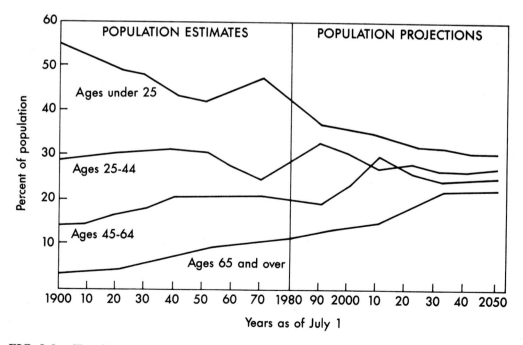

FIG. 1-1   Trend in age distribution of U.S. population (including Armed Forces overseas).
From Insel PM, Roth WT: *Core concepts in health,* ed 5, Mountain View, Calif, 1988, Mayfield Publishing.

TABLE 1-2   *Food and Nutrition Board, National Academy of Sciences: National Research Council Recommended Dietary Allowances,[a] Revised 1989*

		Weight[b]		Height[b]		Protein	Fat-Soluble Vitamins			
Category	Age (years)	(kg)	(lb)	(cm)	(inches)	(g)	Vitamin A (μg RE)[c]	Vitamin D (μg)[d]	Vitamin E (mg α-TE)[e]	Vitamin K (μg)
Infants	0.0-0.5	6	13	60	24	13	375	7.5	3	5
	0.5-1.0	9	20	71	28	14	375	10	4	10
Children	1-3	13	29	90	35	16	400	10	6	15
	4-6	20	44	112	44	24	500	10	7	20
	7-10	28	62	132	52	28	700	10	7	30
Males	11-14	45	99	157	62	45	1000	10	10	45
	15-18	66	145	176	69	59	1000	10	10	65
	19-24	72	160	177	70	58	1000	10	10	70
	25-50	79	174	176	70	63	1000	5	10	80
	51+	77	170	173	68	63	1000	5	10	80
Females	11-14	46	101	157	62	46	800	10	8	45
	15-18	55	120	163	64	44	800	10	8	55
	19-24	58	128	164	65	46	800	10	8	60
	25-50	63	138	163	64	50	800	5	8	65
	51+	65	143	160	63	50	800	5	8	65
Pregnant						60	800	10	10	65
Lactating										
1st 6 months						65	1300	10	12	65
2nd 6 months						62	1200	10	11	65

[a]The allowances, expressed as average daily intakes over time, are intended to provide for individual variations among most normal persons as they live in the United States under usual environmental stresses. Diets should be based on a variety of common foods in order to provide other nutrients for which human requirements have been less well defined. See text for detailed discussion of allowances and of nutrients not tabulated.

[b]Weights and heights of Reference Adults are actual medians for the US population of the designated age, as reported by NHANES II. The use of these figures does not imply that the height-to-weight ratios are ideal.

[c]Retinol equivalents. 1 retinol equivalent = 1 μg retinol or 6 μg β-carotene.

[d]As cholecalciferol. 10 μg cholecalciferol = 400 IU of vitamin D.

[e]α-Tocopherol equivalents. 1 mg d-α tocopherol = 1 α-TE.

[f]1 NE (niacin equivalent) is equal to 1 mg of niacin or 60 mg of dietary tryptophan.

Water-Soluble Vitamins							Minerals						
Vitamin C (mg)	Thiamin (mg)	Riboflavin (mg)	Niacin (mg NE)[f]	Vitamin B$_6$ (mg)	Folate (µg)	Vitamin B$_{12}$ (µg)	Calcium (mg)	Phosphorus (mg)	Magnesium (mg)	Iron (mg)	Zinc (mg)	Iodine (µg)	Selenium (µg)
30	0.3	0.4	5	0.3	25	0.3	400	300	40	6	5	40	10
35	0.4	0.5	6	0.6	35	0.5	600	500	60	10	5	50	15
40	0.7	0.8	9	1.0	50	0.7	800	800	80	10	10	70	20
45	0.9	1.1	12	1.1	75	1.0	800	800	120	10	10	90	20
45	1.0	1.2	13	1.4	100	1.4	800	800	170	10	10	120	30
50	1.3	1.5	17	1.7	150	2.0	1200	1200	270	12	15	150	40
60	1.5	1.8	20	2.0	200	2.0	1200	1200	400	12	15	150	50
60	1.5	1.7	19	2.0	200	2.0	1200	1200	350	10	15	150	70
60	1.5	1.7	19	2.0	200	2.0	800	800	350	10	15	150	70
60	1.2	1.4	15	2.0	200	2.0	800	800	350	10	15	150	70
50	1.1	1.3	15	1.4	150	2.0	1200	1200	280	15	12	150	45
60	1.1	1.3	15	1.5	180	2.0	1200	1200	300	15	12	150	50
60	1.1	1.3	15	1.6	180	2.0	1200	1200	280	15	12	150	55
60	1.1	1.3	15	1.6	180	2.0	800	800	280	15	12	150	55
60	1.0	1.2	13	1.6	180	2.0	800	800	280	10	12	150	55
70	1.5	1.6	17	2.2	400	2.2	1200	1200	320	30	15	175	65
95	1.6	1.8	20	2.1	280	2.6	1200	1200	355	15	19	200	75
90	1.6	1.7	20	2.1	260	2.6	1200	1200	340	15	16	200	75

TABLE 1-3   *Dietary Guidelines for Americans*

Eat a variety of foods
Maintain desirable body weight
Choose a diet low in fat, saturated fat, and cholesterol
Choose a diet with plenty of vegetables, fruits, and grain products
Use sugars in moderation
Use salt and sodium in moderation
If you drink alcoholic beverages, do so in moderation

From *Report of the Dietary Guidelines Advisory Committee for Americans,* Washington, DC, 1990, USDA.

contrast to younger children, adolescents themselves most often determine their food intake. Their food choices reflect various factors including family eating patterns, peer influence, media, appetite, and food availability. Some of these factors can be positive for nutritional quality and others may leave a lot to be desired. Body image plays a very important role in the eating behaviors of adolescents. Eating disorders account for a large number of nutritional concerns during adolescence.[3,4]

Adulthood. The adult years span a number of decades during which nutritional needs change very little, but family circumstances and lifestyle often undergo substantial change. Marital status, living environment, job setting and responsibilities, income, and a variety of other factors significantly affect specific food choices and long-term dietary patterns. Ideally, a major focus during these years is health promotion and disease prevention. This goal entails, among other things, establishing nutritional practices that will maximize health and minimize risk for developing preventable chronic diseases. Appropriate practices vary somewhat among individuals due in large part to differences in genetic bases. Of primary concern, however, is maintaining desirable body fatness by eating moderate amounts of a wide variety of wholesome foods.[5-7]

Older adults. Persons who are 65 years of age or older comprise the fastest-growing segment of the population in most developed countries (Fig. 1-1). Of these older individuals, 95% live within the community, many of them on incomes barely sufficient for survival. Financial limitations adversely affect food purchasing power. However, an assortment of other factors also contribute to the increased prevalence of malnutrition in this age group. Important contributors to the problem include loneliness, depression, oral discomfort, and chronic diseases, all of which lead to poor appetite. Physical and mental handicaps may limit the ability to shop for food or to prepare it. Use of an assortment of drugs, both prescription and over-the-counter, may further interfere with the maintenance of satisfactory nutritional status. The aging process itself may reduce nutrient absorption, increase urinary loss, and interfere with normal pathways of nutrient utilization.[8]

GUIDELINES FOR HEALTH MAINTENANCE AND DISEASE PREVENTION

During the past 10 years, understanding of the role of nutrition in health promotion and disease prevention has improved. Relationships between specific nutrient deficiencies and inferior health status have long been recognized. But in recent years, diet has been associated with a number of chronic diseases such as cardiovascular disease, cancer, and diabetes. The focus of concern about human nutrition has moved from the issues of nutritional deficiencies toward increased emphasis on chronic disease prevention and health maintenance in all phases of the life cycle.

The American public has been presented with a variety of dietary recommendations for health maintenance and disease prevention. The federal government of the United States has provided the Recommended Dietary Allowances, the most recent issue of which is shown in Table 1-2.[9] This famous directive, now in its tenth edition, specifies its guidelines in gram and milligram amounts. For professionals, this series of recommendations is useful in evaluating the quality of diets of groups of people. More understandable directions are presented by the U.S. Department of Agriculture (USDA) and the U.S. Department of Health and Human Services (USDHHS) in the Dietary Guidelines for Americans listed in Table 1-3, and by the National Academy of Sciences in their publication *Diet and Health,* summarized in Table 1-4.[10,11]

In 1980, the Surgeon General of the United States included specific nutrition objectives in his recommendations for the health promotion of Americans.[12] In 1990, these objectives

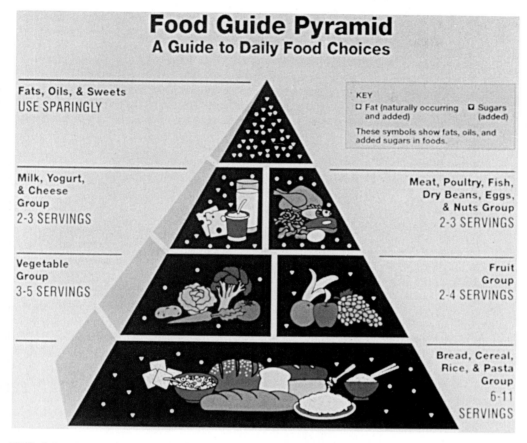

FIG. 1-2 USDA's Food Guide Pyramid — A Guide to Daily Food Choices. This guide lists the food groups and the number of servings of each to consume.

TABLE 1-4 *1989 National Academy of Sciences Recommendations (Diet and Health)*

- Reduce total *fat* intake to 30% or less of kcalories. Reduce saturated fatty acid intake to less than 10% of kcalories, and the intake of cholesterol to less than 300 mg daily.
- Increase intake of starches and other *complex carbohydrates.*
- Maintain *protein* intake at moderate levels.
- Balance food intake and physical activity to maintain appropriate *body weight.*
- For those who drink *alcoholic beverages,* limit consumption to the equivalent of less than 1 oz of pure alcohol in a single day. Pregnant women should avoid alcoholic beverages.
- Limit total daily intake of *salt* (sodium chloride) to 6 g or less.
- Maintain adequate *calcium* intake.
- Avoid taking dietary *supplements* in excess of the RDA in any one day.
- Maintain an optimal intake of *fluoride,* particularly during the years of primary and secondary tooth formation and growth.

Reprinted with permission from *Diet and health,* © 1989 by the National Academy of Sciencies, National Academy Press, Washington, DC.

The Public Health Service National Nutrition Objectives for 2000

Looking to the year 2000, the U.S. Surgeon General has identified 21 specific nutrition-related objectives to improve the nation's health.

1. Reduce coronary heart disease to no more than 100 per 100,000 people.
2. Reverse the rise in cancer deaths to achieve a rate of no more than 130 per 100,000 people.
3. Reduce overweight to a prevalence of no more than 20% among people aged 20 and older and no more than 15% among adolescents aged 12 through 19.
4. Reduce growth retardation among low-income children aged 5 and younger to less than 10%.
5. Reduce dietary fat intake to an average of 30% of calories or less, and average saturated fat intake to less than 10% of calories among people aged 2 and older.
6. Increase complex carbohydrates and fiber-containing foods in the diets of adults to five or more daily servings for vegetables and fruits, and to six or more daily servings for grain products.
7. Increase to at least 50% the proportion of overweight people aged 12 and older who have adopted sound dietary practices combined with regular physical activity to attain an appropriate weight.
8. Increase calcium intake so at least 50% of youths aged 12 through 24 and 50% of pregnant and lactating women consume three or more servings daily of foods rich in calcium, and at least 50% of people aged 25 and older consume two or more servings daily.
9. Decrease salt and sodium intake so at least 65% of home meal preparers prepare foods without adding salt, at least 80% of people avoid using salt at the table, and at least 40% of adults regularly purchase foods modified or lower in sodium.
10. Reduce iron deficiency to less than 3% among children aged 1 through 4 and among women of childbearing age.
11. Increase to at least 75% the proportion of mothers who breastfeed their babies in early postpartum period and to at least 50% the proportion who continue breastfeeding until their babies are 5 to 6 months old.
12. Increase to at least 75% the proportion of parents and caregivers who use feeding practices that prevent baby bottle tooth decay.
13. Increase to at least 85% the proportion of people aged 18 and older who use food labels to make nutritious food selections.
14. Achieve useful and informative labeling for virtually all processed food and at least 40% of fresh meats, poultry, fish, fruits, vegetables, baked goods, and ready-to-eat carry-away food.
15. Increase to at least 5000 brand names the availability of processed food products that are reduced in fat and saturated fat.
16. Increase to at least 90% the proportion of restaurants and institutional food service operations that offer identifiable low-fat, low-calorie food choices, consistent with the *Dietary Guidelines for Americans.*
17. Increase to at least 90% the proportion of school lunch and breakfast services and child care food services with menus that are consistent with the nutrition principles in the *Dietary Guidelines for Americans.*
18. Increase to at least 80% the receipt of home food services by people aged 65 and older who have difficulty in preparing their own meals or are otherwise in need of home-delivered meals.
19. Increase to at least 75% the proportion of the nation's schools that provide nutrition education from preschool through 12th grade.
20. Increase to at least 50% the proportion of work sites with 50 or more employees that offer nutrition education and/or weight management programs for their employees.
21. Increase to at least 75% the proportion of primary care providers who provide nutrition assessment and counseling and/or referral to qualified nutritionists or dietitians.

From US Dept of Health and Human Services, Public Health Service: *Healthy people 2000: national health promotion and disease prevention objectives,* Washington, DC, 1990, US Government Printing Office.

TABLE 1-5 *Recommended Servings From the Food Guide Pyramid*

	Many Women, Older Adults	Children, Teen Girls, Active Women, Most Men	Teen Boys, Active Men
Kcal level*	1600	2200	2800
Bread group	6	9	11
Vegetable group	3	4	5
Fruit group	2	3	4
Milk group	2-3†	2-3†	2-3†
Meat group	2, totaling 5 oz.	2, totaling 6 oz.	3, totaling 7 oz.
Total fat (grams)	53	73	93
Added sugar (teaspoons)	6	12	18

*These kcal levels are based on a diet that uses low-fat, lean foods from the five major food groups and uses fats, oils, and sweets sparingly.
†Women who are pregnant or breast feeding, teenagers, and young adults to age 24 need three servings per day.
From Dupuy NA, Mermel VL: *Focus on nutrition,* St Louis, 1995, Mosby.

have been updated to define the nation's goals for the year 2000, as shown in the box on p. 12.[13] Among the broad goals to be achieved by 2000 are:
- Increase the number of healthy years for Americans
- Reduce health disparities among segments of Americans
- Achieve equal access to preventive health services for all Americans

Among the major nutrition objectives identified are reducing overweight and dietary fat intake. Just how each of these objectives should be addressed during the various stages of the life cycle will be examined throughout this text.

In April 1992, the U.S. Department of Agriculture replaced the old concept of the Basic Four Food Groups with the Food Guide Pyramid: A Guide to Daily Food Choices. It provides useful directions to people about choosing the best foods by presenting a visual picture of recommendations in the Food Guide Pyramid (Fig. 1-2). The plan offers five food groups instead of four, but many of the original concepts still apply. The foods in each group are notable contributors of certain key nutrients but they assure a good supply of many of the other nutrients as well. A minimum number of servings is recommended from each part of the pyramid. The plan makers suggest that to meet additional energy needs, a person should choose more servings of food from the very same groups. Table 1-5 lists recommended servings from the Food Guide Pyramid for various categories of diets and people.

Some foods—such as butter, margarine, cream, salad dressing, potato chips, jelly, coffee, tea, alcoholic beverages, and others—don't fit into any of the food groups. Some of these contribute a few nutrients, but most primarily contribute energy. Fat, sugar, alcohol, and water are largely provided in these foods; they are grouped together into a miscellaneous category of extras. The originators of the plan suggest they should be used sparingly. The beauty of the Food Guide Pyramid is its simplicity; with proper choices it can satisfactorily meet the needs of those who choose to be vegetarians.

DIET THERAPY AS A COMPONENT OF DISEASE MANAGEMENT

Although the maintenance of health and prevention of disease is a priority focus throughout the life cycle, circumstances arise in every stage of life when dietary interventions are required to treat disease, trauma, or other undesirable situations. The basic principles governing diet therapy are simple: meet nutritional needs while modifying the diet to satisfy the health problem under treatment. Some changes in diet may be easily implemented, but others require special planning and in some cases major changes from established food habits. The degree to which an individual—with the help of family, friends, health care providers, and others—is able to follow short-term or permanent changes in diet varies in each case. The needed diet changes may impact significantly on quality of life and in some cases even on chances of survival. While the focus of this book is health maintenance and disease prevention, some discussion of necessity will include selected problems that require diet and nutrition intervention.

Summary

Growth, development, reproduction, and the maintenance of health require that the human organism satisfy basic biologic needs. Nutrition is a basic need that can be met minimally to prevent death or optimally to help achieve maximum genetic potential. The goal of this book is to approach the issue of optimum nutrition from the developmental framework of specific stages of the life cycle. Attention to normal needs and feeding practices will predominate but management strategies for selected special problems will be addressed. For more detailed coverage of special problems requiring diet therapy, the reader is referred to other available clinical texts.

Review Questions

1. Outline key functions of the basic nutrients.
2. Describe major influences on food choices of Americans.
3. Define key nutritional concerns at each stage of the life cycle.

4. Summarize the National Nutrition Objectives for the year 2000.
5. Describe the new Food Pyramid concept.

References

1. Worthington-Roberts B, Williams SR: *Nutrition in pregnancy and lactation,* ed 5, St Louis, 1993, Mosby.
2. Lawrence RA: *Breastfeeding: a guide for the medical profession,* ed 3, St Louis, 1989, Mosby.
3. Pipes P: *Nutrition in infancy and childhood,* ed 4, St Louis, 1989, Mosby.
4. Mahan LK, and Rees JM: *Nutrition in adolescence,* St Louis, 1984, Mosby.
5. Pennington JAT: Dietary patterns and practices, *Clin Nutr* 5(1):17, Jan/Feb, 1986.
6. Crosetti AF, Guthrie HA: Alternate eating patterns and the role of age, sex, selection, and snacking in nutritional quality, *Clin Nutr* 5(1):34, Jan/Feb, 1986.
7. Lecos C: America's changing diet, *FDA Consumer,* p. 4, October 1985.
8. Schlenker ED: *Nutrition in aging,* St Louis, 1984, Mosby.
9. National Research Council: *Recommended dietary allowances,* ed 10, Washington, DC, 1989, National Academy Press.
10. US Departments of Agriculture and Health and Human Services: *Dietary guidelines for Americans,* Washington, DC, 1990, US Government Printing Office.
11. National Research Council: *Diet and health: implications for reducing chronic disease risk,* Washington, DC, 1989, National Academy Press.
12. US Department of Health and Human Services, Public Health Service: *Promoting health/ preventing disease: objectives for the nation,* Washington, DC, 1980, US Government Printing Office.
13. US Department of Health and Human Services, Public Health Service: *Healthy people 2000: national health promotion and disease prevention objectives,* Washington, DC, 1990, US Government Printing Office.

2

Nutrition and Assessment Basics

Sue Rodwell Williams

Basic Concepts

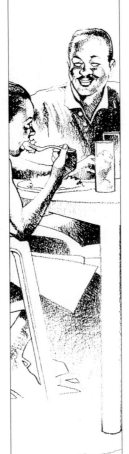

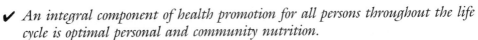

✔ *An integral component of health promotion for all persons throughout the life cycle is optimal personal and community nutrition.*

✔ *Through their specific and interdependent physiologic roles, certain nutrients in the food we eat are essential to life, health, and well-being.*

✔ *Changing nutrient needs throughout the life cycle relate to normal growth and development and resulting changes in body composition.*

✔ *The overall process of nutrition assessment reflects individual and community nutritional status and provides an important basis for personal health care plans and public nutrition intervention programs.*

We live in a rapidly changing world, one of changing environment, food supply, scientific knowledge, and population. Our numbers are increasing not only in total population and age distribution, but also in ethnic diversity. Within individual environments and communities, physical growth and development through the life cycle bring personality changes and with them come changing personal needs and goals. These *constant changes* of life must be in *balance* to produce healthy living at any age.

Thus to be realistic, within these life concepts of change and balance our study of life-cycle nutrition focuses on health promotion through good food and its basic nutrients and continued assessment of nutritional status and health needs. Because the background nutrition knowledge of students using this book varies widely and to set the overall learning focus, we provide a brief overview of nutrient and assessment basics in terms of the three most fundamental physiologic components that must be present for the human body to survive and remain healthy: (1) *energy* to do its work, (2) *building materials* to maintain its form and functions, and (3) *control agents* to regulate these processes efficiently.

NUTRIENTS: PHYSIOLOGIC ROLES
Macronutrients and Energy

Carbohydrate: basic fuel source. All three of the macronutrients in our food—carbohydrate, fat, and protein—can be **metabolized** to yield body **energy.** However, the body uses carbohydrate as its basic fuel supply, along with fat, and reserves protein mainly for its unique tissue-building role. In the human energy system, this major carbohydrate fuel comes from the two forms of carbohydrate foods we eat—starches and sugars. To produce energy from a basic fuel supply, a successful energy system must be able to do three things: (1) change the basic "raw" fuel to a refined fuel form that the system is designed to use, (2) carry this refined fuel to the places that need it, and (3) burn this refined fuel at these energy production sites in the special equipment set up there to do it. Far more efficient than any machine, the body easily does these three things. It digests its basic food fuel, carbohydrate, changing it to the refined fuel **glucose,** then absorbs this refined fuel and transports it through blood circulation to the cells that constantly need it. There glucose is broken down in the cell's highly specific equipment, releasing energy through its intricate biochemical pathways, **glycolysis** and the **citric acid cycle,** of cell metabolism. In this overall process, glucose is broken down to its basic carbon and hydrogen atoms and combined with oxygen, yielding energy as the cell's energy currency compound **adenosine triphosphate (ATP),** with its high-energy phosphate bonds, and releasing carbon dioxide and water as end products.

The classes of food carbohydrates vary from simple to complex structures and thus

Metabolism
(Gr *metaballein,* to change) Sum of all the various biochemical and physiologic processes by which the body grows and maintains itself (anabolism) and reshapes tissues (catabolism), transforming energy to do its work.

Glycolysis
Initial energy production pathway by which 6-carbon glucose is changed to active 3-carbon fragments of acetyl CoA, the fuel ready for final energy production.

Citric acid cycle
Final energy production pathway in the cell mitochondria that transforms the ultimate fuel acetyl CoA from carbohydrate and fat, capturing energy for cell metabolism in high-energy phosphate bonds.

Adenosine triphosphate (ATP)
The energy currency of the cell, binding energy in its high-energy phosphate bonds for release as these bonds are split.

TABLE 2-1 *Summary of Carbohydrate Classes*

Chemical Class Name	Class Members	Sources
Polysaccharides Multiple sugars, complex carbohydrates	Starch	Grains and grain products
		Cereal, bread, crackers, and other baked goods
		Pasta
		Rice, corn, bulgar
		Legumes
		Potatoes and other vegetables
	Glycogen	Animal tissues, liver and muscle meats
	Dietary fiber	Whole grains
		Fruits
		Vegetables
		Seeds, nuts, skins
Disaccharides Double sugars, simple carbohydrates	Sucrose	"Table" sugar: sugar cane, sugar beets
		Molasses
	Lactose	Milk
	Maltose	Starch digestion, intermediate Sweetener in food products
Monosaccharides Single sugars, simple carbohydrates	Glucose (dextrose)	Starch digestion, final Corn syrup (large use in processed foods)
	Fructose	Fruits, honey
	Galactose	Lactose (milk)

From Williams SR: Basic nutrition and diet therapy, ed 10, St Louis, 1995, Mosby.

Complex carbohydrates
Main dietary carbohy-
drate, the
polysaccharide starch in
varied foods such as
legumes, grains, breads,
cereals, and potatoes.

Glycogen
Briefly stored form of
carbohydrate in the
body cells, available for
energy fuel during
fasting periods of sleep;
built up in larger
amounts by high starch
meals prior to endur-
ance athletic events for
sustained energy.

Dietary fiber
Nondigestible form of
carbohydrate; of
nutritional importance in
gastrointestinal dis-
ease such as diverticu-
losis and management
of serum lipid and
glucose levels in risk-
reduction related to
chronic conditions such
as heart disease and
diabetes.

differ in the speed with which they yield energy (Table 2-1). **Simple carbohydrates** — sugars — made up of only one or two sugar (saccharide) units are broken down easily, releasing energy quickly. On the other hand **complex carbohydrates** — polysaccharides — are large, complex compounds of many saccharide units. For example, starch, the most significant polysaccharide in human nutrition, is made up of both straight-chained coiled structure (amylose, 15% to 20% of the molecule) and many branching chains (amylopectin, 80% to 85% of the molecule). Each of the multiple branching chains is composed of 24 to 30 sugar units of glucose, which are gradually split off in digestion to supply a steady source of energy over a period of time. **Glycogen,** the body's small amount of stored carbohydrate, sometimes called *animal starch,* has a similar, large "tree-like" structure and sustains energy during the brief fasting periods such as sleep hours.

Certain other carbohydrate compounds, fibrous polysaccharides, are nondigestible because humans lack the necessary enzymes to split their particular saccharide links. However, these compounds, especially those that are water-soluble, contribute valuable **dietary fiber** essential to health (Tables 2-2 and 2-3).[1,2] A list of some major food sources of dietary fiber is provided in Appendix K.

TABLE 2-2   *Summary of Dietary Fiber Classes*

Class	Source	Function
Cellulose	Main cell wall constituent of plants	Holds water; reduces elevated colonic intraluminal pressure; binds zinc
Noncellulose polysaccharides Gums Mucilages	Secretions of plants Plant secretions and seeds	Slows gastric emptying; provides fermentable material for colonic bacteria with production of gas and volatile fatty acids; binds bile acids and cholesterol
Algal polysaccharides Pectin substances	Algae, seaweeds Intercellular cement plant material	
Hemicellulose	Cell wall plant material	Holds water and increases stool bulk; reduces elevated colonic pressure; binds bile acids
Lignin	Woody part of plants	Antioxidant; binds bile acids, cholesterol, and metals

From Williams SR: Basic nutrition and diet therapy, ed 10, St Louis, 1995, Mosby.

TABLE 2-3   *Summary of Soluble and Insoluble Fibers in Total Dietary Fiber*

Insoluble	Soluble
Cellulose Most hemicelluloses Lignin	Gums Mucilages Algal polysaccharides Most pectins

Fat: concentrated energy. Fats supply a concentrated fuel source for the body's energy system, yielding over twice the energy value of carbohydrate. Because the body can easily convert carbohydrate to fat and store it in various body **adipose tissues,** fat is an important form of body fuel for energy reserves. Food fats from both animal and plant sources yield the same amount of energy, but have significantly different relationships to health. Excess dietary fat, especially fat from animal sources, and excess dietary cholesterol, which is synthesized only by animals and can only be supplied in the diet by animal food sources, are health risk factors.[1] The dietary guidelines for Americans recommend that we lower our daily dietary fat intake to 30% of the total kcalories.[3] Do you know how much fat you are eating? Try calculating it by the directions given in the box below.

Adipose tissue
Fat storage sites composed of adipocytes (fat cells).

Protein: available energy if needed. As indicated, carbohydrate and fat are primary fuel sources in the body's energy system. However, sometimes protein may furnish additional body energy, but it is a less efficient source. The fuel value of protein is the same as that of carbohydrate.

Measurement of nutrient energy value. The energy yielded by the macronutrients is measured in **kilocalories** (kcalories or kcal). Carbohydrate yields 4 kcal/g, fat 9 kcal/g, and protein 4 kcal/g. These values are called their respective fuel factors. The energy values of various foods, therefore, are based on their carbohydrate, fat, and protein composition. Any portion of these macronutrients not used for energy is restructured for body tissue storage as glycogen or fat for fuel use between meals, or for use in synthesizing other metabolic compounds needed in the body. Excess energy intake (kcalories) over energy use by the body to do its work results in weight gain. Insufficient energy intake to meet body needs results in weight loss. Any beverage alcohol is also metabolized by the body to yield 7 kcal/g. Excess alcohol intake, therefore, is harmful in terms of both weight gain (when it is converted to fat and stored) and its toxic effects.

Kilocalorie (kcalorie, kcal)
Unit of measure of energy produced in the body by the energy-yielding macronutrients carbohydrate, fat, and protein.

How Much Fat Are You Eating?

- Keep an accurate record of everything you eat or drink for 1 day. Be sure to estimate and add amounts of all fat or other nutrient seasonings used with your foods. (If you want a more representative picture and have a computer available with nutrient analysis programming, keep a 1-week record and calculate an average of the 7 days.)
- Calculate the total kilocalories (kcal) and grams of each of the energy nutrients (carbohydrate, fat, and protein) in everything you eat. Multiply the total grams of each energy nutrient by its respective fuel value:

$$
\begin{aligned}
\text{fat} &\underline{\hspace{1cm}} \text{g} \times 9 = \underline{\hspace{1cm}} \text{kcal} \\
\text{protein} &\underline{\hspace{1cm}} \text{g} \times 4 = \underline{\hspace{1cm}} \text{kcal} \\
\text{carbohydrate} &\underline{\hspace{1cm}} \text{g} \times 4 = \underline{\hspace{1cm}} \text{kcal}
\end{aligned}
$$

- Calculate the percentage of each energy nutrient in your total diet:

$$
\frac{\text{Fat kcal}}{\text{Total kcal}} \times 100 = \% \text{ fat kcal in diet}
$$

- Compare with fat in American diet (40% to 45%); with the U.S. dietary goals (25% to 30%).

From Williams SR: *Basic nutrition and diet therapy,* ed 10, St Louis, 1995, Mosby.

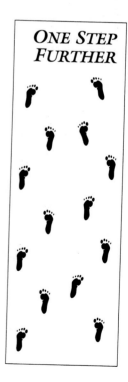

ONE STEP FURTHER

Amino Acids and Protein Metabolism

Amino acids: basic building material. All protein, whether in our bodies or in the food we eat, is made up of its building units, the **amino acids.** These amino acids are joined by peptide linkages in unique chain sequence to form specific proteins. When we eat protein foods, the protein (for example, casein in milk and cheese, albumin in egg white, or gluten in wheat products) is broken down into its constituent amino acids in the digestive process. According to need, from the body's overall metabolic "pool" of amino acids (Fig. 2-1) specific ones are then reassembled in the body in the *specific* order to form *specific* tissue proteins (for example, collagen in connective tissue, myosin in muscle tissue, hemoglobin in red blood cells [see Fig 2-2], cell enzymes, or insulin) that are required by the body.

Role as nitrogen supplier. Amino acids are named for their chemical nature. The word *amino* refers to the monovalent chemical group—NH_2. Like carbohydrates and fats, proteins have a basic structure of carbon, hydrogen, and oxygen. But unlike fats and carbohydrates, which contain no nitrogen, protein is about 16% nitrogen. In addition, some proteins contain small but valuable amounts of minerals such as sulfur.

Essential amino acids. Nine amino acids are now classed as **essential amino acids** because the body cannot manufacture them, or cannot do so in sufficient amounts. Thus the term *essential* as used here means that they are necessary in the diet. In the strict physiologic sense, all amino acids are essential in overall body metabolism. Although the ninth amino acid added to the essential list, histidine, has previously been known as essential for infants, it has now been demonstrated to be required also by adults.[4] The nine essential amino acids are histidine, isoleucine, leucine, lysine, methionine, phenylalanine, threonine, tryptophan, and valine (Table 2-4). (See the box on p. 21.) Applying this concept of essentiality to our dietary food choices, we would need to obtain all of these nine essential amino acids in our diet to meet our protein needs for tissue growth and maintenance throughout the life cycle. A protein food that supplies all of these essential amino acids in sufficient quantities to meet human needs is called a **complete protein.** Since only foods of animal source—milk, cheese, egg, and meat—are complete proteins, a person following a vegetarian food pattern would need to plan carefully to obtain sufficient

Amino acids
Structural units of protein that supply essential nitrogen.

Essential amino acid
An amino acid that the body cannot synthesize in sufficient amounts to meet body needs so it must be supplied by the diet, hence a *dietary* essential for nine such specific amino acids.

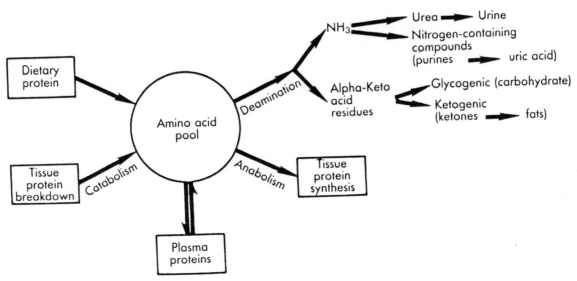

FIG. 2-1   Balance between protein compartments and amino acid pool.

TABLE 2-4 *Amino Acids Required in Human Nutrition, Grouped According to Nutritional (Dietary) Essentiality*

Essential Amino Acids	Semiessential Amino Acids*	Nonessential Amino Acids
Histidine	Arginine	Alanine
Isoleucine	Cystine (cysteine)	Asparagine
Leucine	Tyrosine	Aspartic acid
Lysine		Glutamic acid
Methionine		Glutamine
Phenylalanine		Glycine
Threonine		Hydroxyproline
Tryptophan		Hydroxylysine
Valine		Proline
		Serine

*These are considered semiessential because the rate of synthesis in the body is inadequate to support growth; therefore these are essential for children.
From Williams SR: Nutrition and diet therapy, ed 7, St Louis, 1993, Mosby.

Essential Amino Acids—Nine or Eleven?—and Their Complementary Food Proteins

All of the nine essential amino acids must be supplied by the diet. But two of them, phenylalanine and methionine, have helpers as interactive backup. The body makes the amino acid tyrosine, which can spare some of the phenylalanine, and cystine, which can interact with methionine. So although there are only 9 essential amino acids the body cannot make, some may speak of 11 when they add the two helpers tyrosine and cystine.

The real life concern in a vegetarian diet is to get a balanced amount of the essential amino acids to complement one another and make complete food combinations. Only three of these nine essential amino acids are critical, however, because if persons eat foods to supply enough of these three in a combined pattern, they will get sufficient amounts of the others too. These three amino acids are thus called the *limiting amino acids*—lysine, methionine, and tryptophan. Of these three, lysine is the most limiting.

The answer lies in mixing families of foods like grains, legumes, and milk products to make complementary food combinations to balance these needed amino acids. For example, grains are low in lysine and high in methionine, while legumes are just the opposite—low in methionine and high in lysine. Basically, grains and legumes will always balance one another and additions of milk products and eggs will enhance their adequacy. Here are a few sample food combination dishes to illustrate:

Rice + black-eyed peas—a Southern United States dish called "Hopping John"
Whole wheat or bulgur + soybeans + sesame seeds—protein enhanced by the addition of yogurt
Cornmeal + kidney beans—a combination in many Mexican dishes, protein enhanced by the addition of cheese
Soybeans + peanuts + brown rice + bulgur wheat—an excellent sauce dish served over the rice and wheat

Prepared with a variety of herbs, spices, onions, and garlic, to suit your taste, such dishes can supply needed nutrients and good eating.

ONE STEP FURTHER

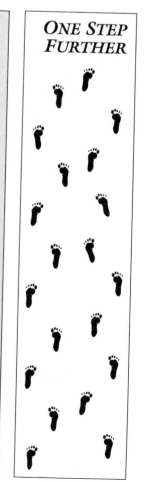

quantities of essential amino acids by using combinations of complimentary plant proteins, as described in the box on p. 21. During the growth years, arginine is also essential to meet normal childhood growth demands. Although arginine is synthesized by the body, it may not be made in sufficient amounts to meet the rapid growth of infants, especially premature infants, and young children.[4]

Nonessential amino acids. All amino acids have essential tissue-building and metabolic functions. However, as used here, the nonessential amino acids are 12 amino acids that the body can synthesize in sufficient amounts to meet needs, so they are not essential in the diet.

Protein balance. The term *balance* refers to the relative intake and output of substances in the body to maintain normal levels needed for health in various circumstances during the life cycle. We can apply this concept of balance to life-sustaining protein and the nitrogen it supplies. The body's tissue proteins are constantly being broken down, a process called **catabolism**, and then resynthesized into tissue protein as needed, a process called **anabolism.** To maintain nitrogen balance, the nitrogen-containing amino part of the amino acid may be removed by a process called **deamination,** converted to ammonia (NH^3), and the nitrogen excreted as urea in the urine, as shown in Fig 2-1. The remaining non-nitrogen residue can be used to make carbohydrate or fat, or reattached to an amino group ($—NH^2$) make another amino acid according to need. The rate of this protein and nitrogen turnover varies in different tissues, according to their degree of metabolic activity. This process involves a continuous reshaping and rebuilding, adjusting as needed to maintain overall protein balance within the body. Also, the body maintains an internal balance between tissue protein and plasma protein. Then, in turn, these two body protein stores are further balanced with dietary protein intake. With this finely balanced system, a metabolic "pool" of amino acids from both tissue protein and dietary protein is always available to meet construction needs.

Nitrogen balance. The body's **nitrogen balance** indicates how well its tissues are being maintained. The intake and use of dietary protein is measured by the amount of nitrogen intake in the food protein and the amount of nitrogen excreted in the urine. Total 24-hour urinary urea nitrogen excretion measure is used with calculated dietary nitrogen intake over the same time period to determine a person's nitrogen balance:

$$\text{Nitrogen balance} = \text{Protein intake} \div 6.25 - (\text{Urinary urea nitrogen} + 4)$$

The formula factor of 4 in the equation represents the additional nitrogen loss through feces and skin. Urinary urea nitrogen excretion reflects metabolism of dietary protein, as the nitrogen balance formula indicates, and is a measure of the adequacy of the protein nutriture. For example, 1 g of urinary nitrogen results from the digestion and metabolism of 6.25 g of protein. Therefore, if for every 6.25 g of protein consumed 1 g of nitrogen is excreted in the urine, the body is said to be in nitrogen balance. This is the normal pattern in adult health, but at different times during the life cycle, or in states of malnutrition or illness, this balance may be either positive or negative.

1. Positive nitrogen balance. A positive nitrogen balance exists when the body takes in more nitrogen than it excretes. This means that the body is storing nitrogen by building more tissue than it is breaking down. This situation occurs normally during periods of rapid growth such as infancy, childhood, adolescence, and during pregnancy and lactation. It also occurs in persons who have been ill or malnourished and are being "built back up" with increased nourishment. In such cases protein is being stored to meet increased needs for tissue building and associated metabolic activity.

2. Negative nitrogen balance. A negative nitrogen balance exists when the body takes in less nitrogen than it excretes. This means that the body has an inadequate protein intake and is losing nitrogen by breaking down more tissue than it is building up. This situation

Catabolism
Metabolic process by which tissue is broken down.

Anabolism
Metabolic process by which tissue is built up.

Deamination
Process by which the nitrogen radical (NH_4) is split off from amino acids; important in maintaining nitrogen balance.

Nitrogen balance
Metabolic balance between nitrogen intake in dietary protein and output in urinary nitrogen compounds such as urea and creatinine.

occurs in states of malnutrition and illness. For example, this nitrogen imbalance is seen not only in underdeveloped countries but also in America in cases where specific protein deficiency exists, even when kcalories from carbohydrate and fat may be adequate, causing the classic protein deficiency disease **kwashiorkor.**[5] Failure to maintain nitrogen balance may not become apparent for some time, but it will eventually cause loss of muscle tissue, impairment of body organs and functions, and increased susceptibility to infection. In children, negative nitrogen balance will cause growth retardation.

Primary tissue building. Protein is the fundamental structural material of every living cell in the body. In fact, the largest portion of the body, excluding the water content, is made up of protein. Body protein, mainly the lean body mass of muscles, accounts for about three-fourths of the dry matter in most tissues other than bone and adipose fat.[1] Protein not only makes up the bulk of the muscles, internal organs, brain, nerves, skin, hair, and nails, but also is a vital part of regulatory substances such as enzymes, hormones, and blood plasma. All of these tissues must be constantly repaired and replaced. The primary functions of protein are to repair worn-out, wasted, or damaged tissue and to build up new tissue. Thus protein meets growth and development needs during early life and maintains tissue health during adult years.

Micronutrients and Metabolic Control

As indicated, the body uses the macronutrients carbohydrate, fat, and protein to solve its two major problems of energy production and tissue building and rebuilding to maintain life and health, processes that require thousands of interrelated physiologic and metabolic activities. However, meeting these two basic needs creates another major overall problem, that of metabolic regulation and control. To maintain life and health, all of these multiple physiologic tasks must proceed in a highly organized and orderly fashion, without which metabolic chaos, illness, and death would occur. Such order requires specific control agents. In harmony with hormones and specific partnerships with key cell enzymes, the remaining nutrients, the micronutrients vitamins and minerals, operate mainly in the key role of **coenzyme factors,** as is the case with some vitamins, or essential enzyme components, as with some minerals, required in a specific enzyme system for a particular metabolic reaction to occur.

Vitamins

From 1900 to 1950, as the discoveries of the **vitamins** occurred, two characteristics marked a compound for assignment to the vitamin group: (1) it must be a vital organic dietary substance, which is neither carbohydrate, fat, or protein (hence noncaloric), and is necessary in only very small quantities to do special metabolic jobs or to prevent its deficiency disease; and (2) it cannot be manufactured by the body, and therefore must be supplied in food. With current knowledge, however, it has become evident that one of these organic substances—vitamin D—has been misassigned to the vitamin group. It is now known to behave as a hormone in its active form, now called vitamin D hormone, or *calcitriol,* but is still generally discussed with the vitamins in most source materials for the sake of convenience. Vitamins are usually grouped according to solubility in a medium. The fat-soluble vitamins—A, D, E, and K—are closely associated with lipids in their fate in the body. The water-soluble vitamins—B-complex and C—have fewer problems in absorption and transport throughout.

Fat-soluble vitamins. Vitamin A enters the body in two forms: (1) the preformed vitamin A from animal food sources, usually associated with lipids, and (2) the **precursor** beta-carotene pigment from plant food sources, which actually supplies about two-thirds of the vitamin A necessary in human nutrition. Its major physiologic roles relate to the eye's vision cycle adaptation to light and dark and to a more generalized role in the formation

Kwashiorkor
Classic protein deficiency disease, frequently encountered in children in developing countries, but also seen in the United States in poverty areas and in metabolically stressed and debilitated hospitalized patients.

Coenzyme factors
Major metabolic role of the micronutrients vitamins and minerals as essential partners with cell enzymes in a variety of reactions in both energy and protein metabolism.

Vitamin
A nonenergy-yielding micronutrient required in very small amounts for specific metabolic tasks that cannot be synthesized by the body so must be supplied in the diet.

Precursor
Substance from which another substance is produced.

and maintenance of healthy functioning epithelial tissue, the body's primary barrier to infections.

Vitamin D hormone is produced in the body, first by sunlight irradiation of a precursor cholesterol compound in the skin, intermediate product synthesis in the liver, and subsequent formation in the kidneys of the physiologically active form, *calcitriol*—1,25-dihydroxycholecalciferol [1,25 $(OH)_2D_3$]. Its major physiologic role is in regulation of bone and mineral metabolism. A more widespread tissue role relates to controlling basic cell processes associated with cellular proliferation and differentiation.

Vitamin E has a single vital physiologic role relating to its action in many tissues as an

ONE STEP FURTHER

Vitamin E and Premature Infants

A medical problem found in infants, especially those born prematurely, has responded positively to vitamin E therapy. This problem is *hemolytic anemia*.

Anemia is a blood condition characterized by loss of mature functioning red blood cells. Different types of anemia are usually named according to cause, or to the nature of an abnormal nonfunctioning cell produced instead of the normal cell. In this case the name comes from the cause. The word *hemolysis* has two roots, *hemo* referring to blood and *lysis* meaning dissolving or breaking. Hemolysis is the bursting or dissolving of red blood cells and the resulting condition is hemolytic anemia.

Vitamin E can help prevent this destruction of red blood cells and the loss of their vital oxygen-carrying hemoglobin because it is one of the body's foremost antioxidants. An oxidant is a compound, or oxygen itself, that oxidizes other compounds and in the process breaks them down or changes them. Vitamin E is readily oxidized. When there is plenty of vitamin E among other compounds exposed to an oxidant, it can take on the oxidative attack and thus protect the others. Vitamin E is fat soluble so it is found in fat-rich tissues of the body among the polyunsaturated fatty acids that make up the core of the cell membranes. The cell membranes of red blood cells are particularly rich in these polyunsaturated lipids and they are exposed to concentrated oxygen because they constantly circulate through the lungs. This would be a destructive situation were it not for the vitamin E present. It takes the oxygen itself, protecting the polyunsaturated fatty acids and preserving the red blood cells intact, to continue their life-sustaining journey throughout the body. Thus vitamin E acts as nature's most potent fat-soluble antioxidant. It interrupts the oxidative breakdown by free radicals (parts of compounds broken off by cell metabolism) in the cell, protecting the cell membrane fatty acids from the oxidative damage.

Infants fed formulas rich in polyunsaturated fatty acids and supplemented with iron (an oxidant) may develop hemolytic anemia as the fragile red blood cell membranes break down due to the high cell oxidative process and the induced deficiency of vitamin E. This protective need for increased vitamin E is especially great with small premature infants fed formulas containing iron, which acts as an oxidant, and high concentrations of polyunsaturated fatty acids, which are vulnerable to oxidative breakdown. To avoid this problem and comply with American Academy of Pediatrics recommendations, manufacturers have increased the vitamin E and lowered the iron in formulas for premature infants. Now the improved formula ratio of vitamin E, polyunsaturated fatty acids, and iron no longer makes additional supplement necessary to prevent hemolytic anemia.

Modified from Bieri JG, et al: Medical uses of vitamin E, *N Engl J Med* 308(18):1063, 1983; and National Research Council, Food and Nutrition Board: *Recommended dietary allowances*, ed 10, Washington, DC, 1989, National Academy Press.

antioxidant, an agent that prevents tissue breakdown by oxygen—the process of oxidation. It acts as nature's most potent fat-soluble antioxidant, protecting the cell membrane fatty acids from damage. For example, vitamin E can protect fragile red blood cell membranes in premature infants from breaking down and causing *hemolytic anemia* (see the box on p. 24). It is interesting that vegetable oils, the richest sources of vitamin E, are also the richest sources of polyunsaturated fatty acids, which vitamin E protects.

Vitamin K has a basic physiologic role relating to the body's vital blood-clotting process through its essential presence in the formation of several proteins involved, including *prothrombin*. In this role it can serve as an antidote for excess effects of anticoagulant drugs and is often used in the control and prevention of certain types of hemorrhages. A more recently discovered function of vitamin K relates to bone development.[7] Specific proteins found in bone and bone matrix depend on vitamin K for their synthesis and are involved with calcium in bone development. Since intestinal bacteria usually synthesize adequate vitamin K, supporting food sources such as green leafy vegetables, a deficiency is unlikely except in clinical conditions related to blood clotting. For example, patients treated with antibiotics that kill intestinal bacteria and who are then placed on poor diets after surgery are susceptible to vitamin K deficiency with resulting blood loss and poor wound healing.[8] A more detailed summary of the fat-soluble vitamins is given in Table 2-5 for review.

Water-soluble vitamins. Nine vitamins, eight B-complex vitamins and vitamin C, comprise the water-soluble group. The letter name "B" remains loosely attached, from the

Hemolytic anemia
(Gr *haima,* blood; *lysis,* dissolution) An anemia (reduced number of red blood cells) caused by breakdown of red blood cells and loss of their hemoglobin.

TABLE 2-5   A Summary of Fat-Soluble Vitamins

Vitamin	Functions	Results of Deficiency	Food Sources
A (retinol); provitamin A (carotene)	Vision cycle—adaption to light and dark; tissue growth, especially skin and mucous membranes; toxic in large amounts	Night blindness, xerophthalmia, susceptibility to epithelial infection, changes in skin and membranes	Retinol (animal foods): liver, egg yolk, cream, butter or fortified margarine, fortified milk; carotene (plant foods): green and yellow vegetables, fruits
D (chole-calciferol)	Absorption of calcium and phosphorus, calcification of bones; toxic in large amounts	Rickets, faulty bone growth	Fortified or irradiated milk, fish oils
E (tocopherol)	Antioxidant—protection of materials that oxidize easily; normal growth	Breakdown of red blood cells, anemia	Vegetable oils, vegetable greens, milk, eggs, meat, cereals
K (phylloquinone)	Normal blood clotting	Bleeding tendencies, hemorrhagic disease	Green leafy vegetables, milk and dairy products, meat, eggs, cereals, fruits, vegetables

From Williams SR: *Basic nutrition and diet therapy,* ed 10, St Louis, 1995, Mosby.

TABLE 2-6   *A Summary of B-Complex Vitamins*

Vitamin	Functions	Results of Deficiency	Food Sources
Thiamin	Normal growth; coenzyme in carbohydrate metabolism; normal function of heart, nerves, and muscle	Beriberi; GI: loss of appetite, gastric distress, indigestion, deficient hydrochloric acid; CNS: fatigue, nerve damage, paralysis; CV: heart failure, edema of legs especially	Pork, beef, liver, whole or enriched grains, legumes
Riboflavin	Normal growth and vigor; coenzyme in protein and energy metabolism	Ariboflavinosis; wound aggravation, cracks at corners of mouth, swollen red tongue, eye irritation, skin eruptions	Milk, meats, enriched cereals, green vegetables
Niacin (precursor: tryptophan)	Coenzyme in energy production; normal growth, health of skin, normal activity of stomach, intestines, and nervous system	Pellagra; weakness, lack of energy, and loss of appetite; skin: scaly dermatitis; CNS: neuritis, confusion	Meat, peanuts, legumes, enriched grains
Pyridoxine	Coenzyme in amino acid metabolism: protein synthesis, heme formation, brain activity; carrier for amino acid absorption	Anemia; CNS: hyperirritability, convulsions, neuritis	Grains, seeds, liver and kidney meats; milk, eggs, vegetables
Pantothenic acid	Coenzyme in formation of coenzyme A: fat, cholesterol, and heme formation and amino acid activation	Unlikely because of widespread occurrence	Meats, cereals, legumes; milk, vegetables, fruit
Biotin	Coenzyme A partner; synthesis of fatty acids, amino acids, purines	Natural deficiency unknown	Liver, egg yolk, soy flour, cereal (except bound form in wheat), tomatoes, yeast
Folic acid	Part of DNA, growth and development of red blood cells	Certain type of anemia: megaloblastic (large, immature red blood cells)	Liver, green leafy vegetables, legumes, yeast
Cobalamin	Coenzyme in synthesis of heme for hemoglobin, normal red blood cell formation	Pernicious anemia (B_{12} is necessary extrinsic factor that combines with intrinsic factor of gastric secretions for absorption)	Liver, kidney, lean meats, milk, eggs, cheese

GI, gastrointestinal; *CNS,* central nervous system; *CV,* cardiovascular.
From Williams SR: Basic nutrition and diet therapy, ed 10, St Louis, 1995, Mosby.

initial name *water-soluble B* given to the food factor in rice polishings used by early investigators to cure beriberi. When an increasing number of water-soluble vitamins were discovered, however, their distinct and unique natures led to a new naming system, now in common use, based on individual chemical structure or function, and we now know that initial "water-soluble B" as *thiamin,* a name based on its ring-like chemical structure. These eight initial "B" vitamins are now recognized as unique individual compounds and so named (although the previous letter name "B" is still commonly used for two of them): thiamin, niacin, riboflavin, pyridoxine (B_6), pantothenic acid, biotin, folate, cobalamin (B_{12}). Discovered later than the initial "B" vitamins, the remaining water-soluble vitamin, C, still carries its common letter name, although its true chemical name *ascorbic acid,* based on its function in curing scurvy, is more precise.

Despite their remarkable diversity of chemical structure and physiologic roles, the water-soluble vitamins are alike in many ways. Aside from sharing enough likeness in chemical structure to have the common chemical characteristic of water-solubility, all these vitamins—with one exception in each case—share three additional characteristics significant in human nutrition:

1. **Food source.** All are synthesized by plants and are supplied in the diet by plant foods (as well as by animal foods)—except *cobalamin (vitamin B_{12}).*
2. **Storage.** All have no stable body "storage" form and must therefore be provided regularly in the diet—except *cobalamin (vitamin B_{12}).*
3. **Function.** All serve as coenzyme factors in cell enzyme reactions—except *ascorbic acid (vitamin C),* which serves mainly as a structural agent in building connective tissue.

Tables 2-6 and 2-7 provide water-soluble vitamin reviews for reference. Note that food sources of vitamin B_{12} are only animal foods. A nutrition concern centers on possible B_{12} deficiency states among vegans, strict vegetarians who use no animal foods (meat, milk, cheese, egg). A supplement of vitamin B_{12} may be needed when the demand is greater, especially in periods of rapid growth through the life cycle, such as pregnancy, infancy, childhood, and adolescence.

Minerals

The remaining micronutrients, the minerals, are single inorganic elements that are widely distributed in nature. During the eons in which the earth was forming, shifting oceans and mountains deposited a large number of minerals into earth materials. Over time these minerals have moved from rocks to soil, then to plants, to animals, and to humans.

TABLE 2-7   A Summary of Vitamin C (Ascorbic Acid)

Functions	Clinical Applications	Food Sources
Intercellular cement substance; firm capillary walls and collagen formation Helps prepare iron for absorption and release to tissues for red blood cell formation	Scurvy (deficiency disease) Sore gums Hemorrhages, especially around bones and joints Tendency to bruise easily Stress reactions Growth periods Fevers and infections Wound healing, tissue formation Anemia	Citrus fruits, tomatoes, cabbage, leafy vegetables, potatoes, strawberries, melons, chili peppers, broccoli, chard, turnip greens, green peppers, other green and yellow vegetables

From Williams SR: *Basic nutrition and diet therapy,* ed 10, St Louis, 1995, Mosby.

Ions

(Gr *ion*, wanderer) Activated form of certain minerals, such as sodium (NA$^+$), potassium (K$^+$), and chloride (Cl$^-$), that carry an electrical charge and perform a variety of essential metabolic tasks.

As a result, the mineral content of the human body is quite similar to that of the earth. Of the 54 known earth elements in the periodic table of elements, 25 have been shown to be essential to human life. In comparison with the vitamins, which are large, complex organic compounds, minerals—single inert elements—may seem very simple. However, in their activated form of **ions** (carrying a positive or negative charge) they perform a wide, fascinating variety of essential metabolic tasks. Minerals differ from vitamins in the variety of their physiologic roles and in the amounts, relatively large to exceedingly small, needed for these tasks.

Variety of physiologic roles. These seemingly simple, single elements, in comparison with the much larger organic structure of vitamins, perform an impressive variety of metabolic tasks. They build, activate, regulate, transmit, and control. For example, sodium and potassium control water balance. Calcium and phosphorus are building materials that structure body framework. Iron helps build the vital oxygen carrier hemoglobin in red blood cells (Fig. 2-2). Cobalt is the central core of cobalamin (vitamin B$_{12}$). Iodine helps structure thyroid hormone, which in turn regulates the overall rate of all body metabolism. Thus, far from being static and inert, minerals are active essential participants, helping to control many of the body's overall metabolic processes.

Variety in amount needed. As indicated, all vitamins are required in very small amounts for their specific metabolic tasks. On the contrary, minerals occur in varying amounts in the body. For example, calcium forms a relatively large amount of the body weight—about 2%. Most of this amount is in bone tissue. An adult who weighs 150 lb has about 3 lb of calcium in the body. On the other hand, iron occurs in very small amounts. This same adult has only about 3 g (about 1/10 oz) of iron in the body. In both cases, the amount of each mineral is essential for its specific task. This varying amount of individual minerals in the body provides the basis for classifying them into two main groups, major minerals and trace elements.

1. Major minerals. Certain elements are referred to as major minerals not because they are more important in metabolism, but simply because they occur in larger amounts in the body; thus, their requirement is greater. On this basis, seven elements for which the

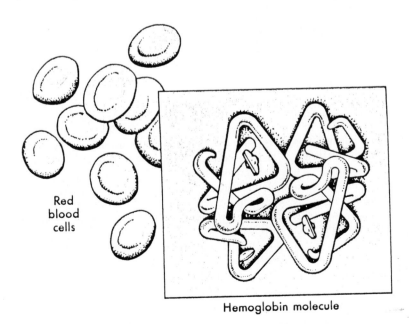

Red blood cells

Hemoglobin molecule

FIG. 2-2 Hemoglobin is an oxygen-carrying protein of red-blood cells.

requirement is greater than 100 mg/day are classed as **major minerals.** They contribute from 60% to 80% of the inorganic material in the human body. These seven major minerals are calcium, phosphorus, sodium, potassium, magnesium, chloride, and sulfur (Table 2-8). A review of their physiologic roles is given in Table 2-9. Our major food source of calcium for bone growth through the life cycle (see p. 30) is milk and other dairy products.

    2. Trace elements. The remaining 18 elements in Table 2-8 make up the group of **trace elements.** These minerals are no less important, but they occur in very small traces or amounts in the body, contributing only 20% to 40% of all the inorganic material in the human body. For example, the human body contains only about 45 mg of iron per kilogram body weight. Nonetheless, each of these trace elements is necessary for its specific metabolic task. A review of the main physiologic roles of the trace elements is given in Table 2-10.

The concept of essentiality. Note in Table 2-8 that the trace elements are divided into two subgroups on the basis of essentiality in human nutrition. In the first subgroup labeled essential, 10 trace elements have been deemed definitely essential on the basis of defined function and requirement determined from research. The remaining group of eight elements is probably essential also, but a more complete understanding of their status requires finer means of analysis and tests for function.

    By the simplest definition, an essential element is one required for the existence of life and, conversely, its absence brings death. However, for components that occur in very small amounts in the body, this determination of essentiality is not easy to make. Most living matter, as we know it, is made up of five fundamental elements, carbon (C), hydrogen (H), oxygen (O), nitrogen (N), and sulfur (S), which make up the macronutrients. We know these elements well because their concentrations are relatively large, hence more easily studied, and their requirements for human function can be expressed in multiples of grams per kilogram body weight. We have means for analysis of such quantities and can easily see that these are essential elements. Also, the major minerals occur in respectable quantities in the body, and their essentiality has been more easily studied and determined. However, the much larger number of trace elements occur in biologic matter in very small amounts, and we know less about them. It is harder to determine essentiality of these trace elements because we require so little of them in the face of relatively large amounts found in our diet and environment. This makes it experimentally difficult to demonstrate essentiality, which

Major minerals
  Minerals that occur in relatively large quantities in the body and hence have greater dietary requirements.

Trace elements
  Minerals that occur in small amounts, or traces, in the body, and hence are required in very small amounts.

TABLE 2-8   *Major Minerals and Trace Elements in Human Nutrition*

Major Minerals (Required Intake Over 100 mg/day)	Trace Elements	
	Essential (Required Intake Under 100 mg/day)	Essentiality Unclear
Calcium (Ca)	Iron (Fe)	Silicon (Si)
Phosphorus (P)	Iodine (I)	Vanadium (V)
Sodium (Na)	Zinc (Zn)	Nickel (Ni)
Potassium (K)	Copper (Cu)	Tin (Sn)
Magnesium (Mg)	Manganese (Mn)	Cadmium (Cd)
Chlorine (Cl)	Chromium (Cr)	Arsenic (As)
Sulfur (S)	Cobalt (Co)	Aluminum (Al)
	Selenium (Se)	Boron (B)
	Molybdenum (Mo)	
	Fluorine (Fl)	

From Williams SR: Basic nutrition and diet therapy, ed 10, St Louis, 1995, Mosby.

TABLE 2-9   *A Summary of Major Minerals*

Mineral	Metabolism	Physiologic Functions	Clinical Application	Requirements	Food Sources
Calcium (Ca)	Absorption according to body need, aided by vitamin D; hindered by binding agents (oxalates), or excessive fiber. Parathyroid hormone controls absorption and mobilization	Bone formation Teeth Blood clotting Muscle contraction and relaxation Heart action Nerve transmission	Tetany—decrease in ionized serum calcium Rickets Osteoporosis	Adults: 1200 mg Pregnancy and lactation: 1200 mg Infants: 400-600 mg Children: 800-1200 mg	Milk Cheese Whole grains Egg yolk Legumes, nuts Green leafy vegetables
Phosphorus (P)	Absorption with calcium aided by vitamin D; hindered by excess binding agents (aluminum)	Bone and tooth formation Overall metabolism Energy metabolism (enzymes) Acid-base balance	Bone loss Poor growth	Adults: 1200-800 mg Pregnancy and lactation: 1200 mg Infants: 300-500 mg Children: 800-1200 mg	Milk Cheese Meat Egg yolk Whole grains Legumes, nuts
Sodium (Na)	Readily absorbed	Major extracellular fluid control Water balance Acid-base balance Muscle action; transmission of nerve impulse and resulting contraction	Fluid shifts and control Buffer system Losses in gastrointestinal disorders Dehydration	Limit to 2.4 g or less	Table salt (NaCl) Milk Meat Egg Baking soda Baking powder Carrots, beets, spinach, celery
Potassium (K)	Secreted and reabsorbed in digestive juices	Major intracellular fluid control Acid-base balance Regulates nerve impulse and muscle contraction Glycogen formation Protein synthesis Energy metabolism	Fluid shifts Heart action—low serum potassium (cardiac arrest) Insulin release Blood pressure factor	About 2000-3500 mg Diet adequate in protein, calcium, and iron contains adequate potassium	Fruits Vegetables Meats Whole grains Legumes

Mineral	Metabolism	Physiologic functions	Clinical applications	Requirement	Food sources
Magnesium (Mg)	Absorption increased by parathyroid hormone	Aids thyroid hormone secretion, normal BMR; Activator and coenzyme in carbohydrate and protein metabolism; Muscle, nerve action	Tremor, spasm; low serum level following gastrointestinal losses or renal losses from alcoholism; convulsions	Adults: 280-350 mg; Pregnancy and lactation: 320-355 mg; Deficiency in humans unlikely	Whole grains; Nuts; Legumes; Green vegetables (chlorophyll)
Chlorine (Cl)	Absorbed readily	Acid-base balance—chloride shift; Gastric hydrochloric acid—digestion	Hypochloremic alkalosis in prolonged vomiting, diarrhea, tube drainage	Parallel requirement of sodium	Table salt
Sulfur (S)	Absorbed as such and as constituent of sulfur-containing amino acid methionine	Essential constituent of cell protein; Hair, skin, nails; Vitamin structure; Collagen structure; High-energy sulfur bonds in energy metabolism	General protein malnutrition	Diet adequate in protein contains adequate sulfur	Meat; Egg; Cheese; Milk; Nuts, legumes

From Williams SR: Basic nutrition and diet therapy, ed 10, St Louis, 1995, Mosby.

TABLE 2-10 *A Summary of Selected Trace Elements*

Element	Metabolism	Physiologic Functions	Clinical Application	Requirements	Food Sources
Iron (Fe)	Absorption according to body need; aided by vitamin C Heme and nonheme forms Excretion from tissue in minute quantities; body conserves then reuses	Hemoglobin formation Cellular oxidation of glucose Myoglobin in muscle Antibody production Drug detoxification Carotene conversion to vitamin A Collagen synthesis	Growth Pregnancy demands Deficiency—anemia	Men: 10 mg Women: 15 mg Pregnancy: 30 mg Lactation: 15 mg Children: 10-15 mg	Liver Meats Egg yolk Whole grains Enriched bread and cereal Dark green vegetables Legumes, nuts
Iodine (I)	Absorbed as iodides, taken up by thyroid gland under control of thyroid-stimulating hormone (TSH) Excretion by kidney	Synthesis of thyroxine, the thyroid hormone, which regulates cell oxidation BMR regulation	Deficiency—endemic colloid goiter; cretinism Hypothyroidism Hyperthyroidism	Men: 150 µg Women: 150 µg Infants: 35-45 µg Children: 70-150 µg	Iodized salt Seafood
Zinc (Zn)	Transported with plasma proteins Excretion largely intestinal Stored in liver, muscle, bone, and organs	Essential enzyme constituent Combined with insulin for storage of the hormone Immune system leukocytes Associated with iron in	Wound healing Taste and smell acuity Retarded sexual and physical development	Men: 15 mg Women: 12 mg Children: 10-15 mg Infants: 5 mg	Meat Seafood, especially oysters Eggs Milk Whole grains Legumes
Copper (Cu)	Stored in muscle, bone, liver, heart, kidney, and central nervous system Iron twin	Energy production Hemoglobin synthesis Absorption and transport of iron	TPN deficiency Anemia	Adults: 1.5-3.0 mg Children: 1.0-2.5 mg (estimated)	Liver Seafood Whole grains Legumes, nuts

				Requirements	Food sources
(Mn)	Excretion mainly by intestine	Urea formation, Protein metabolism, Glucose oxidation, Lipoprotein clearance and synthesis of fatty acids	(...) protein-energy malnutrition, Inhalation toxicity in miners	Adults: 2-5 mg (estimated), Children: 1-5 mg	Cereals, whole grain, Soybeans, Legumes, nuts, Tea, Vegetables, Fruits
Chromium (Cr)	Improves faulty uptake of glucose by body tissues as part of glucose tolerance factor	Associated with glucose metabolism; raises abnormally low fasting blood sugar levels	Possible link with cardiovascular disorders and diabetes	Adults: 50-200 µg (estimated), Children: 20-200 µg	Whole grains, Cereal products
Cobalt (Co)	Absorbed chiefly as constituent of vitamin B_{12}	Constituent of vitamin B_{12}; essential factor in red blood cell formation	Deficiency associated with deficiency of vitamin B_{12}—pernicious anemia	Unknown	Supplied by preformed vitamin B_{12}
Selenium (Se)	Active as cofactor in cell oxidation enzyme systems	Associated with vitamin E as antioxidant; protects lipid in cell membrane	Keshan disease, heart muscle failure, TPN deficiency	Men: 70 µg, Women: 55 µg, Children: 20 µg	Seafoods, Kidney, Liver, Meats
Molybdenum (Mo)	Minute traces in the body	Constituent of specific enzymes involved in purine conversion to uric acid		Adults 75-250 µg (estimated)	Whole grains, Organ meats, Milk
Fluorine (Fl)	Deposited in bones and teeth	Aldehyde oxidation, Associated with dental health	Small amount prevents dental caries, Excess causes endemic dental fluorosis	Adults 1.5-4 mg (estimated), Children 0.5-2.5 mg	Whole grains, Leafy vegetables, Legumes, Fluoridated water (1 ppm Fl)

From Williams SR: Basic nutrition and diet therapy, ed 10, St Louis, 1995, Mosby.

of course requires removing it from the diet and the environment—an almost impossible task.

Essential function. Nonetheless, despite the difficulties in determining essentiality of these small amounts of trace elements in our bodies, studies have indicated that essentiality can be determined on the basis of function and deficiency effect. Studies in trace element metabolism have indicated that in the simplest terms an element is essential when a deficiency causes an impairment of function and when supplementation with that substance, but not with others, prevents or cures this impairment. However, in relation to health care today, Mertz, a leading researcher in trace elements, also reminds us that major modern disease is often multifactorial and a complex of nutritional interventions is often required.[9] His studies of human metabolism have identified the function of trace elements in terms of catalytic and structural components of larger molecules.

1. Catalytic components. Small amounts of various trace elements may act as an enzyme component in a catalytic manner in essential cell metabolic reactions.

2. Structural components. Additional elements act as a structural molecule component in building materials used in cell and tissue formation.

These trace elements carry out their function in three ways: (1) they may amplify the full function of the larger molecule of which they are a part, (2) they are specific to the particular function involved, and (3) they contribute to homeostatic regulation through their absorption-excretion balance and the degree of their carrier transport situation. Stages of research concerning trace element needs can be compared in terms of how far advanced our knowledge is: (1) longstanding knowledge, as is the case with iron and iodine; (2) recent history and questions, as for elements such as chromium, copper, zinc, and selenium; and (3) newer but incomplete knowledge, such as exists for silicon, vanadium, nickel, and arsenic. For example, metabolic studies of vanadium in laboratory cultured cells and test animals have shown that, among other actions, this ultratrace element may affect glucose metabolism by altering or mimicking the action of insulin, possibly by altering membrane function for ion transport processes.[10-12] These continuing studies, as well as knowledge of its food sources and nutritional requirement, suggest that vanadium may have an essential functional role in human beings,[10] which in turn may yet indicate possible future clinical roles, for example, in diabetes management.

Water

The final basic nutrient, water, underlies all the functions of the other nutrients and, next to air, is the most essential substance to our survival. It creates the water-based environment necessary for the vast array of chemical actions and reactions that comprise body metabolism and sustain life. Also, it provides the means for maintaining a stable body temperature and helps give structure and form to our bodies through the turgor it provides for the tissues. We obtain this life-giving water in fluids we drink, including water and other beverages; in foods we eat, and the water of oxidation created within from the end products of cell metabolism. The average adult metabolizes from 2.5 to 3 L of water/day in a constant turnover balanced between intake and output. This water enters and leaves the body by various routes, controlled by basic mechanisms such as thirst and hormonal activity.

THE HUMAN LIFE CYCLE AND CHANGING NUTRIENT NEEDS
Growth and Development

Physical growth. Growth may be defined as an increase in size, but it encompasses far more than that. Biologic growth of an organism occurs through cell multiplication.

Catalyst

(Gr *katalysis,* dissolution) A substance, such as enzymes and their component trace elements, that controls specific cell metabolism reactions but is not changed or consumed itself in the reaction as are the specific substances on which it works.

Development is the associated process in which growing tissues and organs take on an increased complexity of function. Both processes combine to form a unified whole in the many aspects of human growth and development throughout the life cycle. This dual concept indicates the magnitude and quality of maturational changes that establish early embryonic cells through cell multiplication and differentiation, set the pattern for subsequent rapid fetal growth and development, produce a fully formed, small, dependent newborn, and transform this newborn infant through successive childhood growth periods into a fully functioning, independent adult.

Physiologic and psychosocial development. Physiologic growth depends on a variety of nutrients in the food a child eats. It also depends on the vast number of biochemical processes of metabolism that supply the right materials in the right place at the right time for forming and maintaining unique body tissues. Human growth and development, however, involves far more than the physical process alone. It takes in social and psychologic influences and relationships—indeed, the entire environment and culture that promotes individual growth potential. Food and feeding, especially during the early formative childhood years but also throughout the life cycle, do not and cannot exist apart from this broader, overall personal growth and development. Although we are concerned about necessary nutrients at any age, we do not eat nutrients; we eat food, with all the uniquely different social, cultural, and personal meanings it holds for each of us.

Changing nutrient needs. Through the successive age groups of the life cycle, changing nutrient needs reflect an increasing differentiation based on age and sex as the physical body grows and develops. There is a general steady increase in nutrient and energy needs through early age groups to about age 10-12 years, with individuals within any age group often having different needs according to individual growth patterns. With the onset of puberty and the differing sexual development of boys and girls, nutrient needs for the two sexes begin to vary. During this adolescent period, the final growth spurt of childhood occurs. Maturation during this period varies so widely that chronological age as a reference point for discussing growth ceases to be useful (if indeed it ever was, for individual differences occur at all ages). **Physiologic age** becomes more important in dealing with individual adolescent girls and boys (see Chapter 8). It accounts for wide fluctuations in metabolic rates, food requirements, scholastic capacity, and even illness. These capacities can be more realistically viewed in individual physiologic growth terms. The profound growth period of adolescents requires increases in energy, protein, minerals, and vitamins. Boys usually eat well enough to receive all necessary nutrients, whereas girls often do not.

Body Composition

Individual variation. Throughout the life cycle the physical composition of the human body is changing. From conception and birth, throughout childhood growth and adult aging, to old age decline and death, the human body and its basic components change and adapt in a remarkable fashion to meet physiologic needs. Given the genetic imprint of its heritage and the physical and psychosocial nature of its environment, the human body, in the most literal sense, is the product of its nutrition throughout life. Through profound and fascinating transformations, food makes possible the living body and all its functions, and the varying mass of tissue it produces and maintains. There is no precise "ideal" or "standard" **body composition** except for purposes of study in the laboratory. In reality this is a hazardous assumption, for within the limits of genetic potential, individuals differ widely. There is great variability among healthy persons in both body composition and body response to internal and external environmental influences and to disease. However, a general knowledge of body composition components and their interrelatedness provides an important basis for measuring and determining the nutritional status of specific individuals of all ages, as well as the many influences that shape it.

Physiologic age
Rate of biologic maturation in individual adolescents that varies widely and accounts for more than does chronologic age for wide and changing differences in their metabolic rates, nutritional needs, and food requirements.

Body composition
The relative sizes of the four body compartments that make up the physical body-lean body mass, fat, water, and mineral mass.

Basic concepts of compartments and balance. With the two basic physiologic concepts of body compartments and balance for a foundation, we can identify and describe the gross components of body composition, especially in relation to body changes and nutritional needs through the life cycle. The concept of *balance* provides a dynamic view of the body, ever changing and adjusting to its internal and external environments. The biologic term **compartment** is used to describe the body's internal collection of a given vital substance. The concept of compartments gives a comprehensive view of the human body, not of static mechanical parts, but of **homeostasis,** a state of dynamic equilibrium within an interdependent whole. The nutritional needs of individuals throughout growth and development can be understood through the application of these two basic concepts.

Body compartment
The collective quantity of a particular vital substance in the body; for example, the mineral compartment, composed mainly of the skeletal bone mass.

Body Composition Compartments Based on Metabolic Activity

Nutritional scientists, who are interested in nutritional status as a means of determining nutritional needs throughout life, usually use the criterion of metabolic activity to define the gross components of body composition. On this basis many researchers commonly distinguish four main components in two divisions: (1) those parts that are most active in energy metabolism—*lean body mass*—and (2) those parts that are relatively inactive—*body fat, extracellular water,* and the *mineral mass of bones and smaller structural parts.* The remaining body compartment most active in energy metabolism is the **lean body mass.**

Lean body mass compartment. The body's lean cell mass is the primary determinant of its energy requirements and thus its overall nutrient needs. Its relative size and metabolic activity, as well as its relation to weight changes, are important considerations.

1. Compartment size and metabolic activity. In various individuals the lean body mass, as a collective compartment of the body's active fat-free mass of cells, will account for anything from 30% to 65% of the total body weight. However, in any person it accounts for almost all the energy consumption. As a percentage of body weight, for example, the values for this lean cell mass will range from low levels in very fat, sedentary persons to higher levels in very muscular persons.

2. Relation to weight changes. When persons gain or lose weight because of diet changes, it is not merely a reflection of changes in the body fat mass but also in the lean body mass. The density of the tissue added or lost is never that of pure fat. The density of the nonfat lean part also changes with nutritional status. Added exercise enhances its relative size.

Body fat compartment. The gross amount of the body fat compartment can vary widely and affect individual health status. In general, it reflects the number and size of fat cells—**adipocytes**—making up the adipose tissue. However, adipose tissue is not pure fat. It also contains parts of other compartments such as blood vessels, connective tissue, cell membranes, and water.

Adipocytes
(L *adipis,* fat; Gr *kytos,* hollow vessel, cell) Fat cells.

1. Compartment size. In relation to a standard "reference body" and from body water measurements, the body fat compartment has been variously estimated in healthy persons to range in an adult man, for example, from about 14% to 28% of the total body weight. The woman's "reference body" would have a somewhat larger fat compartment, about 15% to 29% of total body weight. These percentages vary with factors such as age, climate, exercise, and fitness. About half of the total body fat is in the subcutaneous fat layers, which serve the important task of helping to maintain body temperature.

2. Relation to health. Extremes in size of the body fat compartment can affect individual health status. For example, some athletes, especially compulsive runners, may strive for a very low level of body fat, even in some cases to an unhealthy deficit. Conversely, at the other extreme, massively obese sedentary persons carry increased health risks from an excessively large body fat mass. However, common beliefs that even moderate overweight brings poorer health and a shorter life span seem unfounded. Studies of various populations, such as the classic data from the long-standing Framingham study as well as later work, appear to indicate that it is the extremes of both underweight and obesity that increase health risks and contribute to higher mortality rates, concluding that moderate amounts of overweight, especially in older adults, may actually be a health protection.[13-15]

Body water compartment. The total body water content varies widely with relative body composition in terms of leanness and fatness, since lean muscle tissue contains more water than any other body tissue except blood. It also varies with age, being relatively higher in infants, and with hydration status, being lower in conditions causing dehydration and higher in conditions causing edema or ascites. In pregnancy the total maternal body water increases normally to support the increased metabolic work, and sometimes abnormally in complications of pregnancy-induced hypertension.

1. Total body water compartments. The total body water is divided into two subcompartments—the collective water inside the cells and the remaining collective water outside of cells. The water inside of cells is part of the active cell mass or lean body mass. So it is the remaining collective water outside of cells, the **extracellular fluid (ECF)**, that makes up this designated water compartment of gross body composition.

2. ECF compartment. The size of the ECF compartment varies with individual fatness or leanness, being higher in thin persons and lower in fat persons. In average weight adults, the collective water outside cells makes up about 20% of the total body weight; in fat persons, about 15%; in thin persons, about 25%. The ECF consists of four parts: (1) *blood plasma,* which accounts for about 25% of the ECF and 5% of body weight; (2) *interstitial fluid,* water surrounding the cells; (3) *secretory fluid,* circulating secretions in transit; and (4) *dense tissue fluid,* water in dense connective tissue, cartilage, and bone (Fig 2-3).

Body mineral compartment. The body's major mineral content by far is found in its large skeletal mass, with much smaller amounts in teeth, nails, and hair. Of all the minerals in the human body, calcium is present in far greater amounts than any other, comprising about 2% of the total body weight.

Extracellular fluid (ECF)
The total body water compartment composed of the collective water outside of cells.

Mineral compartment
Smallest part of the body composition, found mainly in the skeletal bone mass.

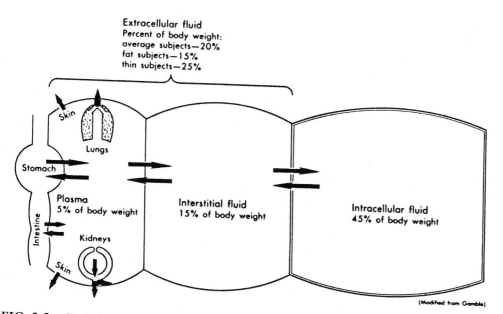

FIG. 2-3 Body fluid compartments. Note the relative total quantities of water in the intracellular compartment and in the extracellular compartment.

1. Skeletal mass. The human skeleton is a relatively large structure, comprising in the living body about one-sixth of the total body mass. Most of the body calcium—about 99%—is in the skeleton, accounting for most of the total body mineral compartment. Other minerals occur in varying lesser amounts.

2. Mineral ash. Only a small part of the skeletal mass, however, is comprised of mineral matter. The other components of bone—water, protein, and fat—are accounted for in their respective body composition compartments. In its dried, defatted state, the skeleton represents only about 6% of the gross body weight. Bone mineral mass as estimated from bone ash values is about 5% of total body weight.

To meet these human nutrition needs, most developed countries of the world have created nutrient standards and food guides for health promotion. The United States guides are discussed in the preceding chapter and may be reviewed there.

ASSESSMENT OF NUTRITIONAL STATUS
Nutritional Status of Persons and Populations

Nutritional assessment
Process of determining individual or group nutritional status as a basis for identifying needs and goals and planning personal health care or community programs to meet these identified goals.

Throughout the life cycle, in the health care of individuals or communities, **nutritional assessment** is the first step in developing nutritional care plans and programs. At both levels of care, individual clinical care plans and Public Health programs, although the scope of the work may vary from a simple conversation with a clinic patient or parent to a complex nationwide survey including all ages, the basic principles of the assessment process remain the same—to identify nutritional status and needs on which to base care plans and programs designed to meet these identified needs.

Person-Centered Clinical Care

Levels of care. Nutrition is essential to individual health on two levels:

1. Tissue level. Nutrients and energy from the food we eat build and maintain body tissues and it is on the integrity of these tissues that the physiologic functioning and health of the body depend.

2. Personal level. Food has many meanings that help fulfill personal needs and it is on the integrity of these personal psychosocial and cultural values that health as a human being depends.

In personal health care or clinical nutrition, assessment of individuals helps health care providers, together with the patient or client, determine nutritional and health status on both physiologic tissue level and psychosocial personal level, and plan nutritional care according to personal needs and goals. The overall goal is health promotion and disease prevention, or treatment of disease. If an underlying chronic disorder such as diabetes mellitus is present, or if risk factors for potential health problems such as heart disease have begun to develop, the goal is healthy control of the disorder or prevention of the health problem by reduction of risk factors. All of these nutrition and health goals involve personal health and nutrition education and skills in self-care, as well as collaboration of a skilled and sensitive team of health care professionals, including the clinical nutritionist.

Clinical care process
Interactive process of planning personal health care through five phases of assessment and data collection, analysis of findings, planning care according to a written individual care plan, implementing the plan, and evaluating and recording results.

Phases of the clinical care process. Five distinct yet interactive phases are essential in the clinical care process:

1. Assessment. A broad base of information about the person's body composition, nutrition and health status, food habits, and personal living situation provides necessary knowledge for assessing initial nutritional status and needs. Useful background information will come from various sources, primarily the individual and family, as well as health care records and other health care team members.

2. Analysis. The data collected must be analyzed carefully to determine specific needs. Some will be evident immediately. Others will develop as the situation unfolds. On the basis of this analysis, a list of problems forms.

3. Planning care. As problems are identified, valid care can be planned with the individual and family to solve them. This plan must be based on personal needs and goals, as well as any health problem involved.

4. Implementing the plan. Realistic and appropriate action plans are carried out. In nutritional care and education this will involve decisions and actions about the diet, mode of feeding as needed, and training of the person, staff, and family to carry out the plan.

5. Evaluating and recording results. As the plan is carried out, results are monitored carefully to see if the needs are being met, or if revisions in the plan must be made. Records of data, plans, procedures, and progress guide actions and instructions for continuing self-care.

Community-Centered Public Health

Changing population patterns and health goals. As the 1990 census reports, the U.S. population continues to increase, reflecting rapid change not only in total numbers but also in greater ethnic diversity, especially in border states such as California and Texas, and in increasing age (see Chapter 9). In community nutrition, assessment of population groups helps Public Health officials determine health goals and allocation of resources according to priority of need. Often the focus of this nutrition and health assessment is on groups of people bearing higher health risks: pregnant women, infants and children, adolescents, and elderly adults, especially those under the added stress of poverty, malnutrition, and illness.

Phases of the community care process. At whatever level of community nutrition work—national, state, or local—nutrition is an integral component of health and health care. The program-planning process to identify and meet these needs involves four basic areas of activity.

Community care process
Program planning to meet defined community health needs through assessment procedures, objectives, program plan, and evaluation.

1. Assessment. The two-fold process of assessment includes (1) data collection about the population of concern, and (2) analysis of the information to identify nutrition needs and problems.

2. Objectives. In relation to the identified needs or problems, both general goals and specific contributory objectives are determined to meet these needs. These goals involve staff and agency decisions about what actions are to be accomplished and a projected timeline for doing the work.

3. Program plan. To reach the established objectives, a specific plan of action is developed and carried out as projected. The program plan must consider such items as staff, tools and documents required, sources of funding, and budget for cost control.

4. Evaluation. Assessment of program activities and results continues throughout the nutrition project for health promotion or disease prevention. On the basis of this monitoring information, revisions may be made for study purposes or for conversion to a regular, continuing program status.

Community groups with special life-cycle needs. Several high-risk groups in the general population will require special nutritional attention, especially if their normal growth and development needs are compounded by such basic problems as poverty.

1. Pregnant women. During a woman's pregnancy, she must meet increased nutrient and energy needs to support this period of rapid fetal growth and bring the pregnancy to a successful outcome. At best this period is one of physiologic stress. In poor circumstances this normal stress is compounded by inadequate nutrition, bringing increased stress to both mother and baby. Continued nutrition assessment can identify specific needs, help prevent problems and complications, and promote a healthy pregnancy for both mother and baby.

2. Infants and children. The highest nutrient requirements per kilogram of body weight during the entire life cycle occur during infancy, when rates of growth and metabolism are at their highest point. Because of this direct relation between growth and

STRATEGIES FOR NUTRITION EDUCATION

Nutrition Counseling: An Important Dimension of Nutrition Education

Nutrition education is the process of helping children or adults develop the knowledge, skills, and motivation needed to make appropriate food choices throughout life. Nutrition counseling is a method of nutrition education that is being used in a variety of settings to assist individuals in adjusting their food intake to meet their personal or health needs. Nutrition counseling is often used in a hospital or clinic setting to help patients who must modify their current diet or adopt a therapeutic diet for the treatment of a medical condition such as diabetes mellitus or hypertension. Health or exercise clubs often provide dietary counseling as one of their services to members. Nutrition counseling is an important component of public health programs such as the Special Supplemental Foods Program for Women, Infants, and Children (WIC) and the National Cholesterol Education Program (NCEP). Treatment strategies for teenagers with eating disorders include nutrition counseling.

Dietary counseling must be client-centered. The nutritionist or dietitian must develop a diet strategy that will not only meet the nutrition and health objectives of the client but also be consistent with his/her lifestyle, ethnic food pattern, food preferences, and socioeconomic realities. For example an adult who must carry a lunch and has no access to a refrigerator at the work site must choose foods that meet both dietary recommendations and are safely held at room temperature. A child who receives lunch in the school cafeteria must be assisted in making appropriate choices from the foods available.

Successful nutrition counseling includes the following components.

1. *Involve the client.* The counselor and client must develop a trusting relationship if the client is to feel comfortable talking about personal needs and goals.
2. *Explore the problem.* The counselor and client should identify the problem and discuss related details and issues of importance to the client.
3. *Examine the alternatives.* The counselor and client should review possible solutions; the counselor should help the client identify and select goals.
4. *Develop a plan.* The counselor and client should form a plan of action and set up a series of steps to enable changes over time.
5. *Review progress.* The counselor and client should meet regularly to review progress, modify the plan as needed, and set new goals.

Clients must be active participants in all stages of this process. An individual is not likely to implement dietary changes if merely told what to eat. Including a family member in the counseling session who can assist in food selection and preparation and provide social support can contribute to successful dietary intervention.

nutritional status, close nutrition assessment is required to monitor progress. Over the following period of young childhood, the growth pattern slows and becomes erratic with alternating small growth spurts and plateaus. Continued assessment of progress is essential to promote health.

3. Adolescents. With puberty comes the second large growth spurt for the child. In both sexes intensive growth and hormonal changes profoundly affect nutritional needs. Continued monitoring of growth, changing body composition, and nutritional status helps ensure foundations for a healthy adulthood.

4. Adults and the elderly. With our increasing life span the gradual aging process through adulthood requires a sound nutritional base to maintain health and prevent or control chronic diseases, which account for 75% of all deaths in the United States. Nutritional risk factors are associated with most all of these chronic diseases of aging.

Methods of Assessment: Clinical and Population

Whether the assessment is being done in a clinical or community setting, four basic methods are used—anthropometric, biochemical, clinical, and dietary. Community assessment centers mainly on dietary intake surveys and nutrient analyses, but comparative data from biochemical tests, body measurements, and various clinical observations are also used to evaluate individual nutritional status as well as provide practical information about response to nutrition intervention programs. Clinical assessment may include a broader focus on related disease processes with more extensive biochemical and clinical assessment. Whatever the situation, all four methods together provide essential information to identify needs and plan health care. The American Dietetic Association has developed comprehensive guidelines and components for appropriate nutrition screening and assessment and determination of nutritional risk.[16] To review assessment basics here, a few of the commonly used measures in each method category are briefly outlined.

Anthropometry. Anthropometry is the process of measuring various dimensions of the human body. Several of these body measures provide valid estimates of muscle and fat components of body composition. They have the advantage of being inexpensive and simple to obtain. Skill gained through careful practice will minimize the margin of error. Selection and maintenance of proper procedures and equipment, as well as attention to careful technique, will help secure accurate data.

1. Weight. For accuracy, use regular clinic beam balance scales with nondetachable weights, with an additional weight attachment for use with very obese persons. Metric scales with readings to the nearest 20 g provide specific data, but the standard clinic scale is satisfactory. Read and record the person's weight, obtain information about usual body weight, and check standard weight-height tables for comparison. However, approach these tables with caution in applying them to individuals as specific ideals, remembering that wide *normal* variations occur in healthy bodies. Keeping this in mind, interpret present weight in terms of percentage of the person's usual body weight, with general reference to standard tables. Check for any significant weight loss.

2. Height. Use a true vertical bar, such as a flat wall-attached measuring stick or the movable measuring rod on the platform clinical scales. Have the person put his back to the measuring rod, stand as straight as possible, without shoes or hat, heels together, looking straight ahead. The heels, buttocks, shoulders, and head should be touching the vertical measuring surface. Read and record the measure. Compare it with previous recordings to detect possible errors, and to note growth of children or diminishing height of older adults.

3. Body mass index (BMI). The weight and height measures can be used to calculate the person's body mass index (BMI), a value often used in clinical assessment:

$$\text{BMI} = \text{Weight (kg)} \div \text{Height (meters)}^2$$

The metric conversion factors involved are 1 kg equals 2.2 lb and 1 m equals 39.37 in. This weight:height ratio is commonly used in evaluating obesity states in relation to risk factors. The desired health maintenance BMI range for adults is 20 to 25 kg/m^2. Health risks associated with obesity begin in the range of 25 to 30 kg/m^2. Values above 40 kg/m^2 indicate severe obesity.

4. Mid-upper-arm circumference (MAC). On the nondominant arm, unless it is affected by edema, use a nonstretchable centimeter tape to locate the midpoint of the upper arm. Measure the circumference at this midpoint. Read this measure accurately to the nearest tenth of a centimeter and record. Compare this result with previous measurements to note possible changes and with standard reference tables.

5. Triceps skinfold thickness (TSF). With thumb and forefinger, grasp a vertical pinch of the skin and subcutaneous fat at this previously marked upper-arm midpoint and gently pull away from the underlying muscle. Using a standard millimeter skin-

Anthropometry
(Gr *anthropos,* man, human; *metron,* measure) The process of measuring various dimensions of the human body to help determine basic body composition and needs.

Body mass index (BMI)
A calculated assessment of body mass based on weight and height: BMI = weight (kg) ÷ height (m)^2.

fold caliper and avoiding excessive pressure, measure the skinfold thickness quickly, within 2 or 3 seconds, to the nearest full or fraction of a millimeter. For increased accuracy take three measures and use the mean for calculations. Record results and compare with standard reference tables. This measure provides a good estimate of the subcutaneous fat reserves.[17]

Mid-upper arm muscle circumference (MAMC)
Indirect measure of body's skeletal muscle mass based on mid-arm muscle circumference (MAMC) and triceps skinfold (TSF): MAMC (cm) = MAC (cm) − [π × TSF (mm)].

6. Mid-upper-arm muscle circumference (MAMC). Using the two previous measures, calculate this value to provide a good indirect measure of the body's skeletal muscle mass:

$$MAMC(cm) = MAC(cm) - [\pi \times TSF(cm)]$$

If desired, the TSF can be left in millimeters as measured and the value of the mathematical factor *pi* in the formula changed accordingly to 0.314. The formula then is:

$$MAMC(cm) = MAC(cm) - [0.314 \times TSF(mm)]$$

Standard reference tables for all of these body measures are given in the Appendix. **Biochemical tests.** Numerous biochemical tests are available for assessing nutritional status. The most commonly used ones are listed here. Further description, formulas, and reference standards are given in the Appendix.

1. Plasma protein. Basic measures of plasma protein include serum albumin, hematocrit, and hemoglobin. Also, for persons with diabetes the standard monitoring tool, especially during an intensive insulin therapy program, is the **glycosylated hemoglobin A_{1c}.** Additional general tests may include serum transferrin or total iron-binding capacity (TIBC) and ferritin.

2. Protein metabolism. Basic 24-hour urine tests are used to measure urinary creatinine and urea nitrogen levels. These materials are products of protein metabolism. The 24-hour excretion of creatinine is interpreted in terms of ideal creatinine excretion for height, the creatinine-height index (CHI). The 24-hour urea nitrogen excretion is used with the calculated dietary nitrogen intake (6.25 g protein = 1 g nitrogen) over the same 24-hour period to calculate nitrogen balance:

$$\text{Nitrogen balance} = (\text{Protein intake} \div 6.25) - (\text{Urinary urea nitrogen} + 4)$$

3. Immune system integrity. Any diminished capacity of the immune system (*anergy*) is reflected in basic measures such as lymphocyte count and by additional skin-testing, observing for any delayed sensitivity to common recall antigens such as mumps or purified protein derivitive of tuberculin (PPD).

Clinical observations. Careful observations of physical signs of nutritional status provide an important added dimension to the overall assessment of individuals. Using a general examination guide for such physical signs, such as in Table 2-11, check for any possible evidence of malnutrition. Also, other physical data may include such vital signs as pulse rate, respiration, temperature, and blood pressure. A study of the common procedures of a normal physical examination will provide useful background orientation.

Dietary evaluation. Information about food intake of different groups of people or individuals is usually obtained by use of several basic tools. Choices among these procedures are guided by purposes of the assessment, available staff, and funds. More than one tool may be used for cross-checking or expanding the data received. For example, an initial nutrition history to learn basic food patterns may be followed by specific food records to provide some examples of actual food choices, quantities, and meal/snack schedule. A brief review of commonly used diet evaluation methods is outlined here.

1. Diet history. Depending on the assessment needs, information about food habits may be obtained by a comprehensive nutrition interview or a tested questionnaire filled out by the individual or parent and followed up by a brief personal review as needed by the nutritionist. Whatever its form a careful nutrition history, including related living situation

TABLE 2-11 *Clinical Signs of Nutritional Status*

	Good	Poor
General appearance	Alert, responsive	Listless, apathetic; cachexia
Hair	Shiny, lustrous; healthy scalp	Stringy, dull, brittle, dry, de-pigmented
Neck glands	No enlargement	Thyroid enlarged
Skin, face and neck	Smooth, slightly moist; good color, reddish pink mucous membranes	Greasy, discolored, scaly
Eyes	Bright, clear; no fatigue circles	Dryness, signs of infection, increased vascularity, glassiness, thickened conjunctiva
Lips	Good color, moist	Dry, scaly, swollen; angular lesions (stomatitis)
Tongue	Good pink color, surface papillae present, no lesions	Papillary atrophy, smooth appearance; swollen, red, beefy (glossitis)
Gums	Good pink color; no swelling or bleeding; firm	Marginal redness or swelling; receding, spongy
Teeth	Straight, no crowding; well-shaped jaw, clean, no discoloration	Unfilled cavities, absent teeth, worn surfaces, mottled, malpositioned
Skin, general	Smooth, slightly moist, good color	Rough, dry, scaly, pale, pigmented, irritated; petechiae, bruises
Abdomen	Flat	Swollen
Legs, feet	No tenderness, weakness, or swelling; good color	Edema, tender calf; tingling, weakness
Skeleton	No malformations	Bowlegs, knock-knees, chest deformity at diaphragm, beaded ribs, prominent scapulae
Weight	Normal for height, age, body build	Overweight or underweight
Posture	Erect, arms and legs straight, abdomen in, chest out	Sagging shoulders, sunken chest, humpback
Muscles	Well developed, firm	Flaccid, poor tone; undeveloped, tender
Nervous control	Good attention span for age; does not cry easily; not irritable or restless	Inattentive, irritable
Gastrointestinal function	Good appetite and digestion; normal, regular elimination	Anorexia, indigestion, constipation, diarrhea
General vitality	Good endurance; energetic, vigorous; sleeps well at night	Easily fatigued, no energy, falls asleep in school, looks tired, apathetic

and other personal, psychosocial, and economic problems, as well as any drugs being used, is a fundamental base of nutrition assessment.

2. 24-hour recall. Individuals are asked to recall the specific food items they ate during the previous day, describing the nature and amount of each. Sometimes this method is used because it is simpler and less costly than a longer diet history, but it has disadvantages in some groups such as elderly persons whose memory may be limited. Also, there are measurement problems in determining portion sizes.

3. Food records. When a full dietary analysis of all nutrient and energy values is needed, a 3 to 7-day food record supplies the detailed information. Individuals are asked to record their food intake for a brief period, or on certain days periodically. Each person is taught how to describe food items used singly and in combination, and how to measure amounts eaten. Studies indicate that a 3-day record is usually sufficient and the best choice to provide accurate information for nutrition analysis.[18] Currently, computer analysis of these daily food records is common, using a computer program with a large data base of food values for analysis of the person's intake of kcalories (energy) and nutrients as compared with the Recommended Dietary Allowances. A simple food analysis may be made by comparison with the five food groups of the Food Guide Pyramid.[19]

4. Food frequency questionnaire. This assessment tool provides information about an individual's food intake over an extended period of time, useful data when studying a group's disease risk and incidence. It has two basic parts: (1) a list of foods, and (2) a scale for checking frequency of use over a given period of time.

Assessment Evaluation Criteria

Well-nourished persons. Throughout the life cycle, nutritional status monitoring, guided by reference growth standards for each age group and general signs of good or poor nutrition as outlined in Table 2-11, helps to assure sound nutrition and healthy development. The rapid growth and development of the early years of life and the stress of later adult years of aging carry risks and require special attention.

1. Pregnancy. During a woman's pregnancy, she must meet increased nutrient and energy needs to support this period of rapid fetal growth and bring the pregnancy to a successful conclusion. Sufficient weight gain to meet maternal-fetal-placental demands during the pregnancy must be assured. Recent criteria for this weight gain, which reflects a positive nutritional status, have been established by the National Academy of Sciences' Institute of Medicine and can serve as a general guide.[21] Optimal nutrient and energy intake to meet both pregnancy and lactation needs can be monitored in general terms by the Recommended Dietary Allowances (see inside book covers) and guidelines discussed in Chapters 4 and 5. At best pregnancy is a period of physiologic stress, and in poor circumstances this normal stress is compounded by inadequate nutrition, bringing increased stress to both mother and baby. Continued nutrition assessment can identify specific needs, help prevent problems and complications, and promote a healthy pregnancy for both mother and baby.

2. Early growth and childhood. The highest nutrient requirements per kilogram body weight during the entire life cycle occur during infancy, when rates of growth and metabolism are at their highest point. Because of this direct relation between growth and nutritional status, close nutrition assessment is required to monitor progress. Over the following period of young childhood, the growth pattern slows and becomes erratic as the child grows in spurts and plateaus. Continued assessment of progress is essential to promote health. Commonly used monitoring tools are the age-specific growth charts from birth through adolescence, such as the National Center for Health Statistics percentile charts included in the Appendix. Age-specific RDA nutrient and energy levels can serve as general criteria, with reference to Chapters 6 and 7 for interpretations and guidance.

3. *Adolescence.* With puberty comes the second large growth spurt for the child. In both sexes intensive growth, under control of hormonal changes, profoundly affects nutritional needs. Continued monitoring of growth, changing body composition, and nutritional status helps ensure foundations for a healthy adulthood. In addition to the growth charts through age 18, extensive height-weight tables for the adolescent years are included in the Appendix. The RDA reference standard provides general evaluation criteria for monitoring nutrient and energy needs. Refer to Chapter 8 for specific monitoring guidelines.

4. *Aging and the aged.* With our increasing life span, the gradual aging process through adulthood requires a sound nutritional base to maintain health and prevent or control chronic diseases, which account for 75% of all deaths in the United States. Nutritional risk factors are associated with most all of these chronic diseases of aging. The age-adjusted weight-height table (see Appendix) serves as better evaluation criteria for older adults than the regular standard tables. Also, alternate measures of height and weight for stooped or nonambulatory older adults are included in the Appendix. The RDA provides general nutrient-energy standards, although more specific individual analysis of needs may be required for elderly persons. These needs are discussed in detail in Chapter 9.

Malnourished persons. Poorly nourished persons may be found at both extremes of the nutrient-energy intake range. On one hand, gross deficits are obvious in children suffering from protein-energy malnutrition, while at the other extreme nutrient deficits may be masked by obesity from excess caloric intake.

1. *Protein-energy malnutrition.* The high risk of malnutrition in low-income families caught in a cycle of poverty, as well as among the "new poor," is well known and documented. There is also a growing awareness of the extent of various degrees of malnutrition among persons in hospitals, rehabilitation centers, and other long-term care facilities, especially among elderly patients or residents. Assessment procedures in Public Health Services and medical/nursing facilities are designed to identify persons at risk for malnutrition. This assessment can provide the base for planning community intervention programs or individual care plans for needed nutrition support and family food assistance programs, especially for pregnant women, infants, and young children to meet crucial growth needs.

2. *Obesity.* In real terms, obesity, especially extreme forms, is a dangerous form of malnutrition because it carries increased risk of chronic disease, such as hypertension, heart disease, and diabetes. Weight assessment and early monitoring, especially of children in high-risk families for obesity and chronic disease, is an important health promotion and disease prevention practice.

Importance of Nutrition Assessment to Health Care and Public Policy

Nutritional care management. In both preventive health care and clinical care of disease, nutrition assessment is the essential first step in identifying individual nutritional needs and planning valid care to meet these needs. Careful assessment in health care can detect underlying risk factors early so that programs for reducing these risks and thus helping to prevent related disease can be initiated. In clinical care, assessment of nutrition needs can identify and help change lifestyle factors and food habits that contribute to the disease process and thus control its progress. A number of these health promotion and disease prevention or management approaches are discussed in Chapters 3 and 9.

Public nutrition intervention programs. In a similar manner, Public Health intervention programs must include careful assessment of community need and resources, identifying those persons with problems that hinder care, and the higher cost in the long run of unmet needs. For example, the community cost of simple supportive prenatal care for poor pregnant women is far more cost-effective public policy than is the high long-term cost of neonatal medical technology for salvaging tiny low-birth-weight babies, premature and with multiple medical problems, who then die in infancy or require continuous disability care. Similar situations exist in care of young children and older adults. Poor childhood nutrition, especially during important early growth and development years, contributes to learning disabilities and educational problems. Unmet older-adult nutritional needs contribute to progressive chronic disease and long-term costly care.

Summary

Human life and health depends on an appropriate supply of basic nutrients for body energy and tissue building. Of the macronutrients, carbohydrate is the primary fuel to produce energy, with fat as an additional concentrated fuel. Protein provides the amino acids necessary for building tissue. The micronutrients, vitamins and minerals, serve as control agents for biochemical reactions of body metabolism and structural material for certain tissues. The most basic nutrient, water, provides the life-sustaining solvent base for all the body's metabolic work. Nutrient needs change through the life cycle according to requirements for growth and maintaining body composition and are supplied by a balanced diet based on variety and moderation.

Nutrition is an integral component of both health and health care. Thus, nutrition assessment, both community and clinical, is basic to meeting these nutritional needs. This assessment process includes a variety of methods, including anthropometric, biochemical, clinical, and dietary procedures, and is important to both health care and public policy.

Review Questions

1. Compare the roles of each of the macronutrients in meeting energy needs of the body. How is this energy measured?
2. What are the amino acids? Describe their role in tissue growth and maintenance.
3. What are the two major types of metabolic tasks that the micronutrients perform? Give several examples of each type of task.
4. Describe the basic functions of water, the fundamental nutrient, in maintaining the human body.
5. Describe each of the two major forms of growth and development during the human life cycle. Give examples of how each relates to nutrition and changing nutrient needs.
6. Describe each of the four compartments of body composition based on metabolic activity. What part is most active metabolically? Why?
7. What basic role does assessment play in meeting nutritional needs? Compare this role in both clinical and community nutrition.
8. Identify the four basic methods of nutrition assessment and give examples of each.
9. Describe the importance of this basic assessment to nutritional health care and public policy.

References

1. Committee on Nutrition and Health, Food and Nutrition Board, National Research Council: *Diet and health: implications for reducing chronic disease risk,* Washington, DC, 1989, National Academy Press.
2. Slavin JL: Dietary fiber: mechanisms or magic on disease prevention? *Nutr Today* 25(6):6, 1990.
3. US Department of Agriculture and US Department of Health and Human Services: *Nutrition and your health: Dietary guidelines for Americans,* ed 3, Home and Garden Bull No 232, Nov 1990.
4. National Research Council, Food and Nutrition Board: *Recommended dietary allowances,* ed 10, Washington, DC, 1989, National Academy Press.

5. Rossouw JE: Kwashiorkor in North America, *Am J Clin Nutr* 49:588, April 1989.
6. DeLuca HD: Vitamin D: 1993, *Nutr Today* 28(6):6, 1993.
7. Suttie JW: Vitamin K and human nutrition, *J Am Diet Assoc* 92(5):585, 1992.
8. Usui Y et al: Vitamin K concentrations in the plasma and liver of surgical patients, *Am J Clin Nutr* 51:846, May 1990.
9. Mertz W: A balanced approach to nutrition for health: The need for biologically essential minerals and vitamins, *J Am Diet Assoc* 94(11):1259, 1994.
10. Harland BF, Harden-Williams BA: Is vanadium of human nutritional importance yet? *J Am Diet Assoc* 94(8):891, 1944.
11. Neilsen FH: Nutritional requirements for boron, silicon, vanidium, nickel, and arsenic: Current knowledge and speculation, *FASEB J* 5:2661-2667, 1991.
12. Shils ME, Olson JA, Shike M, editors: *Modern nutrition in health and disease,* vol 1, ed 8, Philadelphia, 1994, pp 282-286.
13. Kannel WB, Gordon T: *Physiological and medical concomitants of obesity: the Framingham study.* In Bray GA, editor: *Obesity in America,* Department of Health, Education, and Welfare, Pub No (NIH) 79-359, Washington, DC, 1979, US Government Printing Office.
14. Committee on Diet and Health, Food and Nutrition Board, National Research Council: *Diet and health: implications for reducing chronic disease risk,* Washington, DC, 1989, National Academy Press.
15. Bray GA: Pathphysiology of obesity, *Am J Clin Nutr* 55:448S, 1992.
16. Posthauer ME et al: ADAs definitions for nutrition screening and nutrition assessment, *J Am Diet Assoc* 94(8):838, 1994.
17. Orphanido C et al: Accuracy of subcutaneous fat measurement: comparison of skinfold calipers, ultrasound, and computed tomography, *J Am Diet Assoc* 94(8):855, 1994.
18. Crawford PB et al: Comparative advantage of 3-day food records over 24-hour recall and 5-day food frequency validated by observations of 9- and 10-year-old girls, *J Am Diet Assoc* 94(6):626, 1994.
19. Achterberg C et al: How to put the Food Guide Pyramid into practice, *J Am Diet Assoc* 94(9):1030, 1994.
20. Peters JR et al: The Eating pattern assessment tool: a simple instrument for assessing dietary fat and cholesterol intake, *J Am Diet Assoc* 94(9):1008, 1994.
21. Institute of Medicine, Food and Nutrition Board, National Academy of Science: *Nutrition during pregnancy,* Washington, DC, 1990, National Academy Press.

Further Reading

Dodd J et al: ADA supports USDA school meals initiative for healthy children but recommends more improvements for child nutrition, *J Am Diet Assoc* 94(8):841, 1994.

This report reviews current school feeding programs and identifies key areas for improving child nutrition programs through combining classroom nutrition education and lunchroom nutrition, improving nutritional food quality through principles of balance, variety, and moderation.

Dwyer J, Havala S: Position of the American Dietetic Association: vegetarian diets, *J Am Diet Assoc* 93(11):1317, 1993.

This helpful guide discusses the values of vegetarian diets, if they are well planned to provide complementary proteins and other balanced nutrients, especially if they are used by groups with special needs, such as infants, children, adolescents, and pregnant women. A regular source of vitamin B_{12} is needed for vegans, especially during pregnancy and lactation, and use of a variety of foods providing adequate energy.

Greene GW et al: Stages of change for reducing dietary fat to 30% of energy or less, *J Am Diet Assoc* 94(10):1105, 1994.

These authors descibe a gradual change process for help in changing habits of fat use to meet the Healthy People 2000 objective of reducing fat intake to 30% of the diet's kcalories, to reduce risks of cancer and cardiovascular diease.

3

Nutrition and the Adult:
THE YOUNG AND MIDDLE YEARS

Sue Rodwell Williams
Eleanor D. Schlenker

Basic Concepts

+++

✔ *A healthy lifestyle based on health promotion and disease prevention will delay development of chronic disease in young men and women.*

✔ *A variety of national and community health promotion programs assist individual efforts toward positive health maintenance and disease prevention.*

✔ *The human life cycle begins with a good nutritional status and healthy lifestyle that young parents bring to their children.*

✔ *Although genetic factors influence adult health and longevity, personal lifestyle choices determine 50% of an adult's health status.*

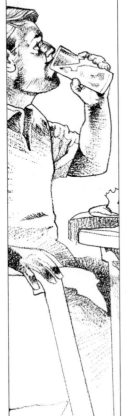

*E*stablishing lifestyle patterns that promote personal health and reproductive capacity and a state of well-being and fitness for a lifetime should be a priority for the young adult. Following the tumultuous teen years, when physical growth and development have reached their adult goal, nutrition education and patterns of living focus on food and exercise behaviors that will maintain optimal physical and mental health. Health promotion for adults is often directed toward particular physical problems. Rising medical costs associated with long-term treatment of chronic disorders such as heart disease and diabetes mellitus have led to our current emphasis on health education for disease prevention. Our goals are to help individuals identify and adopt those practices that will support optimum health and wellness throughout their adult years.

This chapter looks at some of the ways we can meet these health goals during the adult years. We focus on the nutritional needs of adults with attention to the particular health issues of young women and young men, and appropriate health promotion strategies for planning a healthy lifestyle. If signs of chronic disease do become apparent, nutrition intervention can arrest their development and help individuals maintain the highest possible level of personal well-being.

ADULT HEALTH, WELLNESS, AND LIFESTYLE
The Concept of Wellness

Health and *wellness* are words that cannot be used interchangeably. Health is most simply defined as the absence of disease, although the World Health Organization has expanded this definition to include complete physical, mental, and social well-being, and not merely the absence of disease or dysfunction. The concept of wellness carries this state of being one step further. It seeks to develop the maximal potential of individuals within their own environments. This implies a balance between activities and goals, work versus leisure, personal needs versus the expectations and goals of others, and lifestyle choices versus health risks. Wellness indicates a positive dynamic state as a person strives toward a higher level of function.

Wellness represents a continuum from high-level wellness and optimum health to low-level wellness, illness, and death. Various body functions will differ in their level of wellness from time to time. As one system or function is improving, another may be deteriorating. However, an area of strength may compensate for an area of weakness or stress. For example, excellent physical health may help an individual cope with severe emotional stress that occurs with the death of a family member, job loss, dissatisfaction with a job, or the disapproval of one's peer group.

Approaches to Health and Well-Being

Every day individuals are bombarded with messages that encourage actions to improve their health. However, people approach personal health decisions in many different ways and these approaches may differ at different stages in the life cycle. A healthy child may see little need for appropriate health behavior whereas an overweight man with above-normal serum lipid levels may be concerned about his risk of heart disease and consider changing his lifestyle to modify predisposing factors. In general, persons use one of three approaches to health care: the traditional, preventive, or wellness approach.

Traditional approach. The traditional approach to health leads to change only when the symptoms of illness or disease already exist and the individual seeks out a physician to diagnose and cure the condition. This is the pattern usually followed for acute illnesses that develop suddenly and are cured with specific drugs or treatment. Because major chronic problems like heart disease or cancer develop over a period of years, long before overt signs become apparent, this approach is of little value for lifelong positive health.

Preventive approach. The **preventive approach** to health focuses on identifying risk factors that increase a person's chances of developing a particular health problem and making behavior choices that will prevent or minimize such risks. Preventive measures may include screening programs to detect the development of a problem while it is still asymptomatic and thus allow early intervention. Health fairs, for example, emphasize blood pressure screening and intervention to reduce risk of stroke. The disadvantage of this approach is that it tends to be negative in style, emphasizing disease risk and "do not" rules of care.

Preventive approach
Approach to health that seeks to identify and reduce risk factors for disease.

Wellness approach. The **wellness approach** emphasizes positive lifestyle choices that will enhance physical and mental well-being. On this basis persons may choose to consume more vegetables and whole-grain cereals and fewer foods high in fat, salt, or sugar. The wellness approach begun early in life allows the development of full personal potential while retarding the onset of degenerative changes and chronic disease.

Wellness approach
Approach to health that promotes positive planning of a healthy lifestyle for physical and mental well-being.

Determinants of Health Status

Good or poor health is determined by five factors: heredity, environment, health outlook, health care, and lifestyle. The first of these factors, heredity, is beyond the individual's control. But the remaining four factors can, at least to some extent, be modified if the person wishes to achieve better health.

Environment. Our environment has two dimensions: the physical environment and the social environment. The *physical environment* encompasses both the near environment and the extended surrounding area. Families living in poor housing with ineffective plumbing and no refrigerator are highly susceptible to infection and disease. Poor air and water quality or contaminated food influences health status. The *social environment* can be friendly or hostile. A person may have family or friends for emotional support or be essentially alone. A person may be in a fast-paced environment with high expectations for performance or be in a setting that has low expectations and few demands.

Health outlook. Health outlook relates to personal perception of one's own health and well-being, although perception and reality may not necessarily agree. Individuals who rate their health as excellent or good have a longer life expectancy than those who rate their health as fair or poor.[1] In fact, self-rating of health is a stronger predictor of life expectancy than actual physical status based on a medical examination. Positive feelings about one's health usually reflect a similar attitude toward life in general that supports positive adjustment and adaptation.

Health care. Health care may or may not be under a person's control. People in lower socioeconomic groups do not always have access to the same level or quality of medical care as those in higher income groups. Poor reading skills, limited education, or a language barrier may hinder an individual who is attempting to carry out instructions from a health professional about a change in health habits or steps in the treatment of disease. Health care also includes wise self-care such as seeking medical care when symptoms so indicate, following directions when using medications (including over-the-counter drugs) or exercising regularly.

Lifestyle. The term **lifestyle** refers to a person's unique pattern of living. These patterns reflect our values and beliefs. They involve what, how much, and when an individual chooses to eat, whether or not an individual exercises regularly, or whether an individual uses addictive drugs. Use of time is a lifestyle choice. One person may spend leisure time watching television and consuming large amounts of alcohol and snack foods high in sodium and fat. Another person of similar age may spend leisure time practicing tennis or choose to walk rather than drive to a nearby store. A young adult may relieve stress in harmful ways by overeating, smoking, or abusing alcohol. For another, appropriate outlets involving exercise, counseling, or relaxation techniques may be the choice.

> **Lifestyle**
> A person's unique pattern of living, which depending on its form can be negative or positive in its health results.

Health and wellness throughout adulthood are to a great extent the result of lifestyle choices. When we consider what determines health status, we find that over 50% of this influence is under our personal control. Diet, exercise, smoking habits, use of addictive substances, and stress management all contribute to this total. For those exhibiting early signs of chronic disease, or for those at risk because of genetic background, adoption of positive health behaviors can slow or interrupt the degenerative disease process.

Health Promotion

Definitions. Public attention began to focus on health promotion in 1979 with the publication of *Healthy People: The Surgeon General's Report on Health Promotion and Disease Prevention*.[2] The goal was to help people maintain and enhance their well-being by making use of preventive health services and lifestyle modification strategies. Although lifestyle changes are a major component of health promotion, health strategies might also include educational, economic, and environmental adjustments that support behavior conducive to good health.[3] An individual with poor reading skills attempting to select a diet lower in saturated fat and cholesterol may need help to understand food labels or could benefit from meal planning materials that emphasize pictures. Health promotion requires a combination of intervention strategies to bring about behavior change.

Models for behavior change. Health and nutrition educators are learning more about the social and psychological factors that influence behavior change. By understanding how people choose to alter their behavior we can best develop programs that will encourage positive change. Several ideas have emerged that have been successful in helping people change their behavior and adopt better health practices. These include the health belief model, the **locus of control** model, and the idea of self-efficacy.

Health belief model. The health belief model was developed to explain how a person who does not have a disease chooses to change behavior and alter risk factors to prevent future development of this disease.[3] This model suggests that the decision for action is based on three factors: (1) the individual's perception of vulnerability to the disease, (2) the seriousness of the disease, and (3) the degree of difficulty in implementing the lifestyle changes required. A young woman whose mother is confined to a wheel chair as a result of osteoporosis and bone fractures (see p. 86) may begin to exercise regularly and select calcium-rich foods.

Locus of control model. People perceive the world and their ability to control events occurring around them in different ways. Some individuals perceive the day to day events in their lives as being under their (internal) control. They assume responsibility for their life choices and the physiologic and psychologic components of their well-being. Individuals with an internal locus of control tend to be more successful in weight management as they assume responsibility for their body weight.[4] In a study of 309 men and women enrolled in a weight-reduction program, those participants with the highest self-assurance scores were most likely to complete the 10-week program.[5] Self assurance was defined as a person's perceived ability to alter daily food and exercise habits affecting body weight. Individuals with an external locus of control consider their health status to be the result of outside forces beyond their control. Consequently, they take less responsibility for their lifestyle behaviors. This individual may view his elevated blood pressure as caused by his genetic sensitivity to sodium and decide that reducing sodium intake will not be effective in reducing his risk. Some persons consider all life happenings to be a matter of chance with no particular basis of control. It may be difficult to motivate these individuals to alter lifestyle behavior to improve well-being.

Concept of self-efficacy. The concept of self-efficacy relates to an individual's belief that he or she will be able to make and maintain the health-related changes desired. This feeling of empowerment is based on the facts or skills provided to the individual that support behavior change. Using role play to enable a man at high risk of heart disease to ask diplomatically for juice or a carbonated beverage when offered an alcoholic beverage at a business party will increase his confidence when placed in the situation. As nutritionists, registered dietitians, or other health team members who become involved in health promotion, we must learn to recognize our client's beliefs and attitudes relating to behavior change and develop programs to address these needs.

Health Care Reform

Health and nutrition education has as its primary goal the optimum health status of individuals in all population groups. This public health approach, designed to assure each member of our society appropriate access to health assessment and intervention, is receiving increased attention within the framework of proposals for health care reform. At present health care issues are a matter of much debate at the state and national level. A major concern is the fact that many Americans have very limited access to health care. Although most people receive health insurance coverage as a fringe benefit through their employer, many people who work for small companies or are self-employed do not have health insurance. It is estimated that nearly 37 million people in the United States have no health

Locus of control
(L *locus,* place, site) A person's perceived control center over his/her life.

insurance and about one fourth of these are children.[6] Consequently, health care services are less available to them. Because they must pay directly for all services they often postpone seeking care with the result that their condition worsens. Uninsured persons also have less access to preventive health services such as nutrition counseling to facilitate weight loss and a possible reduction in elevated blood pressure levels.

A second concern with the current health care delivery system is our emphasis on the treatment of existing medical problems with very limited attention to health promotion strategies. As a result Americans are not nearly as healthy as they could be. At the same time health care costs are escalating rapidly, by more than 10% per year, and considerably faster then personal income.[6] The high cost of technological improvements in medical care such as open heart surgery or kidney transplantation has in part contributed to these rising costs. Targeted programs that address prevention of diseases including breast cancer, heart disease, or stroke will not only decrease long-term health care costs but also contribute to an increased level of wellness and quality of life. A nutritious and prudent diet combined with regular physical activity is the cornerstone for public health intervention.

COMPONENTS OF A PRUDENT HEALTHY LIFESTYLE

Health promotion activities should focus on those lifestyle behaviors known to influence long-term health. These behaviors include dietary and exercise patterns, ability to manage stress, and addictive behaviors related to smoking and use of alcohol. This section discusses current recommendations in these areas.

Dietary Recommendations

Assessing risks and benefits. Absolute proof of a relationship is especially difficult to establish when evaluating a multifaceted issue such as diet and associated health risks. When developing dietary recommendations policy makers must balance the potential benefits of the dietary pattern recommended against the possible adverse effects. Another consideration when developing dietary recommendations is the practicality of the diet for implementation by the public. For example, the production of leaner animal products may be as important as public education in lowering dietary fat levels.

In 1989 an expert panel was commissioned by the Food and Nutrition Board of the National Research Council to develop dietary recommendations that would assist people in reducing their risk of chronic disease.[7] These recommendations for use by nutritionists, government policy makers, and the public are outlined in the box on page 53.

Basis for recommendations. These recommended nutrient and energy guides are based on their relation to established chronic disease risks.

1. **Fats.** Diets high in saturated fat and cholesterol are associated with increased incidence of atherosclerosis and coronary heart disease. Also, high fat diets contribute to the development of obesity and increase cancer risk. One issue related to reducing dietary fat centers on the fact that red meat, an important source of bioavailable iron and zinc, and dairy foods, important sources of calcium and riboflavin, can be high in total fat, saturated fat, and cholesterol. But fats and cholesterol can be limited by using lean meat, poultry without skin, fish, and low-fat or nonfat dairy products without sacrificing intakes of other important nutrients. Total fat and saturated fat can be reduced further by using polyunsaturated vegetable oils and margarines and fewer fried foods. New research findings suggest that regular consumption of cold water fish such as herring and mackerel, high in omega 3 polyunsaturated fatty acids, may be beneficial to health; however, ingesting fish oil capsules is not recommended.[8] It also appears that monounsaturated fats (e.g., oleic

---

Recommendations for Healthy Eating

- Reduce total fat to 30% or less of total kilocalories, saturated fat to less than 10% of total kilocalories, and cholesterol to less than 300 mg per day; polyunsaturated fatty acids should not exceed 10% of total kilocalories.
- Each day eat five or more servings of fruits and vegetables, especially dark green and deep yellow vegetables and citrus fruits; eat six or more servings from breads, cereals, or legumes.
- Maintain protein intake at a moderate level, not more than two times the RDA.
- Balance energy intake and physical activity to maintain appropriate weight; avoid diets that are either excessive or severely restricted in kilocalories.
- Limit alcohol consumption to less than one ounce per day (the equivalent of two 12 ounce cans of beer, two 3.5 ounce glasses of wine, or two average cocktails).
- Limit daily intake of salt (sodium chloride) to 6 g or less, including salt added in cooking or at the table and that found in highly processed foods or pickled items.
- Maintain adequate calcium intake with servings of low-fat and nonfat dairy products and dark green vegetables; use of calcium supplements by healthy people to raise intake above the RDA is not justified.
- Avoid taking dietary supplements that contain any nutrient in amounts above the RDA.
- Maintain an optimal intake of fluoride particularly during the years of tooth formation and growth.

Modified from Committee on Diet and Health, Food and Nutrition Board: *Diet and health: Implications for reducing chronic disease risk,* Washington, DC, 1989, National Academy Press.

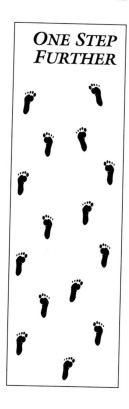

ONE STEP FURTHER

---

acid) present in nuts, canola oil, and olive oil have a favorable effect on serum lipoprotein patterns and might be a prudent substitute in part for polyunsaturated fatty acids. Trans fatty acids produced in the processing of polyunsaturated fats, albeit present at very low levels, are believed to enhance atherosclerotic damage to the arterial wall.

2. **Complex carbohydrates.** The kilocalories lost from the diet when fat is reduced can be replaced by eating more vegetables, fruits, grains, and legumes. Plant foods rich in complex carbohydrates and fiber reduce chronic disease risk in several ways. First, a diet high in plant foods is likely to be low or moderate in fat. Also, soluble fiber found in plant foods independently lowers blood lipid levels and thereby lowers cardiovascular risk. Fruits and vegetables are good sources of potassium, which seems to play a role in moderating blood pressure levels in some persons and thereby may reduce the risk of stroke. **Carotenoids** present in dark green and deep yellow fruits and vegetables offer some protection against particular forms of cancer. Dark green, leafy vegetables and citrus fruits, particularly oranges, are rich in folacin, a vitamin of special importance to young women planning a pregnancy. Finally, the insoluble fiber component of plant foods assists in maintaining proper function of the large bowel and lower gastrointestinal tract and decreases risk of colon cancer.

3. **Proteins.** Protein intakes among most age groups in the United States are well in excess of the RDA.[9] Protein intakes greater than two times the Recommended Dietary Allowance (RDA) are associated with increased incidence of certain cancers and coronary heart disease, mainly as a result of the high levels of saturated fat and cholesterol usually associated with diets high in animal protein. High protein intakes could lead to increased urinary loss of calcium and increased risk of osteoporosis. It has been suggested that long-term consumption of excessive levels of dietary protein might contribute to

Carotenoids
Any of a group of red and yellow pigments chemically similar to and including carotene found in dark green and yellow vegetables and fruits.

degenerative changes in renal function; however, this effect has not been demonstrated in human subjects.

4. Energy. Current trends among young adults include decreased energy intakes among women, decreased physical activity, and increased body fat as defined by body mass index (BMI).[10] Physical activity even at moderate levels will allow an energy intake sufficient to obtain recommended levels of important vitamins and minerals, assist in maintaining reasonable weight for height, and improve fitness. Excess body weight increases risk of coronary heart disease, hypertension, noninsulin-dependent diabetes mellitus (NIDDM), and gallbladder disease. Weight loss will decrease risk, even if desirable weight is not attained. A loss of even 10 pounds of body weight can lower blood pressure and serum lipid levels and improve glucose tolerance.[8] Excessive alcohol consumption, which adds kilocalories that provide few other nutrients, not only undermines energy balance but also increases risk of heart disease, liver disease, high blood pressure, some forms of cancer, and nutrient deficiencies. Pregnant women should totally avoid alcoholic beverages. A diet low to moderate in fat supports energy balance. A daily menu in which fat provides no more than 30% of total energy contains reduced kilocalories as compared to a similar menu comprised of high-fat foods. Women who substituted reduced-fat foods for the food items they normally consumed lost 2.4 kg over a 12-week period although reduced energy intake was not a goal of the program.[11] Moreover, dietary fat in contrast to carbohydrate requires less metabolic energy for conversion to storage in adipose tissue. Thus energy balance may be related to the proportion of energy consumed from fat independent of the total energy content of the diet.

5. Minerals. Intakes of salt (sodium chloride) above 6 g per day (2400 mg sodium per day) are associated with elevated blood pressure in genetically sensitive individuals.[7] However, it is not possible at this time to identify those particular individuals. The recommended level of intake (2400 mg of sodium or less) is likely to prevent the development of high blood pressure in sensitive individuals, and is not deficient for the general population. Foods that are pickled or prepared in brine should be used sparingly. Calcium is receiving increased attention based on the reports associating low calcium intake with elevated blood pressure and increased risk of bone fracture. At the same time there is no strong evidence that calcium intakes above the RDA carry any particular benefit. A recent study in Finland found increased risk of myocardial infarction among men with high-normal body iron stores.[12] This study has not been duplicated by other researchers but does suggest that frequent consumption of food products highly fortified with iron may not be prudent for men.

6. Supplements. Protein, vitamin, and mineral supplements in excess of the RDA have not been shown to be beneficial and excessive intakes of iron and vitamins B_6, A, and D have been shown to be harmful, leading to toxicity or inappropriate interactions with other nutrients.[7] Amino acid supplements proposed to enhance development of lean body mass and fitness can be dangerous to health if amino acid imbalances are created. Long-term health risks and benefits related to supplementation have yet to be identified.

Exercise and Physical Fitness

Positive effects of exercise. Regular physical exercise contributes to health and fitness in many ways. Some of these benefits include improved energy balance, body composition, cardiac efficiency, and serum lipid levels.

1. Energy balance. One of the most obvious health benefits of exercise is its role in energy balance and weight management. Increasing energy expenditure with exercise allows a higher energy intake in food, increasing the likelihood of obtaining adequate amounts of all important nutrients without inappropriate weight gain. An indirect effect of exercise is increased glucose uptake and utilization by muscle cells in the trained versus the untrained individual. Increased uptake of glucose by muscle can help to prevent the development of NIDDM or lower serum glucose levels in those who have this disease.

2. Body composition. Physical exercise strengthens muscle fibers and helps prevent age-related loss of lean body mass and increase in body fat. Exercise strengthens bone by stimulating bone formation and preventing bone loss. Regular physical stress on the bone through exercise that increases the gravity pull of body weight on bone as occurs in walking, jogging, dancing, or bicycling can prevent or retard the onset of osteoporosis, a common bone disorder among older men and women.

3. Cardiovascular efficiency. Regular exercise increases one's ability to do physical work with increased cardiovascular efficiency and decreased recovery time. Maximal oxygen consumption increases while heart rate and blood pressure levels decrease both during exercise and at rest. Improved condition of the heart as a pump as well as reduced fat deposition in the arterial wall contribute to the maintenance of appropriate blood pressure levels in those exercising regularly. Blood pressure levels increase with age among those with sedentary lifestyles.[13]

4. Serum lipid levels. Physical activity retards degenerative changes through its effect on serum lipid levels. Daily exercise increases serum levels of high-density lipoproteins (HDLs), which help protect against coronary artery disease by removing cholesterol molecules from the blood before they can enter the arterial wall. At the same time physical activity assists a low-saturated fat, low-cholesterol diet to significantly lower low-density lipoproteins (LDLs), which carry cholesterol to the cells and increase cardiovascular risk.

Exercise and disease risk. Physically fit persons have a lower risk of death from all causes as compared to their less fit peers. In a study of over 10,000 male Harvard College alumni aged 45 to 84, mortality rates from coronary heart disease and all other causes were 23% lower in those who in the 9 years prior began a moderately vigorous sports program.[14] Those benefited most who expended about 2000 kcal per week in exercise; however, walking at least 9 miles per week or climbing at least 20 flights of stairs per week also reduced risk. This suggests that such simple changes in lifestyle as taking the stairs rather than the elevator or parking your car at a greater distance from a store entrance can improve your level of fitness and general health. A brisk walk of 30 minutes per day, an exercise level within the physical ability of most people, can result in a moderate level of fitness. The duration and resulting energy expenditure of exercise may be more important than the intensity. Regular exercise reduces the incidence of coronary heart disease and death even among those with elevated serum cholesterol and blood pressure levels, and increased BMI. In fact, risk of a coronary death was about half in men with a high level of fitness, despite the presence of other risk factors, as compared to those less fit.[15] Regular exercise may be most critical for those individuals who already suffer from several negative risk factors.

Developing an exercise program. A sedentary individual, regardless of age, should undergo a physical examination before embarking on a strenuous exercise program. Also, people should pay attention to body signals. The appearance of pain suggests that it is time to slow down or stop. To prevent muscular or skeletal injury, or a cardiovascular incident, the progression in both duration and intensity of exercise must be gradual. Cardiovascular exercise requires an increase in heart rate to 70% of maximum (pulse: 220 minus age) continued for at least 20 minutes. However, these levels may need to be achieved over a period of time. For a person with cardiovascular problems, heart rate must be carefully monitored.

An individual may be motivated to initiate an exercise program to improve or maintain health, but long-term adherence is more likely if the activity is enjoyed and family support is provided. Activities of great intensity that are perceived to require great exertion or carry risk of injury are less likely to be begun or continued. Walking is an ideal activity, contributing to energy expenditure and cardiorespiratory fitness and providing a transition to more vigorous exercise if desired. Characteristics of exercise programs that promote continuing participation include:

- No need for specialized facilities or equipment
- Limited discomfort
- Potential for incorporation in the daily routine
- Opportunity for social interaction

Health professionals need to give particular attention to the transitions in lifestyle often associated with a decline in physical activity. These include the transition from high school or college to a work situation, a change in residence, or recovery from an illness or injury. Suggestions for exercise activities are given in Table 3-1.

Stress Management

Stress
Sum of biologic reactions to adverse stimuli, physical, mental, or emotional, internal or external, that disturbs the state of homeostasis and sense of well-being.

Stress is a specific physiologic or psychologic reaction to a life event. The event may be starting a new job, moving to a different city, getting married, or the death of a family member. The stress response is the same whether initiated by a positive or negative event. Stress can result in adverse physiologic symptoms including: (1) gastrointestinal distress, for example, nausea, vomiting, or diarrhea; (2) irregular sleep patterns; (3) increased muscle tension with resulting headache or backache; or (4) cardiovascular responses resulting in constriction of blood vessels and rapid pulse.

Everyone experiences one or more of these symptoms occasionally, but the danger lies in the long-term consequences resulting from continuing, unalleviated stress. Continued gastric upset and inappropriate secretion of stomach acid can lead to peptic ulcers and associated stomach problems. Heart disease is accelerated by high blood pressure that occurs over time as a stress response. Psychologic distress can have a detrimental effect on food intake. This can result in patterns of overeating or binge eating leading to inappropriate weight gain, or at the other extreme, anorexia nervosa or bulimia nervosa, now increasing among young adults.

Because poorly managed stress is a threat to both physical and mental health and occupational safety and productivity, cognitive and behavioral approaches have been developed for stress reduction. Group and individual counseling help people improve understanding and attitude, develop constructive coping mechanisms, and learn positive

TABLE 3-1 *Energy Cost of Various Physical Activities**

Activity	kcal/kg/hr
Aerobic dancing	8.9
Bicycling (moderate speed)	2.5
Bicycling (racing)	7.6
Golf	3.9
Rowing in race	16.0
Running	7.0
Skating	3.5
Skiing (cross country)	5.9
Swimming (2 mph)	7.9
Tennis	5.3
Walking (3 mph)	2.0
Walking (4 mph)	3.4

*Does not include basal metabolism.

approaches to problem solving. Behavioral approaches include reduction in use of alcohol, caffeine, or nicotine, along with increased exercise, rest, and relaxation.

ADDICTIVE BEHAVIORS HARMING HEALTH

Particular personal habits can become **addictions** and harm health. Each year two of these addictive behaviors, cigarette smoking and alcohol abuse, continue to disrupt lives and families, harm health, and cause death. A third form of addictive behavior, eating disorders, poses difficult problems often rooted in earlier adolescent development years (see Chapter 8) and centers on misuse of food, an agent necessary for life but when misused can become life threatening and cause death. We discuss these addictive behaviors in terms of their incidence, associated health problems, and treatment programs.

Cigarette Smoking

Incidence. Cigarette smoking is considered the greatest single preventable cause of illness and premature death in the United States.[16] A current U.S. Department of Health and Human Services report examining underlying causes of death indicated that although heart disease and cancer may be listed as the nation's leading killers, tobacco use was the largest underlying culprit, followed by poor diet.[17] A major concern of health professionals is the prevalence of cigarette smoking among teenagers and young adults. By the age of 16, 21% of teenagers have begun to smoke. Most adult smokers started to smoke by age 20.[18] In the general population smoking peaks by age 25, with 33% of men and 28% of women smoking.[19] Use of cigarettes differs according to ethnic and socioeconomic group. More black men than white men smoke and more black women than white women smoke, probably contributing to the higher incidence of heart disease, hypertension, and stroke in the black population.[19] Young adults who did not complete high school are more likely to smoke than their better-educated peers.[18]

Health problems. Cigarette smoking is a major risk factor for many chronic conditions accounting for 87% of lung cancer deaths, 21% of coronary heart disease deaths, and 18% of stroke deaths.[16] Use of cigarettes accelerates the development of atherosclerotic lesions, leading to the estimate that more than 40% of deaths from coronary heart disease occurring among men and women less than 65 years of age are attributable to smoking.[16] Smoking exacerbates the risk associated with alcohol use, high blood pressure, and diabetes mellitus.

Mortality risk for both sexes increases with the number of cigarettes smoked and is higher for those who began smoking at younger ages. By age 30, a person smoking two packs of cigarettes a day has a life expectancy 8 to 9 years shorter than a nonsmoker of similar age.[16] Until recently, prevalence of lung cancer was lower among women, as relatively fewer women were smoking. Lung cancer has now passed breast cancer as the leading cause of death in women.[19] Smokers who quit smoking experience both immediate and long-term benefits. Risk of coronary heart disease is reduced within the first few years. Risk of lung cancer drops substantially in 5 to 9 years, but still remains two times that of the lifelong nonsmoker after 20 years.[16] Although further deterioration of the lungs is arrested, smokers with obstructed air passages cannot anticipate major improvement despite cessation of smoking.

Treatment programs. A positive result of smoking cessation programs has been the overall decline in adult smokers from 40% to 27% of the population over the past 25 years.[16] Nearly half of all living adults who ever smoked have quit. Smoking cessation programs have focused on behavior modification techniques and coping strategies to assist with physiologic, psychologic, and social factors related to nicotine addiction. Fear of unwanted weight gain may deter some young people from joining a smoking cessation program. Contrary to common belief, average weight gain was found to be only 2.8 kg

Addiction
(L *addictio*, a giving over, surrender) State of being enslaved to some undesirable practice that is physically or psychologically habit-forming to the extent that its cessation causes severe trauma.

(6 lb) in men and 3.8 kg (8 lb) in women.[20] Major weight gain of 13 kg (28 lb) or more occurred in only 10% of the men and 13% of the women. Black persons, persons under the age of 55, and those who smoked at least 15 cigarettes a day were more likely to gain weight. Attention to weight control is usually included in such health education programs.

Alcohol Abuse

Incidence. In the United States alcohol consumption is highest among persons aged 25 to 44.[19] About 80% of the men in this age group are current drinkers and 13% are heavy drinkers, consuming 14 or more drinks per week and assuming 0.5 ounces of ethanol per drink.[19] Sixty percent of women in this age range drink but only 3% drink heavily. Fewer black and Hispanic men and women are current drinkers compared with white men and women. Among Native Americans the rate of alcohol abuse remains high. The U.S. Indian Health Service (IHS) has identified alcoholism as the most significant health problem of American Indians and Alaska Natives.[21] Alcohol abuse is more frequent in youth and middle age.

Health problems. Inappropriate use of alcohol has a negative effect on nutritional status and enhances risk of chronic disease. Alcohol has a toxic effect on the gastrointestinal tract and reduces the absorption of many nutrients including vitamins B_6 and B_{12}, folate, and zinc. Alcohol further contributes to malnutrition by adding kilocalories (7 kcal/g) to the diet that provide no protein or essential vitamins or minerals. This problem of nutrient density is evident in the diets of some young adults for whom alcohol kilocalories replace about one third of the nonalcohol food kilocalories. Although this practice is intended to avoid weight gain, it further decreases intakes of iron and calcium, nutrients already low in the diets of young adult women.

Continuing alcohol abuse contributes to deteriorating health through its association with elevated serum LDL-cholesterol and triglyceride levels, hypertension, and liver disease. Although it was believed that liver damage resulted from a lack of food and nutrients rather than from a direct toxic effect of alcohol itself, studies have found the development of liver abnormalities in well-nourished alcohol abusers. Regular use of alcohol increases risk of stroke and cancer of the oral cavity and esophagus. Depletion of liver stores of vitamin A is a consequence of alcohol abuse and may contribute to the relationship observed between alcohol consumption and cancer of the liver, breast, and pancreas.

The paradox of alcohol consumption lies in its effect on serum levels of HDL-cholesterol, the so-called "good cholesterol." Increased levels of HDL-cholesterol are associated with *low to moderate* drinking, often defined as no more than 1 to 2 drinks per day. This is likely the basis for the epidemiologic findings that coronary heart disease risk is lower in persons consuming these low to moderate levels of alcohol. At the same time the potentially devastating effects of excessive alcohol intake on health and overall mortality preclude any recommendation that individuals increase their alcohol intake or start to drink if they do not already.

Screening tests. The cost of alcoholism is high, in both lives lost and the financial burden of care. The United States' combined lifetime prevalence of addiction and dependence ranges from 11% to 16%, with hospitalized medical patients showing even greater numbers of 15% to 60%, depending on the population studied. In one year alone—1990—more than 65,000 Americans lost their lives because of alcohol abuse, 22,000 of them on the highways.[22] Estimates of the National Center for Health Statistics indicate that the financial burden of alcohol abuse will reach $150 billion by 1995 (up from $128 billion in 1986), more than the total cost of cardiovascular disease.[22] Thus screening tests to identify early signs of alcohol abuse before it becomes so lethal an addiction become crucial medical tools. Two basic types of tests are used, questionnaires and biochemical tests.

1. **Questionnaires.** An example of a commonly used screening tool is the **CAGE** questionnaire included as part of a history-taking interview. It can be used to help detect a suspected alcoholic, even if he is in denial.[22,23] Its name is an **acronym** that indicates its focus: Cutting down, Annoyance by criticism, Guilt feelings, and Eye-openers. It is short, easy to use, and relatively nonintimidating. Nonalcoholics are distinguished from alcohol abusers by answering three of the four questions in the negative:

- **C** Have you ever felt you should **C**ut down on your drinking?
- **A** Have people **A**nnoyed you by criticizing your drinking?
- **G** Have you ever felt bad or **G**uilty about drinking?
- **E** Have you ever taken a drink first thing in the morning to get rid of a hangover or steady your nerves (**E**ye opener)?

2. **Biochemical tests.** Because alcohol abuse affects many body systems and metabolites, a single marker does not provide an effective screening tool. Screening test strategies involve combinations of tests, which can be arranged in parallel, in series, or both, according to what kind of computer analysis is needed. A combination of tests is interchangeably called a *battery, panel,* or *profile* of tests, such as the classic clinical test battery in the standard automated *sequential multiple analyzer* (SMA-6, SMA-12).[22,23] The SMA-6 is essentially a panel of renal tests; the SMA-12 can include renal tests, electrolytes, and commonly used clinical chemistry tests. For example, a battery of tests used to screen for alcohol abuse may include standard hematologic values, liver enzymes, and serum lipid concentrations.[22]

Treatment programs. Alcohol addiction programs have two phases—initial detoxification treatment and maintenance of behavior change.[24] At times, physicians may prescribe disulfiram (Antabuse) to help alcoholics abstain from drinking. This drug does not cure alcoholism. It acts to interfere with the normal metabolic breakdown in the liver of **acetaldehyde,** the highly toxic initial substance ordinarily produced from alcohol metabolism. Powerful reactions to the buildup of unmetabolized acetaldehyde toxicity occur when the person drinks even small amounts of alcohol. These serious and highly unpleasant toxic reactions can include throbbing headache, flushing, breathlessness, nausea, thirst, palpitations, dizziness, and fainting. Fear of such events may deter the alcohol abuser from drinking even small amounts of alcohol but does not solve the underlying problem of addiction.

By its nature, a chemical dependency such as alcoholism has biologic, psychologic, and social components that require a health care team approach to meet comprehensive needs and problems.[25] These care needs are:

- **Biologic.** Chronic alcohol (drug) poisoning causes brain and liver dysfunction.
- **Psychologic.** Progressive brain dysfunction creates personality disorganization—the "addictive personality."
- **Social.** Secondary relationship problems interfere with functioning and support systems at home, on the job, and with friends.

Experienced leaders in the field of addictive behavior indicate that in terms of maintaining the behavior change all paths lead to the difficult job of relapse prevention.[24] This self-control task requires training in stress-coping skills and lifestyle changes. Such training helps addicted persons deal with guilt and self-blame by recognizing that their addictive behavior has certain negative consequences and that these behaviors can be changed.[24] In the team approach to health care of persons with alcohol abuse problems, an experienced registered dietitian with special training in rehabilitative care is needed to provide comprehensive nutrition care[21,25,26] that includes the following:

- Initial and ongoing nutritional assessment
- Nutritional management of meals and supplements that help develop normal eating patterns

Acronym
(Gr *acros,* topmost, foremost; *-onym,* word, name) A word or name formed from the initial letters or groups of letters of words in a set series.

Acetaldehyde
Chemical compound, intermediate metabolic product in the breakdown of alcohol by liver enzymes.

- Nutrition education and counseling that help develop an eating plan to support stable recovery

Eating Disorders

Incidence. Health care professionals working in the field of eating disorders estimate that some form of addictive eating disorder affects the lives of nearly 8 million American adolescents and young adults (see Chapter 8 for discussion of early beginnings in the adolescent years).[27] Eating disorders have been most prevalent in white females in the middle and upper social classes, but the incidence is rising in all socioeconomic and ethnic groups; 90% to 95% of the total cases are women.[27] Studies indicate that the incidence in men may be higher than 5% to 10%, but a true number is unknown because many of these men do not seek treatment.[28] Also, persons at risk for developing eating disorders are those involved in activities that stress body and form, such as ballet, gymnastics, or any highly competitive sport with pressures that make them vulnerable. When such eating disorders develop in young persons with insulin-dependent diabetes, the situation can become even more life threatening and difficult to manage.[29]

The American Psychiatric Association's newly revised fourth edition of the *Diagnostic and Statistical Manual of Mental Disorders (DSM-IV)* describes the two classic types of eating disorders, anorexia nervosa and bulimia nervosa, and identifies two new subtypes of each.[30] In addition, the new manual now recognizes and describes a third type, the binge eating disorder.

Anorexia nervosa. Persons with this severe disturbance in eating behavior have an intense fear of gaining weight or becoming fat, a fear fed in susceptible young women by social and fashion ideals of the "perfectly thin body" and by family dynamics of conflict that devalue individuality.[31] They refuse to maintain a minimally normal body weight, develop a mental distortion of body image and see themselves as fat when they are emaciated, and impose a self-starvation pattern that becomes life threatening. The two new subtypes described in DSM-IV are (1) *restricting type,* in which the anorexic does not regularly use binge eating or purging behavior, and (2) *binge eating/purging type,* in which the anorexic does use these behaviors.[32]

Bulimia nervosa. Persons with this type of eating disorder regularly consume large amounts of food, often as much as 15,000 kilocalories worth within any 2-hour period, with a feeling of lack of control during that time. They then compensate for this huge food intake by inappropriate behaviors to prevent weight gain such as self-induced vomiting; use of laxatives, diuretics, enemas, or other medications; fasting; or excessive exercise. These behaviors occur, on average, at least twice a week for extended periods of time.

Binge eating disorder. Persons with this newly recognized type of eating disorder described in DSM-IV have recurrent episodes of eating binges in which they sense a loss of control over eating and feel that they cannot stop. These episodes occur, on average, at least 2 days a week and are characterized by eating much more rapidly than normal until feeling uncomfortably full, eating large amounts of food when not feeling physically hungry, eating alone because of being embarrassed by the large quantity consumed, and then feeling disgusted with oneself, depressed, or very guilty. This type of binge eating disorder is not associated with the use of inappropriate compensatory behaviors such as purging, fasting, or excessive exercise.

Treatment programs. Eating disorders are complex addictive behaviors that relate directly to food and body weight and involve relationships within oneself and with others. Thus they require a multidisciplinary health team approach to care by specially trained professionals, including physician, psychotherapist, and registered dietitian with advanced course work, clinical experience, additional training in counseling, and experience in the treatment of eating disorders.[33]

HEALTH PROMOTION AND CHRONIC DISEASE

Within this century nutrition research has shifted from the identification of nutrients and deficiency symptoms to the study of the effect of diet and lifestyle on the diseases of civilization such as heart disease and cancer. An abundant food supply along with the decrease in physical activity made possible by modern technology have contributed to the widespread prevalence of chronic diseases. Chronic diseases, in contrast to acute conditions, are lifelong and can only be managed, not cured. The long-term health care costs associated with these diseases have led policy makers and health professionals to identify risk factors associated with these conditions and develop public education approaches that support risk reduction.

Atherosclerotic Heart Disease

Prevalence and impact. The major cause of death in the United States and other Western societies is disease of the heart and blood vessels, accounting for nearly half of all deaths. Nearly 18% of these deaths occur in people under 65 years of age.[18] Risk is low in early adulthood but increases rapidly with age. Mortality rates from cardiovascular disease have declined by one fourth over the past two decades as a result of better medical care following a heart attack, therapeutic intervention such as development of drugs to lower serum lipids and blood pressure, and changes in diet and exercise patterns. Unfortunately, improvement has not been equal across ethnic groups. Black men are twice as likely to die of stroke and black women have higher death rates from heart disease as compared to the general population.[10]

Development of atherosclerosis. Atherosclerosis, a pathological series of events occurring in the coronary arteries supplying blood to the heart muscle and the cerebral arteries supplying blood to the brain, actually begins in childhood. Lipid deposits appearing as fatty streaks in children may regress or progress to form fibrous plaques of accumulated fat and debris. Ulceration or hemorrhage into the plaque, causing swelling, can occlude the lumen of the artery resulting in tissue breakdown as blood supply is interrupted. Arterial injury in the coronary arteries results in coronary heart disease. This most commonly occurs in middle age and carries risk of myocardial infarction or heart attack. Occlusion or hemorrhage in a cerebral artery usually occurs 10 to 20 years later, resulting in a stroke with possible paralysis or loss of speech, vision, hearing, or memory. Elevated serum total cholesterol or LDL-cholesterol levels and high blood pressure levels increase the severity of atherosclerosis, although high blood pressure is more closely associated with problems in the cerebral arteries.

Risk factors and coronary heart disease. Genetic, dietary, and lifestyle factors as described in Table 3-2 influence the development of atherosclerosis and heart disease. Intervention strategies have been directed toward diet- or drug-induced reductions in LDL-cholesterol levels, smoking cessation, weight loss, limited use of alcohol, and increases in physical activity. High dietary cholesterol and saturated fatty acids lead to increased LDL-cholesterol levels, whereas polyunsaturated fatty acids when substituted for saturated fats lower both HDL- and LDL-cholesterol concentrations. Monounsaturated fatty acids appear to decrease LDL-cholesterol levels without lowering HDL-cholesterol levels. Soluble fiber, commonly found in oat bran and starchy vegetables, also appears to lower serum LDL-cholesterol levels. Physical activity increases HDL-cholesterol levels as does moderate use of alcohol. The effect of the omega-3 polyunsaturated fatty acids on serum LDL-cholesterol levels is uncertain although these fatty acids do interfere with the formation of unwanted blood clots in the coronary arteries.

Intervention trials for coronary heart disease. Several large-scale diet-heart trials

TABLE 3-2 *Factors Contributing to Cardiovascular Disease Risk*

Personal Characteristics (No Control)	Lifestyle Behaviors (Intervene and Change)	Background Conditions (Screen and Treat)
Sex	Stress/ability to cope	Hypertension
Age	Smoking cigarettes	Diabetes mellitus
Family history	Abuse of alcohol	Hyperlipidemia (especially hypercholesterolemia)
	Sedentary lifestyle	
	Obesity	
	Food habits	
	Excess fat	
	Excess salt	
	Excess sugar	
	Excess kilocalories	
	Low fiber	

have been conducted with middle-aged hypercholesterolemic men to evaluate strategies for reducing mortality from coronary heart disease. Interventions to reduce serum cholesterol levels included diets low in fat and saturated fat and lipid-lowering drugs. A general finding was that reduction in coronary risk was directly proportional to the decrease in serum cholesterol levels. Over the short term a 1% decrease in serum cholesterol levels resulted in a 2% decrease in coronary risk; over the long term a 1% decrease in serum cholesterol levels may result in as much as a 3% decrease in coronary risk. Other nutrients now receiving attention regarding a possible role in cardiovascular risk are vitamins C and E and beta carotene. Men and women who consumed vitamin E supplements containing 10 to 100 times the RDA over several years had decreased risk. Further research is needed to determine the safety and effectiveness of long-term consumption of vitamin E before this can be recommended to the general public.

A study in San Francisco evaluated the influence of lifestyle changes without surgical or drug intervention on atherosclerotic damage.[34] After one year a measurable decrease in fatty plaques in the coronary arteries was observed in men and women who exercised regularly, stopped smoking, and followed a vegetarian diet with less than 10% of energy coming from fat. Such a diet could be deficient in essential fatty acids, vitamin B_{12}, zinc, and iron, and should not be followed without close medical supervision. However, this study provided evidence that lifestyle changes over a long-term period not only retard but may actually reverse coronary artery disease. A diet less restrictive in fat, combined with other positive lifestyle changes may also lead to significant reduction in coronary risk.

Hypertension

Hypertension or sustained elevated arterial blood pressure increases risk of stroke, coronary heart disease, and kidney damage. Obesity is associated with elevated blood pressure levels that decrease during periods of active weight loss. It appears that regular exercise can prevent the usual age-related increase in blood pressure levels and also lead to a decrease in elevated levels.[13]

Risk reduction and hypertension. Dietary factors associated with hypertension are alcohol, calcium, and various electrolytes including sodium and potassium. Excessive ingestion of alcohol, more than one ounce of alcohol each day, can raise blood pressure.[13] The effect of particular nutrients on hypertension is less well understood. Epidemiologic data suggest that a habitual intake of more than 6 g of salt or 2400 mg of sodium per day increases the risk of hypertension in salt-sensitive individuals.[13] Dietary calcium has been associated with high blood pressure in some but not all U.S. surveys. On the other hand, a liberal potassium intake (from food sources) may protect against developing hypertension and play an ameliorative role in those with blood pressures above normal. When dietary intakes of fruits and vegetables were increased by middle-aged people with hypertension, 38% of them were able to reduce their antihypertensive medication and their blood pressure remained well-controlled.[35]

Individual response. The impact of sodium restriction or calcium or potassium supplementation on blood pressure levels is a highly individual response. Clinical trials resulting in no significant change in mean blood pressure among all participants have produced striking decreases in blood pressure levels in particular individuals. Diets limited in sodium but generous in food sources of potassium and calcium may be of general benefit. Reductions in dietary sodium should be strongly encouraged for black Americans among whom salt sensitivity and hypertension are highly prevalent.[13] Potassium supplementation with potassium chloride, unless medically supervised, is not recommended, and is especially dangerous for those using potassium-sparing diuretics or with compromised kidney function.

Overweight and Obesity

Incidence of overweight. In the United States 32% of white and black men, 32% and 49% of white and black women, and 40% and 48% of Mexican-American men and women, respectively, are overweight, and these numbers are increasing.[36] Between 1976 and 1991 the prevalence of overweight increased 8% among adults and mean body weight increased 3.6 kg. Americans in all social and ethnic groups are attempting to lose weight but most gain it back. The diets chosen are often low in protein, vitamins, and minerals, as well as kcalories, and lead to nutrient depletion. Very low calorie diets (VLCD) containing 500 to 800 kcal have been used in medical clinics to bring about rapid weight loss, however such diets are dangerous when unsupervised. Moreover, extremely low energy diets do not help the dieter develop new eating patterns; consequently, when the diet is discontinued and the usual eating pattern resumed the weight is likely to be regained. This can establish a cycle of weight gain, weight loss, and weight gain that over a period of years can be more detrimental to health than the initial overweight. An approach to weight loss that includes an increase in energy expenditure in the form of physical activity along with a reasonable decrease in energy intake is more effective than either strategy alone (see box on p. 64).

Obesity and disease risk. Obesity is an independent risk factor for cardiovascular disease in addition to contributing to the development of elevated blood pressure and serum cholesterol levels.[37] Obesity promotes degenerative **osteoarthritis** and bone-joint disease, reducing flexibility and hindering mobility. In a 15-year follow-up of 698 older women, those considered to be overweight (BMI > 27) when first measured were twice as likely to become disabled and unable to carry groceries or perform housekeeping chores as those who had been normal weight.[38] Because physical exercise is difficult, the obese individual is more likely to be sedentary, which sustains the obesity and further contributes to degenerative changes. Obesity is a significant factor in the development of maturity-onset non–insulin-dependent diabetes mellitus (NIDDM) as enlarged fat cells resist the action of insulin.

The influence of obesity and overweight on mortality risk is controversial. Life insurance statistics indicate that individuals greatly above or below average weight are more likely to die at younger ages. In early reports underweight persons had an even greater mortality rate than overweight persons. This led to the assertion by some health professionals that being slightly overweight might actually be protective, particularly in the

Osteoarthritis
(Gr *osteon* + *arthron*, joint; *-itis*, inflammation) A form of arthritis in which joints undergo degenerative changes resulting in stiffness, pain, and swelling; arthritis in the hip, knee, or spine can result in some degree of disability.

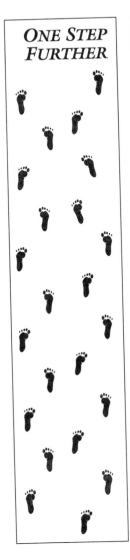

Weight Reduction: The High Cost of False Hope

At any given time 65 million Americans are trying to lose weight. It is estimated that they spend at least $51 billion a year on weight loss products and services. The weight loss industry has continued to market new diets, formulas, and gimmicks to those who are desperate to shed unwanted pounds. Unfortunately, many of these efforts end in failure, and the obese dieter is again left in despair or worse. At present the weight loss industry is largely unregulated, and advertisements present a false hope of success. Very low calorie diets may be a threat to health when followed without medical supervision. Even hospital-based programs with appropriate nutrition counseling and social support may impose unrealistic weight goals on individuals who have never achieved ideal weight despite a lifetime of effort.

A more successful and appropriate approach is weight management without dieting. This non-dieting approach involves five steps.

1. Provide counselor and peer support. Many overweight individuals are socially isolated and failure at dieting reinforces these feelings. Group interaction with peers who have similar problems provides acceptance and understanding.
2. Develop normal eating patterns. Chronic dieters often restrict intake by skipping meals or fasting. Encourage eating of three meals each day even though energy intake may increase.
3. Increase exercise gradually. Exercise will burn calories and allow more flexibility in food choices. Walking is an appropriate activity. Begin with short sessions (5 minutes if necessary) to avoid pain or stiffness.
4. Reduce dietary fat gradually. Over time help the dieter reduce current fat intake to 20% to 30% of kilocalories. High fat diets are more likely to lead to weight gain than low fat diets.
5. Accept the body weight achieved through appropriate diet and exercise. A lower body weight that does not approach ideal weight still contributes to functional benefits in blood pressure, serum lipid, and serum glucose levels.

A weight loss of even 10% sustained for a lifetime will be of greater benefit than extensive weight lost that is promptly regained.

From Begley CE: Government should strengthen regulation in the weight loss industry, *J Am Diet Assoc* 91:1255, 1991; and Foreyt JP and GK Goodrick: Weight management without dieting, *Nutr Today* 28(2):4, 1993.

presence of severe illness or disease. Long-term follow-up of participants in the Framingham Heart Study revealed that high mortality among underweight men was related to cigarette smoking.[37] Eighty percent of the underweight men were cigarette smokers as compared to only 55% of the overweight men.

The age when an individual becomes obese also influences mortality from cardiovascular disease. Individuals who become obese before age 55 have a higher risk of mortality than those who become obese after age 55. Regardless of body weight at age 25, excess weight gain during the adult years increases cardiovascular risk whereas voluntary weight loss among those who are overweight can reduce their risk.[39] Men appear to be more sensitive than women to the detrimental effects of weight gain and overweight. The location of body fat also influences risk (see p. 84). Men with thick layers of body fat in the abdominal region have higher risk of coronary heart disease and death than those with similar amounts of fat about their hips. In fact the site of accumulated fat, abdominal area versus the hips, may explain in part the increased mortality risk of men versus women with similar BMI. Even mild overweight can be detrimental to the maintenance of good health. A weight loss of 10 to 15 pounds can bring about a significant drop in elevated blood pressure and reduction in serum LDL-cholesterol levels.[40]

Cancer

Cancer development. Cancer is the second leading cause of death in the United States. One researcher suggests that one third of all cancers are diet related.[7] Dietary fat, fiber, the antioxidant vitamins A, C, and E, and the vitamin A precursor beta carotene have been evaluated as to their influence on cancer risk. Dietary components may interact at various stages in cancer development. They may also influence the development of cancer in particular organs or tissues. Three stages of abnormal cell growth transform a normal cell into cancerous tissue.

  1. **Initiation.** An irreversible genetic alteration in a normal cell is brought about by a carcinogen that makes the cell capable of uncontrolled growth.
  2. **Promotion.** The abnormal cell is stimulated to grow and produce a cancer.
  3. **Progression.** The tumor cells invade healthy tissues and spread throughout the body.

Linoleic acid has been shown to interact at all stages to promote carcinogenesis. In contrast naturally occurring compounds present in the cruciferous vegetables (e.g., broccoli, cauliflower, brussels sprouts) block both the initiation and promotion of cancer development in the cell. Dietary antioxidants may destroy **free radicals** that can initiate carcinogenesis or actually reverse the process after it has begun.

Free radical
An unstable, high-energy cell molecule with an unpaired electron that causes oxidation reactions in unsaturated fatty acids and may act as a carcinogen.

Diet and cancer. Dietary fat, particularly saturated fat, has been implicated in the development of breast, prostate, and colon cancer, although findings differ according to where and how the study was performed. For example, fat intakes per person are higher in countries with generally higher rates of breast cancer. However, studies that have examined the fat intakes of large groups of women in relation to their subsequent development of breast cancer have found no direct relationship. Incidence of breast cancer is higher among obese women. Possibly, the high caloric density of foods containing a high proportion of fat contribute to development of obesity and thereby influence cancer risk. Epidemiologic studies have related high intakes of red meat with increased incidence of colon cancer.[41]

Consumption of dark green and deep yellow vegetables and fruits may offer some protection against cancer death. Dietary intakes of vitamins A, C, and E, and beta carotene tend to be inversely related to human cancer risk; however, unknown compounds present in food sources of these nutrients may be responsible for the effects observed. It has been suggested that these naturally occurring antioxidants reduce the risk of lung cancer among smokers but this is not true in all cases.[41]

The strongest evidence associating a dietary component with reduced cancer risk exists for fiber and cancer of the colon. It has been proposed that colon cancer risk would decrease by 31% if fiber intake would increase by 13 g (the amount of fiber in one apple and ½ cup of cooked legumes).[42] The protective effect of fiber against colorectal cancer may relate to its bulk, which dilutes the bile acids that are present. Fiber also hastens the passage of the food bolus through the digestive tract thereby shortening the time during which ingested carcinogens are in contact with the intestinal wall. Finally, diets high in fiber may be low in other dietary constituents such as fat that promote carcinogenesis.

Diabetes Mellitus

Diabetes mellitus is a metabolic disorder characterized by high blood glucose levels and abnormal carbohydrate utilization caused by inappropriate levels of insulin. Insulin-dependent diabetes mellitus (IDDM) results from destruction of the beta cells of the pancreas. Because no insulin is secreted by the pancreas, insulin must be supplied by injection or death will result. Destruction of the beta cells is believed to occur through an autoimmune reaction of genetic origin. Age of onset is usually in childhood.

Non–insulin-dependent diabetes mellitus (NIDDM), formerly referred to as adult-onset diabetes, usually occurs after age 40 and is generally associated with obesity. It is more likely caused by secretion of an inappropriate form of insulin or resistance of oversize adipose cells to the action of insulin, rather than a deficiency of insulin. Treatment usually involves weight reduction and dietary intervention. The dietary pattern most commonly prescribed in the past was high in carbohydrate (50% to 60% of kcalories) and low in fat (less than or equal to 30% of kcalories). Ongoing studies have indicated that moderating this nutrient ratio may be beneficial in controlling serum glucose and lipid levels in some patients with NIDDM. Recent guidelines indicate that fat intake may increase up to 40% if monounsaturated fat is emphasized (20% of total kcalories).[43] Regular exercise is important, and, if necessary, oral hypoglycemic drugs are prescribed. Atherosclerotic coronary disease is a frequent complication of this disorder; thus diets high in soluble fiber and low in cholesterol and saturated fat are advisable. Maintenance of appropriate weight for height and avoiding alcohol intake are important preventive measures for lowering individual risk.

NUTRITION AND HEALTH PROMOTION PROGRAMS

National Health Promotion Programs

National cholesterol education program. The National Cholesterol Education Program (NCEP) sponsored by the National Heart, Lung, and Blood Institute was begun in 1985 in response to the published findings from large scale intervention studies that reducing elevated blood cholesterol levels reduces the rate of heart attacks and associated mortality. Revised guidelines released in 1993 have added standards for serum HDL-cholesterol levels to be used in evaluation and treatment.[8] The NCEP encourages a team approach with physicians, dietitians, nurses, and pharmacologists in developing intervention strategies and materials to educate health professionals, patients, and the public. The guidelines presented in Table 3-3 emphasize dietary intervention as a primary treatment and present a rational approach applicable to persons of different ages and health status. Use of drugs to lower serum cholesterol levels is reserved for persons with the following:

- Known coronary heart disease
- Risk factors in addition to elevated serum cholesterol
- Serum cholesterol levels that remain high despite dietary intervention

Since diagnosis of high blood cholesterol depends on the accuracy of a blood test, standardized procedures for cholesterol testing have been established. The NCEP has defined intervention strategies for children and adolescents whose blood cholesterol levels or family history places them at risk. Findings from national surveys conducted between 1960 and 1991 indicate that mean serum cholesterol levels in adults ages 20 to 74 years have declined from 221 to 206 mg/dl.[44] More than 50% of this decrease has occurred since 1976.

Dietary counseling and drug intervention requiring professional supervision usually take place in a physician's office or health care facility. But public education to promote preventive dietary changes and encourage screening of those at high risk must target the community. The overall goal is to provide practical dietary information "wherever people eat." Major supermarkets can distribute heart healthy recipes, provide shelf markers noting

TABLE 3-3 *Classification of Blood Cholesterol Levels and Recommended Follow-Up for Persons With No Evidence of Coronary Heart Disease*

Total Blood Cholesterol	HDL-Cholesterol	Recommended Action
<200 mg/dl (desirable)	≥35 mg/dl	Provide general guidelines for diet, physical activity, and risk reduction.
<200 mg/dl (desirable)	<35 mg/dl	Do fasting lipoprotein analysis (total, HDL- and LDL-cholesterol). Recommendation based on LDL-cholesterol results (see below).
200-239 mg/dl (borderline high)	≥35 mg/dl and fewer than 2 risk factors*	Provide information on dietary modification, physical activity, and risk factor reduction. Reevaluate in 1-2 years.
200-239 mg/dl (borderline high)	<35 mg/dl or 2 or more risk factors*	Do fasting lipoprotein analysis (total, HDL- and LDL-cholesterol). Recommendation based on LDL-cholesterol results (see below).
≥240 mg/dl		Do fasting lipoprotein analysis (total, HDL- and LDL-cholesterol).

Recommendation based on LDL-cholesterol levels:

LDL-cholesterol <130 mg/dl (desirable)
  Provide general guidelines for diet, physical activity, and risk reduction. Reevaluate within 5 years.

LDL-cholesterol 130-159 mg/dl (borderline-high-risk); fewer than two risk factors.*
  Provide information on Step I diet (fat ≤ 30% total kcal; saturated fat 8%-10% total kcal). Encourage physical activity. Reevaluate annually.

LDL-cholesterol 130-159 mg/dl (borderline-high-risk); 2 or more risk factors *or*
LDL-cholesterol ≥160 mg/dl (high risk)
  Initiate intensive dietary therapy. Evaluate for other CHD risk factors.*

*Positive risk factors:
  age: male ≥45 year
      female ≥55 years or early menopause without estrogen replacement
  family history of premature coronary heart disease
  cigarette smoking
  hypertension
  diabetes mellitus
  HDL-cholesterol <35 mg/dl
HDL-cholesterol ≥60 mg/dl is a negative risk factor that protects against coronary heart disease.
From US Department of Health and Human Services: Second report of the expert panel on detection, evaluation, and treatment of high blood cholesterol in adults, NIH Publication No. 93-3095, Washington, DC, 1993, US Government Printing Office.

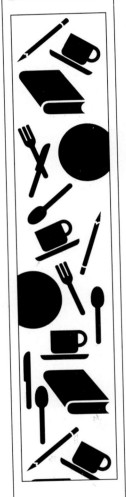

Nutrition Information for the Adult: Point of Choice

An educational intervention used to encourage adults to make appropriate food choices has been nutrition information at the point of purchase. Such programs are conducted at sites where people purchase food to eat immediately or to prepare at a later time. To bring about behavior change it is necessary to make the target population aware of a new idea or practice and then provide an opportunity for them to implement the new practice. Supermarkets, grocery stores, worksite cafeterias, and restaurants all provide such opportunities for point of choice nutrition education.

In-Store Nutrition Information:

A recent survey indicated that 36% of all grocery chains were providing some type of nutrition education in their stores. These activities can take the form of food-tasting booths that provide nutrition information, recipes, and samples of healthy food items. Shelf labels indicating the energy, fat, cholesterol, or sodium content of food items can reinforce the information provided on the nutrition label. Banners and special promotions can direct attention to appropriate food choices for reducing chronic disease risk. Supermarket tours conducted by nutritionists or dietitians can point to heart healthy foods and emphasize the comparison and evaluation of similar products. Store managers consider in-store nutrition education programs to be helpful to their customers and good for their company's image in the community.

Food Service Nutrition Approaches:

Restaurants, cafeterias, convenience stores, and even vending machines can provide materials to educate customers as to the nutrient content of their foods. Colorful signs or posters pointing to the health benefits of a lower fat entree can increase purchases of that item in a fast food restaurant or worksite cafeteria. Labels listing the fat, sodium, or energy content of particular cafeteria or vending machine items might help individuals select a salad dressing with reduced fat or choose a more healthy snack or dessert. Both family restaurants and fine dining establishments have targeted menu items with a heart healthy logo. Culinary institutes now sponsor classes for their students that emphasize high quality food consistent with the Dietary Guidelines for Americans. Community health organizations and local restaurant associations can be targeted as sponsors of in-service classes for food service managers and restaurant chefs that promote food products with appropriate nutrient content. As the number of meals eaten away from home continues to grow, food outlets will become increasingly important sites for community nutrition education.

From Probart CK: In-store consumer nutrition education utilizing student educators, *J Nutr Educ* 25(1):25, 1993.

the cholesterol and sodium contents of important foods, and serve as sites for blood cholesterol screening. Restaurants need to offer menu items carrying a heart healthy logo. School and work-site cafeterias may sponsor contests featuring menu items low in cholesterol and saturated fat. The NCEP has developed sample menus using foods from the traditional American diet as well as items common to Mexican-American, Asian, or vegetarian diets to assist people in making appropriate food choices (Table 3-4).[8] Support from community businesses, local health care agencies, and volunteers can make these programs possible. A multi-faceted, community-based program sponsored by the department of public health in South Carolina resulted in an 8.9% decrease in the use of animal fats among both black and white adults.[45] Thirty-three percent of those interviewed also

TABLE 3-4   *Heart Healthy Sample Menus for Various Food Patterns*

Traditional American Cuisine	Mexican-American Cuisine	Asian-American Cuisine	Lacto Ovo Vegetarian Cuisine

Breakfast
Bagel, plain
  Margarine
  Jelly
Cereal, shredded
  wheat
Banana
Milk, skim
Orange juice
Coffee
  Milk, skim
	Breakfast
	Cantaloupe
	*Farina prepared
	  with skim milk
	White bread
	  Margarine
	  Jelly
	Orange juice
	Hot cocoa pre-
	  pared with skim
	  milk
		Breakfast
		Banana
		Whole wheat bread
		  Margarine
		Orange juice
		Milk, skim
			Breakfast
			Orange
			*Pancakes made
			  w/1% milk &
			  egg whites
			Pancake syrup
			  Margarine
			Milk, 1%
			Coffee
			Milk, 1%

Lunch
Minestrone soup
  canned, low so-
  dium
Roast beef sand-
  wich
  Whole wheat
  bread
  *Lean roast
  beef, unsea-
  soned
  American cheese,
  low fat and
  low sodium
  Lettuce
  Tomato
  Margarine
Apple
Water
	Lunch
	Beef enchilada
	  Tortilla, corn
	  *Lean roast
	  beef
	  Vegetable oil
	  Cheddar cheese
	  low fat and
	  low sodium
	  Onion
	  Tomato
	  Lettuce
	  Chili peppers
	*Refried beans
	  prepared with
	  vegetable oil
	Carrots
	Celery
	Milk, skim
		Lunch
		Beef noodle soup
		  canned low so-
		  dium
		*Chinese noodle
		  and beef salad
		  Sirloin steak
		  Peanut oil
		  Soy sauce, low
		  sodium
		  Carrots
		  Squash
		  Onion
		  Chinese noodles,
		  soft type
		*Steamed white
		  rice
		Apple
		Tea, unsweetened
			Lunch
			Vegetable soup
			  canned, low so-
			  dium
			Bagel
			  Processed Amer-
			  ican cheese,
			  low fat and
			  low sodium
			Spinach salad
			  Spinach
			  Mushrooms
			  *Olive oil
			  dressing,
			  regular
			  calorie
			Apple
			Iced tea

Dinner
*Flounder
  Vegetable oil
*Baked potato
  Margarine
*Green beans sea-
  soned with margarine
*Carrots seasoned
  with margarine
*White dinner
  roll
  Margarine
	Dinner
	Chicken taco
	  Tortilla, corn
	  *Chicken breast
	  without skin
	  Vegetable oil
	  Cheddar cheese
	  low fat and
	  low sodium
	  Guacamole
	  Salsa
		Dinner
		Pork stirfry with
		  vegetables
		  *Pork cutlet
		  Peanut oil
		  Soy sauce, low
		  sodium
		  Broccoli
		  Carrots
		  Mushrooms
		*Steamed
		  white rice
			Dinner
			*Omelette
			  Egg whites
			  Green pepper
			  Onion
			  Mozzarella cheese
			  made from
			  part skim milk
			  Vegetable oil
			*Brown rice sea-
			  soned with marga-
			  rine

*No salt is added in recipe preparation or as seasoning. All margarine is low sodium
From US Department of Health and Human Services: Second report of the expert panel on detection, evaluation and treatment of high blood cholesterol in adults, NIH Publication No. 93-3095, Washington, DC, 1993, US Government Printing Office.

Continued

TABLE 3-4 *Heart Healthy Sample Menus for Various Food Patterns — cont'd*

Traditional American Cuisine	Mexican-American Cuisine	Asian-American Cuisine	Lacto Ovo Vegetarian Cuisine
Dinner Frozen yogurt Iced tea unsweetened	**Dinner** *Corn, seasoned with margarine *Spanish rice prepared with margarine Banana Coffee Milk, skim	**Dinner** Milk, skim Tea, unsweetened	**Dinner** *Carrots, seasoned with margarine Whole wheat bread Margarine Fig bar cookies Tea Honey
Snack *Popcorn Margarine	**Snack** Popcorn Margarine	**Snack** Wonton soup prepared with low-sodium broth Tea, unsweetened	**Snack** Corn flake cereal Milk, 1%

reported looking at restaurant nutrition information when making their selections. Such programs encourage participation in screening and follow-up counseling.

National health promotion and disease prevention objectives. Since its beginning, the U.S. Public Health Service has had responsibility for disease prevention and developed programs for the eradication of nutritional deficiency diseases such as pellagra and the control of infectious diseases. In the late 1970s this agency was directed by Congress to establish national goals for health promotion and disease prevention. These goals were publicized nationwide as the 1990 Health Objectives for the Nation. Goals included improved health status, improved health services, improved public awareness of personal health strategies, and improved health and nutrition monitoring. By 1985 there was significant progress toward meeting many of the 1990 objectives with major reductions in illness and death among specific groups of infants, children, and adults.

Based upon this success regional hearings were organized to allow professional organizations, community health groups, and state and local governments to provide input toward the development of new national health objectives for the 1990s targeted for the year 2000. With the findings of these regional hearings, the U.S. Department of Health and Human Services, Public Health Services issued the new goals in 1990: *Healthy People 2000: National Health Promotion and Disease Prevention Objectives.*[10] The target areas are:

- **Health promotion** — Includes behavioral lifestyle factors that influence health and well-being including use of tobacco, alcohol, and drugs; nutrition; physical fitness; and mental health.
- **Health protection** — Includes health problems related to the physical and social environment including violence and abusive behavior, air quality, waste disposal, and occupational safety and health.
- **Preventive health services** — Includes preventive services directed toward specific health problems such as sexually transmitted disease, adolescent pregnancy, heart disease and other chronic conditions, maternal and infant health problems, and human immunodeficiency virus (HIV).

The Year 2000 Objectives will continue to provide a framework for cooperative activities among state, local, and federal government agencies, health care providers, and community groups through this decade.

Community Sites for Health Promotion

The popular emphasis on health and wellness has led community groups in schools, hospitals, and local government agencies to become involved in health promotion. In the private sector health maintenance organizations (HMOs), businesses, and health clubs are providing health education and screening programs for their members and employees.

Hospital-Based Community Programs

The increasing number of hospitals becoming involved in health promotion is reflective of their changing role from institutions providing care for the sick to those providing a continuum of health care, including education for disease prevention, monitoring, and follow-up care when the patient returns home. Hospital programs include community screening programs to identify those at major risk for chronic disease, and educational programs describing lifestyle patterns to reduce risk. Programs may involve blood pressure and cholesterol screening and education, nutrition assessment and counseling, and weight management with support groups for long-term weight loss.

Some hospitals are marketing health promotion services to local employers. These services include employee assistance programs offering counseling and treatment for specific problems such as alcohol and drug dependency, occupational health services for monitoring the safety of the work environment or treating work-related illness or injury, and wellness programs emphasizing improvement of lifestyle habits.

Health Maintenance Organizations

General organization. Health maintenance organizations (HMOs), based on a concept first developed in the early 1900s, operate currently under federal law regulating their practice enacted in the 1960s. They present the option of prepaid medical care, usually by group medical practices. Subscribers pay a set fee per individual or family and in turn are guaranteed all health services required, including visits to physicians and other health-care professionals, hospital care, and related services. HMOs negotiate fees with hospitals, pharmacies, or specialty practice consultants.

As providers of health-care services, HMOs have both advantages and disadvantages. From the consumer's point of view HMOs provide an opportunity to control one's own health-care costs as all services required will be provided for the set fee. Such a system effectively insulates an individual or family against the financial devastation that can result from a catastrophic illness or injury. Also, HMOs have a financial incentive to encourage preventive health care. The traditional fee-for-service system rewards providers for treating illness. One disadvantage of the HMO is that individuals may not be able to choose their care provider, but rather must accept the provider under contract to the HMO. Also, any arrangement that does not provide a fee per unit of service may result in a provider limiting services in an effort to control costs.

Health promotion activities. HMOs have taken a leadership role in health promotion activities, often in response to member requests. Seminars and classes are offered on topics such as diet and weight control, smoking cessation, stress management, and physical fitness. Some provide health education libraries, professional counselors including nutritionists or registered dietitians, extensive printed material from public sources, handouts authored in-house, lists of recommended books, or newsletters. Many HMO members consider health education to be an important component of their membership services.

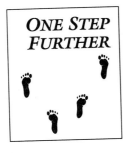

ONE STEP FURTHER

Work Site Wellness Programs

Goals. Work site wellness programs have expanded rapidly in recent years. Now 81% of work sites offer at least one health promotion activity. Companies with more than 50 employees are most likely to sponsor health promotion programs.[46] The incentive for establishing such programs has come at least in part from escalating medical care and insurance costs. Employers have sought to identify causes of this rise and intervene appropriately. Strategies for health promotion programs can be found in the box above.

Health screening programs evaluating blood pressure and serum cholesterol levels, or promoting smoking cessation, nutrition and weight management, physical fitness, and stress management are the most commonly offered. Nutrition programs have been reported to be the most effective wellness program improving health in 59.6% of participants. Stress management training improved productivity and outlook in 46.5% of workers.[46]

Evaluation. Results from many programs indicate that not only do employees lose excess weight, stop smoking, or lower their blood pressure or serum cholesterol levels, but this reduction in risk continues after the formal program has been completed. In one work-site program for treatment and monitoring of elevated blood pressure levels over half of those referred for treatment and follow-up had blood pressure levels below 140/90 mm Hg after three years.[47] Among those referred for treatment outside the work site with no follow-up program, only one fifth maintained blood pressure readings of those levels. The success of the work-site program was attributed to the systematic monitoring that provided employees with information about their condition and offered continued support. A work-site program focusing on dietary changes in middle-aged men reported a mean decrease in serum cholesterol levels from 238 mg/dl to 210 mg/dl that was sustained over a period of one year.[48]

Employer-assisted alterations in the environment that support health promotion are also important to the success of a program. Establishing a smoke-free work place and eliminating cigarette machines, or ensuring low-fat, nutritious food options in the employee cafeteria or vending machines are important when developing a strategy for program evaluation.

Cost effectiveness. Decreasing health risk factors does reduce illness and subsequent health costs, although not immediately. In fact health care costs may rise during the first 6 months following health risk screening when medical intervention needs become apparent. After this initial rise, however, costs decline and this trend continues. In a comparison of work site wellness participants and nonparticipants from the same company, health care costs over a 1-year period were one third lower in those receiving health education. Other companies have reported that physically fit employees had 3.5 fewer sick days each year.[47] Work-site programs offer vast potential for education and intervention in all aspects of health risk.

Health Clubs

Increasing media attention to physical fitness and weight control have fostered the rapid expansion of for-profit health clubs that offer a variety of services for a comprehensive membership fee. Aerobic exercise and use of physical conditioning equipment are the most common activities, although fitness evaluations and development of personal exercise programs may also be provided. Facilities may include a swimming pool, tennis court, or racquetball courts. Nutrition and diet counseling is often available. Unfortunately, in some situations individuals providing dietary evaluations or instruction are not professional nutritionists or registered dietitians.

Health Fairs

Over 2 million people visit health fairs each year. These health fairs are sponsored by service organizations, hospitals, home health agencies, or professional health-related associations. They take place in shopping malls, parking lots, community centers, or parks. They feature displays, posters, hand-out materials, and screening tests for common disorders. Staffed by both professional and lay volunteers, health fairs have as their major purpose health education, and sponsors make an effort to attract both the general population and targeted groups.

Because health fairs are unregulated, little is known about the numbers of persons reached or screening procedures attempted. An organization that offers assistance to health-fair sponsors estimates that over 1.5 million measurements of height and weight and over 20 million blood chemistry tests are performed each year at health fairs. Screening tests to detect health problems may be offered as an incentive to attract participants.

The criteria for those tests and the degree of follow-up within such screening programs concern health professionals. False alarms for the well participants as well as false reassurance for the person at risk are an issue in situations where test conditions and the sheer number of tests performed contribute to error. Despite these limitations blood cholesterol screening does appear to motivate individuals to seek professional care when indicated. In one community 74% of those with identified elevated blood cholesterol levels sought help resulting in a 4.5% decrease in blood cholesterol levels over the next year.[49] Health fairs serve an important role in drawing attention to healthy lifestyle choices and emphasizing personal responsibility for one's own health.

ADULT STAGE OF THE LIFE CYCLE

We start our application of nutrition to the human life cycle with young adults because they are the biologic *progenitors,* the parents who must initiate and nourish each new generation. Worldwide, a healthy beginning for each child depends on the degree that these young adults, especially women, have the opportunity and support to nourish their own state of healthy maturity.[50] A healthy adult maturity depends on physiologic, cultural, and other psychosocial strengths born of individual and societal health values that produce healthy lifestyles.

Adult Homeostasis

After the turbulent physical growth and sexual development of adolescence under control of growth and sex hormones, the human body's growth pattern levels off into a state of adult **homeostasis.** The word was first used by Boston physiologist Walter Cannon (1871-1945) in his now classic book to describe what he called the "wisdom of the body." In a state of gene regulation and feedback, the "body's wisdom" maintains an internal dynamic equilibrium and stability within the ebb and flow of its parts through a balancing system of "homeostatic" mechanisms. Physically, then, the adult body has grown up,

Homeostasis
(Gr *homoios,* same, unchanging; *stasis,* stability) State of the body's internal physiologic balance through constant feedback and adjustment, the operation of homeostatic mechanisms that maintain a dynamic equilibrium within the body in relation to its external environment.

attained its full genetic size and strength, and now leveled off in a stable state of tissue maintenance and function.

This dynamic balance between body parts and functions is life sustaining. All body constituents are in a constant state of flux, although some tissues are more actively engaged than others. This concept of dynamic equilibrium can be seen in carbohydrate and fat metabolism, but it is especially striking in protein metabolism. The adult body's state of metabolic stability or homeostasis results from a balance between the rates of tissue protein breakdown and resynthesis. In earlier growth years, the tissue protein synthesis rate is higher so that the necessary new tissues can be formed. In later adult years, as in the aging process in the elderly, the rate of tissue protein breakdown gradually exceeds that of synthesis, and the older adult body slowly declines.

Body Composition

Adult body composition is maintained within a rather wide range of individual variance according to sex, weight, and age (see Chapter 2). The most metabolically active tissue is the lean body mass compartment. It requires the greatest amount of energy and is larger in men than in women, accounting for 30% to 65% of the total body weight. The lean body mass will be larger in adults who are physically active and consume a low fat diet. The fat compartment is larger in women than in men and may vary in average weight adults from about 14% to 30% of the total body weight. In overweight persons, too prevalent a situation among Americans because of a relatively sedentary lifestyle and a rich diet, the fat compartment is larger. It is smaller in persons who exercise regularly and eat less fat. In general, as adults grow older and become less physically active, the lean body mass decreases and the relative fat tissue increases. The water compartment in adults of average weight accounts for about 20% of the total body weight. It is larger in thin or less fat persons and smaller in fat persons. The mineral compartment, the smallest part of adult body composition, accounts for only about 5% to 6% of the body weight, most of it in the skeleton.

Physiologic Maturity

The young adult reaches physiologic maturity when full genetic body size is attained and tissue growth continues only on a healthy maintenance basis. There is full development of body functions, including sexual **maturation** and reproductive capacity. During middle and older adulthood, however, there is a gradual cell loss and reduced cell metabolism, with a gradual reduction in the performance capacity of most organ systems. Individuals vary widely in the rate and order at which these changes occur. In general, the age-related decline in lean body mass accelerates in later life.

Psychosocial Maturity

Psychosocial development continues in individual and changing patterns throughout adulthood with its unique potentials and fulfillments. Throughout the human life cycle, food not only serves to meet nutritional requirements for physical growth and tissue maintenance but also relates intimately to personal psychosocial development. Over the past 30 years, Erikson's classic structure of human development in relation to society and culture has greatly influenced our view of the human life cycle.[51] In this pattern, the three adult stages—young, middle, and older—of the human life cycle complete the whole and give meaning to human development.

Young adulthood—ages 18-40. In the years of young adulthood every person, now launched as an individual, must resolve the core problem of intimacy versus isolation. If positive development is achieved, the person is able to build intimate relationships leading to self-fulfillment, either in marriage or in other personal relationships. Persons who have

Maturation
(L *maturus,* mature) Process or stage of attaining one's full physical, psychosocial, and mental development. Individual genetic potential guides physical and mental development, which in turn bears the imprint of environmental, psychosocial, and cultural influences.

failed to develop psychosocial strengths in previous years of growing up, however, may become increasingly isolated from others. These are the years of career beginnings, of establishing one's own home, of parenthood, of starting young children on their way through the same life stages, and of early struggles to make one's way in the world.

Middle adulthood—ages 40-60. In the years of middle adulthood the psychosocial problem persons face is **generativity** versus self-absorption. The children have now grown and gone to make their own lives. For some, these are the years of the "empty nest." For others, these years are an opportunity for expanding personal growth—"it's my turn now." There is a coming to terms with what life is all about along with great opportunity to express stored learning and pass on life's teachings. It is a regeneration of one life in the lives of young persons following the same way. To the degree that these inner struggles are not won, there is increasing self-absorption, a turning-in on oneself, and a withering rather than a regenerating spirit of life.

Older adulthood—ages 60-80 +. In the last stage of life the final core psychosocial problem is resolved between integrity and despair. Depending on a person's resources at this point, there is either a predominant sense of wholeness and completeness or a sense of distaste and bitterness and of wondering what life was all about. If the outcome of life's basic experiences and problems has been positive, the individual arrives at old age a person rich in wisdom. Building on each previous level of development, psychosocial growth has reached its individual, positive human resolution. Some elderly persons, however, will not have resolved core psychosocial conflicts and will struggle with conflicts with which they have wrestled in previous stages of life. They arrive at middle and later years poorly equipped to deal with the adjustments and health problems that may face them. Alternatively, many others will have been enriched by life's experiences in their maturing process, and in turn they will bring enrichment to the lives of those around them. The resulting generational relationship is mutually rewarding.

Generativity
(L *generatio,* generation)
The dynamic psychosocial process of renewing a society's values from one generation to the next.

BASIC NUTRIENT NEEDS
Physiologic Differences

Beginning with adolescent growth and development, significant body changes occur between the sexes (see Chapter 8). This profound period of physiologic change brings sexual maturity and biologic reproductive capacity to initiate new life. Distinct differences in growth patterns emerge between the sexes and are strengthened in their young adult bodies.

Males. In the male physical growth is manifested more in an increased muscle mass and in long-bone growth. His rate of growth is slower than that of the female body, but he soon passes her in weight and height and becomes the larger of the two young adult forms.

Females. In the female there is an increasing amount of subcutaneous fat deposit, particularly in the abdominal area. The hip breadth increases and the bony pelvis widens in preparation for reproduction. A pelvic girdle of subcutaneous fat results, often a source of anxiety to many figure-conscious young women.

With such profound physical body changes and individual differences, largely revolving around sexual development and preparation for adult roles in a complex society, it is small wonder that many psychosocial tensions result.

Dietary Recommendations

The physiologic differences between the sexes account for differing energy and nutrient recommendations for adult men and women in the three age groups—young-, middle-, and older-age adults.

TABLE 3-5   *Age and Sex Comparisons of Recommended Dietary Allowances (1989) for Adults*

Age (yrs) or Cond.	Sex	Weight*		Height*		Energy†	Pro	Major Minerals		
								Calcium	Phosphorus	Magnesium
		kg	lb	cm	in	kcal	g	mg	mg	mg
Young adults 19-24	F	58	128	164	65	2,200	46	1200	1200	300
	M	72	160	177	70	2,900	58	1200	1200	350
Middle adults 25-50	F	63	138	163	64	2,200	50	800	800	280
	M	79	174	176	70	2,900	63	800	800	350
Older adults 51+	F	65	143	160	63	1,900	50	800	800	280
	M	77	170	173	68	2,300	63	800	800	350
Pregnancy						+300	60	1200	1200	320
Lactation						+500	65	1200	1200	355
						+500	62	1200	1200	340

RE, retinol equivalents (see full RDAs); α-TE, alpha-tocopherol equivalents (see full RDAs); NE, niacin equivalent (see full RDAs).
*Medians of US population survey figures (NHANES II); does not imply ideal height-weight ratios.
†Light to moderate activity

Adult RDAs. Table 3-5 compares the Recommended Dietary Allowances for males and females during the three age groups.[52]

Energy (kilocalories). The larger male body size and muscle mass accounts for the greater need for energy, especially since the lean body mass is the most metabolically active tissue in the body composition. In adults, the resting energy expenditure (REE) per unit of total body weight, a measure of metabolic rate, differs by approximately 10% between the sexes. The remainder of energy need is for physical activities and is much smaller than that for metabolic needs. In the past, because of occupational differences, men and women often had markedly different energy expenditures, but their occupational activity requirements now are quite similar. Note that these RDA height-weight reference figures are actual **medians** for the U.S. population of the designated age, as reported by the National Health and Nutrition Examination Survey II (NHANES II), and are not meant to imply ideal height-to-weight ratios. Additional kilocalories are required to support pregnancy and lactation (see Chapters 4 and 5).

Protein. The adult protein allowances are based on a daily protein intake of approximately 0.75 to 0.8 g per kg of body weight for both sexes and all three age groups.[52] Because of the difference in older adult body composition with a gradually decreasing lean body mass, this continuing basic protein allowance is higher per unit of lean body mass for older adults and should allow for some decrease in utilization efficiency. An additional allowance of 10 g/day of protein throughout pregnancy and 15 g/day during lactation is required (see Chapters 4 and 5).

Minerals. Adult allowances are sufficient if provided on a continuing basis by a well-balanced diet. Two minerals need emphasis: calcium and iron. The RDA for calcium has been increased from 800 to 1200 mg/day for young adults to ensure peak skeletal bone mass, which is attained roughly by age 35.[52,53] For middle and older adults the allowance remains at 800 mg/day, although there is some evidence that older adults, especially

Median
The middle figure in a rank order listing an individual group of figures; not an average value of all the figures.

Trace Elements				Fat-Soluble Vitamins				Water-Soluble Vitamins						
Iron	Zinc	Iodine	Sele-nium	A	D	E	K	C	Thiamin	Ribo-flavin	Niacin	B$_6$	Folate	B$_{12}$
mg	mg	μg	μg	μg RE	μg	mg α-TE	μg	mg	mg	mg	mg NE	mg	μg	μg
15	12	150	50	800	10	8	60	60	1.1	1.3	15	1.5	180	2.0
10	15	150	70	1000	10	10	70	60	1.5	1.7	19	2.0	200	2.0
15	12	150	55	800	5	8	65	60	1.1	1.3	15	1.6	180	2.0
10	15	150	70	1000	5	10	80	60	1.5	1.7	19	2.0	200	2.0
10	12	150	55	800	5	8	65	60	1.0	1.2	13	1.6	180	2.0
10	15	150	70	1000	5	10	80	60	1.2	1.4	15	2.0	200	2.0
30	15	175	65	800	10	10	65	70	1.5	1.6	17	2.2	400	2.2
15	19	200	75	1300	10	12	65	95	1.6	1.8	20	2.1	280	2.6
15	16	200	75	1200	10	11	65	90	1.6	1.7	20	2.1	260	2.6

postmenopausal women, should have an increased intake to prevent calcium loss from bone and the development of **osteoporosis**[53] (p. 86). Poor adult diets may also be deficient in iron, which is needed to prevent iron-deficiency anemia. During the reproductive years, women require more iron intake to prevent deficiency due to menstrual blood loss, so their iron allowance is 15 mg/day; for men it is 10 mg/day. Iron requirements during pregnancy are 30 mg/day, which is difficult to attain by diet so a supplement is usually needed.[53] No increase is needed during lactation.

Vitamins. Intake of the adult vitamin allowances is usually met by ordinary well-balanced diets. The problem in some individual cases may stem from inadequate normal intake rather than from an increased need. A well-selected, mixed diet usually supplies all the vitamins needed. There may be increased therapeutic needs in illness that should be evaluated on an individual basis.

Dietary pattern. The publication *Nutrition and Your Health: Dietary Guidelines for Americans,* issued in its third edition by the U.S. Departments of Agriculture and Health and Human Services, provides a good basic guide for choosing a diet to promote health.[54] It is discussed in Table 1-3. Other general food guides including the basic five food groups visualized in The Food Pyramid are discussed in Chapter 1.

WOMEN'S NUTRITION AND REPRODUCTIVE FUNCTION

During the reproductive years of the human life cycle, women conceive, nourish, and bear the new life that begins in turn the new life cycle. Thus health promotion and nutritional support over the life cycle begin in preparation for female reproduction. We therefore focus first on the reproductive function of older adolescent young women and young adult women on whose healthy bodies the foundation for life's continuing cycle

Osteoporosis
(Gr *osteon,* bone; *poros,* passage) Abnormal thinning of bone, producing a lattice-like formation of enlarged spaces in bone, which increases the risk of fracture.

depends. We then look briefly at women's special health issues and how they relate to nutritional care and planning a healthy lifestyle.

The Preparation Years

During early childhood in any culture, care of young children involves early psychosocial initiation, consciously or unconsciously, of girls and boys into the cultural pattern of their respective sex roles. Current American cultural diversity allows women an expanded and diverse social role in the world of work and the home, choosing when and if they will have children. Nonetheless, at the same time, physiologic growth and development of young girls during childhood and early adolescence uniquely prepares their bodies and sets the biologic time clock for potential reproduction. Both nutritional status and nutrition education play basic roles in this development (see Chapters 6-8).

Nutrition and the Female Hormones

Development of ova. Adult female reproduction begins with the development of ova. The primary form of ova began their development many years before during fetal life, when **primordial ova** differentiate from the germinal **epithelium** covering the outside of the fetal ovary and migrate into the ovary's cortex, carrying with them a layer of the epithelioid **granulosa cells.** An ovum surrounded by this single layer of special granulosa cells is called a **primordial follicle.** By the thirtieth week of gestation the peak number of ova produced reaches about seven million, but most soon degenerate so that less than two million remain in the two ovaries at birth, and only 300,000 at puberty. During the reproductive years of the female only about 450 of these follicles develop sufficiently to expel their ova; the rest degenerate. Finally, at the end of reproductive capability, the **menopause,** only a few primordial follicles remain in the ovaries, and these last few follicles shortly degenerate.[55]

Female hormonal system. A hierarchy of hormones from three sources comprises the cyclic female hormone system. First, initiating the cycle, the **hypothalamus** secretes a releasing hormone called luteinizing hormone-releasing hormone (LHRH), which is a decapeptide chain of 10 amino acids, targeted for the anterior pituitary gland. Second, in response, the anterior pituitary secretes two specific hormones, named by their ovary-stimulating functions: luteinizing hormone (LH) and follicle-stimulating hormone (FSH), both of which are small glycoproteins. Third, in final sequence response, the ovaries secrete **estrogen** and **progesterone,** steroids synthesized from cholesterol and acetyl coenzyme A and transported in the blood loosely bound with the plasma albumin or specific binding globulins. The cyclic ovarian changes depend entirely on this systematic sequence of female hormones, which in turn depends on nutritional metabolic support.

Estrogen functions. Of the six different natural estrogens only three are present in significant quantities: beta-estradiol, estrone, and their oxidative product, estriol. Beta-estradiol is by far the most potent, and is thus the major estrogen. During childhood, only small quantities of estrogens are secreted, but with the beginning of puberty estrogen secretion increases twenty-fold or more, stimulated by the pituitary gonadotropic hormones. Although the principle function of the estrogens is the growth and development of the sexual organs and other tissues related to reproduction, they have other important effects related to mineral metabolism and bone growth.

Sexual organs. With the onset of puberty and the surge of estrogen secretion, the female sexual organs change from those of a child to those of an adult. The uterine size increases two- to threefold and important changes occur in its lining, the endometrium. Estrogens cause marked proliferation of the endometrial tissue and development of the glands that will later be used to nourish the implanting ovum. A similar effect occurs on the mucosal lining of the fallopian tubes, enhancing the activity of the epithelial cilia that sweep toward the uterus to help propel the fertilized ovum.

Primordial ova
(L *primordia,* the beginning; *ovum,* egg) Primitive ovum cells produced in large life supply number in the female fetal uterus before birth.

Epithelium
(Gr *epi-,* on, upon, over; *thele,* nipple) The covering tissue of internal and external surfaces of the body, including linings of vessels and other small cavities.

Primordial follicle
(L *follis,* a leather bag) Primitive ovarian follicle formed during fetal life; a sac- or pouch-like cavity; a small secretory sac or gland. A mature ovarian follicle is an ovum surrounded by specialized epithelial cells.

Hypothalamus
(Gr *hypo-,* under; *thalamus* inner chamber) A small gland adjacent to the pituitary in the basal mid-brain area. Serves as a collection and dispatching center for information about the internal well-being of the body, using much of this neuroendocrine information to stimulate and control many widespread important pituitary hormones.

Breasts. The estrogens cause fat deposits in the breasts and initiate growth and development of milk-producing apparatus, resulting in the appearance of the mature female breast. But estrogens do not convert the breasts into milk-producing organs. This task is not initiated until pregnancy, when lactation is stimulated by the hormone prolactin (see Chapters 4 and 5).

Skeleton. Estrogens cause increased osteoblastic activity and bone growth. Thus at puberty when a girl enters her reproductive years, her growth rate becomes rapid for several years and she is often taller than boys of the same age. However, estrogens have another effect on skeletal growth. They cause early uniting of the epiphyses with shafts of the long bones, causing female growth in height to cease several years earlier than that of the male. Estrogens affect overall bone growth by promoting increased deposits of bone matrix with the subsequent retention of both calcium and phosphorus.

Metabolism and fat deposits. Estrogens increase the metabolic rate in young girls after puberty but not as much as the male sex hormone *testosterone* does in young boys. Estrogen also causes increased deposits of subcutaneous fat in the female body, especially in the buttocks and thighs, causing a broadening of the hips.

Progesterone. The most important function of the second ovarian hormone, *progesterone,* is to promote important secretory changes in the **endometrium** lining the uterus, preparing it for implantation of the fertilized ovum. These secretions also occur in the mucosal lining of the fallopian tubes and provide necessary nutrition for the fertilized, dividing ovum as it moves through the tube to the uterus. Progesterone also helps promote breast development of milk-producing structures, but actual milk production is stimulated only after pregnancy by prolactin from the anterior pituitary. During pregnancy the mild catabolic effect of progesterone helps mobilize proteins for use by the fetus.

The Female Sexual Cycle

The normal female reproductive years, between puberty at age 11 to 15 and the menopause at age 45 to 55, are marked by monthly rhythmic changes in rates of secretion of female hormones and corresponding changes in the ovaries and sexual organs. This rhythmic pattern is correctly called the *female sexual cycle,* or less accurately, the *menstrual cycle.* **Menstruation** is only the visible end phase of the cycle when conception does not occur and all the tissue preparations and blood supply for this target event are expelled by the uterus. The overall cycle averages 28 days in length. Normally it can be as short as 20 days or as long as 45 days. The purpose of the cycle is twofold: (1) to develop and release a mature ovum from the ovaries each month, and (2) to prepare the uterus lining, the endometrium, to receive and nourish the ovum. The entire cycle requires nutritional support to function. **Amenorrhea,** absence of **menses,** is a common and distinct sign of malnutrition in women. The normal monthly functioning of the female sexual cycle in well-nourished women is accomplished through five specific phases: preovulation, follicular growth, ovulation, postovulation, and menstruation.

Preovulation phase. The ovarian changes that produce a mature ovum depend entirely on initial secretion of the stimulating hormones FSH and LH from the anterior pituitary gland. Unstimulated ovaries remain completely inactive. This is the state during childhood until the young girl is about 8 years old, when these hormones gradually awaken and progressively secrete these essential hormones, initiating monthly sexual cycles between the ages of 11 and 15. This culmination is called puberty.

Follicular growth phase. At puberty when secretions of the pituitary gland hormones FSH and LH increase, the entire ovaries and their primordial follicles within begin to grow. Each **follicle,** dormant since initial development in fetal life, is a sac- or pouch-like cavity lined with secretory cells that encases an ovum and nourishes its growth. The ovum surrounded by these specialized epithelial cells is called an ovarian follicle. Increased surges

Endometrium
(Gr *endon,* within; *metra,* uterus) Inner mucous membrane of the uterus.

Menstruation
(L *mensis,* month) Monthly discharge of blood and mucosal tissues from the nonpregnant uterus. Final phase of the female sexual cycle.

Amenorrhea
(*a-,* negative; Gr *men,* month; *rhoia,* flow) Absence of menses. Nutritional anemorrhea results from extreme weight loss and malnutrition, as in eating disorders such as anorexia nervosa.

Menses
Monthly menstrual period.

Follicle
(L *follis,* leather bag) Sac-like secretory cavity encasing an ovum and nourishing its growth.

Ovulation

Monthly process in female sexual cycle of secreting a mature ovum for transport through the fallopian tubes to the uterus.

Corpus luteum

(L *corpus,* body; *uteum,* yellow) Mass of estrogen and progesterone secretory cells. Produced monthly from the ovarian follicle in the postovulation phase of the female sexual cycle.

of FSH and LH at the beginning of each monthly cycle cause one of the follicles to outgrow the others after 1 or 2 weeks and nourish its ovum to maturity while hormonal signals stop the growth of the remainder, which involute, awaiting stimulation at another monthly cycle.

Ovulation phase. About midway, day 14 of a normal 28-day cycle, **ovulation** occurs, stimulated primarily by a large increase in secretion rate of the anterior pituitary hormone LH assisted by a moderate increase of FSH. This secretion rate peaks about 18 hours before ovulation, causing rapid swelling of the follicle and degeneration of its capsule, allowing final expulsion of the ovum for its transport through the fallopian tubes into the uterus.

Postovulation phase. During the first few hours after ovulation occurs, the remaining secretory cells of the follicle undergo rapid physical and chemical change into a mass of cells called a **corpus luteum.** These lutein cells enlarge and deposit fatty material that gives them a distinctive yellow color and hence their name. The corpus luteum then secretes large quantities of the female hormones estrogen and progesterone, and after another 2 weeks disintegrates. The following decrease in ovarian estrogen and progesterone causes menstruation to follow.

Menstruation phase. Throughout the cycle, marked changes have occurred in the endometrium of the uterus. During the first 11 days of the cycle, estrogen has stimulated a proliferation of tissue, and during the next 12 days progesterone has greatly increased the secretory function. These changes have occurred for the whole purpose of storing large amounts of nutrients to support rapid growth of a fertilized ovum, should it arrive and implant itself. Without such a need, levels of the two hormones decrease sharply, the engorged endometrial tissue detaches along with its blood supply, and contractions of the uterus expel its contents over the final 5 days of the cycle. During normal menstruation about 35 ml of blood and another 35 ml of serous fluid are lost and only the thin initial layer of basic endothelial tissue remains, ready to grow and develop repeatedly in the same sequence during following cycles, supported by the woman's positive nutritional status.[55]

Female Fertility and Contraception

Fertile period. The period of female fertility during each sexual cycle is very short. The ovum remains viable for only about 24 hours, so sexual intercourse and deposit of sufficient viable sperm must occur some time between 1 day before ovulation and 1 day afterward, if fertilization is to take place. The use of some means of contraception helps maintain a mother's health through family planning, thus preventing a high **parity,** that is, frequent pregnancies that drain maternal nutritional resources with no replenishing between.

Parity

(L *parere,* to bring forth, produce) Number of pregnancies a woman has had with viable offspring.

Rhythm method. The rhythm method of contraception, avoiding intercourse over the period of ovulation, is sometimes practiced but is more often than not unsuccessful. It is usually stated that avoidance of intercourse for 4 days before ovulation and 3 days afterward prevents conception. The problem lies in the fact that it is difficult to predict precisely the day of ovulation.

Oral contraceptive agents — the "Pill." This commonly used method of contraception is based on hormonal suppression of fertility by preventing ovulation but allowing menstruation to occur. Most of these oral contraceptive agents (OCAs) contain a combination of synthetic estrogen and synthetic progestins. Because these substances are synthetic they cannot be destroyed by the liver after they are absorbed, as are natural hormones, so they can be taken orally. The pills are usually begun in the early part of the female sexual cycle, continued beyond time of ovulation, and stopped toward the end of the cycle to allow menstruation and a new cycle start. Other low-dose combinations of these synthetic hormones may occasionally allow ovulation but prevent conception by other means, such as (1) delaying fallopian tube transport of the ovum (normal time is 3 days), (2) inadequately developing the endometrium, (3) developing abnormal cervical mucus that blocks sperm entry, or (4) causing abnormal contractions of fallopian tubes and uterus expelling ovum. One prior concern has been the effect of different OCA hormone combinations on lipid and carbohydrate metabolism, elevating serum levels of triglycerides, LDLs, cholesterol, and insulin. Current study and modification of the type and dose of progestin in OCAs, even use of progestin alone, diminishes all of these serum lipid changes.[56]

Barrier methods. An alternate, though sometimes unreliable, method of contraception is use of a **condom** as a sheath or cover for the penis during intercourse to prevent deposit of sperm. With the epidemic incidence of deadly acquired immunodeficiency syndrome (AIDS), however, the condom has an additional function in helping prevent sexually transmitted disease (STD). Also, in the current upsurge of other STDs such as gonorrhea, a condom not only prevents easy entry of the AIDS virus into open gonorrheal lesions or genital tissue, but also spread of the secondary STD. Another barrier device is the diaphragm, vaginally inserted before intercourse as a cover over the cervix entry to the uterus. When used with a spermicidal jelly, the diaphragm may be a helpful but not always reliable method of contraception.

Nutrition and Fertility

Since normal functioning of the female sexual cycle depends on optimal nutritional support, malnutrition greatly reduces fertility. This malnutrition effect may affect whole communities or larger areas in cases of famine from natural disasters such as long-term drought, or from political events such as war and seige. It may also be caused by self-induced starvation, as in eating disorders such as anorexia nervosa or bulimia, occurring in adolescents and young women (see Chapter 8). Whatever the cause, such situations of starvation produce amenorrhea with no conception or poor pregnancy outcomes and high infant mortality.

Menopause

There is a progressive decline in estrogen secretion toward the end of a woman's reproductive life. When she is approximately 50 years of age, her sexual cycles become irregular and ovulation fails to occur during many of them. This period during which the cycles cease altogether and the female sex hormones diminish rapidly to extremely low levels is called the menopause. The cause of the menopause is the "burning out" of the ovaries; few primordial follicles remain and production of estrogen by the ovaries decreases as the number of primary follicles approaches zero and the final ones involute and disappear. For most women, this menopausal period is a normal physiologic process with no marked physical or psychologic symptoms. Approximately 15% of women, however, experience a variety of symptoms such as "hot flashes" with extreme flushing of the skin, sensations of **dyspnea,** irritability, fatigue, anxiety, and in a few cases occasional psychotic states.[55] In such cases, estrogen therapy may be indicated.

Nutrition and Pregnancy Planning

Ideally every pregnancy should be a planned pregnancy. However, for many reasons this is not always the case. Certainly for women with preexisting disease such as insulin-dependent diabetes mellitus (IDDM) or maternal **phenylketonuria (PKU),** it is mandatory to achieve the best control status possible to help ensure a successful outcome. In any case, planning a healthy lifestyle, including both positive nutritional support and physical fitness as described in this chapter, should definitely begin in the early reproductive years of all women. A helpful daily food guide for women that covers the reproductive years, developed by the California Department of Health Services is given in Table 3-6. (See source listing at end of chapter under Further Reading.)

Condom
(L *condus,* receptacle) A penile sheath serving not only as a barrier method of contraception but also as a means of preventing the spread of sexually transmitted diseases.

Dyspnea
(Gr *dysnia,* difficult breathing) Difficult or labored breathing.

Phenylketonuria (PKU)
Genetic disease that, if untreated, results in severe mental retardation. It is caused by a lack of a key enzyme, phenylalanine hydroxylase, that controls the metabolic conversion of the amino acid phenylalanine to tyrosine. Currently newborn screening and special low phenylalanine diets allow girls with PKU to reach adulthood and have families of their own.

TABLE 3-6 Daily Food Guide for Women

Food Group	One Serving Equals	Recommended Minimum Servings		
		Nonpregnant		Pregnant/ Lactating
		11-24 yr	25 + yr	
Protein foods Provide protein, iron, zinc, and B-vitamins for growth of muscles, bone, blood, and nerves. Vegetable protein provides fiber to prevent constipation.	**Animal Protein:** 1 oz. cooked chicken or turkey 1 oz. cooked lean beef, lamb, or pork 1 oz. or ¼ cup fish or other seafood 1 egg 2 fish sticks or hot dogs 2 slices luncheon meat **Vegetable Protein:** ½ cup cooked dry beans, lentils, or split peas 3 oz. tofu 1 oz. or ¼ cup peanuts, pumpkin, or sunflower seeds 1½ oz. or ⅓ cup other nuts 2 tbsp. peanut butter	5 — A half serving of vegetable protein daily	5	7 — One serving of vegetable protein daily
Milk products Provide protein and calcium to build strong bones, teeth, healthy nerves and muscles, and promote normal blood clotting.	8 oz. milk 8 oz. yogurt 1 cup milk shake 1½ cups cream soup (made with milk) 1½ oz. or ⅓ cup grated cheese (such as cheddar, Monterey, mozzarella, or Swiss) 1½-2 slices presliced American cheese 4 tbsp. parmesan cheese 2 cups cottage cheese 1 cup pudding 1 cup custard or flan 1½ cups ice milk, ice cream, or frozen yogurt	3	2	3
Breads, cereals, grains Provide carbohydrates and B-vitamins for energy and healthy nerves. Also provide iron for healthy blood. Whole grains provide fiber to prevent constipation.	1 slice bread 1 dinner roll ½ bun or bagel ½ English muffin or pita 1 small tortilla ¾ cup dry cereal ½ cup granola ½ cup cooked cereal ½ cup rice ½ cup noodles or spaghetti ¼ cup wheat germ 1 4-inch pancake or waffle 1 small muffin 8 medium crackers 4 graham cracker squares 3 cups popcorn	7 — Four servings of whole-grain products daily	6	7

Food group	Examples	Examples			
Vitamin C–rich fruits and vegetables Provide vitamin C to prevent infection and to promote healing and iron absorption. Also provide fiber to prevent constipation.	6 oz. orange, grapefruit, or fruit juice enriched with vitamin C 6 oz. tomato juice or vegetable juice cocktail 1 orange, kiwi, mango 1/2 grapefruit, cantaloupe 1/2 cup papaya 2 tangerines	1/2 cup strawberries 1/2 cup cooked or 1 cup raw cabbage 1/2 cup broccoli; Brussels sprouts, or cauliflower 1/2 cup snow peas, sweet peppers, or tomato puree 2 tomatoes	1	1	1
Vitamin A–rich fruits and vegetables Provide beta-carotene and vitamin A to prevent infection and to promote wound healing and night vision. Also provide fiber to prevent constipation.	6 oz. apricot nectar or vegetable juice cocktail 3 raw or 1/4 cup dried apricots 1/4 cantaloupe or mango 1 small or 1/2 cup sliced carrots 2 tomatoes	1/2 cup cooked or 1 cup raw spinach 1/2 cup cooked greens (beet, chard, collards, dandelion, kale, mustard) 1/2 cup pumpkin, sweet potato, winter squash, or yams	1	1	1
Other fruits and vegetables Provide carbohydrates for energy and fiber to prevent constipation.	6 oz. fruit juice (if not listed above) 1 medium or 1/2 cup sliced fruit (apple, banana, peach, pear) 1/2 cup berries (other than strawberries) 1/2 cup cherries or grapes 1/2 cup pineapple 1/2 cup watermelon	1/4 cup dried fruit 1/2 cup sliced vegetable (asparagus, beets, green beans, celery, corn, eggplant, mushrooms, onion, peas, potato, summer squash, zucchini) 1/2 artichoke 1 cup lettuce	3	3	3
Unsaturated fats Provide vitamin E to protect tissue.	1/8 med. avocado 1 tsp. margarine 1 tsp. mayonnaise 1 tsp. vegetable oil	2 tsp. salad dressing (mayonnaise-based) 1 tbsp. salad dressing (oil-based)	3	3	3

NOTE: The Daily Food Guide for Women may not provide all the calories you require. The best way to increase your intake is to include more than the minimum servings recommended.

Adapted from California Department of Health Services, Maternal and Child Health: Nutrition during pregnancy and postpartum period: A manual for health care professionals, Sacramento, 1990, CDHS.

Active pregnancy planning health promotion should be based on nutritional assessment and counseling, with correction of any nutrient or weight deficits and elimination of such lifestyle health hazards as alcohol abuse, smoking, and drug-related problems. These nutrition assessment procedures are reviewed in Chapter 2 and the factors involved in planning a successful pregnancy outcome are discussed in Chapter 4. Of particular concern are drugs that can cause birth defects initiated in early cell differentiation of embryonic life weeks before a woman even knows she is pregnant. Serious effects have been shown, for example, among women who conceive while taking pharmacologic megadoses of vitamin A or vitamin A-related retinoid drugs.[29,30] One such retinoid-drug, *isotretinoin* (13-cis retinoic acid), trade name Accutane, as well as its related compound etretinate, has been used for treating severe cystic acne.[31,32] Since Accutane has been shown to produce spontaneous abortions of malformed fetuses or those with congenital defects started in early embryonic life, it must carry a warning label against its use by sexually active women who do not use a reliable form of contraception. In addition, physicians prescribing this drug for their adolescent or young adult women patients usually order pregnancy testing before starting the drug and monthly during its use.

WOMEN'S NUTRITION AND HEALTH ISSUES
Women and Weight

The health problem of obesity, defined as an excessive accumulation of body fat, has been regarded traditionally as the result of overeating. However, recent studies of twins have indicated that there is a strong genetic component to body fat accumulation and its distribution.[57,58] Men and women differ genetically in their respective sex chromosomes. Men carry an XY combination pair of X (female) and Y (male) chromosomes, whereas women carry a complete XX combination. Cell division of the male XY chromosomes produces the final mature sperm cells, half male (Y) sperm and half female (X) sperm. The sex of the offspring depends on which of these two types of sperm fertilizes the ovum. Thus, it should not be surprising that women may well differ from men in the prevalence of obesity, its time of onset, and their responses to treatment. This genetic factor in obesity helps to explain the "yo-yo" pattern of dieting that compounds the weight problem for many women, as a successful diet will reduce body weight and fat stores but cannot change individual genetic makeup.

Once a person has expressed this genetic predisposition to gain weight, and for women this occurs most often in the early adult years, the obesity is likely to recur again and again unless major changes that promote health and fitness and a healthy lifestyle are made in lifetime habits and environmental factors.[59] Thus some form of regular exercise and physical activity needs to be a part of that healthy lifestyle. Although effects of exercise on weight loss may be minimal in the short term, long-term followup studies in both men and women show that those who make regular exercise a part of their long-term lifestyle have dramatically better success at keeping weight off with improved food habits based on moderation and variety.[60]

These study results should encourage adolescent and young adult women who face in their early development the twofold gender disadvantage not only of a physiologic propensity for a larger body fat composition but also the social pressure of a society obsessed with thinness as the ideal female form. These results should also encourage middle-age and older adult women whose health concerns include regional body fat distribution, especially abdominal body fat with its association with potential development of chronic disease risks for cardiovascular problems, hypertension, and diabetes. In women, body fat is usually localized in the hips and thighs (*gynoid* or lower body fat distribution). In men, body fat is usually localized in the abdominal region (*android* or upper body fat distribution). However, this sex-related distribution pattern can vary among individual men and women. In both sexes abdominal body fat tends to increase with age, but with the reduction of the female sex hormones at menopause, postmenopausal women experience an acceleration of this upper body fat accumulation.

Coronary Heart Disease

Gender differences. Through earlier adult years, a large gender gap exists between men and women in the incidence of cardiovascular disease, with men at much greater risk, developing the view of heart disease as a "man's disease." However, the gap closes rapidly with menopause and heart disease becomes the leading cause of death for American women aged 50 years and older, accounting for a large number of the nearly 500,000 deaths of men and women annually. Very few women develop cardiovascular disease before menopause due to the protective effect of the female sex hormone estrogen. Thus women develop coronary heart disease at the same rate as men, but approximately 6 to 10 years later.

Risk factors. Postmenopausal women face the same risk factors for cardiovascular disease as do men (see Table 3-2). They are just as vulnerable to the blood lipid factors, especially elevated cholesterol and the LDLs carrying cholesterol to the cells, that are now recognized as major risk factors in the development of coronary heart disease (p 66). A high level of LDL is an independent risk factor in both men and women, but a high serum triglyceride level is an independent risk factor only in women. Women with diabetes and those who are overweight and hypertensive are at higher risk, and those who smoke compound it further. The devastating effects of smoking leading to peripheral vascular disease and coronary heart disease are now experienced by women as well as men. Thus the coronary heart disease risk profile of a woman can be assessed by a few simple indicators: serum cholesterol, blood pressure, serum glucose, weight, and smoking status. The positive approach of planning a healthy lifestyle, as described earlier, will reduce these risk factors and increase general fitness and well-being.

Non–insulin-Dependent Diabetes Mellitus (NIDDM)

Gender differences. NIDDM, the onset of which occurs in adulthood, is closely related in predisposing risk factors for women described above for cardiovascular disease. It occurs mainly in postmenopausal women aged 45 to 60 and has a greater impact on women, sometimes requiring insulin during the initial treatment period to counteract its degree of impaired glucose tolerance. The reasons for this differing gender impact are not entirely clear. It would seem from current studies that obesity (especially an upper body or abdominal pattern of distribution) and elevated serum lipids (especially triglycerides), combined with a low HDL value and the postmenopausal woman's lack of estrogen, help set the stage for impaired glucose tolerance in women.[61,62]

Dietary recommendations. The current standard of dietary guidelines for diabetes management of the American Diabetes Association and the American Dietetic Association, which generally follow guidelines of the American Heart Association's "prudent" diet, provide the present basis for individual care of diabetes. Some interesting initial data from recent NIDDM studies, however, document plasma glucose and lipid response to diets that vary from these current standards in the relative amount and type of dietary carbohydrate and fat. Studies have shown a persistent elevation of serum triglycerides, an independent heart disease risk factor for women, with the usual high-carbohydrate/low-fat ratio of the standard diet guides. Improvement in serum lipid levels has occurred with moderation of dietary fat to include more use of monounsaturated fat. For treatment of adults with NIDDM, it would appear that an adjustment of the nutrient ratios may achieve better control of serum glucose and lipids: (1) carbohydrate lowered from a high of 60% to 45%

to 50% of total kilocalories, mostly complex in form with little, if any, sucrose; (2) fat moderated from 30% to 35% to 40% of total kilocalories, with the small increase in monounsaturated fat; and (3) protein kilocalories remaining the same at 15% to 20%. Researchers and practitioners agree, however, that any general population guideline must always be applied with reasonable common sense to individuals.

Breast Cancer

Breast cancer is a significant health issue for women. At some time during their lives, one out of 10 American women will develop breast cancer, a rate that has not changed despite current advances in detection. Diagnosis of breast cancers at earlier stages is achieved through widespread screening. However, researchers agree that only prevention efforts will decrease cancer incidence and prolong survival because most women with breast cancer do not have a family history or any of the other known risk factors, which include fibrocystic disease, **nulliparity,** or first pregnancy after age 30. Thus, prevention strategies need to be applied to all women. There is an increasing consensus that obesity and the high-fat American diet are primary risk factors, and that weight reduction and maintenance on a low-fat, high-fiber diet provide a valuable and practical strategy for breast cancer prevention. Such long-term maintenance goals require planning for a lifetime of healthy lifestyle.

For some years, a vast body of **epidemiologic** evidence has supported this association of increased dietary fat and subsequent increase in incidence of breast cancer in populations migrating to the United States, but controlled studies to rule out other confounding factors from the analysis are needed. Current studies are examining nutritional, hormonal, and physiologic data in conjunction with dietary and lifestyle change that will clarify these effects for breast cancer prevention.

Osteoporosis

Bone growth and maintenance. The health problem of osteoporosis in women's later adult years has its roots in earlier growth, development, and maintenance of skeletal bone mass. Thus it provides an excellent example of the importance of the life cycle preventive approach of planning for a healthy lifestyle. Skeletal life cycle homeostasis is a sophisticated response to the alternating pattern of the three basic factors involved in building and maintaining bone mass: nutritional state, physical activity, and hormonal status.[53] There is also a strong genetic role in the development of bone mass in women by the age of about 25, independent of calcium and other nutrients, but dietary factors, physical activity, and hormonal factors constantly modulate the genetically predetermined quantity, size, and shape of bone.

Life cycle bone development. Childhood bone growth is gradual in concert with the child's overall body growth and development, but with puberty a rapid growth period begins. During the healthy adolescent growth spurt of young girls after menarche, under the added stimulus of estrogen secretion of the developing ovaries, large quantities of calcium, between 150 and 350 mg/day, are retained by the skeleton.[53] Calcium absorption efficiency is high during this 3 to 5-year period, but dietary calcium must also be sufficient to sustain this high retention rate. Peak adult bone mass is reached by about 35 years of age, although cortical bone tissue, the hard outer layer, may reach its full mass during the early adult decade of the 20s. The smaller **trabecular** bone tissue completes its development later, at age 35 or afterward. These trabecular bones, which are found in the ends of the long arm bones at the wrists, the vertebrae, and the proximal femurs at the hips, are most susceptible to fractures, beginning at the woman's menopause. Men may sustain fractures at these same sites, but their fracture rates are very much lower than female rates, largely

---

Nulliparity

(L *nullus,* none; *parere,* to bring forth, produce) Reproductive status of a woman who has never given birth to a viable child.

Epidemiology

(Gr *epidemios,* prevalent; *-ology,* study) Study of factor determining the frequency and distribution of diseases in population groups.

Trabecular

(L *trabes,* a little beam) Small bones in the ends of long bones at joints such as wrist, vertebrae, and hips.

due to the man's greater bone mass and shorter life span.[53] During the decade before menopause, which now occurs in most North American women in the United States and Canada in their early 50s, bone mass begins to decrease at a very low rate, and the level of calcium intake appears to have no major effect on the status of this bone mass. At the menopause, the rate of estrogen secretion drops sharply and gradually ceases, a physiologic event that has major impact on the turnover of bone in nearly all women, making them more vulnerable to osteoporosis. If such signs do develop, estrogen replacement therapy may be needed. Continuing an appropriate level of regular exercise during older adult years also helps to maintain the bone mass attained in the premenopause years.

Dietary recommendations. Since the current RDA for calcium for young adults aged 19 through 24 has been raised to 1200 mg/day, matching the already established allowance for adolescent girls, the increased demand for calcium to meet rapid bone growth during this period should be ample for skeletal bone mass needs. The calcium allowance for women from 25 to 50 is set at 800 mg/day, which is sufficient for active women. After the menopause, however, rather than the continued 800 mg/day, the calcium intake probably needs to be increased to 1000 mg/day.[53] Additional calcium supplementation cannot overcome the negative calcium balance that follows the loss of ovarian estrogens. Studies of premenopausal and postmenopausal women suggest that a threshold of calcium intake must be met at the different life cycle stages in order to enhance absorption and retention of calcium, independent of other factors. In short, women who practice good nutrition as a healthy lifetime habit, including not only adequate amounts of calcium but also other bone-building nutrients such as protein, phosphorus, and vitamin D, can develop optimal bone mass during adolescence and young adult years and maintain that bone mass at a higher level during their postmenopausal years. Planning for a healthy lifestyle is the young adult woman's health promotion, disease prevention approach to osteoporosis, as well as the other health issues of women discussed.

Summary

Adult health and wellness for both men and women depend upon a healthy lifestyle throughout young, middle, and older adulthood. Although genetic factors play a role in determining level of health, lifestyle choices are the major determinant of well-being and the onset and severity of chronic diseases that begin to appear in middle age. Components of a healthy lifestyle include a sound diet with attention to risk factors associated with excess fat, cholesterol, sodium, and body weight; regular physical exercise; stress management; smoking cessation; and avoidance of alcohol abuse. Addictive behaviors related to cigarette smoking, alcohol abuse, and eating disorders harm health and require special treatment programs. Chronic diseases of the cardiovascular system, hypertension, diabetes mellitus, and cancer have all been related to one or more of these lifestyle behaviors. A number of health programs have been developed at national and community levels to heighten public awareness and encourage appropriate behavior change. These public and professional activities include hospital-based community programs, health maintenance organization (HMO) programs, work-site wellness programs, health clubs, community screening programs, and health fairs.

Comparison of nutrient energy needs of men and women reflect their gender differences in body composition and size, as well as in physiologic function. Women encounter special gender-based health issues in their adult years, including weight concerns and health problems such as heart disease, diabetes, breast cancer, and osteoporosis.

Review Questions

1. Describe various approaches to health promotion. Which do you think has the greatest application to current health issues? Why?
2. List and discuss the five components of a healthy lifestyle. How does each influence risk of the major chronic diseases? Develop a healthy 1-day food plan for an adult of your choice, indicating daily activities that would influence the meal pattern or food selection.
3. Describe three addictive behaviors that harm health. In each case, outline an appropriate treatment program with special attention to nutritional needs.
4. Describe the National Cholesterol Education Program. List five agencies or sites in your community where this program could be implemented and give strategies for bringing about behavior change in each location.
5. How do women's nutritional needs differ from those of men? Account for each gender difference.
6. Relate women's nutrition to their gender difference in response to health issues such as obesity, heart disease, diabetes, and breast cancer.
7. Describe the gender differences in bone mass growth and development over the life cycle that create a greater risk for women of developing osteoporosis.

References

1. Mossey JM, Shapiro E: Self-rated health: a predictor of mortality among the elderly, *Am J Public Health* 72:800, 1982.
2. US Department of Health and Human Services: *Healthy people: the Surgeon General's report on health promotion and disease prevention,* Washington, DC, 1979, US Government Printing Office.
3. Saunders RP: What is health promotion, *Health Educ Q* 19:14, 1988.
4. Holli BB, Calabrese RJ: *Communication and education skills: the dietitian's guide,* ed 2, Philadelphia, 1991, Lea and Febiger.
5. Contento I, Murphy BM: Psycho-social factors differentiating people who reported making desirable changes in their diets from those who did not, *J Nutr Educ* 22:6, 1990.
6. Johnson RK et al: Medical nutrition therapy and health care reform: strategies of the American Dietetic Association, *Pers Applied Nutr* 2(1):3, 1994.
7. Committee on Diet and Health, Food and Nutrition Board: *Diet and health: implications for reducing chronic disease risk,* Washington, DC, 1989, National Academy Press.
8. US Department of Health and Human Services: *Second report of the expert panel on detection, evaluation, and treatment of high blood cholesterol in adults,* NIH Publication Number 93-3095, Washington, DC, 1993, US Government Printing Office.
9. Murphy SP et al: Demographic and economic factors associated with dietary quality for adults in the 1987-88 Nationwide Food Consumption Survey, *J Am Diet Assoc* 92(11):1352, 1992.
10. US Department of Health and Human Services: *Healthy people 2000: national health promotion and disease prevention objectives,* DHHS Publication Number (PHS) 91-50212, Washington, DC, 1991, US Government Printing Office.
11. Kristal AR et al: Long-term maintenance of a low-fat diet: durability of fat-related dietary habits in the Women's Health Trial, *J Am Diet Assoc* 92(5):553, 1992.
12. Salonen JT et al: High stored iron levels are associated with excess risk of myocardial infarction in eastern Finnish men, *Circulation* 86:803, 1992.
13. US Department of Health and Human Services: *The fifth report of the joint national committee on detection, evaluation, and treatment of high blood pressure,* NIH Publication Number 93-1088, Washington, DC, 1993, US Government Printing Office.
14. Paffenbarger RS et al: The association of changes in physical-activity level and other lifestyle characteristics with mortality among men, *N Engl J Med* 328:533, 1993.

15. Sandovik L et al: Physical fitness as a predictor of mortality among healthy, middle-aged Norwegian men, *N Engl J Med* 328:533, 1993.
16. US Department of Health and Human Services: *Reducing the health consequences of smoking, 25 years of progress: a report of the Surgeon General,* DHHS Publication Number (CDC) 89-8411, Washington, DC, 1989, US Government Printing Office.
17. Update: Study finds tobacco and poor diet to cause most deaths, *J Am Diet Assoc* 94(2):138, 1994.
18. US Department of Health and Human Services: *Health United States 1992 and healthy people 2000 review,* DHHS Publication Number (PHS) 93-1232, Washington, DC, 1993, US Government Printing Office.
19. Williamson DF et al: Smoking cessation and severity of weight gain in a national cohort, *N Engl J Med* 324, 739, 1991.
20. Pelican S et al: Nutrition services for alcohol/substance abuse clients: Indian Health Service's tribal survey, *J Am Diet Assoc* 94(8):835, 1994.
21. Speicher CE: *The right test: a physician's guide to laboratory medicine,* ed 2, Philadelphia, 1993, Saunders.
22. Watson RR et al: Identification of alcohol abuse and alcoholism with biological parameters, *Alcoholism: Clinical and Experimental Research* 10(4):364, 1986.
23. Shattuck DK: Mindfulness and metaphor in relapse prevention: an interview with G. Alan Marlatt, *J Am Diet Assoc* 94(8):846, 1994.
24. Beckley-Barrett LM, Mutch PB: Position of the American Dietetic Association: nutrition intervention in treatment and recovery from chemical dependency, *J Am Diet Assoc* 90(9): 1274, 1990.
25. Biery JR et al: Alcohol craving in rehabilitation: assessment of nutrition therapy, *J Am Diet Assoc* 91(4):463, 1991.
26. Lemberg R, ed: Controlling disorders with facts, advice, and resources, Phoenix, 1992, Phoenix Oryx Press.
27. Anderson AE, editor: *Males with eating disorders,* New York, 1990, Brunner/Mazel.
28. Irvin B, editor: *Disordered eating and diabetes, on the cutting edge: Diabetes Care and Education (DCE) practice group of the American Dietetic Association (ADA)* vol 15, No 6, Winter 1994.
29. American Psychiatry Association: *Diagnostic and statistical manual,* ed 4, Washington, DC, 1994, APA.
30. King NL: *Overview of eating disorders in diabetes management, on the cutting edge: diabetes care and education* 15(6):5, 1994.
31. Emerson EN, Stein DM: Anorexia nervosa: empirical basis for the restricting and bulimic subtypes, *J Nutr Educ* 25(6):329, 1993.
32. Reiff DW, Reiff KKL: Position of The American Dietetic Association: nutrition intervention in the treatment of anorexia nervosa, bulimia nervosa, and binge eating, *J Am Diet Assoc* 94(8):902, 1994.
33. Steinberg D: Antioxidant vitamins and coronary heart disease, *N Engl J Med* 328:1487, 1993.
34. Monsen E: Reversing heart disease through diet, exercise, and stress management: an interview with Dean Ornish, *J Am Diet Assoc* 91(2):162, 1991.
35. Siani A et al: Increasing the dietary potassium intake reduces the need for antihypertensive medication, *Ann Intern Med* 115:753, 1991.
36. Kucznarski RJ et al: Increasing prevalence of overweight among US adults, The National Health and Examination Surveys, 1960 to 1991, *JAMA* 272:205, 1994.
37. Simopoulos AP, Van Itallie TB: Body weight, health, and longevity, *Ann Intern Med* 100:285, 1984.
38. Launer LJ et al: Body mass index, weight change, and the risk of mobility disability in middle-aged and older women: The epidemiologic follow-up study of NHANES I, *JAMA* 271:1093, 1994.
39. Kushner RF: Body weight and mortality, *Nutr Rev* 51:127, 1993.

40. D'Eramo-Melkus MG, Hagen JA: Weight reduction interventions for persons with a chronic illness: findings and factors for consideration, *J Am Diet Assoc* 91(9):1093, 1991.

41. Council of Scientific Affairs, American Medical Association: Diet and cancer: where do matters stand? *Arch Intern Med* 153:5056, 1993.

42. Dwyer J: Dietary fiber and colorectal cancer risk, *Nutr Rev* 51(5):147, 1993.

43. Diabetes Care and Education, A Practice Group of the American Dietetic Association: Commentary and translation: 1994 nutrition recommendations for diabetes, *J Am Diet Assoc* 94(5):1994.

44. Johnson CL et al: Declining serum total cholesterol levels among US adults: The National Health and Nutrition Examination Surveys, *JAMA* 269:3002, 1993.

45. Croft JB et al: Community intervention and trends in dietary fat consumption among black and white adults, *J Am Diet Assoc* 94(11):1284, 1994.

46. Kerber BA, editor: *How employers are saving through wellness and fitness programs,* ed 2, Wall Township, NJ, 1994, American Business Publishing.

47. Blair SN et al: A public health intervention model for work-site health promotion, *JAMA* 255:921, 1986.

48. Baer JT: Improved plasma cholesterol levels in men after a nutrition education program at the worksite, *J Am Diet Assoc* 93(6):658, 1993.

49. Maiman LA et al: Public cholesterol screening in the previously diagnosed, misuse of resources or beneficial function, *Am J Prev Med* 10:20, 1994.

50. Holloway M: Trends in women's health: a global view, *Sci Am* 271(2):76, 1994.

51. Erikson E: *Childhood and society,* New York, 1963, Norton.

52. Food and Nutrition Board, National Research Council: *Recommended Dietary Allowances,* ed 10, Washington, DC, 1989, National Academy Press.

53. Anderson JJB: Dietary calcium and bone mass through the life cycle, *Nutr Today* 25(2):9, 1990.

54. US Department of Agriculture, US Department of Health and Human Services: *Nutrition and your health: dietary guidelines for Americans,* ed 3, Washington, DC, 1990, US Government Printing Office.

55. Guyton AC: *Textbook of medical physiology,* ed 8, Philadelphia, 1991, Saunders.

56. Godsland IF et al: The effects of different formulations of oral contraceptive agents on lipid and carbohydrate metabolism, *N Engl J Med* 323:1375, 1990.

57. Stunkard AJ et al: The body mass of twins who have been reared apart, *N Engl J Med* 322:1483, 1990.

58. Bouchard C et al: The response to long-term overfeeding in identical twins, *N Engl J Med* 322:1483, 1990.

59. Williamsson DF et al: The 10-year incidence of overweight and major weight gain in US adults, *Arch Intern Med* 150:665, 1990.

60. Van Dale D et al: Weight maintenance and resting metabolic rate 18-40 months after a diet/exercise treatment, *Ind J Obesity* 14:347, 1990.

61. Golay A et al: Effect of central obesity on regulation of carbohydrate metabolism in obese patients with varying degrees of glucose toleration, *J Clin Endocrinal Metab* 71:1299, 1990.

62. Haffer SM et al: Cardiovascular risk factors in confirmed prediabetic individuals, *JAMA* 263:2893, 1990.

Further Reading

Beckley-Barrett LM, Mutch PB: Position of The American Dietetic Association: nutrition intervention in treatment and recovery from chemical dependency, *J Am Diet Assoc* 90(9):1274, 1990.

Reiff DW, Reiff KKL: Position of the American Dietetic Association: nutrition intervention in the treatment of anorexia nervosa, bulimia nervosa, and binge eating, *J Am Diet Assoc* 94(8):902, 1994.

These two ADA position papers outline clearly the team role of registered dietitians with advanced training and clinical experience in the care of clients with addictive behaviors related to alcohol abuse and eating disorders. Two excellent examples of team care in complex medical-nutrition problems.

Burrows ER et al: Nutritional applications of a clinical low fat dietary intervention to public health change, *J Nutr Educ* 25:167, 1993.

This article describes a study to help women lower their dietary fat and offers practical suggestions for dietary education.

Cotugna N et al: Nutrition and cancer prevention knowledge, beliefs, attitudes, and practices: the 1987 National Health Review Survey, *J Am Diet Assoc* 92:963,1992.

This article presents data from a U.S. survey that addressed health-related dietary changes of the population and barriers that people encountered in trying to make those changes.

McNutt K: Improving the cost effectiveness of nutrition education, *Nutr Today* 27(6):38, 1992.

This article describes an approach for fact-gathering about sources and types of nutrition information in the media to find what consumers already know and what they need to learn.

Pelican S et al: Nutrition services for alcohol/substance abuse clients, *J Am Diet Assoc* 94(8):835, 1994.

This report of the U.S. Indian Health Service's tribal survey provides insight concerning nutritional services and needs related to alcohol/substance abuse and describes a number of useful training materials developed for staff training and client counseling, including nutrition education.

Robinson JI et al: Obesity, weight loss, and health, *J Am Diet Assoc* 93(4):445, 1993.

This article presents a sensitive overview of the causes and types of treatments for obesity. Emphasis is directed toward individual assessment and intervention.

Shattuck DK: Mindfulness and metaphor in relapse prevention: an interview with G. Alan Marlatt, *J Am Diet Assoc* 94(8):846, 1994.

In this JADA staff interview, Dr. Marlatt discusses his work as a professor of psychology and director of the Addictive Behaviors Research Center at the University of Washington, Seattle, and his views on addictive behaviors and their treatment.

US Department of Health and Human Services: *Report of the Expert Panel on Population Strategies for Blood Cholesterol Reduction*, NIH Publication Number 90-3046, Washington, DC, 1990, US Government Printing Office.

This publication presents a review of successful community-based programs and strategies for health education and cholesterol reduction.

4

Maternal Nutrition: The Course and Outcome of Pregnancy

Bonnie S. Worthington-Roberts

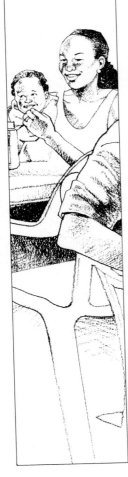

Basic Concepts

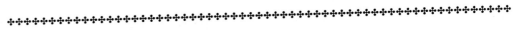

✔ *Data about nutritional influences on fetal growth guide sound maternal nutrition.*
✔ *The physiology of pregnancy determines answers to maternal nutritional issues.*
✔ *Specific nutritional deficiencies and excesses affect fetal development.*
✔ *Prenatal weight gain follows varying individual patterns.*
✔ *Unusual eating behaviors that occur during pregnancy require evaluation.*
✔ *Nonnutrient dietary components affect pregnancy outcome.*

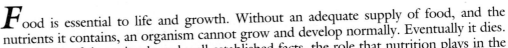

Food is essential to life and growth. Without an adequate supply of food, and the nutrients it contains, an organism cannot grow and develop normally. Eventually it dies.

In spite of these simple and well-established facts, the role that nutrition plays in the course and outcome of pregnancy has not always been recognized. In the controlled conditions of the laboratory, researchers have been able to demonstrate harmful effects of deficient diets on pregnant animals and their offspring in a number of species. However, when studies are made on free-living human populations, direct relationships between what a mother eats during the 9 months of gestation and the course and outcome of her pregnancy are not always evident. Consequently, the emphasis that nutrition has received in prenatal care has varied over the years.

Part of the problem is that the changes occurring during pregnancy, their influence on nutritional needs, and the effects of long-term nutritional status on reproductive performance are not fully understood. The application of nutrition principles to pregnancy has had to depend on progress in scientific knowledge about reproduction itself, and as in any science, one of the most important advances is simply learning to ask the right questions. The emphasis of research has changed as more has become known about nutrition, reproduction, and human growth. It is therefore easy to understand why different dietary recommendations for pregnant women have been made.

NUTRITION AND PREGNANCY: HISTORICAL DEVELOPMENT

Early Beliefs and Practices

During the nineteenth century much of what was known and recommended about diet during pregnancy was based on casual observation rather than controlled studies. Little information was available on the nutrient composition of foods or their biologic values. Dietary advice was influenced by belief in imitative magic: belief that the mother or child would acquire the attributes of the foods in the mother's diet. For example, pregnant women were sometimes forbidden to eat salty, acidic, or sour foods for fear the infant would be born with a "sour" disposition. The beliefs were often colored by the emotional and mystical aura surrounding the pregnant state. Eggs were sometimes restricted because of their association with the reproductive function. On the other hand, certain foods were encouraged for their presumed beneficial effects. Pregnant women were often advised to eat broths, warm milk, and ripe fruits to soothe the fetus and ease the birth process.

Problems in nineteenth century obstetric practice also influenced dietary recommendation. During the Industrial Revolution children in Europe had poor diets and worked long hours in dark factories. Rickets, which impairs normal bone formation during the growth years, was a common disorder. A contracted pelvis resulting from rickets was a major obstetric risk. Physicians did not have the modern means of delivering infants from these mothers. Death of both mother and child during childbirth was common.

Experience with his own patients in the 1880s led a German physician, Prochownick, to advocate a fluid-restricted, high-protein, low-carbohydrate diet for women with contracted pelvises to be followed for 6 weeks before birth. Women following this diet produced smaller infants and had easier deliveries. The diet may have had some justification in the 1880s, but it later gained in popularity and became a standard recommendation throughout pregnancy, even when the original rationale no longer applied. Remnants of the Prochownick diet, restricting fluid and carbohydrate, persist today.

There is very little specific information available about diet and pregnancy before the 1930s, other than reports on effects of food shortages during and after World War I. After the war there was much effort to relate food shortages to the size of the baby, but most of the evidence presented was inconclusive and even contradictory.

Reevaluation and Redirection

It was not until the mid-1960s that renewed interest in infant mortality and morbidity rates led to a reappraisal of the influence of diet on pregnancy. Once attention was redirected toward this problem, a number of significant steps were taken. The resulting progress has been rapid. First, two important events occurred in rapid succession.

The White House conference. The White House Conference on Food, Nutrition, and Health was held in Washington in December 1969. The immediate stimulus was the nationwide shock at the disclosures of widespread hunger and malnutrition in the United States. The determination to do something about it produced the Conference as the first organizational step. Many experts there, involved in the Panel on Pregnancy and Very Young Infants, were also involved with the soon-to-be-published National Research Council (NRC) report on maternal nutrition and the course of pregnancy. They saw the Conference as a priceless opportunity to address the applied issues of diet and pregnancy within the context of their needed health services.

Benchmark NRC report. The NRC report, *Maternal Nutrition and the Course of Pregnancy,*[1] was issued in 1970. It remains today the major source of research information on the role of nutrition in human reproduction. One of the principal findings of that report was the limited and fragmentary nature of studies on diet and pregnancy. The report singled out the need for long-term longitudinal studies on women and their families, a need which still remains.

FOLLOW-UP GUIDELINES AND PROGRAMS
Initial Guidelines for Practice

In 1973, two sets of guidelines appeared as a direct outgrowth of the stimulus given to nutrition services at the White House Conference: (1) the American Public Health Association [2] guidelines and standards issued primarily for public health workers as an aid to assessments and program planning; and (2) the NRC [3] guidelines for uses and limitations of supplementary food provided during pregnancy. Technical issues, practical problems, and political realities were explored, along with the inherent difficulties involved in multidisciplinary and multifactorial studies.

WIC Program

In 1978, the now well-known WIC program — Special Supplemental Food Program for Women, Infants, and Children[4] — was initiated under court order. The purpose of the WIC program was to provide food as an adjunct to health care during critical times of growth and development. Table 4-1 summarizes the main features of this important program. The WIC program has grown from a pilot program costing $40 million in 1973 to one costing over $1 billion in 1991. Many of the same problems addressed in the 1969 White House Conference are still being encountered in the WIC program today, leading to questions of what the program is accomplishing.

ACOG-ADA Guidelines

In 1981, the American College of Obstetricians and Gynecologists (ACOG) and the American Dietetic Association (ADA) issued a joint publication, *Guidelines for Assessment of Maternal Nutrition.*[5] This was indeed a milestone. The report produced the first national consensus on the relevant risk factors before and during pregnancy. This original listing has been updated by the more recent material in the NRC perinatal guide.

NRC Perinatal Guide

In 1981, the NRC produced the highly useful guide *Nutrition Services in Perinatal Care.*[6] This report was particularly timely because it was designed for use with the rapidly growing regional networks for maternal and perinatal services. It is most helpful because it addresses the nutritional issues of infant feeding and the increasingly important concerns about substance abuse — cigarettes, drugs, and alcohol.

TABLE 4-1 *The Special Supplemental Food Program for Women, Infants, and Children (WIC)*

1. Sponsored by the Food and Nutrition Service of the U.S. Department of Agriculture
2. Originally authorized in 1972
3. Target population: pregnant and postpartum women up to 6 months after delivery if not breastfeeding and up to 12 months if breastfeeding; infants; children up to 5 years of age
4. Eligibility criteria: nutritionally at risk and members of low-income families
5. Program administered by state health departments
6. Regulations require that WIC agencies offer nutrition education and that appropriate health services be available directly or by referral.

The Most Recent Landmark Document

The increasing visibility of maternal services in the United States motivated the National Academy of Sciences to appoint an expert committee with a mandate to evaluate data related to prenatal weight gain and nutrient supplements. The committee's final report entitled *Nutrition During Pregnancy: Weight Gain and Nutrient Supplements* was issued in July 1990.[7] Recommendations made in this report are cited throughout this chapter.

Continued Needs

There is increasing realization of the seamless web of variables that together influence the outcome of pregnancy. Within the constellation of income, health, education, family, and fertility, food and nutrition are just one part, but an important and modifiable one. As

---

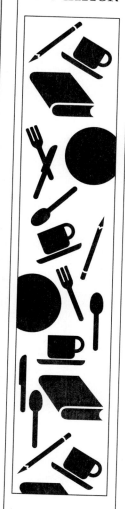

STRATEGIES FOR NUTRITION EDUCATION

WIC: *Providing Supplemental Food With Nutrition Education*

The Special Supplemental Food Program for Women, Infants, and Children (WIC) was established in 1972. Its goal is to improve the diets of pregnant and lactating mothers, and infants and children up to the age of 5 who because of low income or inadequate health care are at high risk. Although all WIC programs must provide foods from each major food group, there is some flexibility at the state and local level. Foods commonly included are:

- Milk: skim, lowfat, whole or buttermilk; infant formula; cheese
- Protein: eggs, peanut butter, dried peas, beans, or lentils; tuna fish
- Fruit/Vegetable: orange, grapefruit, pineapple, tomato, or apple (with added vitamin C) juices; carrots
- Cereal: iron-fortified infant cereal; others for children and mothers (a program may exclude sugar-coated cereals)

The amounts of food provided are intended to include 3 ½ servings from the milk group, 1 serving from the protein group, 2 servings of fruit or vegetable, and 1 to 2 servings of cereal per participant per day.

A major component of the WIC program is the distribution of foods representing all the major food groups; however, an equally important mission is providing food and nutrition education to participating mothers. WIC participants in Ohio considered the nutritionists and dietitians at the WIC clinic to be their major source of nutrition information and over half were interested in additional classes. Surprisingly, the employed mothers were more likely to attend WIC nutrition classes than the unemployed mothers. This points to the need for classes scheduled at other than usual office hours. Teenage mothers and homeless mothers may have a special need for food and nutrition classes. Possible topics for WIC educators are described below.

Food buying: making a shopping list and planning purchases; appropriate use of store specials; unit pricing; using the nutrition label in food selection

Food preparation: easy to prepare recipes using supplemental foods; healthy cooking methods; safe food handling practices

Infant/child feeding: appropriate meal patterns (quantity and selection of food to be provided); nutritious snacks, nutrient dense food choices; meal time behavior; parenting issues (food as a reward, forcing food intake); prevention of baby bottle tooth decay; prevention of inappropriate weight gain

Concerns of homeless mothers: food storage if no refrigeration is available; meal preparation with limited (a hotplate, electric frying pan) or no cooking equipment

Hamilton CV, Schiller MR, Boyne L: Nutrition attitudes, practices, and views of selected Ohio WIC participants, *J Am Diet Assoc* 94:899, 1994.

Siegler MB, Franklin GK, Lynch MA: Lesson plans for WIC homeless, *J Nutr Educ* 25:294A, 1993.

❖

COMPONENTS OF PRECONCEPTION CARE AS PART OF PRIMARY CARE SERVICES

Risk assessment
Individual and social conditions (age, diet, education, housing, and economic status)
Adverse health behaviors (tobacco, alcohol, and illicit drug abuse)
Medical conditions (immune status, medications, genetic illness, illnesses including infection, and prior obstetric history)
Psychological conditions (personal and family readiness for pregnancy, stress, anxiety, and depression)
Environmental conditions (workplace hazards, toxic chemicals, and radiation contamination)
Barriers to family planning, prenatal care, and primary health care

Health promotion
Promotion of behaviors (proper nutrition, avoidance of smoking, alcohol, teratogens, and practice of "safe sex")
Counseling about the availability of social, financial, and vocational assistance programs
Advice of family planning, pregnancy spacing, and contraception
Counseling about the importance of early registration and compliance with prenatal care, including high-risk programs if warranted
Identification of barriers to care and assistance in overcoming them
Arrangements for ongoing care

Interventions
Treatment of medical conditions, including changes in medications, if appropriate, and referral to high-risk pregnancy programs
Referral for treatment of adverse health behaviors (tobacco, alcohol, and illicit drug abuse)
Rubella and hepatitis immunization
Reduction of psychosocial risks that may involve counseling or referral to home health agencies, community mental health centers, safe shelters, enrollment in medical assistance, and assistance with housing
Nutrition counseling, supplementation or referral to improve adequacy of diet
Home visit to further assess and intervene in the home environment
Provision of family planning services

From Jack B, Culpepper L: Preconception care: risk reduction and health promotion, *JAMA* 264:1147, 1990.

one observer stated, "Special efforts to improve prenatal, child, and maternal health showed clear evidence that the services did make a difference. . . . No one has yet teased out the relative effects of different variables."[8] This is the clearest statement of the nature of the problems that need to be addressed in the years ahead.

A NEW THRUST—PRECONCEPTION CARE

A major movement is underway to motivate potential new parents to participate in advanced planning of their pregnancies. This effort, now referred to as "preconception care," allows for preparation of the best possible prenatal environment for the conceptus (see the box above). The components of preconception care include risk assessment, health promotion, and interventions to reduce risk. Risks identifiable prior to conception may involve medical, social, psychological, or lifestyle conditions. Risk assessment provides opportunity to identify social factors related to poor obstetric outcome, including inadequate housing, low income, having less than a high school education, and problems

CASE STUDY

Preconceptional Counseling

A professional woman 35 years of age visits her health care provider for advice. She and her husband are planning a pregnancy and she wishes to approach this project systematically. An interview and physical examination reveals that she:
- Has been using oral contraceptives for 10 years
- Smokes
- Is 10 pounds underweight
- Enjoys wine with her meals
- Has a family history of diabetes
- Has a typical 60-hour work week
- Intends to continue her career during and after pregnancy

Analysis
1. Outline appropriate recommendations for the preconception period.
2. Define those issues that require discussion about the pregnancy period itself.
3. Summarize appropriate anticipatory guidance for the postpartum period.

related to being a single parent. Once risks are known, some women may benefit from counseling and referral to social, mental health, and substance abuse treatment programs or vocational training.

Preconception assessment of nutritional status should identify those individuals who are underweight or overweight; conditions such as bulimia, anorexia, pica, or hypervitaminosis; and special dietary habits such as vegetarianism. Nutrition counseling may prove useful; this may include information about dietary control of chronic diseases like diabetes mellitus. The same applies to phenylketonuria; strict control of maternal serum phenylalanine levels is essential to optimizing chances for normal development of the offspring.

It is hoped that eventually preconception care will be shown to yield such positive results that insurance coverage will routinely be provided and clinicians will urge their clients of reproductive age to prepare for conception in every possible way. This preparation should include a formal preconception evaluation to determine (1) if reproduction is associated with high risk that is not modifiable and thus suggestive that serious consideration should be given to avoiding pregnancy and (2) if modifiable risks exist, if they are identified and addressed, can it be expected that there will be a marked increase in the likelihood of good pregnancy outcome.

PHYSIOLOGY OF PREGNANCY

Normal pregnancy is accompanied by anatomic and physiologic changes that affect almost every function in the body. Many of these changes are apparent in the very early weeks. This indicates that they are not merely a response to the physiologic stress imposed by the fetus but are an integral part of the maternal-fetal system, which creates the most favorable environment possible for the developing child. The changes are necessary to regulate maternal metabolism, promote fetal growth, and prepare the mother for labor, birth, and lactation.

The changes that occur in pregnancy are too complex to be given full treatment here, but a look at some changes that have effects on general metabolism will lay the foundation for interpreting nutritional requirements and dietary allowances (see the box below).

Blood Volume and Composition

Plasma is the fluid component of blood, whereas serum is the part of plasma that remains after its coagulation factors have been removed. Total plasma volume in a non-pregnant woman averages 2600 ml. Near the end of the first trimester of pregnancy,

ONE STEP FURTHER

Key Physiologic Changes During Pregnancy and Nutritional Implications

Cardiovascular changes
Increased cardiac output — a function of increased stroke volume and heart rate
Increased blood volume
Changes in blood flow
Decreases in arterial pressure (first and second trimesters)

Changes in blood volume
Progressive plasma volume expansion occurs from weeks 10 to 12 through weeks 33 to 35
Weekly increments are maximal during mid-gestation
Expansion in red cell mass is proportionally smaller than that in plasma, resulting in the so-called physiologic anemia of pregnancy

Blood pressure during pregnancy
Blood pressure tone decreases and peripheral vascular resistance falls. Arterial pressure falls during the first trimester; it is used as the baseline to evaluate pregnancy-induced hypertension in the third trimester.
Changes occur in regional blood flow. For example, uterine blood flow increases from 15 to 20 ml/min in nonpregnant to 500 to 600 ml/min near term.

Adjustments in the respiratory system
The enlarging uterus results in increased intraabdominal pressure and elevation of the diaphragm by as much as 4 cm. As a result thoracic breathing replaces intraabdominal breathing.
Resting ventilation increases by about 48%; this exceeds increments in either oxygen consumption (21%) or metabolic rate (14%) and expanded title volume.
Since respiratory rate remains constant throughout gestation, there is more efficient exchange of lung gases in the alveoli. The oxygen-carrying capacity of the blood is increased accordingly.

Changes in renal functions
In normal pregnancy, changes include ureteral dilation, slowed velocity of urine, increased susceptibility to urinary tract infections, and uterine compression of the ureters as they go over the pelvic brim.
Renal function is altered considerably. Renal blood flow and glomerular filtration rate are increased to facilitate
the clearance of waste products resulting from fetal and maternal metabolism.
The increase in glomerular filtration rate presents the tubules with greater quantities of nutrients than they can reabsorb, sometimes resulting in proteinuria and glycosuria in healthy women.

Changes in gastrointestinal function
Due to the influence of hormonal changes during pregnancy, it is normal to observe adaptations such as taste changes, heartburn, nausea and vomiting, and constipation.

plasma volume begins to increase, and by 34 weeks it is about 50% greater than it was at conception.

There is considerable variation from these averages. Women who have small volumes to begin with ususally have a greater increase, as do **multigravidae** and mothers with multiple births.

Researchers have shown that the increase in plasma volume is correlated with obstetric performance. They found that women who have a small increase when compared with the average are more likely to have stillbirths, abortions, and **low-birth-weight** babies. Clearly the restriction of a normal expansion of plasma volume is undesirable in pregnancy.

If the availability of nutrients or the synthesis of normal blood constituents does not keep pace with the expansion of plasma volume, their concentrations per 100 ml of blood will decrease, even though the total amount may rise. This is apparently what happens with red blood cells, serum proteins, minerals, and water-soluble vitamins.

Red cell production is stimulated during pregnancy so that their numbers gradually rise, but the increase is not as large as the expansion of plasma volume (Fig. 4-1). The **hematocrit**, which is normally around 35% in women, may be as low as 29% to 31% during pregnancy. The amount of hemoglobin in each red blood cell does not change, but because there are fewer red blood cells per 100 ml of blood, hemodilution occurs. Nonpregnant **hemoglobin** values of 13 to 14 g per 100 ml can drop as low as 10 or 11 g/100 ml in the early months. In a nonpregnant woman this level of hemoglobin would indicate anemia, but in pregnancy the red blood cells are **normochromic** and **normocytic.**

Serum levels of the major nutrients typical for pregnant and nonpregnant women are compared in Table 4-2. The values for pregnant women must be interpreted with caution. Investigators have obtained different values depending on the laboratory methods used. Moreover, levels of certain nutrients can be influenced by a number of maternal factors such as age, parity, smoking, and the use of various medications before or during pregnancy. Even the sex of the fetus can influence the mother's blood levels of some nutrients. The levels will also fluctuate at different times during **gestation.**

Multigravida
(L *multus,* many; *gravida,* pregnant) A woman who has had two or more pregnancies.

Low birth weight
Birth weight less than 2500 g (5.4 lb). Very low birth weight: birth weight less than 1500 g (3.3 lb).

Hematocrit (HCT)
(Gr *haima,* blood; *krinein,* to separate) The volume percentage of red blood cells (RBCs) in whole blood; normally about 35% in women. Shows the ratio of RBC volume to total blood volume.

Hemoglobin
(Gr *haima,* blood; L *globus,* a ball) Oxygen-carrying pigment in red blood cells; a conjugated protein containing four heme groups combined with iron and four long globin polypeptide chains; formed by the developing RBC in bone marrow.

Normochromic
Normal red blood cell color.

Normocytic
Normal red blood cell size.

Gestation
(L *gestare,* to bear) Intrauterine fetal growth period (40 weeks) from conception to birth.

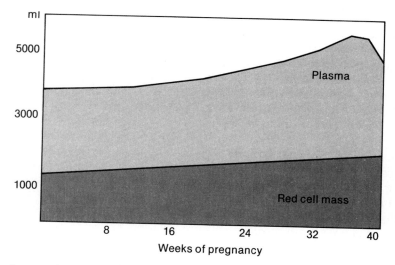

FIG. 4-1 Increase in plasma volume and red cell mass during the course of human pregnancy.
From Worthington-Roberts BS, Williams SR: *Nutrition in pregnancy and lactation,* ed 5, St. Louis, 1993 Mosby.

TABLE 4-2   *Serum Nutrient Levels in Pregnant and Nonpregnant Women*

Nutrient	Normal Nonpregnancy Range	Values in Pregnancy
Total protein	6.5-8.5 g/100 ml	6.0-8.0
Albumin	3.5-5.0 g/100 ml	3.0-4.5
Glucose	<110 mg/100 ml	<120
Cholesterol	120-190 mg/100 ml	200-325
Vitamin A	20-60 µg/100 ml	20-60
Carotene	50-300 µg/100 ml	80-325
Ascorbic acid	0.2-2.0 mg/100 ml	0.2-1.5
Folic acid	5-21 ng/100 ml	3.15
Calcium	4.6-5.5 mEq/L	4.2-5.2
Iron/iron-binding capacity	>50/250-400 µg/100 ml	>40/300-450

Modified from Aubry RH, Roberts A, Cuenca V, *Clin Perinatol* 2:207, 1975.

The Cardiovascular System

Extensive anatomic and physiologic changes occur in the cardiovascular system during the course of pregnancy. These adaptations serve to protect the woman's normal physiologic functioning to meet the metabolic demands pregnancy imposes on her body, and to provide for fetal development and growth needs.

The slight cardiac **hypertrophy** or dilation is probably secondary to the increased blood volume and cardiac output. As the diaphargm is displaced upward, the heart is elevated upward and to the left. The degree of shift depends on the duration of pregnancy and the size and position of the uterus.

During the first half of pregnancy, there is a decrease in both systolic and diastolic pressure of 5 to 10 mm Hg. The decrease in blood pressure is probably the result of peripheral **vasodilation** from the hormonal changes during pregnancy. During the third trimester, maternal blood pressure should return to the values obtained during the first trimester (Fig. 4-2).

Cardiac output increases from 30% to 50% by week 32 of pregnancy; it declines to about a 20% increase at week 40. The elevated cardiac output is largely a result of increased stroke volume and is in response to increased demands for oxygen (normal value is 5 to 5.5 L/min). The cardiac output decreases with the woman in the supine position and increases with any exertion such as labor and delivery. The circulation time decreases slightly by week 32. It returns to near normal near term.

Respiration

Respiration adaptations occur during pregnancy to provide for both maternal and fetal needs. Maternal oxygen requirements increase in response to the acceleration in metabolic rate and the need to add to the tissue mass in the uterus and breasts. The fetus requires oxygen and a way to eliminate carbon dioxide.

As mentioned previously, the level of the diaphragm is displaced by as much as 4 cm during pregnancy. With advancing pregnancy thoracic breathing replaces abdominal breathing and descent of the diaphragm with respiration becomes less possible.

The pregnant woman breathes deeper (greater **tidal volume,** the amount of gases exchanged with each breath) but increases her respiratory rate only slightly (about two breaths per minute). There is a more efficient exchange of lung gases in the **alveoli;** the oxygen-carrying capacity of the blood is increased accordingly.

Hypertrophy

(Gr *hyper,* above; *trophe,* nutrition) Enlargement of an organ or part due to the process of increasing cell size.

Vasodilation

(L *vas,* vessel; *dilatare,* to spread out) Expansion or stretching of a blood vessel.

Tidal volume

The amount of gases passing into and out of the lungs in each respiratory cycle.

Alveoli

(L *alveus,* hollow) Small sac-like formations; thin-walled chambers in the lungs surrounded by networks of capillaries through whose walls exchange of carbon dioxide and oxygen takes place.

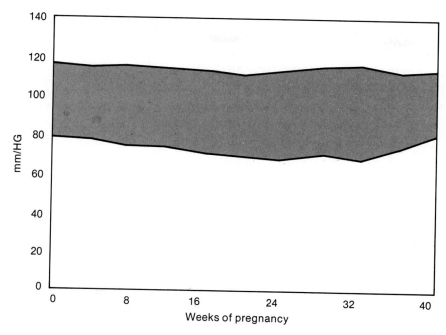

FIG. 4-2   Change in blood pressure during the course of human pregnancy.
From Worthington-Roberts BS, Williams SR: *Nutrition in pregnancy and lactation,* ed 5, St. Louis, 1993 Mosby.

Renal Function

In normal pregnancy, renal function is altered considerably. The woman's kidneys must manage the increased metabolic and circulatory demands of the maternal body as well as excretion of fetal waste products. Changes in renal function are caused by pregnancy hormones, an increase in blood volume, the woman's posture, and nutritional intake.

To facilitate the clearance of creatinine, urea, and other waste products of fetal and maternal metabolism, blood flow through the kidneys and the glomerular filtration rate are increased during pregnancy. The change in glomerular filtration rate is partially caused by the lower osmotic pressure, which results from the fall in serum albumin. This is one adaptation that appears to be purely mechanical, since no effects of hormones on this aspect of kidney function have been shown. However, there are consequences for nutrition.

Normally most of the glucose, amino acids, and water-soluble vitamins that are filtered by the nephrons are reabsorbed in the tubules to preserve the body's balance. However, in pregnancy substantial quantities of these nutrients appear in the urine. The most satisfactory explanation at present is that the higher glomerular filtration rate offers the tubules greater quantities of nutrients than they can feasibly reabsorb. Because the change in filtration rate is largely mechanical, there may not be an accompanying mechanism by which the tubules can readjust.

Gastrointestinal Function

The functioning of the gastrointestinal system undergoes a number of interesting changes during the course of pregnancy. The appetite increases, nausea and vomiting may occur, motility is diminished, intestinal secretion is reduced, sense of taste is altered, and absorption of nutrients is enhanced.

Peristalsis
　(Gr *peri*, around; stalsis, contraction) A wave-like progression of alternate contraction and relaxation of the muscle fibers of the gastrointestinal tract.

Hemorrhoids
　(Gr *haima*, blood; *rhoia*, to flow) Enlarged veins in the mucous membranes inside or outside of the rectum; causes pain, itching, discomfort, and bleeding.

Flatulence
　(L *flatus*, a blowing) Excessive formation and expulsion of gases in the gastrointestinal tract.

Increased progesterone production causes decreased tone and motility of the smooth muscles of the gastrointestinal tract. This leads to esophageal regurgitation, decreased emptying of the stomach, and reverse **peristalsis.** As a result, the pregnant woman may experience heartburn. The decreased smooth muscle tone also results in an increase in water absorption from the colon, and constipation may result. In addition, constipation is secondary to hypoperistalsis, unusual food choices, lack of fluids, abdominal pressure by the pregnant uterus, and displacement of intestines with some compression. **Hemorrhoids** may be everted or may bleed during straining at stool.

Decreased emptying time of the gallbladder is typical. This feature, together with slight hypercholesterolemia from increased progesterone levels, may account for the frequent development of gallstones during pregnancy.

Intraabdominal alterations that can cause discomfort include pelvic heaviness or pressure, **flatulence,** distention and bowel cramping, and uterine contractions. In addition to displacement of intestines, pressure from the expanding uterus increases venous pressure in the pelvic organs. Although most abdominal discomfort is a consequence of normal maternal alterations, occasional bowel obstruction or an inflammatory process may be present.

Insofar as taste is concerned, a recent study[9] examined the ability of the pregnant woman to discriminate among different concentrations of salt and sucrose solutions. Results of tests with salt solutions showed that pregnant women were significantly less able to identify concentration differences correctly and preferred significantly stronger salt solutions than did nonpregnant women. The researchers suggest that these observations may reflect a physiologic mechanism for increasing salt intake during pregnancy.

Hormones

The pregnant woman secretes more than 30 different hormones throughout gestation. Some, like those just mentioned, are only present in pregnancy, whereas others that are normally present have altered rates of secretion that are modified by the pregnant state.

Most hormones are proteins or steroids that are synthesized from precursors such as amino acids and cholesterol in endocrine glands throughout the body. Their production is influenced by the mother's general health and nutritional status. Under normal circumstances they are controlling factors in a complex feedback system that maintains homeostatic between cellular and extracellular constituents and metabolism. During pregnancy many of these homeostatic mechanisms are "reset" so that changes occur in the retention, utilization, and excretion of nutrients. Some of the hormones that exert important effects on nutrient metabolism are summarized in Table 4-3. Only those that have more general implications for nutritional management are singled out for discussion here.

Progesterone and estrogen are two hormones that have major effects on maternal physiology during pregnancy. The chief action of progesterone is to cause a relaxation of the smooth muscles of the uterus so that it can expand as the fetus grows, but it also has a relaxing effect on other smooth muscles in the body. Relaxation of the muscles of the gastrointestinal tract reduces motility in the gut, allowing more time for the nutrients to be absorbed. The slower movement is also a cause of the constipation commonly experienced by pregnant women. General metabolic effects of progesterone are to induce maternal fat deposition, reduce alveolar and arterial P_{CO_2} (partial pressure or tension of the gas carbon dioxide, facilitating exchange of lung gases in respiration and ensuring buffer capacity), and increase renal sodium excretion.

The secretion of estrogen is lower than that of progesterone during the early months of pregnancy, but it rises sharply near term. Its role is to promote the growth and control the function of the uterus, but it too has generalized effects on nutrition. One effect that

TABLE 4-3   *Hormonal Effects on Nutrient Metabolism in Pregnancy*

Hormone	Primary Source of Secretion	Principal Effects
Progesterone	Placenta	Reduces gastric motility; favors maternal fat deposition; increases sodium excretion; reduces alveolar and arterial P_{CO_2}; interferes with folic acid metabolism
Estrogen	Placenta	Reduces serum proteins; increases hydroscopic properties of connective tissue; affects thyroid function; interferes with folic acid metabolism
Human placental lactogen (HPL)	Placenta	Elevates blood glucose from breakdown of glycogen
Human chorionic thyrotropin (HCT)	Placenta	Stimulates production of thyroid hormones
Human growth hormone (HGH)	Anterior pituitary	Elevates blood glucose; stimulates growth of long bones; promotes nitrogen retention
Thyroid-stimulating hormone (TSH)	Anterior pituitary	Stimulates secretion of thyroxine; increases uptake of iodine by thyroid gland
Thyroxine	Thyroid	Regulates rate of cellular oxidation (basal metabolism)
Parathyroid hormone (PTH)	Parathyroid	Promotes calcium resorption from bone; increases calcium absorption; promotes urinary excretion of phosphate
Calcitonin (CT)	Thyroid	Inhibits calcium resorption from bone
Insulin	Beta cells of pancreas	Reduces blood glucose levels to promote energy production and synthesis of fat
Glucagon	Alpha cells of pancreas	Elevates blood glucose levels from glycogen breakdown
Aldosterone	Adrenal cortex	Promotes sodium retention and potassium excretion
Cortisone	Adrenal cortex	Elevates blood glucose from protein breakdown
Renin-angiotensin	Kidneys	Stimulates aldosterone secretion; promotes sodium and water retention; increases thirst

From Worthington-Roberts BS, Williams SR: *Nutrition in pregnancy and lactation,* ed 5, St Louis, 1993, Mosby.

has caused some difficulties for clinicians is the alteration of the structure of mucopolysaccharides in connective tissue. This alteration is beneficial because it makes the tissue more flexible and therefore assists in dilating the uterus at birth, but it also increases the affinity of connective tissue to water. This **hydroscopic** effect of estrogen and the sodium-losing effect of progesterone produce a confusing clinical picture of the pregnant woman's fluid and electrolyte balance. Because of estrogen, many pregnant women complain of excess

Hydroscopic
(Gr *hydro,* water; *skopein,* to measure or examine) Possessing tendency to take up and hold water readily.

Edema
(Gr *oidema*, swelling)
Accumulation of fluid in
the intercellular tissue
spaces of the body.

Preeclampsia
(L *prae*, before; *ek-lampein*, to shine forth)
Condition in late
pregnancy in which hypertension and edema
occur, with or without proteinuria.

Juxtaglomerular apparatus
(L *juxta*, near; *glomus*, ball) Complex of special
cells located near or
adjoining a nephron at
the head of a glomerulus of the kidney, responsible for sensing
the level of sodium
in the blood.

fluid retention in the skin. Their faces and fingers become puffy, and there are other indications of generalized **edema.** In addition, changes in cardiovascular dynamics cause extracellular fluid to accumulate in the feet and legs.

Since excess fluid retention is one of the hallmarks of **preeclampsia,** some clinicians view these changes with alarm, and may initiate rather rigorous treatment with diuretics and a sodium-restricted diet to promote water loss. The evidence, however, weighs strongly against this practice. It is now apparent that while the incidence of generalized and peripheral ankle edema is high, it is not associated with an increase in perinatal mortality when the two other symptoms of preeclampsia—hypertension and proteinuria—are absent. In fact, women with mild edema have slightly larger babies and a lower rate of premature births.

The propensity of women to lose sodium from the action of progesterone is compensated for by an increased secretion of aldosterone from the adrenal glands and renin from the **juxtaglomerular apparatus** of the kidneys. If sodium restriction is imposed, this renin-aldosterone system must work harder to maintain normal sodium concentrations in the body. Pushed beyond the stress naturally induced by pregnancy, the system could become exhausted so that, in the long run, less aldosterone and renin are produced. The sodium and water depletion that would result is more dangerous than the mild degree of edema that the treatment is supposed to prevent. This effect has been demonstrated in pregnant rats that are placed on sodium-restricted diets that would be equivalent to 1 g/day of sodium or "no added salt" diet in humans.

Although hormonal effects on fluid and electrolyte balance need more research, the mechanisms that are understood to date suggest that a mild degree of edema is physiologic in pregnancy and that the measures commonly used to prevent it impose an unnecessary risk.

Metabolic Adjustments

The basal metabolic rate (BMR) usually rises by the fourth month of gestation, although small increments may occur before that time. It is normally increased by 15% to 20% by term. The BMR returns to nonpregnant levels by 5 or 6 days postpartum. The elevation in BMR reflects increased oxygen demands of the uterine-placental fetal unit as well as oxygen consumption from increased maternal cardiac work. Peripheral vasodilation assists in the release of the excess heat production, though some women may continue to experience heat intolerance. Lassitude and fatigability after only slight exertion are described by many women in early pregnancy. These feelings may persist along with a greater need for sleep.

A complex series of adjustments in carbohydrate, protein, and fat metabolism occur during gestation to ensure that the fetus receives a continuous supply of fuel when the needs are maximal in late pregnancy. These adjustments are induced by changes in the endocrine milieu and by development of new endocrine tissue, the placenta.

Approximately 50% to 70% of the kilocalories required daily by the fetus in the third trimester (43 kcal/kg/day) is derived from glucose; about 20% of the kilocalories are derived from amino acids, and the remainder from fat. When maternal blood glucose levels fall, the rate of glucose transfer to the fetus declines and fatty acids may become a more dominant fuel source. The net effect of maternal fuel adaptations is to increase the use of fat as a fuel source by the mother to conserve glucose for the fetus. During the second trimester, the mother prepares for the anticipated fetal glucose demand by storing fat. Then in the third trimester, when the fetal glucose demand causes maternal plasma glucose levels to fall, **lipolysis** increases in the maternal compartment.

During a brief fast, such as overnight, maternal plasma glucose concentrations in pregnant women fall significantly below that of nonpregnant women because of continual

Lipolysis
(Gr *lipus*, fat; *lysis*, dissolution) The breakdown of fat.

placental uptake of glucose and impaired hepatic gluconeogenesis. The reduced capacity for gluconeogenesis is related in part to the reduced availability of alanine; the latter is the result of increased placental alanine uptake and restrained maternal muscle breakdown. Lipolysis is enhanced and mild ketosis may occur. In the postprandial period, maternal glucose uptake is lower than in nonpregnant women, despite increased plasma insulin concentrations. More of the glucose removed by the liver is converted to triglycerides; these are stored in maternal adipose tissue to be available for later fasting periods.

Overall, the major adjustment in energy utilization during pregnancy is a shift in the fuel sources. Fat becomes the major maternal fuel whereas glucose is the major fetal fuel. Since the size of the maternal tissue is considerably greater than the size of the fetal mass, lipolysis dominates, causing the respiratory quotient to fall in fasting women. Pregnant women gain weight readily without appreciable changes in energy intake, because water normally comprises about 65% of the weight gain, not because energy is utilized more efficiently. However, there is still some question about the efficiency of energy utilization, especially in the pregnant woman exposed to severe food deprivation.

Role of the Placenta

The **placenta** is not a passive barrier between the mother and the fetus. Rather, it plays an active role in reproduction. The placenta is the principal site of production for several important hormones that regulate maternal growth and development. For the fetus it is the only way that nutrients, oxygen, and waste products can be exchanged.

Structure and development. Evolving from a tiny mass of cells in the first weeks of pregnancy, the placenta becomes a complex network of tissue and blood vessels weighing about 1.4 lb (650 g) at term. The vital role it plays as a link between mother and child is represented by the two principal parts of the placenta—one uterine and the other fetal.

On the maternal side the placenta is part of the uterine mucosa. When the tiny **blastocyst** implants itself in the uterus 6 to 7 days after fertilization of the **ovum,** the uterine tissue and blood vessels break down to form small spaces called **lacunae** that fill with maternal blood. These spaces are eventually bounded on the maternal side by the decidua or basal plate. Blood begins to circulate in the spaces at about 12 days gestation.

Meanwhile the **trophoblast** grows and sends out rootlike villi into the pools of maternal blood. The villi contain capillaries, which will exchange nutrients and metabolic waste products between the mother and the fetus. In the early weeks of pregnancy the villi are thick columns of cells, but as they subdivide throughout gestation the villi become thinner and produce numerous branches. Some branches become anchored in the maternal tissue, and others remain free or floating in the intravillous spaces. The multiple villus branches provide a large surface membrane area for efficient exchange of nutrients and metabolic waste products between mother and fetus (Fig. 4-3). Even though uterine and embryonic tissues are intermingled, the blood of the mother and the embryo never mix because they are always separated by the placental membrane (Fig. 4-4).

Mechanisms of nutrient transfer. The efficiency of placental nutrient transfer is a determinant of fetal well-being. Reduced surface area of the villi, insufficient vascularization, or changes in the hydrostatic pressure in the intervillous space can limit the supply of nutrients available to the fetus and inhibit normal growth.

Nutrient transfer in the placenta is a complex process. It employs all the mechanisms used for the absorption of nutrients from the gastrointestinal tract: simple diffusion, facilitated diffusion, active transport, and **pinocytosis** (Table 4-4). The difference, however, is that in the placenta two completely separate blood supplies are maintained. The maternal circulation remains in the intervillous space. The fetal capillaries are separated from the maternal blood by two layers of cells. Their thickness is approximately 5.5 μm (Fig. 4-4).

Although the same nutrient may be simultaneously transferred by more than one

Placenta
(L *placentas*, a flat cake) Characteristic organ of mammals during pregnancy joining mother and offspring, providing supportive nourishment and endocrine secretions for embryonic-fetal development and growth.

Blastocyst
(Gr *blastos*, germ; *kystis*, sac, bladder) A stage in the development of the embryo in which the cells are arranged in a single layer to form a hollow sphere.

Ovum
(L *ovum*, egg) The female reproductive cell (egg) that develops into a new organism.

Lacunae
(L *lacuna*, small pit or hollow cavity) Blood spaces of the placenta in which the fetal villi are found.

Trophoblast
(Gr *trophe*, nutrition; *blastos*, germ) Extraembryonic ectodermal tissue on the surface of the cleaving, fertilized ovum, which is responsible for contact with the maternal circulation and supply of nutrients to the embryo.

Pinocytosis
(Gr *pinein*, to drink; *kytos*, cell) Uptake of fluid nutrient material by a living cell by means of incupping and invagination of the cell membrane, which closes off, forming free cell vacuoles.

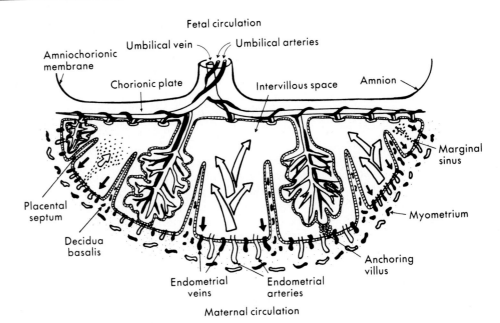

FIG. 4-3 Diagrammatic representation of a section through a mature placenta showing the relationship of the fetal placenta (villous chorion) to the maternal placenta (decidua basalis), fetal placental circulation, and maternal placental circulation. Maternal blood is forced into the intervillous space, and exchanges occur with the fetal blood as the maternal blood flows around the villi. Incoming arterial blood pushes venous blood into the endometrial veins, which are scattered over the surface of the maternal placenta. Umbilical arteries carry deoxygenated fetal blood to the placenta, and the umbilical vein carries oxygenated blood to the fetus.

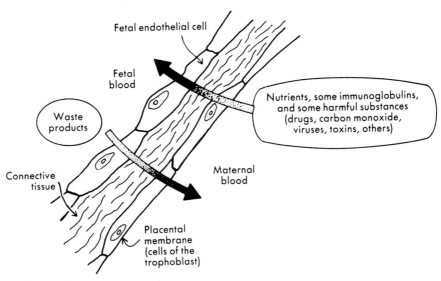

FIG. 4-4 Nutrients, waste products, and other transportable compounds must cross two layers of cells in the process of movement through the placenta.

TABLE 4-4   *Placental Transport Mechanisms and Materials Transported by Each Mechanism*

Transport Mechanism	Substance Transported
Passive diffusion	Oxygen
	Carbon dioxide
	Fatty acids
	Steroids
	Nucleosides
	Electrolytes
	Fat-soluble vitamins
Facilitated diffusion	Most monosaccharides
Active transport	Amino acids
	Some cations (calcium, iron)
	Iodine
	Phosphate
	Water-soluble vitamins*
Solvent drag†	Electrolytes

*At very high concentrations vitamin C has been shown to cross the placenta via diffusion.
†Movement of ions with water as it flows back and forth across the membrane.

mechanism, the major means of transport can be estimated by comparing nutrient concentrations in maternal and cord blood. If the concentrations are equal, the transfer has most likely occurred by simple or facilitated diffusion. Simple diffusion is a passive process in which nutrients move from high concentrations in the maternal blood to lower concentrations in fetal capillaries until equilibrium is reached. Facilitated diffusion differs from simple diffusion in that the rate of transfer is faster than would be expected. The mechanism of facilitated diffusion is not established, but it is thought that a carrier in the membrane is employed. Active transport requires both a carrier protein and metabolic energy to move a nutrient against an electrochemical gradient.

Most proteins do not cross the placenta since their molecular size is too big to allow penetration through the cells of the villi. This protects the fetus from acquiring harmful agents of high molecular weight, but it also means that the fetus must synthesize its own proteins from its supply of amino acids. An exception is the maternal immunoglobulin IgG. It is not known why this particular protein crosses the placenta, but it appears that the selectivity is related to the structure and not to the size of the molecule. IgG is probably transported by pinocytosis. The benefit to the fetus is that it has the same resistance to infectious diseases as the mother.

Respiratory and excretory exchange. Besides serving as a lifeline for nutrients, the placenta functions in the exchange of respiratory gases and waste products between the mother and fetus.

The delivery of oxygen to the fetus is just as important to proper metabolism as an adequate supply of nutrients. The mother makes adjustments in her breathing to meet fetal oxygen needs, but the amount ultimately depends on the blood flow through the uterus to the placental villi. Near term the rate of flow through the intervillous space is 375 to 560 ml/min. Exchange is made between maternal red cells, which characteristically have a lower affinity for oxygen during pregnancy, and fetal red cells, which have a high affinity.

Maternal nutrition can influence oxygen exchange through the production of hemoglobin. Each gram of hemoglobin carries 1.34 ml of oxygen. In normal concentrations it can deliver up to 16 ml of oxygen per 100 ml of blood to the placenta. If maternal hemoglobin levels are depressed from iron deficiency, the supply of oxygen per 100 ml of blood is reduced. Since the fetus can tolerate little variation in the rate at which oxygen is supplied, the mother must compensate by increasing her cardiac output.

Another function of the placenta is to rid the fetus of metabolic wastes. The placenta is freely permeable to carbon dioxide, water, urea, creatinine, and uric acid. **Hyperventilation** by the mother reduces her PCO_2 so that carbon dioxide exchange from the fetus is accomplished by simple diffusion. Urea, creatinine, and uric acid, which are the wastes of fetal amino acid metabolism, move through the placenta by diffusion and active transport.

Placental hormones. The production of hormones to regulate the activities of pregnancy is one of the most interesting special functions of the placenta. From the earliest days of pregnancy the cells of the trophoblast and their successors in the placenta manufacture a large variety of hormones. The first to be manufactured in appreciable amounts is the protein hormone *human chorionic gonadotropin (HCG)*. Early in the differentiation of the trophoblast this hormone is found coating the trophoblasts's outer cell surfaces, where it is believed to act as an immunologically protective layer, preventing the rejection of the blastocyst and thereby facilitating implantation. HCG also stimulates the synthesis of *estrogen* in the placenta. Synthesis of estrogen actually begins in the free-floating blastocyst where it acts to facilitate implantation. The fact that the cells of the small, primitive blastocyst are already equipped to conduct complex steroid manipulation is a measure of the importance of these hormones at this early stage.

As pregnancy proceeds, large amounts of progesterone are synthesized in the placenta, principally from maternal cholesterol. In addition to sustaining pregnancy, this hormone serves as a raw material for the production of estrogens, mainly estrone, estradiol, and estriol, which in turn act on many organs and tissues of both the mother and fetus. Interestingly, the human placenta lacks the enzymes needed for converting the large amounts of progesterone it makes into certain essential estrogens and other steroids. Consequently, these synthetic events are carried out in the *fetal zone* cells, which are clusters of transient cells found in the developing adrenal glands of the fetus. These cells lack the enzymes necessary to manufacture progesterone but possess the requisite ones for its conversion. In this way the fetal and placental tissues complement each other. When the fetus' endocrine glands become sufficiently mature to take over the manufacture of steroid hormones, the fetal zone cells gradually diminish and eventually disappear. Presumably this sophisticated collaboration is organized and timed by precise genetic instructions and is regulated by equally precise releasing hormones.

Because a great variety of regulatory hormones are synthesized in the placenta, including HCG, human placental lactogen (HPL), chorionic somatomammotropin, and human chorionic thyrotropin (HCT), the placental control during pregnancy must be as comprehensive as that maintained by the pituitary gland throughout life. By means of these hormones the placenta not only carries out the functions of the fetus' pituitary until the organ is ready to perform on its own, but also conducts the entire "endocrine orchestra of pregnancy," which performs largely in the placenta itself.

Immunologic Protection

During pregnancy it is absolutely vital that the embryo be protected from immunologic rejection by maternal tissue. One of the mechanisms that seems to play a part in this task is the nonspecific suppression of lymphocytes, the cells that normally mediate the rejection of a graft. Experiments have shown that lymphocytes can be suppressed by HCG, HPL, prolactin, cortisone, progesterone, the estrogens, and a variety of proteins and glycoproteins.

It is also likely that the embryo is protected by the large tightly packed cells that enclose

Hyperventilation

(Gr *hyper,* over; L *ventilatio,* ventilation) Increased respiration with larger consequent air intake and oxygen-carbon dioxide exchange in the lungs above the normal amount.

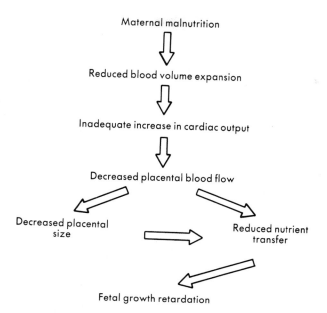

Maternal malnutrition

⇩

Reduced blood volume expansion

⇩

Inadequate increase in cardiac output

⇩

Decreased placental blood flow

Decreased placental size

Reduced nutrient transfer

Fetal growth retardation

FIG. 4-5 Postulated mechanisms responsible for placental and fetal growth retardation as seen with maternal malnutrition in animal models and in human subjects.
Modified from Rosso P: *Fed Proc* 39:250, 1980.

Morula
(L *morus*, mulberry)
Solid mass of cells resembling a mulberry, formed by cleavage of a fertilized ovum.

it soon after the implantation of the blastocyst. This protective barrier prevents the drainage of lymphocytes to maternal tissues. In addition, the maternal blood vessels do not invade the trophoblast of the placenta, so this potential means of graft rejection is blocked. In the early days of the development of the trophoblast further protection is provided by the absence of the expression of antigens. So even though the embryonic tissue is "foreign," it manages to conceal the fact, at least for a while.

Effects of Maternal Malnutrition

Maternal malnutrition has also been found to interfere with normal placental growth and function (Fig. 4-5). This is reflected by lower placental weight, smaller placental size, and reduced deoxyribonucleic acid (DNA) content. Affected placentas also have a reduced peripheral villous mass and villous surface.

STAGES OF HUMAN FETAL GROWTH

After the ovum is released from the mature follicle in the ovary, it enters the fallopian tube (Fig. 4-6). It moves slowly through the tube toward the uterus, encountering potential fertilizing sperm along the way. The stages of human embryonic-fetal growth are illustrated in Fig. 4-7. Fertilization usually occurs in the fallopian tube within 48 hours, after which cell division rapidly proceeds. The resulting solid ball of cells, the **morula,** enters the uterus where it undergoes reorganization into a hollow ball, the *blastocyst.* The blastocyst ultimately buries itself in the endometrial lining of the uterus (5 to 7 days postovulation). Here the precursor cells of the placenta begin to arrange themselves into a functioning placental unit. Nutritional support for the embryo at this time comes from the endometrial lining of the uterus. After its initial development, the placenta grows

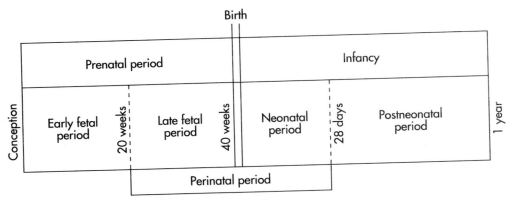

FIG. 4-6   Periods of prenatal and infant life.

rapidly throughout gestation. By 34 to 36 weeks the fetus has completed cell division. From that time until term, growth continues only by increase in size of existing cells.

Embryologic studies indicate three stages of fetal growth:

1. **Blastogenesis stage.** The fertilized egg divides into cells that fold in on one another. An inner cell mass evolves, giving rise to the embryo and an outer coat, the *trophoblast*, which becomes the placenta. This process is complete about 2 weeks after fertilization.
2. **Embryonic stage.** This is the critical time when cells differentiate into three germinal layers. The **ectoderm**, outer layer, gives rise to the brain, nervous system, hair, and skin. The **mesoderm**, middle layer, produces all of the voluntary muscles, bones, and components of the cardiovascular and excretory systems. The **endoderm**, inner layer, forms the digestive and respiratory systems, and glandular organs. By 60 days' gestation all of the major features of the human infant are achieved.
3. **Fetal stage.** This is the period of most rapid growth. From the third month until term, fetal weight increases nearly 500-fold from 6 g (0.2 oz) to 3000-3500 g (6.5 to 7.5 lb) at birth. The average weight curve from 10 weeks to term is shown in Fig. 4-8.

Measurements of DNA and protein in embryonic and fetal tissues show that embryonic growth occurs only by increase in number of cells, **hyperplasia.** Fetal growth continues in cell number, but now also involves increase in cell size, hypertrophy. The stages of cell growth involving hyperplasia and hypertrophy are illustrated in Fig. 4-9.

Growth-Retarded Infants

From the sequence described, it is possible to estimate the effects of malnutrition on growth at different stages of gestation. In the early months of pregnancy a severe limit on supply or transport of nutrients would have to occur to cause retarded growth because the quantitative requirements of the embryo are extremely small. Nevertheless, a restriction of materials and energy needed for cell synthesis and cell differentiation could produce malformations or cause the embryo to die. Malnutrition after the third month of gestation would not have teratogenic effects, but it could interfere with fetal growth. Nutrient requirements are greatest in the last trimester of pregnancy, when cells are increasing rapidly in both number and size. Even a relatively mild restriction could have serious effects at this time.

Ectoderm
(Gr *ektos,* outside; *derma,* skin) Outermost of the three primitive cell layers of the embryo.

Mesoderm
(Gr *mesos,* middle; *derma,* skin) Intermediate layer of embryonic cells developing between the ectoderm and endoderm.

Endoderm
(Gr *endon,* within; *derma,* skin) Innermost of the three primitive embryonic cell layers.

Hyperplasia
(Gr *hyper,* above; *plasis,* formation) Enlargement of tissue due to a process of rapidly increasing cell number.

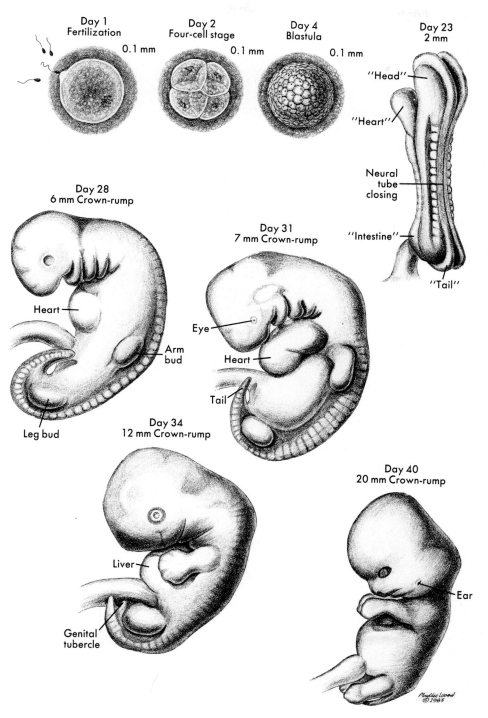

FIG. 4-7 Stages of fetal development.

Continued.

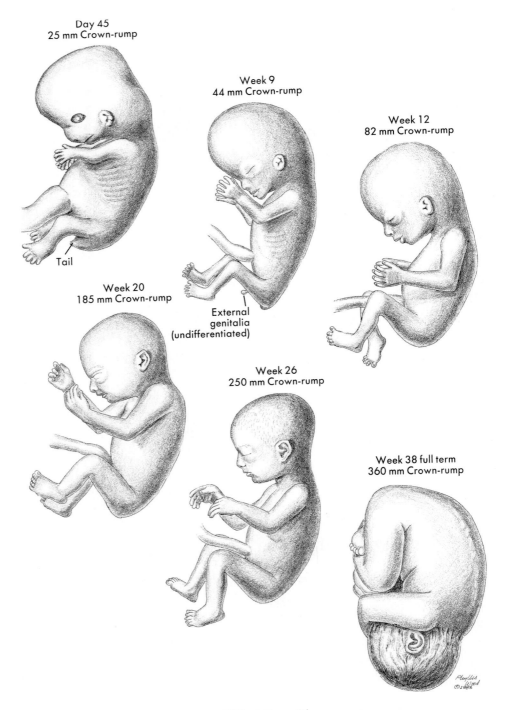

Day 45
25 mm Crown-rump

Week 9
44 mm Crown-rump

Week 12
82 mm Crown-rump

Tail

Week 20
185 mm Crown-rump

External
genitalia
(undifferentiated)

Week 26
250 mm Crown-rump

Week 38 full term
360 mm Crown-rump

FIG. 4-7 cont'd

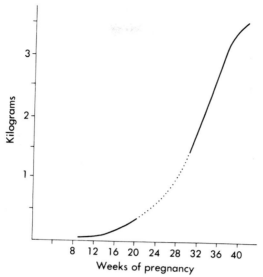

FIG. 4-8 Average curve of fetal growth.

From Hytten FE, Leitch I: *The physiology of human pregnancy,* ed 2, Oxford, 1971, Blackwell Scientific Publications; reprinted from Thompson AM et al: *J Obstet Gynaec Brit Commonw* 75:903, 1965.

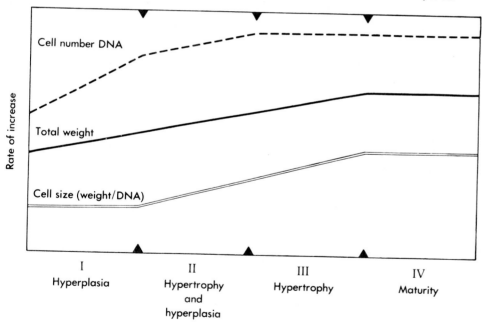

FIG. 4-9 Stages of cell growth.

Modified from Winick M: *Nutr Rev* 26:195, 1968.

Characteristics of SGA Infants

The effects of fetal malnutrition are reflected in the characteristics of small-for-gestational-age (SGA) infants, who though full term are poorly developed. Their conditions are variable, suggesting the multiple causes and importance of timing shown in

Gestational age
Stage of fetal growth and development at birth, varying from a premature delivery to full term.

animal studies. Among those SGA infants that do not have birth anomalies, there are two patterns of growth retardation. One type affects weight more than length; the other affects weight and length equally:

1. **Type I: growth retardation primarily affecting weight.** Head size (circumference) and skeletal growth are about normal, but the infants have poorly developed muscles and almost no subcutaneous fat. The resemblance of these infants to the large head and small body features of animals malnourished during the last weeks of gestation, either by maternal dietary restrictions or uterine ligation, is remarkable.

2. **Type II: growth reduction in both weight and height.** Size of all parts of the body, including head circumference and skeleton, is reduced proportionally. The physical characteristics of these infants are similar to those of rat pups whose mothers had deficient diets throughout all of gestation.

NUTRITIONAL INFLUENCES ON FETAL GROWTH

It is not possible, for obvious reasons, to examine maternal-fetal relationships directly at the cellular and molecular levels in humans. Consequently, work toward understanding how maternal nutrition influences growth and development in utero must be done on animals. The technique has usually been to manipulate the diets of pregnant animals and study the effects on cellular morphology and physiology in the offspring at various stages of gestation. Over the past few years much information has accumulated from studies of this type.

Experiments in Animals

Energy and nutrient restriction. Two types of dietary restrictions have been imposed on laboratory animals to study the effects of maternal nutrition on fetal growth and development. One restriction is simply not giving the animals enough food so that the diet is low in kilocalories. The other restriction holds kilocalories at an adequate level but reduces or completely eliminates one or more essential nutrients. The effects of deficiencies of almost all of the known nutrients have been studied this way, but restrictions of protein and kilocalories have more relevance to humans than restrictions of vitamins or minerals. All animals need energy and use protein in essentially the same way, but the need for vitamins and minerals and their specific functions differ from species to species.

A number of investigators have demonstrated what can happen to fetuses when pregnant animals are fed kilocalorie- or protein-restricted diets. Maternal malnutrition can interfere with the ability of the mother to conceive, it can produce death and resorption or abortion of the fetuses, and it can produce malformations or retarded growth. Of course, the more severe the dietary restrictions are the more serious the effects will be. A reduction of as little as 25% of the total kilocalories without an imbalance in the quality of the maternal diet in rats can reduce both the number of pups born and their ability to survive.

Biochemical studies show why this occurs. One effect of protein-kilocalorie malnutrition is an impairment of cell energy metabolism by interfering with the enzymes involved in glycolysis and the citric acid cycle. Without adequate supplies of amino acids and energy, cell functions break down, and normal processes of growth cannot occur. The effects would be most damaging when cells are normally undergoing rapid division. This implies that the timing of the dietary deficiency, as well as its severity, is important.

Types of growth failure. It is now clear that a number of things can produce growth failure in utero. The cause can be either *"intrinsic"* or *"extrinsic."* In differential diagnosis the condition of the placentas of animals born small for gestational age is considered. In *intrinsic intrauterine growth failure* placentas are usually of normal size. This implies that fetal growth retardation was not caused by inadequate maternal-fetal transport but was the result of other factors. Some examples include chromosomal abnormalities and maternal infections. *Extrinsic intrauterine growth* failure is usually manifested by placentas that are reduced in size. This indicates that they were incapable of supplying the fetus with adequate nutrition.

The principle feature of *intrinsic growth failure* is the presence of multiple malformations in the fetuses. These are absent in growth failure produced experimentally by ligation of blood vessels supplying the placenta. They are variable in maternal malnutrition, depending on the timing of the restriction. In both vascular and nutritional failure, placentas are reduced in proportion to fetal weight. In the ligated animals and in late maternal malnutrition, the reduction is caused by a decrease in the average size of the cells. Maternal protein restriction maintained throughout most of the gestation, however, decreases both the number and size of placental cells.

The fetuses themselves also show different patterns of growth retardation. Those subjected to vascular insufficiency show an asymmetric retardation. The fetuses have relatively normal brain sizes and head circumferences, but their livers are greatly reduced, by as much as 50%, and glycogen reserves are completely absent. Proportionally these animals have bigger brains and heads compared to the rest of their bodies. They are extremely hypoglycemic at birth.

When maternal protein restriction is limited to the last few days of gestation, the fetuses show a pattern of growth retardation similar to that produced by vascular insufficiency — proportionally big heads and small bodies. However, when the restriction is imposed throughout most of the gestation period, the pattern of fetal growth retardation becomes more symmetric. There is a 15% to 20% decrease in cell number in all organs including the brain. Head circumference is also reduced. The reduced cell number is greatest in those regions of the brain that are undergoing the most rapid rates of cell division.

Consequences of growth failure. These findings make it obvious that fetuses are *not* perfect parasites that can survive intrauterine insults without adverse effects. Data suggest that inadequate maternal nutrition can affect the fetus in ways that coincide with the stages of cell growth, and that the body reserves of the mother cannot always insulate the fetus from dietary deficiencies. What happens to animals whose mothers were nutritionally deprived during pregnancy depends to a great extent on how they are fed after birth.

Perhaps the finding of most concern is the effect of continued deprivation on the growth of brain cells. If prenatally malnourished pups are restricted after birth by feeding them in litters of 18 pups per dam, they demonstrate a 60% reduction in brain cell number by the time they are weaned. This contrasts with the 20% to 25% reduction associated with prenatal or postnatal malnutrition alone. Thus it seems that continued malnutrition throughout the entire time the brain cells are dividing produces greater deficits than would be expected if the separate effects were simply added together. Experiments have shown that nutritional rehabilitation will not enable these animals to recover their normal size once the period of cell proliferation has passed. They will continue to be small no matter how well fed they are after weaning. Other data suggest that maternal malnutrition may even have intergenerational effect; brain cell numbers were reduced in rats whose mothers were prenatally malnourished, even though these mothers had adequate diets during gestation and after weaning.

These studies would not be so disturbing if size were not related to function. The fact is, however, that alterations in normal biochemical and developmental processes accompany fetal and neonatal malnutrition in several species of animals. Changes in the usual constituents of cells are observed, as well as the delayed appearance of specific enzyme systems. Depending on the timing of the dietary deficiency, degeneration of the cerebral cortex, the medulla, and the spinal cord occurs. Muscular development is also impaired because of a reduced number of muscle cells and fibers.

What has been learned from animal research. Much can still be learned from experiments with animals about the processes of fetal growth and development and the consequences of maternal malnutrition. However the work to date has produced important results, as summarized below.

1. **Growth failure.** Although a number of prenatal influences affect fetal growth, maternal malnutrition can be one cause of growth failure that results in low birth weight.
2. **Nature of tissue effects.** Animals malnourished from restrictions of their mothers' diets throughout most of gestation are characterized by (1) reduced number and size of cells in the placenta, (2) reduced brain cell number and head size, (3) proportional reductions in the size of other organs, and (4) alterations in normal cell constituents and biochemical processes.
3. **Influencing factors.** The fetal consequences of malnutrition depend on the timing, severity, and duration of the maternal dietary restriction. These consequences may be reversible if the restriction primarily affects growth in cell size. But a reduction in the number of cells may be permanent if the restriction is maintained throughout the entire period of hyperplastic growth.

Human Experience in Fetal Growth

Low birth weight. In view of the risks of early death or permanent disability associated with low birth weight, it is apparent that the animal research on intrauterine failure may have great implications for human problems. Of the annual incidence of low birth weight infants, it is estimated that 10% to 20% is a result of intrauterine growth failure. This means that 80,000 to 120,000 infants who have experienced malnutrition in utero are born each year in the United States. An important thing to understand when interpreting these statistics is that there is no one cause—a number of factors can retard fetal growth. When the term *fetal malnutrition* is applied to human infants, it simply means that there was a reduction in the maternal supply or placental transport of nutrients so that fetal growth is retarded significantly below genetic potential. It does not necessarily mean that the mother's nutrition was at fault. At present there is no way to judge how many growth-retarded infants are the result of maternal malnutrition.

Relation of animal studies. Although the animal experiments are highly suggestive, caution should be taken in making direct applications to humans. A primary reason for doing animal research is to find out what can possibly happen when certain conditions are imposed. The findings do not guarantee that these things actually happen in the course of human events. There are a number of reasons why the dramatic results of maternal malnutrition demonstrated in animals may not occur as readily in human beings. In effect the consequences of maternal malnutrition on fetal growth and development are all magnified in the animal studies. This is because (1) relative rates of growth and development are much slower in humans compared with laboratory animals, (2) the timing of maximum growth also differs, (3) the number and size of fetuses a mother must nourish in utero compared with her own body size and nutritional reserves are much smaller in humans than in laboratory animals, and (4) the magnitude of dietary deprivation used for experimentation is rarely encountered in human populations under ordinary circumstances.

EFFECTS OF MATERNAL MALNUTRITION

Observations described above provide fertile grounds for speculation, but what is the evidence in human populations that maternal malnutrition causes fetal malnutrition? Of necessity much of the information is incidental. Nonetheless, there have been three kinds of studies that have addressed this question with highly significant results: (1) natural experiments in which birth statistics before, during, and after periods of acute famine are studied and compared; (2) measurements of organ size and cell numbers in stillbirths and neonatal deaths in which all causes not related to maternal malnutrition have been ruled out; and (3) epidemiologic studies of the nutritional correlates of birth weights.

Natural Experiments

The hardships of war afford researchers an opportunity to study the effects of severe dietary restrictions during pregnancy under conditions that fortunately are seldom duplicated. Throughout most of Europe at various times during World War II, food shortages were common. Reports were made on the effects of these shortages during the 1940s, but they are being considered with renewed interest today in light of the findings from animal research. Experiences in Russia and Holland provide examples of these effects:

1. **Russia.** During the seige of Leningrad in 1942 and its immediate aftermath, there was an 18-month period of severe starvation. Comparison of statistics for infants born before, during, and after the seige revealed an expected toll in the course and outcome of pregnancy under such desperate conditions. During the famine period there was a twofold increase in fetal mortality, as well as an increase in the number of infants weighing less than 2500 g (5.4 lb) at birth.

2. **Holland.** Similar findings were reported from Holland. Here the results are more insightful because the famine began suddenly and was limited to about 6 months during the winter of 1944 to 1945. It was not accompanied by other deprivations as severe as those experienced during the seige of Leningrad, and the women of Holland had fairly good diets before the food shortage. During the famine period dietary intake dropped to less than 1000 kcal per day, and protein was limited to 30 to 40 g. Since the famine lasted only 6 months, babies conceived before and during that period were exposed for varying lengths of time, but none was exposed for the entire course of gestation. On the average, birth weights of infants exposed to the famine were reduced by 200 g (7 oz). Weights were lowest for babies exposed to the famine during the entire last half of pregnancy. Added exposure before that time did not reduce birth weights further. In fact, babies exposed to the famine during the first 27 weeks of gestation, but finishing their terms after the famine ended, had higher average birth weights than those who were only exposed during the last 3 weeks of gestation. The data for stillbirths and congenital malformations followed a different pattern. The rates were lowest for infants conceived before the famine and highest for those conceived during it.

   The findings are in line with what is anticipated from knowledge of the stages of human growth. Poor nutrition in the latter part of pregnancy affects fetal growth, whereas poor nutrition in the early months affects development of the embryo and its capacity to survive.

3. **Great Britian.** It is interesting to note that, in contrast with the experiences in Russia and Holland, the prenatal mortality rate in Great Britain, which had been fairly constant before the war, actually declined between 1940 and 1945 despite the poor environmental conditions and no discernible improvements in prenatal care. One possible explanation is that pregnant and lactating women were given priority status for food in Britain as a matter of national policy.

Organ Studies

Studies that attempt to relate the size of organs in human infants to maternal nutrition must control for other conditions known to affect fetal growth. One group of researchers looked at the organs of 252 American stillborn infants and infants who died in the first 48 hours of life, excluding all multiple births, maternal complications, and congenital defects. The infants were grouped as coming from poor or nonpoor families according to income. Comparisons of organs between the two groups showed that the mass of adipose tissue and the size of individual fat cells were smaller in the poor infants. These infants also had smaller livers, adrenal glands, thymuses, and spleens. Heart, kidney, and skeleton were also reduced, but the differences were not as great. The ranking in organ size is consistent with reductions noted in animals who have been prenatally malnourished and in humans who have experienced uterine or placental disorders. Since the last two conditions were ruled out of the study, the investigators concluded that undernutrition could be responsible for prenatal growth retardation in infants from low income families.

The organs in infants who survive intrauterine malnutrition cannot be studied to see if cells are reduced in number or size, but one organ is available. This is the placenta. One scientist reported that the size of placentas and the number of placental cells are 15% and 20% below normal when infants experience growth failure.[10] By comparing placentas from different sources, he has shown that those from indigent populations in developing countries have reductions in cell numbers similar to the reductions noted in placentas from American infants with intrauterine growth failure. In one interesting case in the United States, a mother who was severely undernourished from anorexia nervosa during pregnancy gave birth to an infant weighing less than 2500 g (5.4 lb). When the placenta was examined, it was found to have only 50% of the normal number of cells.

Nutritional Correlates of Birth Weight

Studies of the relationship between maternal nutrition and the birth weight of the infant have tended to focus directly on the nutrient composition of the diet during pregnancy. Because of variations in the nutritional requirements of individuals, these studies have produced conflicting results. However, there are two indicators of long-term and immediate nutritional status that have shown consistent associations with birth weight. These are (1) *maternal body size,* height and prepregnancy weight of the mother; and (2) *maternal weight gain,* the amount of weight gained by the mother during the pregnancy itself.

Maternal body size. It should not be surprising that big mothers have big babies. What is less often appreciated is that the size of the infant at birth largely depends on the size of the mother and is not influenced to a great degree by the size of the father. This was shown years ago in a classic experiment in which Shire stallions were bred with Shetland mares and Shetland stallions with Shire mares. The newborn foals were always an appropriate size to the mothers' breeds. No intermediate sizes were ever produced. The same effects have been demonstrated in a number of animals, and there is indirect evidence for the same phenomenon in humans.

It has been further demonstrated in humans that height and prepregnancy weight of the mother have independent and additive effects on the birth weight of a child. In an analysis of 4095 mothers in Aberdeen, Scotland,[11] it was found that, on average, the tallest and heaviest mothers had babies who weighed 500 g (1 lb) more at birth than babies of the shortest and lightest mothers. It is postulated that maternal size is a conditioning factor on the ultimate size of the placenta and thus controls the blood supply of nutrients available to the fetus.

This idea has support in findings from the Collaborative Perinatal Project of the National Institutes of Health. In this project, Naeye[12] analyzed data from nearly 60,000 pregnancies to discover causes of fetal and **neonatal morality** amoung different racial groups. He found that Puerto Ricans experience a higher rate of placental growth retardation than whites. However, this difference disappears when women with prepregnancy weights of 45 kg (101 lb) or less are excluded from the analysis. Naeye

Neonatal mortality
Number of newborn deaths during the neonatal period (birth to 1 month postpartum) per 1000 live births.

concludes that the high rate of placental growth retardation in Puerto Ricans is a result of the greater proportion of women who enter pregnancy with low body weights. Further data from Naeye's study show that, regardless of race or ethnic origin, mothers with low prepregnancy weights have much lighter placentas than heavier mothers.

Maternal underweight. Infants of underweight women show several kinds of morbidity. Edwards and colleagues[13] compared outcomes for women who entered pregnancy at 10% or more below standard weight for height with outcomes for women who entered pregnancy at normal weight (Table 4-5). The women were matched for age, race, parity, and socioeconomic status. The incidence of both low birth weight and prematurity were significantly higher among the underweight mothers. Infants of underweight women also scored lower on the **Apgar scale.** This scale measures the general condition of the neonate as evidenced by heart rate, respiration, muscle tone, reflex irritability, and color at delivery. Differences in Apgar scores were even greater when only those infants of women who were excessive cigarette smokers were compared. Underweight women who smoked more than one pack of cigarettes a day during pregnancy had three times the number of infants with low Apgar scores compared with their normal weight controls.

Underweight women were also subject to different rates of pregnancy complications.[13] Anemia occurred more frequently in the underweight group, and those who were both underweight and anemic had an incidence of low birth weight of 17.4%, compared to 3.6% among women who were anemic but of normal weight. The investigators point out that both underweight status and iron deficiency anemia reflect long-term suboptimum nutritional intake. They suggest this as a possible explanation for the apparent influence of anemic underweight mothers on the incidence of low birth weight.

The condition of underweight is potentially modifiable since it is often related to abusive dieting practices and/or exercise programs. A woman motivated toward improvement of her body weight-for-height status may successfully and healthfully achieve her goal within a relatively short period of time (three to six months).

Maternal Weight Gain

The weight gained in a normal pregnancy is the result of physiologic processes designed to foster fetal and maternal growth. Much of the weight gain can be accounted for by the products of gestation.

The total number of pounds gained in pregnancy will vary among individual women. Young mothers and **primigravidae** usually gain more than older mothers and multigravidae. A normal gain for most healthy women is about 11 to 15 kg (25 to 35 lb), but current guidelines from the National Academy of Sciences specify appropriate ranges for weight gain related to maternal prepregnancy weight-for-height, height, age, and race

Apgar score
Number defining an infant's condition at 1 minute after birth by scoring the heart rate, respiratory effort, muscle tone, reflex irritability, and color; named for its developer, American anesthesiologist Virginia Apgar (1909-1974).

Primigravida
(L *prima*, first; *gravida*, pregnant) A woman pregnant for the first time.

TABLE 4-5 *Infant Morbidity in Underweight Women and Normal Weight Controls*

Infant Morbidity	Low Pregnancy Weight (% of births)	Normal Weight Controls (% of births)
Low birth weight	15.3	7.6
Prematurity	23.0	14.0
Low Apgar score	19.0	12.0

From Edwards LE et al: Pregnancy in the underweight woman: Course, outcome and growth patterns of the infant, *Am J Obstet Gynecol* 135:297, 1979.

(Table 4-6). A chart incorporating these recommendations for underweight, normal weight, and overweight women is provided in Fig. 4-10.

The normal pattern of weight gain is illustrated in Fig. 4-11. Less than half the total weight gain resides in the fetus, placenta, and amniotic fluid. The remainder is found in maternal reproductive tissues, fluid, blood, and "stores." The weight component labeled "maternal stores" is largely composed of body fat, although some increase in the lean body mass, other than reproductive tissue, may also occur. The action of progesterone in the pregnant woman dictates that a fat pad be produced to serve as a caloric reserve for both pregnancy and lactation. Fatfold measurements from 10 to 30 weeks' gestation have shown gradual increases in subcutaneous fat at the abdomen, back, and upper thigh. The pregnant woman who attempts to restrict weight gain to avoid development of the fat pad will simultaneously affect to some degree normal development of the other products of pregnancy (Fig. 4-11).

A sudden weight gain that greatly exceeds this rate is likely to be caused by excess fluid retention,. As stated repeatedly in this chapter, mild generalized edema and some accumulation of fluid in the lower limbs is not unphysiologic. Women with edema can gain as much as 9 liters of fluid and still have clinically normal pregnancies. However, it should be emphasized that this accumulation is gradual. A large shift in water balance reflected by a sudden increase in weight is usually an indication of preeclampsia, particularly if it occurs after the twentieth week.

The more liberal attitude about weight gain during pregnancy that prevails today should not detract from the logic of avoidance of excessive weight gain. While large weight gain may have little or no adverse impact on the developing fetus, it may be detrimental to the mother during pregnancy and afterward.[14] Women who gain excessively large amounts of weight during pregnancy are at greater risk for the development of hypertension and are more likely to require cesarean delivery. Figure 4-12 illustrates the correlation between maternal weight and infant weight. Evidence also suggests, not surprisingly, that excessive weight gain during pregnancy may increase risk of long-term problems in controlling weight gain later in life. Tips for the health professional when evaluating maternal weight loss and weight gain can be found in the box on p. 123.

Maternal obesity. Women exceeding their desirable body weight by more than 35% are at greater risk than normal-weight women for unsatisfactory pregnancy course and outcome. Numerous studies have shown that obese women are at higher risk for antenatal complications, especially pregnancy-induced hypertension, gestational diabetes, urinary

TABLE 4-6 *Recommended Total Weight Gain Ranges for Pregnant Women,* * by Prepregnancy Body Mass Index (weight/height^2)†*

	Recommended Total Gain	
Weight-for-Height Category	**kg**	**lb**
Low (BMI <19.8)	12.5-18	28-40
Normal (BMI of 19.8-26.0)	11.5-16	25-35
High‡ (BMI >26.0 to 29.0)	7-11.5	15-25

*Young adolescents and black women should strive for gains at the upper end of the recommended range. Short women (<157 cm or 62 inches) should strive for gains at the lower end of the range.
†Body mass index (BMI) is calculated using metric units.
‡The recommended target weight gain for obese women (BMI >29.0) is at least 7.0 kg (15 lb).
From Institute of Medicine: *Nutrition during pregnancy: weight gain and nutrient supplements,* Washington, DC, 1990, National Academy Press.

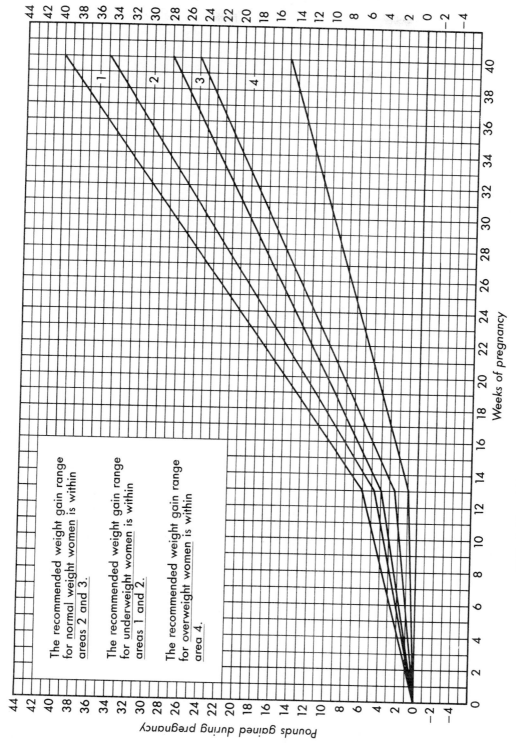

FIG. 4-10 A "modern" weight gain chart for pregnant women. Modified from the National Academy of Science's *Nutrition during Pregnancy*, 1990.

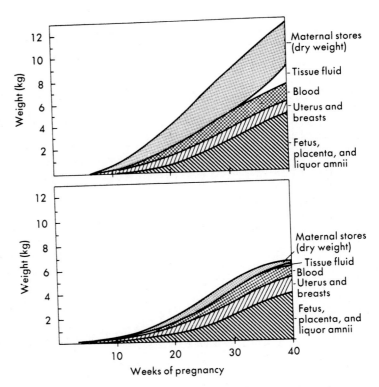

FIG. 4-11 Estimated composition of weight gain during pregnancy for a normal, healthy, Northern European woman *(top)* and a poor, underfed woman from India *(bottom)*. Modified from Hurley LS: *Developmental nutrition,* Englewood Cliffs, NJ, 1980, Prentice-Hall.

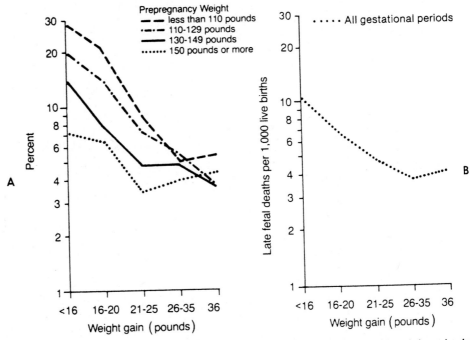

FIG. 4-12 **A,** Percent of live-born infants of low birth weight by maternal weight gain during pregnancy, according to mother's prepregnancy weight: United States, 1980, *National Natality Survey.* **B,** Fetal death ratio by weight gain during pregnancy: United States, 1980, *National Natality and Fetal Mortality Surveys.*

Tips For the Health Professional: Managing Weight Gain and Loss in Pregnancy

What to look for if weight gain is slow or if weight loss occurs:

- Is there a measurement or recording error?
- Is the overall pattern acceptable? Was a lack of gain preceded by a higher than expected gain?
- Was there evidence of edema at the last visit and is it resolved?
- Is nausea, vomiting, or diarrhea a problem?
- Is there a problem with access to food?
- Have psychosocial problems led to poor appetite?
- Does the woman resist weight gain? Is she restricting her energy intake? Does she have an eating disorder?
- If the slow weight gain appears to be a result of self-imposed restriction, does she understand the relationship between her weight gain and her infant's growth and health?
- Is she smoking? How much?
- Is she using alcohol or drugs (especially cocaine or amphetamines)?
- Does her energy expenditure exceed her energy intake?
- Does she have an infection or illness that requires treatment?

What to look for if weight gain is very rapid:

- Is there a measurement or recording error?
- Is the overall pattern acceptable? Was the gain preceded by weight loss or a lower than expected gain?
- Is there evidence of edema?
- Has the woman stopped smoking recently? The advantages of smoking cessation offset any disadvantages associated by gaining some extra weight.
- Are twins a possibility? (A large increase in fundal height may be the earliest sign.)
- Are there signs of gestational diabetes?
- Has there been a dramatic decrease in physical activity without an accompanying decrease in food intake?
- Has the woman greatly increased her food intake? Obtain a diet recall, making special note of high-fat foods. However, rapid weight gain is often accompanied by normal eating patterns, which should be continued. If intake of high-fat or high-sugar foods is excessive, encourage substitutions.
- If serious overeating is occurring, explore why. Does stress, depression, an eating disorder or boredom play a factor? Is there need for special support or a referral?

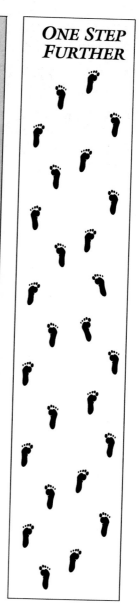

ONE STEP FURTHER

tract infections and pyelonephritis; they also are more likely to demonstrate prolonged labor followed by difficult vaginal delivery and thus are more frequently delivered by cesarean section. Perinatal mortality is likewise higher. Surviving babies of obese mothers may present more challenges in management during the neonatal period since they often demonstrate difficulty in regulating blood glucose. Suffice to say, reducing the degree of maternal obesity prior to conception theoretically should improve pregnancy progress and outcome. Attempts along this line are worth making if time allows and the woman appears to be properly motivated. Unfortunately such motivation may not exist or if it does, ability to follow a prescribed program may be limited. In any case, attempts should be made throughout the reproductive period (if not before) to prevent the development of excessive adiposity.

Supplementation/Intervention Trials

It is now well recognized that the provision of extra food, with or without education, will improve pregnancy outcome in groups of high-risk, low-income pregnant women. The value of supplemental food varies from woman to woman but obviously the severity of the original deficit is predictive of the value of the added food resources. A series of supplementation studies in developing countries have proved the positive impact on birthweight that such interventions can have. Even in developed countries, however, the benefits of nutrition intervention programs for high-risk women have been demonstrated.

The experiences at the Montreal Diet Dispensary in Canada show that the benefits of extra kilocalories and special dietary management during pregnancy are not confined to chronically malnourished women in developing countries.[15,16] They can also improve the pregnancy performance of high-risk mothers in more affluent nations. Knowing the risk of reproductive problems associated with low income, Higgins and colleagues selected the hospital handling the highest percentage of poor patients in Montreal. All patients from two of the hospital's public maternity clinics were enrolled for a total of 1544 women between 1963 and 1970. A unique feature was that dietary needs for kilocalories and protein were individually calculated for each woman based on her body weight for height with adjustments for protein deficiency, underweight, and other stress conditions. Women whose family incomes fell below specified levels (70% of all women in the study) were given supplies of milk, eggs, and oranges every 2 weeks. All of the women received counseling on food selection to meet their individual needs every time they visited the clinic, and nutritionists visited them at home at least once during their pregnancies.

Such intensive nutritional care enabled the women to average 93% of their total kilocalorie needs and 96% of their total protein requirements throughout gestation. Since the majority started out with large average daily deficits, they all showed significant improvements in the quality of their diets. Birth statistics indicate how the mothers and their infants benefited from these measures. The incidence of low birth weight in this high-risk study group decreased to the point that it equaled the all-Canada rate and was lower than the rate for Quebec province. Stillbirths, neonatal mortality, and **perinatal mortality** were also lower than the rates prevailing in Canada and Quebec.

It is impossible to know how much of the improvements in pregnancy performance and outcome demonstrated in this study can be attributed to the diets of the women, the food supplements, or the special attention they received. What is important about the study is that it shows how high-risk mothers, against all odds, can experience successful pregnancies when superior nutritional guidance is a part of their prenatal care.

Other clinicians have made aggressive efforts to improve pregnancy outcome through nutrition intervention for underweight pregnant women and women demonstrating poor weight gain during pregnancy. Between 1984 and 1988, approximately 2000 women receiving prenatal services in Virginia Health Department clinics were provided individualized nutrition interventions based on techniques developed at the Montreal Diet Dispensary. Those responding to the food intake and weight gain guidelines showed a marked reduction in low-birth-weight deliveries (Fig. 4-13).

Similarly, in a large urban clinic, a group of 52 underweight pregnant women who received no counseling were compared with a similar group of 57 underweight and failure-to-gain pregnant women who received extensive nutrition counseling during the course of pregnancy. Women in the counseled group gained significantly more weight during their pregnancies than did the controls. They also delivered babies that averaged 300 g heavier than those born to women in the control group, a difference not related to ethnic background, income status, age, or smoking habit. The percentage of women having low-birth-weight babies was 8% in the counseled group compared with 17% among controls.[18]

Perinatal mortality
(Gr *peri*, around; L *natus*, born) Infant deaths in the perinatal period (before and after birth, from approximately week 20-28 of gestation to 1-4 weeks postpartum) per 1000 live births.

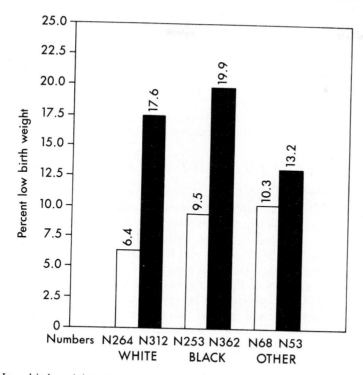

FIG. 4-13   Low birth weight rates of underweight pregnant women enrolled in the Virginia Nutrition Intervention Project, 1984 to 1988, who were ≤90% of expected weight at the initial visit and either >90% *(open bars)* or ≤90% *(solid bars)* of expected weight at the last visit.

From Clements DF: The Nutrition Intervention Project for underweight women, *Clin Nutr* 7:205, 1988. Reprinted with permission from Churchill Livingston Medical Journals.

Orstead and colleagues took the process one step further by estimating the cost effectiveness of individualized nutrition counseling for a group of high-risk women in Chicago. The nutrition services for the counseled group cost about $44,500 more than the usual program, but the cost of caring for the extra low-birth-weight babies in the control group was approximately $230,700. The benefit-to-cost ratio was therefore close to five to one.[19]

Finally, numerous efforts have been made over the years to evaluate the massive Special Supplemental Food Program for Women, Infants, and Children (WIC). In 1986, the U.S. Department of Agriculture published a five volume report based on a nationally representative low-income population.[20] The researchers concluded after 5 years of study that WIC had a significant beneficial effect on the duration of pregnancy, birthweight, head growth, fetal mortality, and neonatal mortality. The program's effects were most clearly seen in high-risk pregnant women.

Not all nutrition intervention programs provided to high-risk pregnant women have demonstrated the degree of positive impact that was shown in the studies cited above. This varied response should certainly be expected, given the different populations served, the different supplements employed, the various methods of supplement administration, and a variety of other differing variables. Overall, however, the findings appear to suggest that *the poorer the nutritional condition of the mother entering pregnancy, the more valuable the prenatal diet and nutritional supplement will be in improving her pregnancy course and outcome.*

NUTRIENT FUNCTIONS AND NEEDS

The nutrients enter into all of the major metabolic processes involving the production of energy, synthesis of cells, maintenance of their structure and function, and the regulation of body processes. First we examine the basis for the Recommended Dietary Allowances (RDA) nutrient and energy standards for pregnancy. Then, in considering each of these nutrient functions, emphasis is given to those nutrients that have major roles in pregnancy and why their requirements during pregnancy increase.

RECOMMENDED DIETARY ALLOWANCES

The Food and Nutrition Board of the National Research Council is well aware of the problems of determining nutrient requirements during pregnancy and considers them when setting dietary allowances and making recommendations about the need for supplementation. Recommended Dietary Allowances are based on the best available evidence from metabolic balance studies and from indirect estimates.[21]

The current 1989 edition of the RDA standards for pregnant and nonpregnant adult women is presented in Table 4-7. The figures in the table indicate the needs of a "reference" woman who is 25 to 50 years of age, 160 cm (64 in) tall, and weighs 63 kg (138 lb) when she conceives. Women may need more or less of the amounts listed for kilocalories and protein depending on body size, activity, and health status. The allowances for vitamins and

TABLE 4-7 *Recommended Dietary Allowances for Women of Reproductive Age (1989)*

	Age				
Nutrient	11-14	15-18	19-24	25-50	Pregnancy
Energy (kcal)	2200	2200	2200	2200	+300*
Protein (g)	46	48	46	50	60
Vitamin A (μg RE)	800	800	800	800	800
Vitamin D (μg)	10	10	10	5	10
Vitamin E (mg α-TE)	8	8	8	8	10
Vitamin C (mg)	50	60	60	60	70
Folate acid (μg)	150	180	180	180	400
Niacin (mg NE)	15	15	15	15	17
Riboflavin (mg)	1.3	1.3	1.3	1.3	1.6
Thiamin (mg)	1.1	1.1	1.1	1.1	1.5
Vitamin B_6 (mg)	1.4	1.5	1.6	1.6	2.2
Vitamin B_{12} (μg)	2.0	2.0	2.0	2.0	2.2
Calcium (mg)	1200	1200	1200	800	1200
Phosphorus (mg)	1200	1200	1200	800	1200
Iodine (μg)	150	150	150	150	175
Iron (mg)	15	15	15	15	30
Magnesium (mg)	280	300	280	280	320
Zinc (mg)	12	12	12	12	15
Selenium (μg)	45	50	55	55	65

*Second and third trimesters.
From Food and Nutrition Board, National Council, National Academy of Sciences: *Recommended Dietary Allowances,* ed 10, Washington, DC, 1989, National Academy Press.

minerals provide sufficient room for individual variation, an important consideration, so that they can be applied to all healthy women. They may not be adequate for women who enter pregnancy in poor nutritional status or who suffer from chronic disease or other complicating conditions. They may not be appropriate for the young pregnant adolescent or the woman who is very overweight.

Energy

Pregnancy requirements. During pregnancy, two factors determine energy requirements: (1) changes in the mother's usual physical activity, and (2) increase in her basal metabolism to support the work required for growth of the fetus and the accessory tissues. The cumulative energy cost of pregnancy has been estimated at 40,000 to 70,000 kilocalories.[22,23] This amount is derived from the kilocalorie equivalents of protein and fat stored in the products of conception and from increased oxygen consumption of the mother. The total 40,000 to 70,000 kilocalories break down to an addition of only 200 to 300 extra kilocalories during the second and third trimesters of pregnancy to the daily allowance of the nonpregnant reference woman. A portion of the energy increment may be offset by the tendency of pregnant women to reduce their physical activity in the last trimester.

Protein

Pregnancy requirements. Requirements for protein during pregnancy are based on the needs of the nonpregnant reference woman plus the extra amounts needed for growth. The easiest way to determine how much extra protein is needed daily to support the synthesis of new tissue is to divide the amounts contained in the products of conception and maternal body by the average length of gestation. About 925 g of protein are deposited in a normal-weight fetus and in the maternal accessory tissues.[22] When this is divided by the 280 days of pregnancy, the average is 3.3 g of protein that must be added to normal daily requirements. The rate at which new tissue is synthesized, however, is not constant throughout gestation. Maternal and fetal growth does not accelerate until the second month, and the rate progressively increases until just before term. The need for protein follows this growth rate. Only about an extra 0.6 g of protein is used each day for new tissue synthesis in the first month of pregnancy, but by 30 weeks gestation protein is being used at the rate of 6.1 g per day. If this is added to the normal maintenance needs of the reference woman, 18.6 to 24 g of protein per day are required.

Protein utilization. These calculations of protein need would equal dietary allowances if 100% of the protein eaten could be used in the body. Actually, however, the efficiency of protein utilization depends on its digestibility and amino acid composition. Proteins that do not contain all of the essential amino acids in amounts proportional to human requirements are utilized less efficiently. Even a high quality protein, such as that in eggs, is utilized much less than 100%. Protein utilization from a mixed diet is about 70% and from a totally vegetarian diet it is even less efficient. Protein utilization also depends on kilocalorie intake. It has been shown that an extra 100 kcal during pregnancy will have the same effect on nitrogen retention as an additional 0.28 g of nitrogen itself. This means that kilocalories from nonprotein sources, that is, carbohydrates and fats, have a protein-sparing effect. If these kilocalories are inadequate, protein requirements would increase. Finally, the trials that measure nitrogen loss are conducted on a limited number of subjects. There is a great deal of variation from the averages obtained. Since a dietary allowance must cover the needs of all healthy women, room for individual differences must be built in.

RDA standard. Because of these considerations, RDAs for protein are set much higher than calculated requirements of 18.6 to 24 g per day.[21] The National Research Council allows 50 g of protein a day for the nonpregnant reference woman with an extra 10 g per day starting in the second month of pregnancy. If individual allowances are calculated on the basis of body weight, daily need would be about 1.3 g/kg of pregnant body weight or about 0.6 g/lb. The RDA standard is based on a mixed diet in which at least one third of the protein comes from high-quality animal foods. Thus vegetarian diets that exclude all animal products can only be made adequate when more total protein is consumed, or when foods are selected so that those low in a particular amino acid are complemented by foods in which that amino acid is high.

Protein deficiency. Adverse consequences of protein deficiency during pregnancy are difficult to separate from the effects of kilocalorie deficiency in real life situations. Almost all cases of limited protein intake are accompanied by limitation in availability of kilocalories. Under such circumstances decreased birth weight has been reported. As indicated in a Guatemalan study,[24] provision of supplemental kilocalories alone to pregnant women with deficient levels of protein intake was just as effective as provision of both protein and kilocalories in influencing birth weight of babies.

Protein excess. Adverse effects of excessive protein during pregnancy are poorly understood at the present time. The New York supplementation study[25] has provoked much discussion of this issue, since use of the high protein supplement was associated with an increased number of very prematurely born infants and excessive neonatal deaths. In light of these findings other data have been reviewed. Analysis of a number of past supplementation studies in human populations[26] has suggested that providing a supplement with more than 20% of the kilocalories from protein is associated with retarded fetal growth, whereas supplements providing less than 20% of the kilocalories from protein yield increments in birth weight of offspring. Although these data suggest that too much protein, presented in an unbalanced nutritional package, may have negative effects on pregnancy course and outcome, data are limited and the debate continues about the relevance of the observations.

Micronutrients: General

It is well recognized that food is the optimal vehicle for delivering nutrients. It therefore follows that nutrient supplementation is an intervention that requires justification. This viewpoint was stated in no uncertain terms by the expert committee appointed by the National Academy of Sciences.[7] In essence, there is limited evidence that multivitamin-mineral supplementation significantly improves fertility or pregnancy outcome in most women. There are situations, however, that justify individualized supplement prescription (Table 4-8). These circumstances are defined throughout this section of the chapter.

Folate

The B-complex vitamin folate is required for cell division to proceed. If this vitamin is lacking, detrimental effects are especially great in body tissues that have high turnover rates. One of the first signs of folate deficiency is megaloblastic anemia, caused by the production of abnormal red blood cells. These cells are arrested in their development, so bone marrow contains a large number of immature megaloblasts and hemoglobin levels are reduced. Hemoglobin levels below 11 g/dl during the first and third trimesters or below 10.5 g/dl during the second trimester are criteria for diagnosis of anemia (Table 4-9). Anemia is associated with increased risk of adverse pregnancy course and outcome.

The treatment of anemia with appropriate dietary changes and nutrient supplement is not an issue subject to much debate. There is, however, controversy about the need for folate supplementation by pregnant women who are not anemic. Much of this controversy stems from our limited knowledge base about the impact of folate deficiency on pregnancy outcome. Maternal folate deficiency in experimental animals is associated with increased incidence of problems related to pregnancy and increased delivery of abnormal offspring.[27]

TABLE 4-8 *Current Supplementation Recommendations: National Academy of Sciences (1990)*

Nutrient	Candidates for Supplementation	Level of Nutrient Supplementation
Iron	All pregnant women (2nd and 3rd trimesters)	30 mg ferrous iron daily
Folic acid	Pregnant women with suspected dietary inadequacy of folate	300 µg/day
Vitamin D	Complete vegetarians and others with low intake of vitamin D-fortified milk	10 µg/day
Calcium	Women under age 25 whose daily dietary calcium intake is less than 600 mg	600 mg/day
Vitamin B_{12}	Complete vegetarians	2 µg/day
Zinc/copper	Women under treatment with iron for iron deficiency anemia	15 mg Zn/day 2 mg Cu/day
Multivitamin-mineral supplements	Pregnant women with poor diets and for those who are considered high risk: multiple gestation, heavy smokers, alcohol/drug abusers, other	Preparation containing: iron—30 mg zinc—15 mg copper—2 mg calcium—250 mg vitamin B_6—2 mg folate—300 µg vitamin C—50 mg vitamin D—5 µg

From Institute of Medicine: *Nutrition during pregnancy: weight gain and nutrient supplements,* Washington, DC, 1990, National Academy Press.

TABLE 4-9 *Current Definition of Anemia*

Trimester	Hemoglobin (g/dl)
First	< 11.0
Second	< 10.5
Third	< 11.0

Data from National Academy of Sciences: *Nutrition during pregnancy: weight gain and nutrient supplements,* Washington, DC, 1990, National Academy Press.

Fetal malformations have been reported in offspring of women using drugs that are folate antagonists.[28] Some evidence in humans suggests that deficiency of this vitamin may be associated with abruptio placentae, spontaneous abortion, preeclampsia, fetal malformations, and subnormal infant development. Such reports, however, are not direct proof of association.

The biggest controversy relates to the role of folate deficiency in the etiology of neural tube defects. The work of Smithells[29-32] and Laurence[33] in northern Europe suggests that multivitamin or folate supplementation of women with previous neural tube defect offspring is associated with significant reduction in second occurrence of the problem. Since methodologic details of these projects have been heavily criticized, the merit of these reports has been questioned. A carefully controlled trial is currently underway in northern Europe to examine the possible preventive value of periconceptional vitamin supplementation.[34] If this trial is completed successfully, it will be possible to develop scientifically based recommendations about vitamin supplementation before and during pregnancy.

In the meantime, several research groups have attempted to address the question indirectly. Three surveys have been conducted in the United States to assess periconceptional vitamin supplementation practices of women delivering and having a diagnosed offspring with neural tube defects and selected "control" women.[35-37] The results have been mixed. In two of the three studies, use of vitamin supplements around the time of conception was associated with a reduced risk of neural tube defect in the offspring. In the third study with a similar protocol, the periconceptional vitamin use was not different between mothers of neural tube defect babies and mothers of other infants.

The most impressive study to date was reported recently by the British Medical Research Council (MRC) Vitamin Study Group. This randomized prevention trial began in July 1983 and was halted in April 1991. It involved 33 centers, 17 in the United Kingdom and 16 in six other countries. Study participants were women who had had a previous pregnancy that resulted in an infant or fetus with a neural tube defect and who were planning a subsequent pregnancy. Each participant was randomly assigned to one of four supplementation groups (Groups A, B, C, and D). Group A received 4 mg of folic acid daily; Group B, a multivitamin preparation plus 4 mg of folic acid; Group C, neither the multivitamin preparation nor folic acid; and Group D, the multivitamin preparation without folic acid. All capsules contained two mineral supplements, ferrous sulfate and di-calcium phosphate.

During the study period, complete information was available on 1195 pregnancy outcomes. Folic acid supplementation was associated with a 71% reduction in the recurrence of neural tube defects. Use of multivitamins without folic acid was not associated with a protective effect. Because of the substantial protective effect, the study data monitoring group recommended halting the study early so that all women at risk could receive the potential benefits of supplementation. Because of these and other findings, the Centers for Disease Control and Prevention recommends the use of folic acid supplementation (4 mg per day) for women who previously have had an infant or fetus with spina bifida, anencephaly or encephalocele.

It is obvious that the last word is not yet in. For the time being, the expert panel from the National Academy of Sciences states: "Pending further research, the subcommittee considers it prudent to supplement the diet with low amounts of folate if there is any question of the adequacy of intake of this vitamin."[7]

Vitamin B$_{12}$

Vitamin B$_{12}$, or cobalamine, like folate, is also an important contributor to the process of cell division. Deficiency of this vitamin can therefore lead to the development of megaloblastic anemia with consequences described above. Fortunately, deficiency of vitamin B$_{12}$ is rare; high-risk women include those who choose a strict vegetarian diet. Such women need vitamin B$_{12}$ supplements of 2 µg per day.[7]

Vitamin B$_6$

Vitamin B$_6$, or pyridoxine, is concerned with amino acid metabolism and protein synthesis. In its active form of pyridoxal phosphate the vitamin is a cofactor in reactions involving a group of enzymes known as transaminases. Vitamin B$_6$ requirements increase in pregnancy not only because of the greater need for nonessential amino acids in growth but also because the body is making more niacin from tryptophan.

Fetal needs. Urinary excretion of vitamin B$_6$ metabolites during pregnancy is 10 to 15 times higher than in nonpregnant women, but blood values are typically reduced. Investigators are not sure of the clinical significance of this. There is evidence that the placenta concentrates vitamin B_6 and that levels in cord blood are much higher than in the maternal circulation. This could mean that the reduced maternal blood levels are simply the result of physiologic adjustments. On the other hand, there is also evidence that the fetus takes up more vitamin B_6 and that maternal levels increase when oral supplements are used.[38] Limited animal data suggest adverse pregnancy outcome in the presence of vitamin B_6 deficiency.[39] In addition, European researchers[40] observed that the depth of pregnancy depression correlated negatively with serum vitamin B_6 concentration. Roepke and Kirksey[41] and Schuster's group[42] observed significantly lower Apgar scores in newborns of mothers with evidence of vitamin B_6 deficiency when compared with offspring of controls. The meaning of these observations remains to be determined.

Maternal nausea and vomiting. While the precise etiology of nausea and vomiting during pregnancy remains unknown, interest continues in the possibility that vitamin B_6 status may be important. Vitamin B_6 is known to catalyze a number of reactions involving neurotransmitter production and in that capacity could conceivably affect an assortment of physiologic states. However, a clear connection between vitamin B_6 and pregnancy nausea remains to be observed.[43,44] In one small study[45] relief of symptoms of pregnancy sickness appeared to be superior in women using Bendectin (an anti-nausea drug now off the market) with added vitamin B_6, as compared with women using Bendectin alone. Additional controlled double-blind studies are required to draw any firm conclusions about the value of vitamin B_6 supplements in the management of nausea during pregnancy.

Vitamin C

Vitamin C deficiency has not been shown to affect the course or outcome of pregnancy in humans. But questions have arisen about the possible association of vitamin C with several specific conditions made known through isolated clinical observations. For example, low plasma levels of vitamin C have been reported in association with premature rupture of the membranes[46] and preeclampsia.[47] An extra 10 mg of vitamin C a day is recommended for the pregnant woman. This total recommendation of 70 mg a day is easily met by the U.S. diet. Large intakes of vitamin C supplements may adversely influence fetal metabolism. Metabolic dependency on high doses may develop in the fetus, causing possible scurvy in the neonatal period.[48,49]

Thiamin, Riboflavin, and Niacin

Since thiamin, riboflavin, and niacin are all part of the reactions that produce energy in the body, requirements are related to caloric intake. Since kilocalorie allowances increase during pregnancy, the allowances for thiamin, riboflavin, and niacin automatically increase also. In addition, evidence from urinary excretion studies indicates that pregnant women have higher requirements for thiamin and riboflavin than nonpregnant women. The RDA for these two nutrients therefore include additional adjustments.

In animals, severe deficiencies of thiamin, riboflavin, or niacin during pregnancy have resulted in fetal death, reduced growth, and congenital malformation. The skeleton and organs that arise from the ectoderm appear to be especially susceptible to riboflavin deficiency. Lack of riboflavin in the mother's diet was once thought to be a cause of prematurity in humans, but recent studies have failed to find a correlation.

Researchers have evaluated the thiamin status of pregnant women at various stages of gestation and have found that 25% to 30% have values that would be considered deficient by nonpregnant standards. Although there have been some reported cases of congenital beriberi from maternal thiamin deficiency, there is no evidence of impairment at the levels consumed by women in developed countries. The niacin status of pregnant women has been inadequately investigated. However, there are no cases indicating that niacin deficiency in humans produces the malformations noted in experimental animals.

Vitamin D

Vitamin D has long been appreciated for its positive effects on calcium balance during pregnancy. Evidence suggests that vitamin D may be involved in neonatal calcium homeostasis. Observations in Great Britain indicate that the peak season for neonatal hypocalcemia coincides with the time of least sunlight.[50] In addition, serum vitamin D levels are often low in such infants, suggesting that some cases of neonatal hypocalcemia and enamel hypoplasia may relate to maternal vitamin D deficiency and subsequent limitation in placental transport of vitamin D to the fetus.[51,52] A study of pregnant Asian women showed that vitamin D supplementation during the third trimester was associated with an improved rate of maternal weight gain, higher maternal and newborn serum 25 (OH)D levels at term, a reduced incidence of symptomatic hypocalcemia in newborns, and a lower percentage of small-for-gestational-age infants.[53] However excessive amounts of vitamin D may be harmful during gestation. Severe infantile hypercalcemia and associated problems have been reported in newborn animals and in human infants.

Vitamin A

Both vitamin A and carotene cross the placenta, and fetal storage of vitamin A accounts in part for the recommendation that pregnant women consume an extra 1000 IU of this vitamin daily. An intake of this level can readily be provided by dietary sources, and there appears to be no need for routine supplementation. Although vitamin A deficiency is teratogenic in lower animals, confirmatory evidence in humans is lacking. Excessive use and the toxic effects have posed problems.

Megadose toxicity. Excessive vitamin A consumption is believed to be teratogenic in humans, but most scientific evidence describes developmental anomalies in animals. However, one report has described a human infant with congenital renal anomalies associated with maternal ingestion of large doses of vitamin A, about 10 times the RDA, during pregnancy.[54] Another report[55] from Scandinavia indicated that a **microcephalic** child with multiple malformations of the central nervous system was born to a mother who consumed 150,000 IU of vitamin A daily during gestation days 19 to 40.

Vitamin A analog. The adverse effects of excessive vitamin A intake in early pregnancy have been dramatically illustrated by the recent introduction of isotretinoin (Accutane) into the marketplace.[56-58] This drug, used for the treatment of cystic acne, is an analog of vitamin A. Since its first appearance on pharmacy shelves in the early 1980s, cases of birth defects and spontaneous abortion have been associated with its use. This toxicity syndrome has been called the *isotretinoin teratogen syndrome* and was described by Benke.[56] Major features include prominent **frontal bossing, hydrocephalus, microphthalmia,** and small, malformed, low-set, undifferentiated ears (Fig. 4-14). More cautionary labeling has now been provided with the product and physicians are warned about the possible dangers of prenatal exposure.[58]

Vitamin E

Requirements for vitamin E are believed to increase somewhat during pregnancy, but deficiency in humans rarely occurs and has not been linked with either reproductive causality or reduced fertility. Since vitamin E deficiency in experimental animals has long been associated with spontaneous abortion, interest in the use of vitamin E for prevention of abortion has been a popular idea. In general, however, studies in humans have not supported this preventive measure. Several studies have shown, however, that the fetal vitamin E level is one third to one fourth the maternal concentration in both premature and term infants. Maternal levels of vitamin E rise during pregnancy such that by the third trimester these levels become 60% greater than in the nonpregnant controls. It has been found, however, that the maternal level must be from 150% to 500% of the value of the

Microcephaly
(Gr *mikros,* small; *kephale,* head) Small size of the head in relation to the rest of the body.

Frontal bossing
(ME *boce,* lump, growth) A rounded protuberance of the forehead. In general, a boss is a knob-like rounded protuberance on the body or some body organ.

Hydrocephalus
(Gr *hydro,* water; *kephale,* head) Condition characterized by enlargement of the cranium caused by abnormal accumulation of fluid.

Microphthalmia
(Gr *mikros,* small; *ophthalmos,* eye) Abnormal smallness of one or both eyes.

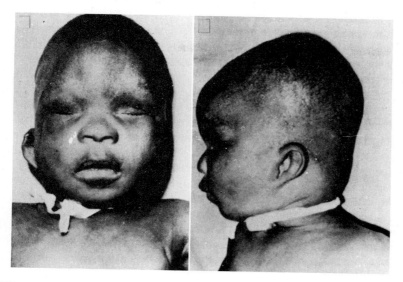

FIG. 4-14   Front and lateral view of a child affected prenatally by isotretinoin. From Benke PJ: *JAMA* 251:3267, 1984.

nonpregnant controls if the cord blood values are to reach the low normal adult vitamin E concentrations.

Although the vitamin E level in the infant at birth is significantly less than in the mother, the infant's level has been shown to correlate directly with the maternal concentration.[59] Attempts to raise the fetal level by supplementing the mother with vitamin E during the last trimester confirmed the direct correlation of fetal and maternal vitamin E concentrations. It has been concluded, however, that parenteral vitamin E administration to the mother before delivery is not enough to prevent an infant from having the hemolytic anemia of vitamin E deficiency. Since this problem develops within 6 weeks after birth, it can best be prevented by oral supplementation of the infant during the postnatal interval.

Vitamin K

Data are insufficient for the RDA committee of experts to establish a standard for vitamin K during pregnancy. Additional increments to usual intakes are not recommended because consumption of this vitamin by adult women exceeds the RDA. Efforts to determine if vitamin K supplementation of pregnant women can improve the vitamin K status of their preterm offspring have yielded conflicting results.[60,61]

Other Vitamins

Little is known about the dietary requirements for biotin and pantothenic acid. Safe and adequate dietary intakes for these vitamins were suggested in the 1989 edition of the RDA (Table 4-10).

Iron

During pregnancy, iron is needed for the manufacture of hemoglobin in both maternal and fetal red blood cells. The fetus accumulates most of its iron during the last trimester. At term a normal-weight infant has about 246 mg of iron in blood and body stores. An additional 134 mg are stored in the placenta. About 290 mg are used to expand the volume of the mother's blood.

Maintenance of **erythropoiesis** is one of the few instances during pregnancy when the

Erythropoiesis
(Gr *erythros*, red; *poiesis*, making) Production of erythrocytes, red blood cells.

TABLE 4-10 *Estimated Safe and Adequate Daily Dietary Intakes of Additional Selected Vitamins and Minerals for Adolescents and Adults*

	Age Group	
	Adolescents	Adults
Age	11+	
Vitamins		
Biotin (µg)	30-100	30-100
Pantothenic acid (mg)	4-7	4-7
Trace elements (mg)		
Copper	1.5-2.5	1.5-3.0
Manganese	2.0-5.0	2.0-5.0
Fluoride	1.5-2.5	1.5-4.0
Chromium	0.05-0.2	0.05-0.2
Molybdenum	0.075-0.250	0.075-0.250

Modified from Food and Nutrition Board, National Research Council, National Academy of Sciences: *Recommended dietary allowances,* Washington, DC, 1989, US Government Printing Office.

fetus acts as a true parasite. It assures its own production of hemoglobin by drawing iron from the mother. Maternal iron deficiency, therefore, does not usually result in an infant who is anemic at birth. The most common cause of iron deficiency anemia in the infant is prematurity. The infant who has a short gestation simply does not have time to accumulate sufficient iron during the last trimester.[62]

Iron deficiency in the mother may have adverse effects on her obstetric performance.[63] A reduction in hemoglobin concentration means that the mother must increase her cardiac output to maintain adequate oxygen use by placental and fetal cells. This extra work fatigues the mother and makes her more susceptible to other sources of physiologic stress. A very low maternal hemoglobin places the mother at risk of cardiac arrest and leads to a poor prognosis for survival should she hemorrhage on delivery.

Setting requirements for iron during pregnancy is complicated by changes in the erythropoiesis system. Even when women have adequate iron status at conception, the plasma volume increases faster than the number of red blood cells so that hemodilution occurs. However, erythropoiesis is stimulated in the last half of pregnancy, and the rate of red blood cell production goes up. If sufficient iron is available, hemoglobin levels should rise to at least 11 mg/100 ml by term.

Generally, the initial drop in hemoglobin is a normal physiologic phenomenon, but there is concern that the usual iron intakes of pregnant women may not support increased erythropoiesis and fetal demands in the last half of pregnancy.[64] Iron absorption increases during pregnancy (to as much as 30%) compared with the usual 10% absorption from the diet. Also working in the mother's favor is the 120 mg or so that she saves over the course of gestation because she is not menstruating. However, even when these adjustments are taken into account, the pregnant woman still may need to consume about 30 mg of iron each day to maintain iron reserves. This amount could be supplied if large servings of iron-rich foods were eaten, but unfortunately, such foods are limited to organ meats, oysters, clams, and prune juice. These are not foods that people typically consume. From an average mixed diet, about 6 mg of iron are obtained from each 1000 kcal of food. At this rate a pregnant woman would have to eat 3000 to 5000 kcal of food per day to meet her iron needs. Furthermore, studies have shown that most women enter pregnancy with low iron stores so they have little to draw on to maintain normal hemoglobin.

For this reason, the expert panel from the National Academy of Sciences[7] concluded:

"Iron is the only nutrient for which requirements cannot be met reasonably by diet alone. To meet the increased need for iron during the second and third trimesters of pregnancy, the average woman needs to absorb approximately 3 mg of iron per day in addition to the amount of iron usually absorbed from food. Evidence from iron supplementation studies indicates that low-dose supplements (e.g., 30 mg of ferrous iron daily during the second and third trimesters) can provide this amount of extra iron." The committee went on to say that since low doses of iron pose no known dangers to the mother or fetus, the potential benefits of iron supplementation outweigh the risks.

Calcium

The fetus acquires most of its calcium in the last trimester when skeletal growth is maximum and teeth are being formed. Widdowson[65] has calculated that the fetus draws 13 mg per hour of calcium from the maternal blood supply, or 250 to 300 mg per day. At birth the infant has accumulated approximately 25 g. Additional calcium is stored in the maternal skeleton as a reserve for lactation.

Extensive adjustments in calcium metabolism are routinely observed in the pregnant woman.[66] Hormonal factors are largely responsible.

1. **Human chorionic somatomammotropin** (from placenta). Progressively enhances the rate of bone turnover throughout pregnancy.
2. **Estrogen** (largely from placenta). Inhibits bone resorption and thus provokes a compensatory release of parathyroid hormone (PTH), which maintains the serum calcium level while enhancing intestinal calcium absorption and decreasing its urinary excretion.

The net effect of this hormonal action is the promotion of progressive calcium retention. The prenatal changes begin well ahead of the time when fetal mineralization starts. It thus appears that anticipatory adjustments prepare the maternal organism for the increased calcium demands later on. Mineralization of the fetal skeleton is ultimately stimulated, largely through active placental calcium transport, leading to fetal hypercalcemia and subsequent endocrine adjustments. Vitamin D and its metabolites also cross the placenta and appear in fetal blood in the same concentration found in maternal circulation.

The current RDA standard for calcium during pregnancy is 1200 mg daily, a level 400 mg higher than recommended for the nonpregnant woman. Some argue that this allowance is set too high, since apparently successful pregnancies occur in many other cultures with calcium intakes substantially below those recommended. The explanation likely relates to the large calcium reservoir in the maternal skeleton, of which the total requirements of pregnancy amounts to about 2.5%. Also, in many other cultures diets contain less protein and this factor might serve to reduce the degree of calcium loss in the urine. Researchers[67] have reported data from balance studies suggesting that if maternal intake of calcium is low, stores of calcium will be depleted to meet fetal needs. If this is the case, frequent pregnancies and consistently low calcium intakes throughout the childbearing years could contribute to suboptimal bone density in later life. Clinical osteomalacia in **multiparous** women has been observed.[68]

Whether or not calcium status is etiologically related to the development of pregnancy-induced hypertension is currently the subject of much debate. Several studies have been conducted to determine if calcium supplementation reduces the incidence of this problem.[69-72] Results to date are highly suggestive of beneficial effects from calcium supplementation. A large, multicenter trial is scheduled in the United States to further explore the role that calcium might play in this mysterious prenatal condition.

Multiparous
(L *multus*, many; *parere*, to bring forth) Referring to women who have had two or more pregnancies resulting in live births.

Phosphorus

The RDA standard for phosphorus is the same as that for calcium, 800 mg with an extra 400 mg during pregnancy. It is so widely available in foods that a dietary deficiency is rare.

In fact, it is possible that many problems may be caused by too much phosphorus rather than too little. Most adults can tolerate relatively wide variation in dietary calcium-phosphorus ratios when vitamin D is adequate.

Calcium-phosphorus balance relates to maintenance of normal neuromuscular action. Twenty years ago it was suggested that sudden clonic or tonic contractions of the *gastrocnemius muscle* (posterior "calf" muscle that flexes knee and ankle joints), occurring often at night, was caused by a decline in serum calcium. Prevention or relief was proclaimed to come from reduction of milk intake, a high phosphorus and calcium beverage. Supplementation with nonphosphate calcium salts was also recommended, along with regular use of aluminum hydroxide to form insoluble aluminum phosphate salts in the gut. While anecdotal reports have suggested benefit of these measures, controlled and double blind studies have failed to show any correlation between leg cramps and either intake of dairy products or the type of calcium supplement used.

Magnesium

Magnesium is much like calcium and phosphorus in that most of it is stored in the bones. The amounts that are biochemically active are concentrated in nerve and muscle cells. Deficiencies of magnesium produce neuromuscular dysfunction characterized by tremors and convulsions. Magnesium-deficient pregnant rats show impaired abdominal contractions during parturition. Not a great deal is known about the need for magnesium during pregnancy. The RDA standard is based on estimates of the amounts accumulated by the mother and the fetus.

Zinc

Zinc has an active role in metabolism for several reasons: (1) it is a component of insulin, (2) it is part of the carbonic anhydrase enzyme system that helps maintain acid-base balance in the tissues, and (3) it acts in the synthesis of DNA and RNA, which gives it a very important role in reproduction.

Much recent interest has centered on the significance of zinc deficiency in adversely affecting pregnancy course and outcome.[73-76] Zinc is a known constituent of a number of important metalloenzymes and a necessary cofactor for other enzymes. Zinc deficiency in rats leads to development of congenital malformations (Table 4-11).[77] Nonhuman primates also are affected. Abnormal brain development and behavior have been described in offspring of zinc-deficient monkeys.[78] Evidence from human populations suggests that the malformation rate and other poor pregnancy outcomes may be higher in populations where zinc deficiency has been recognized.[79-81] For example, Jameson[82] observed in Scandinavia that women with low serum levels of zinc had higher incidence of abnormal deliveries, including congenital malformations. However, since conflicting reports also appear in the literature[83-85] and questions remain about satisfactory measures of zinc status, the true role of zinc deficiency in adverse course and outcome of human pregnancy remains unknown. The potential hazard of prenatal zinc supplements has not been determined in human populations. Haphazard use of such supplements, however, has no role in wise prenatal care.

Iodine

For many years it has been understood that maternal iodine deficiency leads to cretinism in offspring. It is still seen in some parts of the world today. Recent data also suggest that suboptimum iodine nutrition of the mother may compromise development of her fetus, even when cretinism does not occur. Several research groups[86] have evaluated the performance of children born to mothers living in iodine-deficient regions of New Guinea and India. Children born to mothers given adequate iodine were significantly faster and more accurate in tests of mental and manual function than children of control mothers.

TABLE 4-11 *Types and Incidence of Congenital Malformations in Zinc-Deficient Rat Fetuses**

Malformations	Percent of Fetuses
Cleft lip	7
Cleft palate	42
Brain†	47
Micro- or *anophthalmia*	42
Micro- or *agnathia*	14
Spina bifida	3
Clubbed legs	38
Fore	10
Hind	35
Syndactyly	64
Tail	72
Dorsal herniation	1
Diaphragmatic herniation	8
Umbilical herniation	7
Heart‡	2
Lungs§	54
Urogenital	21

From Hurley LS, Gowan J, Swenerton H: Teratogenic effects of short term and transitory zinc deficiency in rats, *Teratology* 4:199, 1971.
*Based on 101 full-term fetuses from 14 litters.
†Hydrocephalus, anencephalus, hydrencephalus, and some exencephalus.
‡Primary transposition of great vessels and abnormal position of heart.
§Small or missing holes.

These findings indicate that iodine deficiency may lead to a spectrum of subclinical deficits that place children at a developmental disadvantage.

Fluoride

The role of fluoride in prenatal development is poorly understood at present. Some questions have existed over the past 50 years about the degree of fluoride transport across the placenta. Should it cross the placenta, questions still remain about its value in the development of caries-resistant permanent teeth.

Development of the primary dentition begins at 10 to 12 weeks of pregnancy. From the sixth to ninth months of pregnancy, the first four permanent molars and eight of the permanent incisors begin to form. Thus 32 of the ultimate teeth are forming and developing during human pregnancy. Since there is no indication that color of the teeth is adversely affected and some evidence that caries resistance and morphologic characteristics are improved, prenatal fluoride supplementation may be justified. *It should be recognized, however, that this issue is highly controversial and to date formal support for routine prenatal fluoride supplementation has not been voiced by any established medical or dental organization.*

Sodium

The metabolism of sodium is altered during pregnancy under the stimulus of a modified hormonal milieu. Glomerular filtration increases markedly over time to "clean up" the increased maternal blood volume. An additional filtered sodium load of 5000 to 10,000 mEq daily is typically seen during pregnancy. Compensatory mechanisms come into play to maintain fluid and electrolyte balance.

Restriction of dietary sodium has been common in the past among pregnant women with edema, but moderate edema is normal during pregnancy and should not be combated with diuretics and low-sodium diets. The increased fluid retained normally during pregnancy actually somewhat increases the body's demand for sodium. Rigorous sodium restriction in pregnant animals stresses the renin-angiotensin-aldosterone system to the point of breakdown. Such animals show reduced weight gain and altered fluid consumption patterns.[87] They also tend to develop water intoxication along with renal and adrenal tissue degeneration.[88] Neonatal hyponatremia (low blood sodium) has been observed in offspring of women who unduly restricted sodium intake before delivery.[89] The damage potential to the maternal renin-angiotensin-aldosterone system also exists. Although moderation in the American habit of excessive salt use is appropriate for all people, aggressive restriction is unwarranted during pregnancy. No less than 2 to 3 g of sodium should be consumed daily.

Other Minerals

One of the more recent advances in nutrition research is the discovery that many other trace elements are necessary for human growth, general health, and reproduction. Chromium, manganese, copper, selenium, molybdenum, vanadium, tin, nickel, and silicon have all been shown to be needed by the body. Like iodine, calcium, and phosphorus, these elements (and likely others as well) participate in reactions that control body processes. Studies in animals have revealed that deficiencies produce widespread and serious metabolic defects. Limited knowledge of requirements in humans makes it impossible to establish RDA standards for the majority of these minerals. The current RDA does, however, list estimated safe and adequate daily dietary intakes for copper, manganese, fluoride, chromium, and molybdenum (see Table 4-10). No figures are available for pregnant women. Since toxic levels for many of the trace elements may be much higher than usual intakes, pregnant women should not take supplements that would greatly exceed the upper limits recommended.

FOOD BELIEFS, CRAVINGS, AVOIDANCES, AND AVERSIONS

Most women change their diets during the course of pregnancy. Some changes are based on medical advice, others on folk medical beliefs, and others on changes in preference and appetite that may be idiosyncratic or culturally patterned. Since those changes that are culturally sanctioned will affect a woman's willingness to follow prescribed dietary regimens, the health care provider should be sensitized to their existence.

Food Beliefs and Food Behaviors

Many beliefs have been recorded about prenatal diet, such as the idea that the mother can mark her child before birth by eating specific foods. Overuse of a craved food during pregnancy is thought to explain physical or behavioral peculiarities of the infant. More often, unsatiated cravings are thought to explain birthmarks that mimic the shape of the desired food (such as strawberry- or drumstick-shaped marks). Behavioral markings have also been thought to derive from the prenatal diet; that is, the mother's consumption of many foods has been said to cause the child to like such foods after birth.

Another important group of beliefs concerns dietary means by which the mother can ensure an easier delivery. Most important, from the biomedical viewpoint, are beliefs that

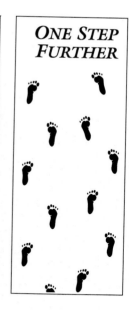

ONE STEP FURTHER

Should Supplements be Recommended for all Women With Childbearing Potential?

Potential supplement benefits
1. Improved nutritional status
2. Reduced risk of some developmental defects
3. Improved antioxidant and immune status
4. Lower incidence and slower progression of some diseases
5. Harmonization of government and health professionals' dietary recommendations for optimal health.

Questions:
1. Will the supplement reduce the women's motivation to maintain and/or improve dietary quality?
2. Will the supplement result in excessive nutrient intakes and adverse nutrient/nutrient interactions?
3. Will supplement use encourage the perception that all women are, by definition, well nourished?

lead a woman to avoid animal protein foods or to avoid "excessive" weight gain. Most lay people know very well that a smaller weight gain during pregnancy produces a smaller infant. Thus, since a smaller baby may be "easier to deliver," low weight gain has been proposed as desirable, especially since it is commonly believed that the baby can "catch up" after birth.

Food avoidances are those foods that the mother consciously chooses not to consume during her pregnancy, usually for a reason she can articulate and that seems reasonable to her. The four most commonly avoided foods are sources of animal protein: milk, lean meats, pork, and liver. Cravings and aversions are powerful urges toward or away from foods, including foods about which women experience no unusual attitudes outside of pregnancy. The most commonly reported craved foods are sweets and dairy products. The most common aversions are reported to be alcohol, caffeinated drinks, and meats. However, cravings and aversions are not limited to any particular food or food groups.

The nutritional significance of these food-related behaviors is difficult to evaluate. Available information has often been collected in an anecdotal or one-sided manner. Thus there is limited detailed information on dietary alterations that appear to be detrimental and little knowledge of total subcultural prenatal dietary intakes. As a result, it is difficult to quantify the nutritional effect of restrictive beliefs, avoidances, cravings, or aversions. The nutritional importance of such practices cannot be assessed without reference to the rest of the woman's diet. Overall, however, most cravings result in increased intakes of calcium and energy, whereas aversions often result in decreased intake of animal protein. Such cravings and aversions are not necessarily deleterious.

Pica

One type of compulsive food behavior or craving during pregnancy, however, does carry potential danger.[90-92] This practice is termed *pica* (from the Latin word for magpie, with reference to the bird's **omnivorous** appetite). Human pica refers to the compulsion for persistent ingestion of unsuitable substances having little or no nutritional value. Pica of pregnancy most often involves consumption of dirt or clay (geophagia) or starch (amylophagia). However, compulsive ingestion of a variety of nonfood substances such as ice, burnt matches, hair, stone or gravel, charcoal, soot, cigarette ashes, mothballs, antacid

Omnivorous
(L *omnis*, all; *vorare*, to eat) Eating all kinds of foods, both animal and plant.

tablets, milk of magnesia, baking soda, coffee grounds, and tire inner tubes has been noted. The practice of pica is not new nor is it limited to any one geographic area, race, creed, culture, sex, or status within a culture.

The medical implications of pica are not well understood, although several speculations have been made. The displacement effect of pica substances could result in reduced intake of nutritious foods, leading to inadequate dietary intakes of essential nutrients. Alternatively, substances that provide kilocalories, for example, starch, could lead to obesity if ingested in large amounts above the usual dietary intakes. Some pica substances may contain toxic compounds or quantities of nutrients not tolerated in disease states. Some pica substances interfere with the absorption of certain mineral elements, such as iron. Other less commonly reported complications of pica include:

1. **Lead poisoning.** Congenital lead poisoning secondary to maternal pica for wall plaster.
2. **Irritable uterus.** Tender, irritable uterus with dystocia associated with fecal impaction from clay ingestion.
3. **Anemia.** Fetal hemolytic anemia caused by maternal ingestion of mothballs and toilet air fresheners.
4. **Obstruction.** Parotid enlargement and gastric and small bowel obstruction from ingestion of excessive laundry starch.
5. **Infection.** Parasitic infection from ingestion of contaminated soil or clay.

The etiology of pica is poorly understood, although several proposals have been made. One theory suggests that the ingestion of nonfood substances relieves nausea and vomiting. Another theory suggests that the deficiency of an essential nutrient such as calcium or iron results in the eating of nonfood substances that contain these nutrients. When pregnant women were questioned about the practice of pica, they gave a variety of answers:

- A taste for clay existed.
- Clay kept the baby from being marked at birth.
- Nervous tension was relieved.
- Starch made the newborn lighter in color.
- Starch helped the baby "slide out" more easily during delivery.
- Clay quieted hunger pains.
- Clay and starch were pleasant to chew.
- Pica carries social approval.

Many of these reasons given are based on superstition, customs and traditions, or practices passed from mother to daughter over generations. Two examples of pica, one of which caused maternal death, are described in the box above.

EFFECTS OF POTENTIALLY HARMFUL FOOD COMPONENTS

A number of food components have shown harmful effects on the course and outcome of pregnancy. Several of these agents and their effects are described here, including alcohol, caffeine, food additives, and food contaminants.

Alcohol

Fetal alcohol syndrome (FAS). During the past 15 years health researchers have become aware of the adverse effect of excessive consumption of alcohol on fetal development. In 1973 pediatricians in Seattle, Washington, described a unique set of characteristics of infants born to women who were chronic alcoholics. These infants exhibited specific anomalies of the eyes, nose, heart, and central nervous system that were accompanied by growth retardation, small head circumference, and mental retardation (Fig. 4-15). The investigators named the condition *fetal alcohol syndrome* (Table 4-12). The condition does not necessarily lead to death but is associated with permanent disabilities (Fig. 4-16).

There is a high rate of prenatal mortality among infants with FAS. Infants who survive are generally irritable and hyperactive after birth. These symptoms are attributed to alcohol withdrawal. Physical and mental development is impaired. FAS infants exhibit poor rates of weight gain and failure to thrive despite concerted efforts at nutritional rehabilitation. The box on p. 144 illustrates the occurrence of FAS due to maternal ingestion of alcohol, in this instance in the unusual form of large amounts of cough syrup.

Fetal alcohol effects. The impact of more moderate levels of alcohol consumption on fetal development has been the focus of much research during the past decade. It is now well recognized that moderate drinkers may produce offspring with "fetal alcohol effects" showing more subtle features of FAS. Such women also demonstrate a higher rate of spontaneous abortion, abruptio placentae, and low-birth-weight delivery.

General actions of alcohol. At present, the mechanisms by which alcohol produces such widespread effects on the fetus are not completely understood. Since alcohol can cross the placenta, the current hypothesis is that high alcohol levels build up in the fetus and produce direct toxic effects that are most severe in the early phases of pregnancy during blastogenesis and cell differentiation. Another theory is that some of the effects of alcohol may be caused by maternal malnutrition. We may not think of alcohol as a food, but it yields 7 kcal/g. Alcohol is considered an "empty kilocalorie" food because most alcoholic beverages supply little or no nutrients. Women who derive a substantial portion of their

CASE STUDY

Pica Cases
Case 1

In England a 21-year-old woman was hospitalized at 38 weeks gestation because of severe anemia. She was generally tired, occasionally dizzy, and had edema of the ankles and mild anorexia. After 3 weeks of concentrated treatment with iron and folic acid she showed no improvement. Through further questioning it was found that throughout her pregnancy she had been eating toilet air freshener blocks at the rate of one to two per week. Cessation of this practice led to immediate improvement.

Case 2

A 31-year-old black woman was admitted to a rural emergency room with extreme weakness, severe nausea and vomiting, and fever. The patient reported no bowel movements during the preceding 2 weeks. On examination she was lethargic and appeared critically ill. Within 10 minutes of arrival she experienced a grand mal seizure followed by cardiorespiratory arrest. Efforts at resuscitation were unsuccessful and the woman died. Autopsy findings included 3 L of pus within the peritoneal cavity and a 4 cm perforation of the sigmoid colon. Free within the cavity were stones measuring 2.5 cm in diameter and a clay ball measuring 5 cm in diameter. Near the site of perforation, the colon was impacted with hardened claylike material. Subsequent inquiry of the family revealed that clay ingestion in the rural area was commonplace, and the husband noted that three of the patient's four children occasionally ate clay from the same bank their mother had used.

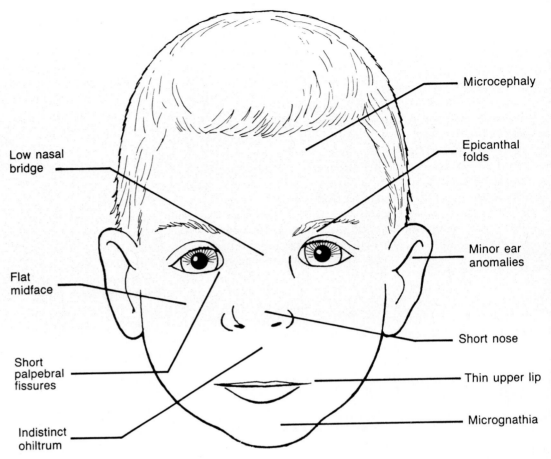

Microcephaly

Epicanthal folds

Minor ear anomalies

Short nose

Thin upper lip

Micrognathia

Low nasal bridge

Flat midface

Short palpebral fissures

Indistinct ohiltrum

FIG. 4-15   Facial characteristics in fetal alcohol syndrome.

TABLE 4-12   Facial Characteristics in Fetal Alcohol Syndrome

	Features Necessary to Characteristic Face	**Associated Features**
Eyes	Short palpebral fissures	
Nose	Short and upturned in early childhood, hypoplastic philtrum	Flat nasal bridge; epicanthal folds
Maxilla	Flattened	
Mouth	Thinned upper vermilion	Prominent lateral palatine ridges, cleft lip with or without cleft palate; small teeth
Mandible		Retrognathia in infancy; micrognathia or relative prognathia in adolescents
Ears		Posterior rotation, abnormal concha

From Clarren and Smith, *N Engl J Med* 298:1063-67, 1978. Reprinted with permission from *The New England Journal of Medicine*.

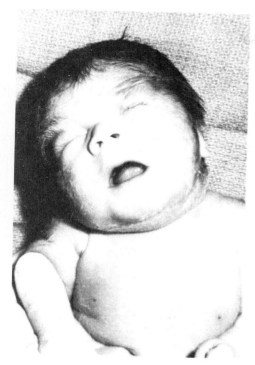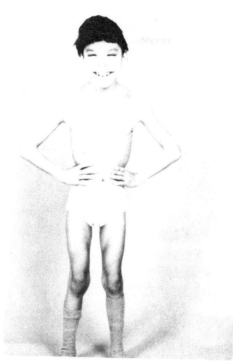

FIG. 4-16   Child with FAS at day 1 and 8 years of age. This child was diagnosed at birth and has spent all his life in a foster home where the quality of care has been excellent. His IQ has remained stable at 40 to 45. Although he is more seriously retarded than most children with FAS, he demonstrates the resistance of the disability to environmental intervention.

Courtesy of Dr. Ann P. Streissguth, University of Washington, Seattle.

daily caloric needs from alcohol may not have an appetite for more nutritious foods. Deficiencies of folic acid, magnesium, and zinc have been shown to be highly teratogenic in animals, so it is reasonable to suspect that deficiencies of these nutrients could play a role in FAS.

Alcohol used by pregnant women. Although the adverse effects of maternal alcohol consumption on fetal development have been known for over a decade, a significant number of women still choose to drink alcohol while they are pregnant (see box on p. 144.). One research team[93] reported that among women delivering in a large urban hospital in Massachusetts, 82% had consumed alcohol during pregnancy: 3% consumed alcoholic beverages more than 20 times per month, and 3% consumed more than 20 oz (600 ml) per month. Streissguth and coworkers[94] reported patterns of alcohol use among pregnant women in a large urban area who had been exposed to a heavy media campaign aimed at preventing fetal alcohol effects. Looking at precampaign and postcampaign data (1974 to 1975 and 1980 to 1981), the number of women who reported any alcohol use around the time of the first prenatal visit dropped from 81% to 42%, but among drinkers, there was no decrease in the proportion of women who reported heavier drinking. As these authors suggest, the relative constancy in the proportion of "heavier" drinkers and binge drinkers, particularly around the time of conception, indicates the need for more attention to this important period of gestation in advice to women who are planning a pregnancy.

Prenatal care for alcoholic mothers. According to Rosett and colleagues,[95,96] pregnancy course and outcome can be significantly improved if problem drinkers agree to

CASE STUDY

Fetal Alcohol Syndrome

An infant with typical features of FAS, including a head circumference below the tenth percentile on the National Center for Health Statistics growth chart, was born at term to a 24-year-old mother who reported consumption of 480 to 840 ml per day of a nonprescription cough syrup. The alcohol content of the syrup was 9.5%, or 36.5 to 63.8 g per day, equivalent to the alcohol content of 1 to 2 L of 4% beer or 0.5 to 1.0 L of wine.

Intensive prenatal care had been instituted with entry into an addiction treatment program at an undefined point in pregnancy. No evidence of distortion of truth was found with urinary test for substance abuse. Whether pregnancy outcome was related to alcohol, to other drugs, or to their interactive effects is not clear. The case emphasizes the need for awareness of the full content of over-the-counter drugs used in pregnancy.

ALCOHOL INTAKE AND PREGNANCY OUTCOME IN THE UNITED STATES:

• THE FACTS

1. There is no established safe level of alcohol intake during pregnancy.
2. The incidence of fetal alcohol syndrome is estimated at 1 to 3 per 1000 live births. Among Native American groups the rate is as high as 10 per 1000. However, for every child born with FAS, 10 times more suffer from alcohol-related problems.
3. In 1989, the Surgeon General reported that there were at least 5000 infants born each year with fetal alcohol syndrome and 50,000 with fetal alcohol effects.
4. Alcohol abuse is a major preventable cause of low birth weight among infants.
5. Alcohol intake is the primary preventable cause of mental retardation.

change their habits after conception has occurred. These workers reported that infants born to women who reduced their heavy drinking did not differ in growth from offspring of rare and moderate drinkers. They did, however, show a higher frequency of abnormalities. This group urges that facilities providing routine prenatal care integrate therapy for heavy drinking into their counseling sessions. Since the desire to have a healthy baby is a powerful motivating force, therapeutic success can be achieved with some of the heaviest drinkers.

Caffeine

Animal studies. The danger of caffeine to the developing fetus has been studied in several animal models. Massive doses appear to be teratogenic in mice, but the effects of smaller quantities have not been satisfactorily examined. One research group[97] did observe that offspring of rats fed coffee during pregnancy had reduced body, liver, and brain weight at birth. By 39 days, these animals had recovered in size but demonstrated increased locomotion, decreased grooming time, and decreased time spent with a novel object. Another research team[98] reported that when caffeine was introduced into the diet of rats throughout pregnancy and lactation, offspring of successive pregnancies showed growth reductions, although teratogenic effects were not seen with this moderate level of caffeine exposure.

A 1980 report from the Food and Drug Administration (FDA) suggested that rather modest amounts of caffeine provided to pregnant rats may increase the incidence of defects in development of the digits.[99] Pregnant rats provided an amount of caffeine (per unit size) equivalent to about 12 to 40 cups of coffee per day for humans produced offspring with an increased incidence of partial or complete absence of the digits of the paws. A Virginia woman subsequently claimed that her 15-year-old child with no fingers or toes was damaged in utero by her daily consumption of 10 to 12 cups of coffee. Although data were limited in relation to human use of caffeine in pregnancy, a general warning was voiced to the public in 1981 to avoid unnecessary caffeine consumption during pregnancy.

Conclusions. Since this warning was released in the early 1980s, systematic observations of large groups of pregnant women have not provided cause for alarm.[100-102]

During the past decade, at least eight studies have dealt with the incidence of birth defects in children and caffeine consumption of their mothers. No associations have been found. In one study, more than 12,000 women were questioned soon after delivery about coffee and tea consumption. No relationship was found between coffee and tea consumption and excess malformations among their babies. Another study published the same year involved 2,030 infants, examined for a relationship between their mother's caffeine intake during pregnancy and six specific birth defects (inguinal hernia, cleft lip with and without cleft palate, isolated cleft palate, cardiac defects, pyloric stenosis and neural tube defects). The findings were negative and the authors concluded that maternal ingestion of caffeine in tea, coffee, and cola has a minimal, if any, effect on incidence of those six birth defects.

However, another recent report suggested that a rather low level of daily caffeine consumption (about 150 mg) is associated with greater risk of late first and second trimester spontaneous abortion.[103]

A prospective cohort study involved over 3,000 women in Connecticut. Almost 80% of these pregnant women used some caffeine daily and 28% consumed ≥ 150 mg caffeine each day. This latter group of moderate to heavy users of caffeine was significantly more likely to experience late first and second trimester spontaneous abortion when compared with nonusers and light users (0 to 149 mg daily) of caffeine. While this report does suggest some cause for concern, the authors wisely point out that confirmation of these findings through additional research is essential before implicating caffeine in the etiology of spontaneous abortion.

Since available data from observations of human populations are inconclusive, common sense suggests that caution should be exercised and pregnant women should be advised to use caffeine in moderation, if at all.

Food Additives

The teratogenicity of common food additives is largely unknown in human situations. Metabolism of cyclamate and red dye no. 2 reportedly damage developing rat embryos,[104] but both of these additives have now been banned for use in the U.S. food supply. Saccharin, mannitol, xylitol, aspartame, and other artificial sugar substitutes have come under careful scrutiny in the last several decades. Kline and co-workers[105] have reported, however, that incidence of spontaneous abortion in a human population was not associated with ingestion of any sugar substitute.

Saccharin. Because saccharin has been shown to be weakly carcinogenic in rats, moderation in its use seems appropriate. This is especially true for women of reproductive age, since studies in rats indicate that saccharin can most effectively initiate bladder cancer when the mother is exposed to high doses before pregnancy and the offspring are exposed in utero and throughout their lives. Saccharin can also markedly promote or enhance the potential of other carcinogens in rats, providing another reason for moderation in use.[106]

Aspartame. The increasing use of aspartame in the American food supply has been associated with outcries from a minority of scientists who propose that one or more of the breakdown products of aspartame may interfere with normal fetal development. Chemically, aspartame is L-aspartyl-L-phenylalanine methyl ester. The dipeptide ester is metabolized into three moieties in the small intestine, so that studies of the safety of aspartame are essentially studies of aspartic acid, phenylalanine, and methanol.

Human studies with pregnant women. Human subjects have been fed up to six times the 99th percentile of the projected daily intake (6 × 34 = 200 mg/kg). No evidence of risk to the fetus has been observed. Aspartate does not readily cross the placenta. Small elevations of blood methanol following the above abuse doses of aspartame have not led to measurable increases in blood formic acid, which is the product responsible for the acidosis and ocular toxicity of methanol poisoning. Phenylalanine is concentrated on the fetal side of the placenta.

Phenylalanine and PKU. The phenylalanine component of aspartame has raised the most concern due to the unknown damaging impact of phenylalanine on brain tissue of children with phenylketonuria (PKU). Individuals with this genetic disease lack the liver enzyme that converts phenylalanine to tyrosine. Thus blood levels of phenylalanine rise to high levels and mental retardation is the ultimate result. Aspartame in abuse doses up to 200 mg/kg in normal subjects, or to 100 mg/kg in PKU **heterozygotes** (carriers of the gene for PKU), have not been found to raise blood phenylalanine levels to the range generally accepted to be associated with mental retardation in offspring.

Conclusions. One might conclude that, under foreseeable conditions of use, aspartame poses no risk for use in pregnancy. However, since limited data are available to date on pregnancy course and outcome in heavy aspartame users, it may be wise to recommend moderation in aspartame use during pregnancy, especially in women known to be PKU heterozygotes.

Heterozygote
(Gr *hetero,* other; *zygotos,* yoked together) Individual possessing different *alleles* (gene forms occupying corresponding chromosome sites) in regard to a given trait.

Food Contaminants

General toxicity. A number of "contaminants" are found in food. Some of these may adversely affect pregnancy course and outcome if consumed in sufficient amounts. Most heavy metals are embryotoxic but only mercury, lead, cadmium, and possibly nickel and selenium have been implicated in this regard. Lead toxicity has long been known to be associated with abortion and menstrual disorders. Evidence as to whether lead is teratogenic is conflicting. Some authors report a correlation between atmospheric lead levels and congenital malformations, whereas others deny these associations. In sheep, prenatal lead exposure has also been shown to affect the offspring's learning ability.

Mercury poisoning. Probably the earliest instance of massive, unplanned exposure of a local population to an environmental toxicant occurred in 1953 in and around Minamata, a town located on a bay in southern Japan. Unusual neurologic problems (for example, mental confusion, convulsions, and coma) began afflicting villagers. Over one third of the affected individuals died, and many infants and children suffered permanent brain damage from prenatal and neonatal exposure. Mercury was transported across the placenta and also appeared in breast milk of mothers consuming contaminated fish. Eventually the source of the mercury was traced to the effluent discharged from a local plastics factory into Minamata Bay. A similar incident occurred in Niigata, Japan in 1964.

Another massive methylmercury disaster occurred in Iraq during the winter of 1971 to 1972. In this case barley and wheat grain treated with methylmercury as a fungicide had been purchased from Mexico. The grain sacks carried a written warning—but only in Spanish. Thirty-one pregnant women who ate the grain were hospitalized with methylmercury poisoning. Almost half of them died. Infants born to surviving mothers showed evidence of cerebral palsy, blindness, and severe brain damage. Similar outbreaks have occurred in Russia, Sweden, and elsewhere.[107]

CASE STUDY

Fetal Arrhythmia Caused by Excessive Intake of Caffeine by Pregnant Women
Case 1

A 26-year-old woman experienced preterm labor from 34 to 36 weeks' gestation. Ten days later she gave birth to a boy who weighed ~3100 g; his Apgar score at 5 minutes was 8. Management of this infant was "touch and go" from the beginning, but the ultimate result was that this baby seemed fine when released from the hospital. The only remarkable finding was that the woman had drunk 10 cups of coffee during the last hours before delivery. The baby's urine contained caffeine.

Case 2

A 23-year-old woman was admitted to a hospital at 40 weeks' gestation to deliver her first baby. The fetal heart rate was very irregular but laboratory tests of cardiac performance were fine. During and after delivery, the fetal heart rate remained irregular. The point of interest is that the woman reported that she had drunk 1.5 L of cola each day during the past 2 weeks because of the hot weather. While the baby was small, she did well, even though cardiac performance was abnormal. However, caffeine could have taken its toll.

Case 3

A 22-year-old woman was admitted to the hospital at 23 weeks' gestation because of fetal arrhythmia. The fetal heart seemed fine but the heart rate was totally irregular. Laboratory tests were normal. The woman reported that she had drunk more than 1.5 L of cola, two cups of coffee, and one cup of cocoa daily. She was told not to drink anything that contained caffeine; 1 week later, the arrhythmias stopped and the pregnancy continued without problems.

From Oei S, Vosters RPL, van der Hagen NLJ: Fetal arrhythmia caused by excessive intake of caffeine by pregnant women, *BMJ* 298:568, 1989.

Other heavy metals. Several other heavy metals probably affect the fetus and infant. Cadmium (which is derived accidentally from tobacco smoke, the electroplating industry, and deterioration of rubber tires) is a known cause of developmental malformations in rodents. Low doses of nickel cause embryotoxicity and eye malformations in the progeny of rats. Selenium is also a suspect teratogen.

Pesticides. A number of pesticides have been a major concern among public health professionals for quite some time. The Environmental Protection Agency reports that about one third of the 1500 active ingredients in registered pesticides are toxic, and one fourth are mutagenic and carcinogenic. Although the agency has established limits on the amounts of pesticide residues that are allowed in foods, it has restricted the use of only five: heptaclor, chlordane, DDT, Mirex, and DBCP. Once deposited in the food chain, they are almost impossible to eliminate. The effects of exposure to low concentrations of these toxins is not only unknown but also difficult to investigate because of the problem of finding pesticide-free control populations.

PCBs. Polychlorinated biphenyls (PCBs), used as plasticizers and heat exchange fluids, comprise another group of chemicals that endanger health. In Kyushu, Japan in 1968, a number of pregnant and lactating women ingested cooking oil contaminated with PCBs. As a result, they had small-for-gestational-age infants with dark skin, eye defects, and other abnormalities. Although prenatal exposure was probably significant, evidence indicated that transfer of PCBs through breast milk was the most significant route of exposure. Polybromated biphenyl (PBB), produced commercially as a fire retardant, also provoked attention after its accidental entry into cattle feed in Michigan in 1973 to 1974. Over 30,000 cattle and many sheep, swine, and poultry died or were slaughtered. Contaminated meat, milk, and eggs were identified in local food supplies, and stillbirths among affected cattle increased. Adverse effects in human pregnancy have not been reported, but considerable concern still exists.

EFFECTS OF RIGOROUS PHYSICAL ACTIVITY

For many years questions have been raised about the effect of heavy maternal physical activity during pregnancy on fetal growth. Some insight may be gained from studies related to heavy physical labor, modern fitness programs, and athletic training.

Heavy Physical Labor

In a study conducted in Ethiopia, trained nutritionists visited pregnant women in their homes for a period of 3 consecutive days. During this time dietary surveys were conducted. Two groups of women who had similar energy and protein intakes during pregnancy were then compared. One group of mothers was forced by circumstances beyond their control to engage in hard physical work throughout pregnancy. The second group of mothers had servants to do such physical labor. Mothers in both groups ate on the mean about 1550 kcal a day.

When the two groups of Ethiopian women were compared, the women who engaged in hard physical labor had significantly lower pregnancy weight gains and smaller babies than did mothers who did not have to engage in such work. Kilocalorie deficiency was likely involved in the etiology of fetal growth retardation that was seen. In addition, however, the oxygen debt incurred by moderate exercise is increased in human pregnancies, and this may lead to fetal hypoxia. This response is also evident in animal studies where uterine blood flow decreases during maternal exercise.

Fitness Programs

The circumstances of mandatory physical labor described above, further imposed on an underlying state of moderate undernutrition, may seem far removed from today's modern fitness-conscious woman who opts to engage in a rigorous exercise program during pregnancy. But some useful comparisons can be made.

The fitness-conscious pregnant woman often gets conflicting advice from her physician and other health professionals. The obstetric textbooks rarely offer more than a single paragraph concerning physical activities during pregnancy. Obstetricians tend to form their own philosophies about various physical activities or athletic participation during pregnancy, and their recommendations often are based on their own (or their wives') experiences. Traditional advice to women from the obstetric community has been to decrease activity and increase periods of rest during pregnancy, particularly in the third trimester.

Over the past 15 years, a number of studies have been conducted to examine the true relationship between physical activity programs and pregnancy course and outcome. A variety of fitness and training regimens have been evaluated.[108] Most studies have reported no difference in pregnancy outcome related to physical activity. However, most pregnant women followed by these investigators decreased frequency, duration, or intensity of exercise in the latter part of pregnancy. One research group at the University of Vermont was able to compare a group of women who maintained frequent vigorous endurance exercise routines throughout the third trimester with other less active pregnant women.[109]

While the incidence of antenatal and neonatal complications was similar in all groups, those exercising vigorously in the third trimester had babies with a mean birth weight of 2633 g (5.5 lb); mean birth weights of offspring from both control groups exceeded 3000 g (6.25 lb).

More recently, this group from Vermont[110-112] examined pregnancy course and outcome in women who continued a regular running or aerobics program during pregnancy at or above 50% of preconceptional levels; active control women were also observed. As can be seen in Table 4-13, the vigorously exercising women had somewhat fewer spontaneous abortions, superior labor and delivery characteristics, better fetal condition at birth, and no greater level of preterm delivery or premature rupture of membranes. However, babies of the vigorously exercising women demonstrated growth restriction; they were clearly born with reduced levels of body fat (Table 4-14). While the authors speculate that this difference in fat mass at birth may have long-term beneficial effects on health of the offspring, one might also wonder if this smaller kilocaloric reserve increases the risk of an infant not successfully combatting a major nutritional or medical insult during infancy. Until additional data are available, it seems prudent to advise women not to engage in very rigorous conditioning exercise during the third trimester.

Some high-risk women, such as those with diabetes, heart disease, or history of spontaneous abortion, may be well advised to be particularly cautious about the selection of exercise programs. The American College of Obstetricians and Gynecologists provides exercise guidelines for all pregnant women that go well beyond discouraging endurance training in the third trimester (Table 4-15).[113] While these guidelines may be overly restrictive for many pregnant women, they provide a common sense base from which to start.

TABLE 4-13   *Features of Pregnancy Course and Outcome in Runners and Aerobic Dancers Versus Active Control Women*

Characteristic	Controls (%)	Exercisers (%)
Spontaneous abortion	25	17 (runners)
		18 (aerobic dancers)
Onset of labor		
Preterm (263 days)	9	8
Premature rupture of membranes	29	30
Induction of labor	13	13
Labor management		
Artificial rupture of membranes	50	23
Stimulation for abnormal labor pattern	20	13
Second stage arrest	14	2
Method of delivery		
Spontaneous	50	88
Forceps	20	6
Cesarean section	30	6
Fetal condition and outcome		
Meconium in fluid	25	14
Abnormal heart rate	25	14
1 min Apgar score less than 7	25	14

From Clapp JF: The effects of maternal exercise on early pregnancy outcome, *Am J Obstet Gynecol* 161:1453, 1989; and Clapp JF: The course of labor after endurance exercise during pregnancy, *Am J Obstet Gynecol* 163:1799, 1990.

TABLE 4-14 *Characteristics of Infants Born to Runners and Aerobic Dancers Versus Active Control Women*

Characteristics	Controls	Exercisers	Significant Difference
Birth weight (g)	3691	3381	Yes
Birth weight percentile	65th	45th	Yes
Length (cm)	51.3	51.4	No
Head circumference (cm)	35.2	35.0	No
Placental weight (g)	456	449	No
Indices of soft tissue growth restriction			
Skinfolds (sum of triceps and subscapular) (mm)	11.8	9.3	Yes
Skinfold percentile	58	28	Yes
Calculated body fat (%)	16.2	11.2	Yes
Calculated fat mass (g)	603	382	Yes

From Clapp JF and Capeless EL: Neonatal morphometrics after endurance exercise during pregnancy, *Am J Obstet Gynecol* 163:1805, 1990.

TABLE 4-15 *American College of Obstetricians and Gynecologists' Guidelines for Exercise During Pregnancy and Postpartum*

1. Regular exercise (at least three times per week) is preferable to intermittent activity. Competitive activities should be discouraged.
2. Vigorous exercise should not be performed in hot, humid weather or during a period of febrile illness.
3. Ballistic movements (jerky, bouncy motions) should be avoided. Exercise should be done on a wooden floor or a tightly carpeted surface to reduce shock and provide a sure footing.
4. Deep flexion or extension of joints should be avoided because of connective tissue laxity. Activities that require jumping, jarring motions, or rapid changes in direction should be avoided because of joint instability.
5. Vigorous exercise should be preceded by a five-minute period of muscle warm-up. This can be accomplished by slow walking or stationary cycling with low resistance.
6. Vigorous exercise should be followed by a period of gradually declining activity that includes gentle stationary stretching. Because connective tissue laxity increases the risk of joint injury, stretches should not be taken to the point of maximum resistance.
7. Heart rate should be measured at times of peak activity. Target heart rates and limits established in consultation with the physician should not be exceeded.
8. Care should be taken to gradually rise from the floor to avoid orthostatic hypotension. Some form of activity involving the legs should be continued for a brief period.
9. Liquids should be taken liberally before and after exercise to prevent dehydration. If necessary, activity should be interrupted to replenish fluids.
10. Women who have led sedentary life styles should begin with physical activity of very low intensity and advance activity levels very gradually.
11. Activity should be stopped and the physician consulted if any unusual symptoms appear.

Pregnancy only

1. Maternal heart rate should not exceed 140 beats/minute.
2. Strenuous activities should not exceed 15 minutes in duration.
3. No exercise should be performed in the supine position after the fourth month of gestation is completed.
4. Exercises that employ the Valsalva maneuver should be avoided.
5. Caloric intake should be adequate to meet not only the extra energy needs for pregnancy, but also of the exercise performed.
6. Maternal core temperature should not exceed 38° C.

Reprinted with permission from the American College of Obstetricians and Gynecologists: Exercise during pregnancy and the postnatal period (ACOG Home Exercise Programs), Washington, DC, 1985, American College of Obstetricians and Gynecologists.

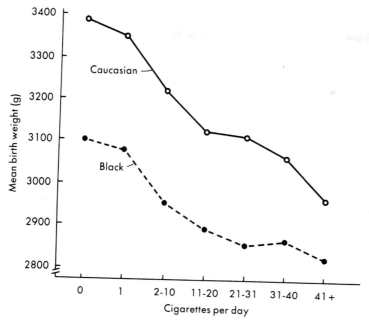

FIG. 4-17   Maternal cigarette use and infant birth weight.

Modified from Niswander KR, Gordon M: *The women and their pregnancies*, Philadelphia, 1972, WB Saunders. In Martin J: *Neurobehav Toxicol Teratol* 4:421, 1982.

EFFECTS OF CIGARETTE SMOKING

Fetal growth retardation is often seen in offspring of cigarette smokers, as shown in Fig. 4-17. It has been postulated that this condition is due to the reduced food intake of the mother. Observations have shown that this is not true. Women who smoke often consume more kilocalories per day than women who do not smoke.[114]

The growth retarding impact of smoking relates to the effects of carbon monoxide, nicotine, and possibly other compounds on placental perfusion and oxygen transport to the fetus. It is also likely that efficiency of kilocalorie utilization is reduced in women who smoke. Whether or not encouraging greater weight gain among smoking mothers will increase the infant's size is as yet an unanswered question. However, several reports have suggested that greater maternal weight is directly related to greater infant birth weight in this population.[114,115] In any event, the wisest counsel to mothers who smoke is to stop—at least during the pregnancy.

COMMON COMPLAINTS WITH DIETARY IMPLICATIONS

General nutritional guidance may also be needed during pregnancy for common functional gastrointestinal difficulties encountered. These complaints are highly individual in form and extent. They will therefore require individual counseling and assurances for control. Usually these difficulties are relatively minor. But if they persist or become extreme, they will need medical care. In most cases general investigation of food practices will reveal some areas where diet counseling may help relieve gastrointestinal problems. Some of the more common difficulties include nausea, constipation, hemorrhoids, or heartburn.

Nausea and Vomiting

Difficulty with nausea and vomiting is usually mild and limited to early pregnancy. It is commonly called "morning sickness" because it tends to occur early in the day, but it can come at any time of day. Usually it lasts only a brief period at the beginning of the pregnancy, but in some women it may persist longer.

A number of factors may contribute to the usual mild condition. Some are physiologic, based on normal hormonal changes that occur early in pregnancy. Other factors may be psychologic, such as various tensions and anxieties concerning the pregnancy itself. Simple treatment generally improves food toleration. Small frequent meals, fairly dry and consisting chiefly of easily-digested energy foods such as carbohydrates, are more readily tolerated. Cooking odors should be avoided as much as possible. Liquids are best taken between meals instead of with food. If the condition persists and develops into hyperemesis—severe, prolonged, persistent vomiting—medical attention is required to prevent complications and dehydration. However, such an increase in symptoms is rare. Most conditions pass early in the pregnancy and respond to the simple dietary remedies given here. Women should be reassured that mild short-term nausea is common in early pregnancy and will not harm the fetus.

Constipation

The condition of constipation is seldom more than minor. Hormonal changes in pregnancy tend to increase relaxation of the gastrointestinal muscles. Also, the pressure of the enlarging uterus on the lower portion of the intestine, especially during the latter part of the pregnancy, may make elimination somewhat difficult at times. Increased fluid intake, use of naturally laxative foods and fiber, such as whole grains with added bran, fibrous fruits and vegetables, dried fruits (especially prunes and figs), and other fruits and juices generally induce regularity. Laxatives should be avoided. They should only be used in special situations under medical supervision.

Hemorrhoids

A fairly common complaint during the latter part of pregnancy is that of hemorrhoids. These are enlarged veins in the anus, often protruding through the anal sphincter. This vein enlargement is usually caused by the increased weight of the fetus and the downward pressure it produces. The hemorrhoids may cause considerable discomfort, burning, and itching. Occasionally they may rupture and bleed under the pressure of a bowel movement, therefore causing more anxiety. The difficulty is usually remedied by the dietary suggestions given above to control constipation. Also, observing general hygiene recommendations concerning sufficient rest during the latter part of the day may help to relieve the pressure of the uterus on the lower intestine.

Heartburn or Full Feeling

The related complaints of "heartburn" or "full feeling" are sometimes voiced by pregnant women. These discomforts may occur especially after meals, usually caused by the pressure of the enlarging uterus crowding the adjacent digestive organ, the stomach, thereby causing some difficulty after eating. Food mixtures may sometimes be pushed back into the lower part of the esophagus, causing a "burning" sensation from the gastric acid mixed with the food mass. This burning sensation is commonly called heartburn simply because of the proximity of the lower esophagus to the heart. Obviously, however, it has nothing to do with the heart and its action. A full feeling comes from general gastric pressure, caused by a lack of normal space in the area, and is accentuated by a large meal or gas formation. These complaints are generally remedied by dividing the day's food intake into a number of small meals during the day. Attention may also be given to relaxation, adequate chewing, eating slowly, and avoiding tensions during meals. Comfort is also improved by wearing loose-fitting clothing.

SELECTED EXAMPLES OF HIGH-RISK PREGNANCY
General Comments

A number of risk factors may contribute to a poor pregnancy outcome. In a joint report, the American College of Obstetricians and Gynecologists and the American Dietetic Association have issued a set of risk factors to identify women with special nutritional and health care needs during pregnancy.[116] These factors, summarized in Table 4-16, relate to nutritional status, habits, needs, and problems. The nutritional factors identified in this report are based on clinical evidence of inadequate nutrition. A better approach, suggested by King,[117] provides useful criteria for predicting nutritional risk, instead of waiting for clinical signs of poor nutrition to appear. Three types of dietary patterns, she summarizes, would not support optimal maternal and fetal nutrition: (1) insufficient food intake, (2) poor food selection, and (3) poor food distribution through the day. These patterns, added to the list of risk factors in Table 4-16, would be much more sensitive for nutritional risk. On this basis, paractitioners can plan personal care and provide for special counseling needs.

Pregnancy-Induced Hypertension (PIH)

Formerly labeled *toxemia,* PIH is a risk factor related to nutrition and treated according to its symptoms:

1. **Clinical symptoms.** PIH is generally defined according to its manifestations, which usually occur in the third trimester toward term. Among these symptoms are hypertension, abnormal and excessive edema, albumuria, and in severe cases, convulsions or coma—*eclampsia.*
2. **Treatment.** Specific treatment varies according to the patient's symptoms and needs. In any case, optimal nutrition is a fundamental aspect of therapy. Adequate dietary protein is essential. Correction of plasma protein deficits stimulates normal

TABLE 4-16 Nutritional Risk Factors in Pregnancy

Risk Factors Present at the Onset of Pregnancy	Risk Factors Occurring During Pregnancy

Age
  15 years or younger
  35 years or older
	Low hemoglobin or hematocrit
	  Hemoglobin less than 12.0 g
	  Hematocrit less than 35.0 mg/dl

Frequent pregnancies: three or more during a 2-year period	Inadequate weight gain Any weight loss
Poor obstetric history or poor fetal performance	Weight gain of less than 2 lb per month after the first trimester
Poverty	Excessive weight gain: greater than 1 kg (2.2 lb) per week after the first trimester)
Bizarre or faddist food habits	
Abuse of nicotine, alcohol, or drugs	
Therapeutic diet required for a chronic disorder	

Inadequate weight
  Less than 85% of standard weight
  More than 120% of standard weight	

❖
GUIDELINES FOR POSITIVE TEACHING TO CORRECT NUTRIENT DEFICIENCIES

- *General counseling approach*
  Reinforce good habits
  Encourage needed changes in food practices
- *Basic counseling actions*
  Identify unmet needs
  Clarify reasons for increased nutrient needs
  Identify reasons for dietary deficiencies
    1. Low income
    2. Food aversions or intolerances
    3. Cultural food pattern
    4. Vegetarian food patterns
  Evaluate need for nutrient supplements
    1. Kilocalories/protein
    2. Vitamins
    3. Minerals

Hypovolemia
(Gr *hypo*, under; ME *volu(me)*, volume; Gr *haima*, blood) Low blood volume.

operation of the capillary fluid shift mechanism and restores circulation of tissue fluid, inducing subsequent correction of the **hypovolemia.** In addition, adequate salt and sources of vitamins and minerals are needed for correction and maintenance of metabolic balances.

Preexisting Disease

Preexisting clinical conditions complicate pregnancy and increase risks. They are managed according to the general principles of care related to pregnancy and to the particular disease involved. Examples of these preexisting conditions include hypertension, diabetes mellitus, and phenylketonuria (PKU).

Hypertension Preventive screening and monitoring of blood pressure are essential. The hypertensive disease process begins long before any signs and symptoms appear and later symptoms are inconsistent.[118] Risk factors for hypertension before and during pregnancy are given in Table 4-17. Nutritional care centers on prevention of weight extremes, either underweight or obesity, and correction of any dietary deficiencies by maintaining optimal nutrition. Sodium intake can be moderate but should never be unduly restricted because of its relation to fluid and electrolyte balances during pregnancies.

Diabetes mellitus The management of diabetes in pregnancy presents special problems. Routine screening is therefore necessary to detect gestational diabetes, and team management is required for control of pre-existing insulin-dependent diabetes mellitus (IDDM Table 4-18)[119,120]

Screening. Most prenatal clinics do routine screening for diabetes and provide careful followup for every patient who shows glycosuria. Risk factors detected in initial history include (1) family history of diabetes, (2) previous unexplained stillbirths, (3) large babies weighing 4 kg (9 lb) or more, (4) recurrent miscarriage, (5) births of babies with multiple congenital anomalies, and (6) excessive obesity.

Gestational diabetes. During pregnancy glycosuria is not uncommon because of the increased circulating blood volume and its load of metabolites. However, only 20% to 30% of women showing glycosuria or somewhat abnormal glucose tolerance subsequently develop diabetes. Nonetheless, identification of women with this condition

TABLE 4-17   Risk Factors in Pregnancy-Induced Hypertension

Before Pregnancy	During Pregnancy
Nulligravida	Primigravida
Diabetes mellitus	Large fetus
Preexisting condition (hypertension, renal or vascular disease)	Glomerulonephritis
Family history of hypertension or vascular disease	Fetal hydrops
Diagnosis of pregnancy-induced hypertension in a previous pregnancy	Hydramnios
Dietary deficiencies	Multiple gestation
Age extremes	Hydatidiform mole
20 years or younger	
35 years or older	

TABLE 4-18   Classification of Diabetes Mellitus During Pregnancy*

New Classifications	Former Names	Clinical Characteristics
Type I insulin-dependent diabetes mellitus (IDDM)	Juvenile diabetes Juvenile-onset diabetes Brittle diabetes Ketosis-prone diabetes	Ketosis prone: insulin deficient because of loss of islet cells; often associated with human leukocyte antigen types, with predisposition to viral insulitis or autoimmune (islet-cell antibody) phenomena; can occur at any age, but more common in youth
Type II non-insulin-dependent diabetes-mellitus (NIDDM) Nonobese Obese	Adult diabetes Adult-onset diabetes Maturity-onset diabetes Stable diabetes Ketosis-resistant diabetes Maturity-onset diabetes of youth	Ketosis resistant: occurs at any age but more frequent in adults; majority are overweight; may be seen in families as an autosomal dominant genetic trait; may require insulin in times of stress; usually requires insulin during pregnancy
Gestational diabetes	Gestational diabetes	Classification retained for women whose diabetes begins (or is recognized) during pregnancy; carries increased risk of perinatal complications; transitory glucose intolerance, which frequently recurs; diagnosis: at least two abnormal values on a 3-hour oral glucose tolerance test (100 g glucose) Fasting plasma glucose 105 mg/100 ml 1 hour 190 mg/100 ml 2 hour 160 mg/100 ml 3 hour 145 mg/100 ml

*This classification replaces the White classification for pregnancy, which was based on age at onset, duration of the disease, and complications.

and their close followup observation are important because of the higher risk of fetal damage during this period. Most of these women revert to normal glucose tolerance after delivery.

Preexisting IDDM. Because of the course of diabetes during pregnancy, as well as the altered course of pregnancy in the presence of diabetes, a team of specialists is necessary for sound management and prevention of problems to reduce risk of fetal death and increase the probability of a successful outcome. Close personalized nutritional care by the team nutritionist is mandatory throughout. The insulin requirement increases during pregnancy and drops dramatically upon delivery.

The woman with IDDM must control blood glucose levels through careful food selection and scheduled meal timing in concert with the administration of insulin. In a nonrandomized study of diabetic women in Europe, preconceptional control of IDDM was associated with a reduction in the incidence of congenital malformations to that of the nondiabetic control population.

	Malformation rate
Nondiabetic women (*n* = 420)	1.4%
IDDM women (*n* = 420)	5.5%
—with early counseling (*n* = *128*)	0.8%
—counseling after 8 weeks' gestation (*n* = 292)	7.5%

In a large multicenter study in the United States during the early 1980s, very early prenatal intervention for management of IDDM was associated with a marked reduction in the congenital malformation rate but not to the low level of the control population.

	Malformation rate
Nondiabetic women (*n* = 468)	3.5%
IDDM women with late counseling (*n* = 296)	13.0%
IDDM women with counseling at 15-21 days post-conception (*n* = 409)	6.0%

The incidence of spontaneous abortion was also significantly reduced in this early-counseled population, presumably due to the improved metabolic control.

Maternal phenylketonuria (MPKU). Mandatory screening of all newborns for the genetic disease PKU and low phenylalanine diet have supported normal growth in PKU children. Now a generation of young women with childhood PKU are having children of their own. Maternal PKU presents potential fetal hazards associated with increased abortions and stillbirths, congenital anomalies often causing death, and intrauterine and postnatal growth and development retardation in surviving infants. A planned pregnancy, with careful management of the mother's diet *before* conception, and close followup care *throughout* the pregnancy itself, can improve the outcome of these high-risk pregnancies (see the box on p. 157). A strict diet low in phenylalanine and a special formula of other amino acids are required.

It makes sense, therefore, that efforts should be made preconceptionally to motivate women with controllable diseases to prepare themselves for conception by initiating those dietary and other necessary lifestyle changes that will allow each of them to offer to her conceptus the optimum maternal metabolic milieu. This can certainly be said for women with IDDM and PKU but it also applies to women with other chronic diseases. Not only will such efforts reduce morbidity and mortality of offspring but they may also improve the health and wellbeing of the mother during the prenatal period.

❖
GUIDELINES FOR NUTRITIONAL MANAGEMENT FOR THE PREGNANT WOMAN WITH PHENYLKETONURIA

The goals of nutritional management are to:

1. Maintain serum phenylalanine levels as low as possible. The U.S. Maternal Collaborative Study recommends concentrations between 2 and 6 mg/dl, or 120 and 360 μmol/L.
2. Maintain adequate and consistent weight gain.
3. Maintain serum tyrosine in the normal range.
4. Meet nutrient requirements for protein, energy, vitamins and minerals using the 1989 RDA as a guide.

The tasks of nutritional management are to:

1. Stress the special nutritional needs during pregnancy.
2. Stress the importance of strictly following the phenylalanine prescription to achieve the necessary rigid control of blood phenylalanine levels.
3. Calculate a food pattern to provide adequate energy, protein, phenylalanine, vitamins, and minerals.
4. Provide a food pattern for the individual that is based on a phenylalanine-free protein source (one of the medical foods).
5. Provide a meal guide and serving lists that indicate protein, energy, and phenylalanine content of foods.
6. Provide education on food selection, food purchasing, food preparation using low phenylalanine recipes, and recording food intake as needed.
7. Review and calculate diet records for accuracy.
8. Compare recorded and calculated food intake with blood phenylalanine levels and weight gain.
9. Adjust the food pattern and meal guide as necessary to meet the individual's needs.

Summary

The relative importance of nutrition in prenatal development has been studied and debated for a number of years. Available evidence strongly supports a key role for maternal nutrition in significantly affecting the fate of both mother and child. Animal data convince, and human observations clearly suggest, that maternal prepregnancy weight and weight gain during pregnancy positively correlate with birth weight of the offspring.

Supplementation programs for pregnant women are successful when they are properly administered and focused on needy populations. The benefit of such programs may also be substantial even when health care workers or food program administrators are unable to measure that benefit with available tools. With limited time and resources in prenatal settings, priority should be given to those women with greatest need. Dietary recommendations must be tailored to meet the specific needs of each woman served.

Review Questions

1. Describe significant historic observations about the relationship between maternal diet and pregnancy outcome.
2. Discuss current dietary recommendations during pregnancy and justify each of them.

3. Define appropriate weight gain guidelines for pregnancy.
4. Define known effects of specific nutrient deficiencies and excesses in human pregnancy.
5. Summarize current information about the impact of alcohol, caffeine, and other food substances on pregnancy course and outcome.
6. Outline appropriate management recommendations for the common gastrointestinal complaints of pregnancy.

References

1. Committee on Maternal Nutrition, Food and Nutrition Board, National Research Council: *Maternal nutrition and the course of pregnancy,* Washington, DC, 1973, National Academy of Sciences.
2. Christakis G, editor: Maternal nutrition assessment, *Am J Public Health* 63(Suppl):1, 1973.
3. Committee on Maternal Nutrition, Food and Nutrition Board, National Research Council: *Nutritional supplementation and the outcome of pregnancy,* Washington, DC, 1973, National Academy of Sciences.
4. Select Panel for the Promotion of Child Health, US Department of Health and Human Services: *Better health for our children: a national strategy,* vols 1-3, Pub No (PHS) 79-55071, Washington, DC, 1981, US Government Printing Office.
5. Task Force on Nutrition: *Assessment of maternal nutrition,* Chicago, 1978, American College of Obstetricians and Gynecologists.
6. Committee on Nutrition of the Mother and Preschool Child: *Nutrition services in perinatal care,* Washington, DC, 1981, National Academy Press.
7. Institute of Medicine, National Academy of Sciences: *Nutrition during pregnancy: weight gain and nutrient supplements,* Washington, DC, National Academy Press.
8. Starr P: *The social transformation of American medicine,* New York, 1982, Basic Books.
9. Brown JF, Toma RB: Taste changes during pregnancy, *Am J Clin Nutr* 43:414, 1986.
10. Winick M: Fetal malnutrition, *Clin Obstet Gynecol* 13:526, 1970.
11. Thomson AM et al: The assessment of fetal growth, *J Obstet Gynaecol Br Commonw* 75:903, 1968.
12. Naeye PL: Causes of fetal and neonatal mortality by race in a selected U.S. population, *Am J Public Health* 69:857, 1979.
13. Edwards LE et al: Pregnancy in the underweight woman: course, outcome, and growth patterns of the infant, *Am J Obstet Gynecol* 135:297, 1979.
14. Shepard MJ et al: Proportional weight gain and complications of pregnancy, labor, and delivery in healthy women of normal prepregnant status, *Am J Obstet Gynecol* 155:947, 1986.
15. Primrose T, Higgins A: A study of human antepartum nutrition, *J Reprod Med.* 7:257, 1971.
16. Higgins AC et al: Impact of the Higgins Nutrition Intervention Program on birth weight: a within mother analysis, *J Am Diet Assoc* 89:1097, 1989.
17. Clements DE: The nutrition intervention project for underweight pregnant women, *Clin Nutr* 7:205, 1988.
18. Bruce L, Tsabo J: Nutrition intervention program in a prenatal clinic, *Obstet Gynecol* 74:310, 1989.
19. Orstead C et al: Efficacy of prenatal nutrition counseling: weight gain, infant birthweight, and cost effectiveness, *J Am Diet Assoc* 85:40, 1985.
20. Rush D: *The National WIC Evaluation: an evaluation of the Special Supplemental Food Program for Women, Infants, and Children,* vols I and II, Research Triangle Park, NC, 1986, Research Triangle Institute and New York State Research Foundation for Mental Hygiene.
21. Food and Nutrition Board, National Research Council, National Academy of Sciences: *Recommended dietary allowances,* ed 10, Washington, DC, 1989, National Academy Press.
22. Hytten FE, Leitch I: *The physiology of human pregnancy,* ed 2, Oxford, 1971, Blackwell Scientific Publications.
23. Durnin JVGA: Energy requirements of pregnancy: an integration of the longitudinal data from

the five-country study, *Lancet* 2:1131, 1987.

24. Lechtig A et al: Effect of food supplementation during pregnancy on birth weight, *Pediatrics* 56:508, 1975.

25. Rush D et al: A randomized controlled trial of prenatal supplementation in New York City, *Pediatrics* 65:683, 1980.

26. Rush D et al: Controlled trial of prenatal nutrition supplementation defended, *Pediatrics* 66:656, 1980.

27. Giroud A: Nutritional requirements of the embryo, *World Rev Nutr Diet* 18:195, 1973.

28. Dansky LV: Anticonvulsants, folate levels and pregnancy outcome: a prospective study, *Ann Neurol* 21:176, 1987.

29. Smithells RW et al: Vitamin deficiencies and neural tube defects, *Arch Dis Child* 51:944, 1976.

30. Smithells RW et al: Possible prevention of neural tube defects by periconceptional vitamin supplementation, *Lancet* 1:339, 1980.

31. Smithells RW et al: Apparent prevention of neural tube defects by periconceptional vitamin supplementation, *Arch Dis Child* 56:911, 1981.

32. Smithells RW et al: Further experience of vitamin supplementation for prevention of neural tube defect recurrences, *Lancet* 1:1027, 1983.

33. Laurence KM et al: Double-blind randomized controlled trial of folate treatment before conception to prevent recurrence of neural tube defects, *Br Med J* 282:1509, 1981.

34. Wald NJ: Neural tube defects and vitamins: the need for a randomized clinical trial, *Br J Obstet Gynaecol* 91:516, 1984.

35. Mulinara J et al: Periconceptional use of multivitamins and the occurrence of neural tube defects, *JAMA* 260:3141, 1988.

36. Milunsky A et al: Multivitamin/folic acid supplementation in early pregnancy reduces the prevalence of neural tube defects, *JAMA* 262:2847, 1989.

37. Mills JL et al: The absence of a relation between periconceptional use of vitamins and neural tube defects, *N Engl J Med* 321:430, 1989.

38. Ejderjamm J, Hamfelt A: Pyridoxal phosphate concentration in blood in newborn infants and their mothers compared with the amount of extra pyridoxal taken during pregnancy and breast-feeding, *Acta Paediatr Scand* 69:327, 1980.

39. Worthington-Roberts BS, Vermeersch J, Williams SR: *Nutrition in pregnancy and lactation,* ed 4, St Louis, 1989, Mosby.

40. Pulkkinen MO et al: Serum vitamin B_6 in pure pregnancy depression, *Acta Obstet Gynecol Scand* 57:471, 1978.

41. Roepke B, Kirksey A: Vitamin B_6 nurtriture during pregnancy and lactation. I. Vitamin B_6 intake, levels of the vitamin in biological fluids, and conditions of the infant at birth, *Am J Clin Nutr* 32:2249, 1979.

42. Schuster K et al: Vitamin B_6 status of the low-income adolescent and adult pregnant women and the condition of their infants at birth, *Am J Clin Nutr* 34:1731, 1981.

43. Schuster K et al: Effect of maternal pyridoxine HCl supplementation on the vitamin B_6 status of mother and infant and on pregnancy outcome, *J Nutr* 114:977, 1984.

44. Schuster K et al: Morning sickness and vitamin B_6 status of pregnant women, *Hum Nutr Clin Nutr* 39C:75, 1984.

45. Wheatley D: Treatment of pregnancy sickness, *Br J Obstet Gynaecol* 84:444, 1977.

46. Wideman CL et al: Ascorbic acid deficiency and premature rupture of fetal membranes, *Am J Obstet Gynecol* 88:592, 1964.

47. Clemetson CAB, Anderson L: Ascorbic acid metabolism in preeclampsia, *Obstet Gynecol* 24:774, 1964.

48. Cochrane WA: Overnutrition in prenatal and neonatal life: a problem? *Can Med Assoc J* 93:893, 1965.

49. Norkus EP, Rosso P: Effects of maternal intake of ascorbic acid on the postnatal metabolism of this vitamin in the guinea pig, *J Nutr* 111:624, 1981.

50. Roberts RA et al: Antenatal factors in neonatal hypocalcemic convulsions, *Lancet* 2:809, 1973.

51. Purvis RJ et al: Enamel hypoplasia of the teeth associated with neonatal tetany: a manifestation of maternal vitamin D deficiency, *Lancet* 2:811, 1973.

52. Delvin EE et al: Vitamin D supplementation during pregnancy: effect on neonatal calcium homeostasis, *J Pediatr* 109:328, 1986.

53. Brooke OG et al: Vitamin D supplements in pregnant Asian women: effects on calcium status and fetal growth, *Br Med J* 1:751, 1980.

54. Bernhardt JR, Dorsey DJ: Hypervitaminosis A and congenital renal anomalies in a human infant, *Obstet Gynecol* 43:750, 1974.

55. Strange L et al: Hypervitaminosis A in early human pregnancy and malformations of the central nervous system, *Acta Obstet Gynecol Scand* 57:289, 1978.

56. Benke PI: The isotretinoin syndrome, *JAMA* 25:3267, 1984.

57. Lammar EJ et al: Retinoic acid embryopathy, *N Engl J Med* 313:837, 1985.

58. Marwick C: More cautionary labeling appears on isotretinoin, *JAMA* 251:3208, 1984.

59. Haga P et al: Plasma tocopherol levels and vitamin B-lipoprotein relationships during pregnancy and in cord blood, *Am J Clin Nutr* 36:1200, 1982.

60. Kazzi NJ et al: Placental transfer of vitamin K1 in preterm pregnancy, *Obstet Gynecol* 75:334, 1990.

61. Morales WJ et al: The use of antenatal vitamin K in the prevention of early neonatal intraventricular hemorrhage, *Am J Obstet Gynecol* 159:774, 1988.

62. Sisson TRC, Lund CJ: The influence of maternal iron deficiency on the newborn, *Am J Clin Nutr* 6:376, 1958.

63. McFee JG: Anemia: a high-risk complication of pregnancy, *Clin Obstet Gynecol* 16:153, 1973.

64. Romslo I et al: Iron requirement in normal pregnancy assessed by serum ferritin, serum transferrin saturation and erythrocyte protoporphyrin determinations, *Br J Obstet Gynaecol* 90:101, 1983.

65. Widdowson EM: *Growth and composition of the fetus and newborn.* In Assali NE, editor: *Biology of gestation,* vol 2, New York, 1968, Academic Press.

66. Villar J, Belizan JM: Calcium during pregnancy, *Clin Nutr* 5:55, 1986.

67. Duggin GG et al: Calcium balance in pregnancy, *Lancet* 2:926, 1974.

68. Felton DJC, Stone WD: Osteomalacia in Asian immigrants during pregnancy, *Br Med J* 1:1521, 1966.

69. Villar J, Repke JT: Calcium supplementation during pregnancy may reduce preterm delivery in high-risk populations, *Am J Obstet Gynecol* 163:1124, 1990.

70. Lopez-Jaramillo P: Calcium supplementation reduces the risk of pregnancy-induced hypertension in an Andes population, *Br J Obstet Gynaecol* 96:648, 1989.

71. Belizan JM: The relationship between calcium intake and pregnancy-induced hypertension: up-to-date evidence, *Am J Obstet Gynecol* 153:898, 1988.

72. Villar J: Calcium supplementation reduces blood pressure during pregnancy: results of a randomized controlled clinical trial, *Obstet Gynecol* 70:317, 1987.

73. Allen LH: Trace elements and outcome of human pregnancy, *Clin Nutr* 5:72, 1986.

74. Apgar J: Zinc and reproduction, *Annu Rev Nutr* 5:43, 1985.

75. Solomans NH et al: Zinc needs during pregnancy, *Clin Nutr* 5:63, 1986.

76. Soltan MH, Jenkins MH: Maternal and fetal plasma zinc concentration and fetal abnormality, *Br J Obstet Gynaecol* 89:56, 1982.

77. Hurley LS: Trace metals in mammalian development, *Johns Hopkins Med J* 148:1, 1981.

78. Sandstead HH et al: Zinc deficiency in pregnant rhesus monkeys: effects on behavior of infants, *Am J Clin Nutr* 31:844, 1978.

79. Bergmann KE et al: Abnormalities of hair zinc concentration in mothers of newborn infants with spina bifida, *Am J Clin Nutr* 33:2145, 1980.

80. Cherry FF et al: Plasma zinc hypertension-toxemia and other reproductive variables in adolescent pregnancy, *Am J Clin Nutr* 34:2367, 1981.

81. Meadows NJ et al: Zinc and small babies, *Lancet* 2:1135, 1981.

82. Jameson S: Effects of zinc deficiency in human reproduction, *Acta Med Scand* 593(suppl): 1976.

83. Ghosh A et al: Zinc deficiency is not a cause for abortion, congenital abnormality, and small-for-gestational-age infant in Chinese women, *Br J Obstet Gynaecol* 92:886, 1985.
84. Hunt IF et al: Zinc supplementation during pregnancy: effects on selected blood constituents and on progress and outcome of pregnancy in low-income women of Mexican descent, *Am J Clin Nutr* 40:508, 1984.
85. Mukherjee MD et al: Maternal zinc, iron, folic acid, and protein nutriture and outcome of human pregnancy, *Am J Clin Nutr* 40:496, 1984.
86. Connolly KJ et al: Fetal iodine deficiency and motor performance during childhood, *Lancet* 2:1149, 1979.
87. Bursel RG, Watson ML: The effect of sodium restriction during gestation on offspring brain development in rats, *Am J Clin Nutr* 37:43, 1983.
88. Pike RL et al: Juxtaglomerular degranulation and zona glomerulosa exhaustion in pregnant rats induced by low-sodium intakes and reversed by sodium load, *Am J Obstet Gynecol* 95:604, 1966.
89. Lelong-Tissier MC et al: Hyponatremie maternofetale carentielle par regime desode, *Arch Fr Pediatr* 34:64, 1977.
90. Horner RD et al: Pica practices of pregnant women, *J Am Diet Assoc* 91:34, 1991.
91. National Research Council, Food and Nutrition Board: *Alternative dietary practices and nutritional abuses in pregnancy*, Washington, DC, 1982, National Academy of Sciences.
92. Lackey CJ: *Pica — pregnancy etiological mystery*. In National Academy of Sciences: *Alternative dietary practices and nutritional abuses in pregnancy*, Washington, DC, 1982, National Academy of Sciences.
93. Lillien LJ et al: Diet and ethanol intake during pregnancy, *J Am Diet Assoc* 81:252, 1982.
94. Streissguth AP et al: Comparison of drinking and smoking patterns during pregnancy over a six-year interval, *Am J Obstet Gynecol* 145:716, 1983.
95. Rosett HL et al: Patterns of alcohol consumption and fetal development, *Obstet Gynecol* 61:539, 1983.
96. Rosett HL et al: Treatment experience with pregnant problem drinkers, *JAMA* 249:2029, 1983.
97. Groisser DS et al: Coffee consumption during pregnancy: subsequent behavioral abnormalities of the offspring, *J Nutr* 112:829, 1982.
98. Dunlop M, Court JM: Effects of maternal caffeine ingestion on neonatal growth in rats, *Biol Neonate* 39:178, 1981.
99. Collins TFX et al: A study of the teratogenetic potential of caffeine ingestion in drinking water, *Food Chem Toxicol* 21:763, 1983.
100. Kurppa K et al: Coffee consumption during pregnancy, *N Engl J Med* 306:1548, 1982.
101. Linn S et al: No association between coffee consumption and adverse outcomes of pregnancy, *N Engl J Med* 306:141, 1982.
102. Rosenberg L et al: Selected birth defects in relation to caffeine-containing beverages, *JAMA* 247:1429, 1982.
103. Furuhashi N: Effects of caffeine consumption during pregnancy, *Gynecol Obstet Invest* 19:187, 1985.
104. Streitfeld PP: Congenital malformation: teratogenic foods and additives, *Birth Fam J* 5:7, 1978.
105. Kline J et al: Spontaneous abortion and the use of sugar substitutes, *Am J Obstet Gynecol* 130:708, 1978.
106. Hoover R: Saccharin — bitter aftertaste? *N Engl J Med* 302:573, 1980.
107. Koos BJ, Longo LD: Mercury toxicity in the pregnant woman, fetus, and newborn infant: a review, *Am J Obstet Gynecol* 126:390, 1976.
108. Culpepper L: *Exercise during pregnancy*. In Merkatz IR et al, editors: *New perspectives in prenatal care*, New York, 1990, Elsevier, pp 193-210.
109. Clapp JF, Dickstein S: Endurance exercise and pregnancy outcome, *Med Sci Sports Exer* 16:556, 1984.

110. Clapp JF, Capeless EL: Neonatal morphometrics after endurance exercise during pregnancy, *Am J Obstet Gynecol* 163:1805, 1990.

111. Clapp JF: The effects of maternal exercise on early pregnancy outcome, *Am J Obstet Gynecol* 161:1453, 1989.

112. Clapp JF: The course of labor after endurance exercise during pregnancy, *Am J Obstet Gynecol* 163:1790, 1990.

113. American College of Obstetricians and Gynecologists: *Exercise during pregnancy and the postnatal period* (ACOG Home Exercise Programs). In ACOG Technical Bulletin: *Women and exercise,* no 87, Washington, DC, 1985, ACOG.

114. Picone TA et al: Pregnancy outcome in North American women. I. Effects of diet, cigarette smoking, and psychological stress on maternal weight gain, *Am J Clin Nutr* 36:1205, 1982.

115. Papoz L et al: Maternal smoking and birth weight in relation to dietary habits, *Am J Obstet Gynecol* 142:870, 1982.

116. Task Force on Nutrition: American College of Obstetrics and Gynecology and American Dietetic Association, Chicago, 1978.

117. King JC: *Dietary risk patterns during pregnancy.* In Weinger J, Briggs G, editors: *Nutrition update* 1:206, 1983.

118. National high blood pressure education program working group report on high blood pressure in pregnancy, *Am J Obstet Gynecol* 163:1691, 1990.

119. Summary of recommendations of the second international workshop conferences on gestational diabetes mellitus, *Diabetes* 34(suppl 2), 1985.

120. Nuwayhid BS, Brinkman CR, Leib SM, editors: *Management of the diabetic pregnancy,* New York, 1987, Elsevier.

Further Reading

Allen LH: Recent developments in maternal nutrition and their implications for practitioners, *Am J Clin Nutr* 59 (#25), 1994.
   Summarizes major issues in maternal nutrition of importance today.

Borrud LG et al: Food and nutrient intake of pregnant and lactating women in the United States, *J Nutr Educ* 25:176, 1993.
   Compares nutrient intake with recommended standards.

Brown JE: *Nutrition for your pregnancy,* Minneapolis, 1983, University of Minnesota Press.
   This well-written, popular book on diet and nutrition during pregnancy continues to provide an excellent resource for the general public.

Charbonneau K: Food for labor? food for thought, *IJCE* 8:37, 1994.
   Provides insight into the controversy about what to eat during labor.

Fassman DK: Prenatal fluoridation: a literature review, *Ped Dentist,* Jan. 1994.
   Reviews data on the value of prenatal fluoride supplementation.

Hess MA, Hunt AE: *Pickles and ice cream,* New York, 1982, McGraw-Hill.
   This award-winning book on diet and pregnancy designed to help mothers through their pregnancies continues to be an excellent practical resource.

Hickey, CH et al: Prenatal weight gain, term birth weight, fetal growth retardation among high risk multi-parous black and white women, *Obstet Gynecol* 81:529, 1993.
   Compares weight gain patterns of black and white women.

Infante-Rivard C et al: Fetal loss associated with caffeine intake before and during pregnancy, *JAMA* 270:2940, 1993.
   Compares caffeine intake with fetal loss during pregnancy.

Institute of Medicine, National Academy of Sciences: *Nutrition during pregnancy: weight gain and nutrient supplements,* Washington, DC, 1990, National Academy Press.
   This new report provides detailed background for current recommendations for maternity care in the two areas of concern for both mothers and their care providers, weight gain and nutrient supplements.

Isaacs JD et at: Obstetric challenges of massive obesity complicating pregnancy, *J Perinatal* 14:10, 1994.

Cites problems associated with obesity in pregnancy.

Johnson JWC et al: Excessive maternal weight and pregnancy outcome, *Am J Obstet Gynecol* 167:353, 1992.

Describes birth outcome in women with excessive body weight.

Keppel KG, Taffel SM: Pregnancy-related weight gain and retention: implications of the 1990 Institute of Medicine guidelines, *Am J Public Health* 83:1100, 1993.

Looks at weight gain patterns of pregnant women compared to new standards.

Kusin JA et al: Energy supplementation during pregnancy and postnatal growth, *Lancet* 340:823, 1992.

Discusses an effort to improve postnatal growth through prenatal nutrition supplementation.

Mills JL et al: Moderate caffeine use and the risk of spontaneous abortion and intrauterine growth retardation, *JAMA* 269:593, 1993.

Summarizes large study on prenatal caffeine intake and pregnancy outcome.

Murphy SP, Abrams B: Changes in energy intakes during pregnancy and lactation: a national sample of US women, *Am Public Health* 83:1161, 1993.

Reviews typical dietary intakes of pregnant and lactating women in the United States.

Parker JD, Abrams B: Differences in postpartum weight retention between black and white mothers, *Obstet Gynecol* 81:768, 1993.

Compares weight retention post-partum in black and white women.

Parker JD, Abrams B: Prenatal weight gain advice: an examination of the recent prenatal weight gain recommendations of the Institute of Medicine, *Obstet Gynecol* 79:664, 1992.

Looks at actual weight gains in pregnancy and compares them with new standards.

Perlow, JH et al: Perinatal outcome in pregnancy complicated by massive obesity, *Am J Obstet Gynecol* 167:958, 1992.

Discusses problems of pregnancy in obese women.

Pappitt SD et al: Evidence of energy sparing in Gambian women during pregnancy: a longitudinal study using whole body caloritemetry, *Am J Clin Nutr* 57:353, 1993.

Shows data on how poor pregnant women adapt to the demands of pregnancy.

Smith DE et al: Longitudinal changes in adiposity associated with pregnancy, *JAMA* 271:1747, 1994.

Summarizes measured changes in adiposity through pregnancy.

Suitor CW et al: Nutrition care during pregnancy and lactation: new guidelines from the Institute of Medicine, *J Amer Diet Assoc* 93:478, 1993.

Reviews the Institute of Medicines guidelines for weight gain in pregnancy and postpartum issues.

Villar J et al: Effects of fat and fat-free mass deposition during pregnancy on birth weight. *Am J Obstet Gynecol,* 167:1344, 1992.

Summarizes a study monitoring weight (fat) changes in pregnancy.

Waller DK et al: Are obese women at higher risk for producing malformed offspring?, *Am J Obstet Gynecol,* 170:541, 1994.

Addresses the above questions in detail.

Worthington-Roberts BS, Williams SR: *Nutrition in pregnancy and lactation,* ed 5, St. Louis, 1993, Mosby.

This manual provides detailed background on issues related to nutrition during pregnancy and lactation.

5

Lactation and Human Milk

Bonnie S. Worthington-Roberts

Basic Concepts

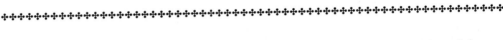

✔ *Specific female anatomy and physiology provide the required structures and functions for normal postpartum lactation.*

✔ *Human milk is designed to meet human infant needs.*

✔ *Successful lactation requires nutritional support.*

✔ *Breastfeeding provides the primary means of supporting growth and development of young infants.*

✔ *Physiologic knowledge and personal skills underlie sensitive counseling for the breastfeeding mother.*

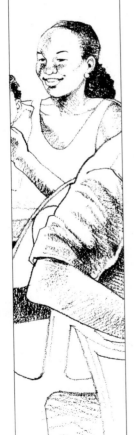

Lactation is a physiologic process accomplished by females since the origin of mammals. Today, as in times past, the process of breastfeeding is successfully initiated by at least 99% of women who try. All that is required of the lactating mother is an intact mammary gland (or preferably two) and the presence and operation of appropriate physiologic mechanisms that allow for adequate milk production and release.

From this basic physiologic view, the establishment and maintenance of human lactation are determined by at least three factors:

1. The anatomic structure of the mammary tissue and the development of milk-producing cells (alveoli), ducts, and nipples to produce and then deliver the milk
2. The initiation and maintenance of milk secretion
3. The ejection or propulsion of milk from the alveoli to the nipple

But the most significant term above is the word "human." This brings an added personal dimension to the physiologic process. Breastfeeding is a very personal process for a mother.

In this chapter, then, we look at lactation, human milk, and breastfeeding in both physiologic and "human" terms. Clear knowledge of the physiologic factors listed above, which includes nutritional needs, is essential for effective lactation management. Furthermore, sensitivity to the personal needs involved is essential for helping mothers have satisfying breastfeeding experiences. Both of these aspects will be explored to provide individual support for today's mother who is largely inexperienced in breastfeeding.

BREAST ANATOMY AND DEVELOPMENT
Anatomy of the Mammary Gland

Basic structure. The **mammary gland** of the human female consists of milk-producing cells (glandular epithelium) and a duct system embedded in connective tissue and fat (Fig. 5-1).[1] The size of the breast is variable, but in most instances it extends from the second through the sixth rib and from the central breast bone (sternum) to the arm pit. The mammary tissue lies directly over the large chest muscle (pectoralis major muscle) and is separated from this muscle by a layer of fat, which is continuous with the fatty tissue of the gland itself.

Areola. The center of the fully developed breast in the adult woman is marked by the **areola,** a circular pigmented skin area from 1.5 to 2.5 cm in diameter. The surface of the areola appears rough because of the presence of large, somewhat modified fluid-producing glands, which are located directly beneath the skin in the thin subcutaneous tissue layer. The fatty secretion of these glands is believed to lubricate the nipple. Bundles of smooth muscle fibers in the areolar tissue serve to stiffen the nipple for a better grasp by the sucking infant.

Nipple and duct system. The nipple is elevated above the breast and contains 15 to 20 **lactiferous ducts** surrounded by modified muscle cell tissues and covered by wrinkled skin. Partly within this compartment of the nipple and partly below its base, these ducts expand to form the short lactiferous sinuses in which milk may be stored. The sinuses are the continuations of the mammary ducts, which extend outward from the nipple toward the chest wall with numerous secondary branches. The duct system ends in masses of milk-producing cells, which form subsections or **lobules** of the breast (Fig. 5-1).

Adolescent-adult development. During adolescence, as indicated in Chapter 3, the female breasts enlarge to their adult size. Frequently, one breast is slightly larger than the other, but this difference is usually unnoticeable. In a nonpregnant woman the mature breast weighs approximately 200 g, the left being somewhat larger than the right. During pregnancy there is some increase in size and weight such that by term the breast may weigh between 400 and 600 g. During lactation this weight increases to between 600 and 800 g.

Variation after childbirth. Wide variation in the structural composition of the human breasts has been observed in women after childbirth. Some breasts contain little secretory tissue; some large breasts contain less glandular tissue than much smaller organs. It is well known, however, that neither size nor structural composition of the breast significantly influences **lactation** success in the average woman. Almost all women who want to breastfeed find that they can.

Breast Development

Infancy and childhood. In the human newborn the mammary glands are developed sufficiently to appear as distinct, round elevations, which feel like movable soft masses. Through the microscope future milk ducts and glandular lobules can be recognized easily. These early glandular structures can produce a milk-like secretion ("witch's milk") 2 or 3 days after birth. All of these **neonatal** phenomena related to the mammary glands probably result from the intensive developmental processes that occur in the last stages of intrauterine life. Usually they subside in the first few weeks after birth. Some shrinkage or involution in the breast takes place by the time the infant is several weeks old, and this is followed by the "quiescent" period of mammary growth and activity during infancy and childhood.

Adolescence. With the onset of puberty and during adolescence, an increased output of estrogenic hormone accomplishes ovarian maturation and follicular stimulation.

Mammary glands
(Gr *mamme,* mother's breast) Milk-producing glands in the females of all mammal species, humans and animals, distinguished from all other animal life by bearing live young and producing milk to nourish them.

Areola
(L *areola,* area, space) Pigmented area surrounding the nipple of the human breast.

Lactiferous ducts
(L *lac,* milk; *ferre,* to bear; *ducere,* to lead or draw) Vessels producing or conveying milk from producing cells to storage and release areas of the breast; tube or passage for secretions.

Lobule
(L *lobus,* lobe, a well-defined area) Smaller branching vessels that make up a lobe of the mammary gland.

Lactation
(L *lactare,* to suckle) Process of milk production and secretion in the mammary glands.

Neonatal
(Gr *,neos,* new; L *natus,* born) Relating to the period surrounding birth, especially the first 4 weeks after birth when the newborn is called a neonate.

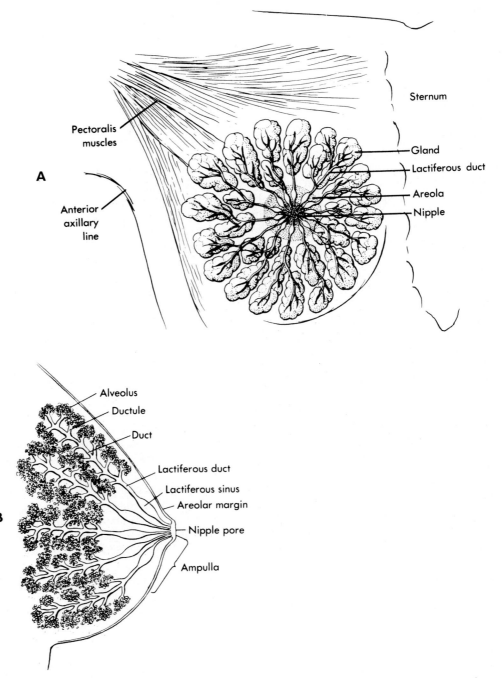

FIG. 5-1 **A,** General anatomic features of the human breast showing its location on the chest, more specifically, the anterior region of the thorax between the sternum and the anterior axillary line. **B,** Detailed structural features of the human mammary gland showing the terminal glandular (alveolar) tissue of each lobule leading into the duct system, which eventually enlarges into the lactiferous duct and lactiferous sinus. The lactiferous sinuses rest beneath the areola and converge at the nipple pore.

As a result of this response, the mammary ducts elongate, and their lining cells reduplicate and proliferate. The growth of the ductal cells is accompanied by growth of fibrous and fatty tissue, which is largely responsible for the increasing size and firmness of the adolescent gland. During this period the areola and nipple also grow and become pigmented.

Breast Maturation

Hormonal effects. As the developing woman matures and ovulation patterns become established, the regular development of progesterone-producing corpora lutea in the ovaries promotes the second stage of mammary development. Lobules gradually appear, giving the mammary glands the characteristic lobular structure found during the childbearing period. This differentiation into a lobular gland is completed about 12 to 18 months after the first menstrual period, but further development continues in proportion to the intensity of the hormonal stimuli during each menstrual cycle and especially during pregnancies.

Functional mammary tissue. Some young women enter reproductive life with insufficient functional mammary tissue to produce enough milk for their baby's total nourishment. In some cases this relates to underdevelopment of the mammary ductwork associated with periodic cessation of menstruation (amenorrhea) or very late menarche. In addition, there are women who have had surgery to remove cysts, tumors, or other growths; others have undergone surgery for breast reduction or reconstruction. For whatever reason, circumstances exist in which functional mammary tissue is insufficient to fully support a nursing infant. Fortunately these situations are rare.

Preparation during pregnancy. The mammary gland of a nonpregnant woman is inadequately prepared for secretory activity. Only during pregnancy do changes occur that make satisfactory milk production possible. In the first trimester of pregnancy the small ducts sprouting from the mammary ducts proliferate to create a maximum number of surface cells for future alveolar cell formation. In the mid-trimester the reduplicated small ductules group together to form large lobules. Their central cavities begin to dilate. In the last trimester the existent clumps of milk-producing cells progressively dilate in the final preparation for the lactation process.

Role of the placenta. The placenta plays an important role in mammary growth in pregnancy. It secretes ovarian-like hormones in large quantities. A number of these hormones have been identified as contributing to mammary gland growth.

Antepartum preparation. Although mammary growth and development occur rapidly throughout pregnancy, additional proliferation of lining cells takes place in the **antepartum** period shortly before delivery of the baby or at **parturition**. The proliferation of these cells that begins just before parturition in response to increasing levels of the hormone **prolactin** results in new cells with a new complement of enzymes.

THE PHYSIOLOGY OF LACTATION
General Activity

Initial postpartum secretions. Full lactation does not begin as soon as the baby is born. During the first 2 or 3 days **postpartum** a small amount of **colostrum** is secreted. In subsequent days a rapid increase in milk secretion occurs, and in usual cases lactation is reasonably well established by the end of the first week. In first-time mothers (primiparas), however, the establishment of lactation may be delayed until the third week or even later. Generally, therefore, the first 2 or 3 weeks are a period of lactation initiation, and this is followed by the longer period of maintenance of lactation.

Antepartum
(L *ante*, before; *partum*, parting, a separate part) Period of gestation before onset of labor and the birth of the infant.

Parturition
(L *parturitio*, to give birth) Act or process of childbirth; labor and delivery.

Prolactin
(Gr *pro-*, before; L *lac*, milk) Hormone of the anterior pituitary gland that stimulates and maintains lactation in postpartum mammals.

Colostrum
(L *colostrum*, bee sting swelling and secretions) Thin, yellowish, milky liquid, mother's initial breast secretion before and immediately after birth of her baby; rich in immune factors and nutrition, especially protein and minerals; foremilk.

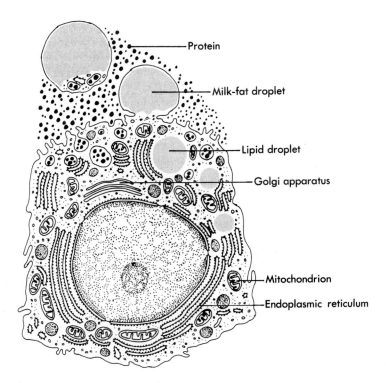

FIG. 5-2 Diagrammatic representation of a mammary gland cell showing the basic square shape with typical wavy surface border and nucleus. Cytoplasmic organization is characteristic of cells undergoing active protein synthesis and secretion. The synthetic apparatus consists of many free ribosomes and an extensive system of rough endoplasmic reticulum. A large Golgi body is located above the nucleus, and associated with it are some vacuoles containing particulate material that condenses into a central core or granule. Toward the top, the granules become progressively larger and contain more dense protein granules. The vacuoles fuse with the surface membrane and liberate their contents intact into the lumen. Fat droplets are found throughout the cell but are largest near the top. They protrude into the lumen and appear to pinch off from the cell proper along with a small bit of cytoplasm. Other cytoplasmic structures include large mitochondria lysosomes, and a small number of smooth membranous tubules and vesicles.

Modified from Lentz TL: *Cell fine structure: an atlas of drawings of whole cell-structure,* Philadelphia, 1971, WB Saunders.

Milk production stages. Initiation and maintenance of lactation comprises a complex process involving both nerves and hormones. It involves the sensory nerves in the nipples, the spinal cord, the hypothalamus, and the pituitary gland with its various hormones. The process of milk production occurs in two distinct stages: (1) secretion of milk and (2) propulsion or ejection whereby the milk passes along the duct system. The two events are closely related and often occur simultaneously in the nursing mother.

The secretion of milk involves both the synthesis of the milk components and the passage of the formed product into the ducts (Fig. 5-2). These events may be under independent control, since the accumulation of both fat and protein reaches a high level during the latter part of pregnancy. Shortly before delivery the accumulated secretory products begin to pass into the duct system. The secretory process is activated again by the sucking stimulus of the infant.

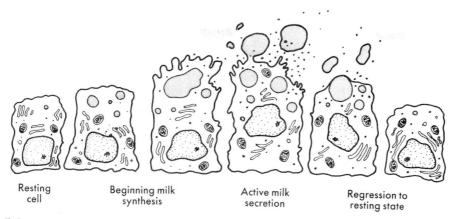

FIG. 5-3   Diagrammatic representation of the cycle of changes that occur in secretory cells of the alveoli from resting stage through milk production and secretion with eventual return to the resting stage.

In general, each milk-producing **alveolar** cell proceeds through a secretory process that is preceded and followed by a resting stage (Fig. 5-3). Milk synthesis is most active during the suckling period but occurs at lower levels at other times. The secretory cells are square but change to a cylindric shape just before milk secretion while cellular water uptake is increased. As secretion commences, the enlarged cell with its thickened surface becomes clublike in shape. The tip pinches off leaving the cell intact. The milk constituents are then free in the secreted solution, and the cell retains a cap of membrane. Between periods of active milk secretion, alveolar cells return to their characteristic resting state.

Fat Synthesis and Release

Initial synthesis. Fat synthesis takes place in the **endoplasmic reticulum** from compounds synthesized intracellularly or imported from the maternal circulation. Alveolar cells are able to synthesize short chain fatty acids, which are derived predominantly from available acetate. Long chain fatty acids and triglycerides are derived from maternal plasma; these fatty acids are predominantly used for the synthesis of milk fat. Synthesis of triglyceride from intracellular carbohydrate also plays a predominant role in fat production for human milk.

Final preparation and release. The process of esterification of fatty acids takes place in the endoplasmic reticulum. The resultant triglycerides accumulate as small fat droplets in the endoplasmic reticulum but eventually coalesce in the basal region of the cell to form large droplets that migrate toward the top of the cell. Ultimately these droplets bulge into the lumen for eventual discharge. Apocrine secretion involves the protrusion of the cell surface into the lumen with eventual pinching off of the protruded unit. This discharged material usually contains fat globules, protein, and a small amount of **cytoplasm,** all of which will appear in human milk.

Protein Synthesis and Discharge

Initial synthesis. The vast majority of proteins present in normal milk are specific to mammary secretions and are not identified in any quantity elsewhere in nature. The formation of milk protein including mammary enzymes is induced by prolactin and further stimulated by other hormones. Studies using sophisticated microscopic techniques have

Alveoli
(L *alveolus,* hollow) Small sac-like out-pouching areas in the mammary gland, secretory units that produce and secrete milk.

Endoplasmic reticulum
(Gr *endon,* within; *plassein,* to form; L *rete,* net) A protoplasmic network of flattened double-membrane sheets in cells; important metabolic cell organelles, some with rough surfaces bearing ribosomes for protein synthesis and other smooth surfaces synthesizing fatty acids.

Cytoplasm
(Gr *kytos,* hollow vessel; *plasma,* anything formed or molded) Protoplasm of the cell outside the nucleus, a continuous gel-like aqueous solution in which the cell organelles are suspended; site of major cell metabolism.

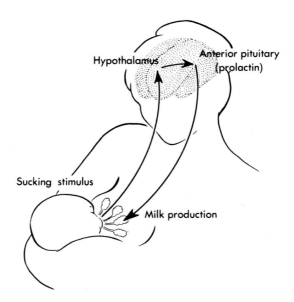

FIG. 5-4 Diagrammatic representation of the basic physiologic features of milk production. The sucking stimulus provided by the baby sends a message to the hypothalamus. The hypothalamus stimulates the anterior pituitary to release prolactin, the hormone that promotes milk production by alveolar cells of the mammary glands.

De novo
(L *anew,* from the beginning) To make a fresh from primary components; "from scratch," as in cooking.

Golgi apparatus
A complex cup-like structure of membranes with associated vesicles first described by Italian Nobel prize-winning histologist Camillo Golgi (1843-1926); synthesis site of numerous carbohydrate metabolic products such as lactose, glycoproteins, and mucopolysaccharides.

Vesicle
(L *vesica,* bladder) A small bladder or sac containing liquid; secretory transport sacs that move out into the cell cytoplasm to aid metabolism.

clearly shown that the abundant rough endothelial reticulum is the site of protein synthesis in the secretory cell.

Final preparation and release. Protein granules accumulate within the Golgi complexes before transport through the cell and release into the lumen by apocrine secretion or reverse pinocytosis. The proteins in milk are derived from two sources: (1) some are synthesized **de novo** in the mammary gland, and (2) others are derived as such from plasma. Inclusion of plasma-derived proteins in the milk secretion occurs primarily in the early secretory product colostrum. Thereafter the three main proteins in milk—casein, alpha-lactalbumin, and beta-lactalbumin—are synthesized within the gland from amino acid precursors. All of the essential and some of the nonessential amino acids are taken up directly from the plasma, but some of the nonessential amino acids are synthesized by the milk-producing cells of the gland.

Carbohydrate Synthesis and Release

Lactose synthesis. The predominant carbohydrate in milk is lactose. Its synthesis occurs within the **Golgi apparatus** of the alveolar cell. The synthesis of lactose combines glucose and galactose. Most of the intracellular glucose is derived continually from circulating blood glucose; galactose is synthesized from glucose.

Final preparation and release. Once synthesized within the Golgi complex, lactose is attached to protein and carried to the cell surface in a **vesicle.** It is then released from the surface of the cell by reverse pinocytosis, as occurs with several other milk components.

The Role of Hormones

Milk secretion. The stimulus for milk secretion derives largely from the hormone prolactin (Fig. 5-4). This hormone acts on alveolar cells and promotes continual milk production and release. Maintenance of milk secretion, however, requires other hormonal

TABLE 5-1   *Nutrient Content of Mature Human Milk*

Constituent (per Liter)	Human Milk	Constituent (per Liter)	Human Milk
Energy (kcal)	680	Minerals	
Protein (g)	10.5	Calcium (mg)	280
Fat (g)	39.0	Phosphorus (mg)	140
Lactose (g)	72.0	Sodium (mg)	180
Vitamins		Potassium (mg)	525
Vitamin A (RE)*	670	Chloride (mg)	420
Vitamin D (μg)	0.55	Magnesium (mg)	35
Vitamin E (mg)	2.3	Iron (mg)	0.3
Vitamin K (μg)	2.1	Iodine (μg)	110
Thiamin (mg)	0.21	Manganese (μg)	6.0
Riboflavin (mg)	0.35	Copper (mg)	0.25
Niacin (mg)	1.5	Zinc (mg)	1.2
Pyridoxine (μg)	93	Selenium (μg)	20
Folic acid (μg)	85	Fluoride (μg)	16
Cobalamine (μg)	0.97	Chromium (μg)	50
Ascorbic acid (mg)	40		

*RE, retinol equivalents.
Data from Institute of Medicine: *Nutrition during lactation,* Washington, DC, 1991, National Academy Press.

The Nature of Human Milk

Variable basic content. Reports during the past 20 years on the biochemical composition of human milk have included over 1000 publications. Large numbers of new components continue to be characterized such that more than a hundred constituents are now recognized. Basically human milk consists of a solution of protein, sugar, and salts in which a variety of fatty compounds are suspended (Table 5-2). The composition varies from one human to another, from one period of lactation to the next, and even hourly during the day. The composition of a given milk sample is related not only to the amount secreted and the stage of the lactation but also to the timing of the withdrawal and to individual variations among lactating mothers. These latter individual variations may be affected by such variables as maternal age, parity, health, and social class. **Gestational age** of the infant also makes a difference.

Milk volume. Observations of completely breastfed babies who appear to be thriving suggest that daily volume of breast consumption ranges from 340 to over 1000 ml/day. The mean falls between 600 and 900 ml/day, at least for representative North American women.[3] Mothers of twins may show an enhanced capacity for milk production (Fig. 5-6). Hartmann, in Western Australia, compared milk outputs of mothers of single infants with that of mothers of twins.[4] The obvious difference in milk production is demonstrated in Fig. 5-6. Severe food restriction may limit the volume of milk production.[3] A lifestyle involving vigorous exercise, however, does not have a detrimental impact on milk output.[5]

Relation to maternal nutrition. Although many data have been recorded on the differences in samples of human milk, the general picture is the same throughout the world. Except for vitamin and fat content, the composition of human milk appears to be largely independent of the state of the mother's nutrition, at least until malnutrition becomes severe. Even after prolonged lactation for 2 years or more, the quality of the milk produced

Gestational age
(L *gestare,* to bear) Period of embryonic-fetal growth and development from ovum fertilization to birth; varying with degree of preterm development to full-term mature newborn.

TABLE 5-2   Classes of Constituents in Human Milk

Protein and nonprotein nitrogen compounds

Proteins
Caseins
α-Lactalbumin
Lactoferrin
Secretory IgA and other immunoglobulins
β-Lactoglobulin
Lysozyme
Enzymes
Hormones
Growth factors

Nonprotein nitrogen compounds
Urea
Creatine
Creatinine
Uric acid
Glucosamine
α-Amino nitrogen
Nucleic acids
Nucleotides
Polyamines

Water-soluble vitamins
Thiamin
Riboflavin
Niacin
Pantothenic acid
Biotin
Folate
Vitamin B$_6$
Vitamin B$_{12}$
Vitamin C
Inositol
Choline

Cells
Leukocytes
Epithelial cells

Carbohydrates
Lactose
Oligosaccharides
Bifidus factors
Glycopeptides

Lipids
Triglycerides
Fatty acids
Phospholipids
Sterols and hydrocarbons
Fat-soluble vitamins
  A and carotene
  D
  E
  K

Minerals
Macronutrient elements
Calcium
Phosphorus
Magnesium
Potassium
Sodium
Chlorine
Sulfur

Trace elements
Iodine
Iron
Copper
Zinc
Manganese
Selenium
Chromium
Cobalt

Modified from National Academy of Sciences: *Nutrition during lactation,* Washington, DC, 1991, National Academy Press.

by Indian and African women appears to be relatively well maintained, although the quantity may be small. Also, it is well known that severely undernourished women during time of famine often manage to feed their babies reasonably well.[3]

Colostrum

In the first few days after birth, the mammary glands secrete a small amount of opaque fluid called colostrum. The volume varies between 2 and 10 ml per feeding per day during

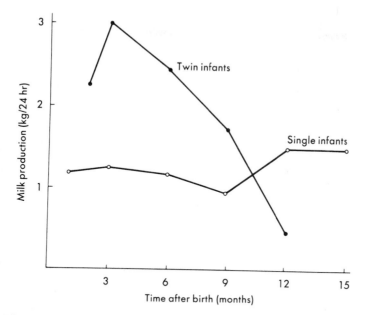

FIG. 5-6　Milk outputs of Western Australian women breastfeeding twins and exclusively breastfeeding single babies.

Based on data from Hartmann PE et al: *Birth Fam J* 8:215, 1981.

the first 3 days, related in part to the parity of the mother. Women who have had other pregnancies, particularly those who have nursed babies previously, usually demonstrate colostrum output sooner and in greater volume than other women. Colostrum is typically yellow, a feature associated with its relatively high carotene content. Also, it contains more protein and less sugar and fat than milk produced thereafter. As might be expected from these composition differences, it is lower in kilocalories than mature milk—67 versus 75 kcal/100 ml. The ash content of colostrum is high, and concentrations of sodium, potassium, and chloride are greater than in mature milk. The few composition analyses of human colostrum that have been reported show striking variability during any one day and from day to day. It is likely that these differences partially reflect the unstable secretory patterns that exist in the mammary apparatus as it begins active production, secretion, and ejection of milk.

Transitional Milk

Colostrum changes to transitional milk between the third and sixth day, at which time the protein content is still rather high. By the tenth day the major changes have been completed, and by the end of the first month the protein content reaches a consistent level that does not fall significantly thereafter. As the content of protein falls, the content of lactose progressively rises. This is also the case for fat, which increases to typical levels as lactation becomes more firmly established.

Preterm Milk

With the renewed interest in the feeding of human milk to preterm infants, substantial attention has been focused on the composition of milk produced by mothers who deliver prematurely.[6] Early reports suggested that the protein and nonprotein nitrogen content of **preterm milk** was higher than that of term milk. Additional observations revealed that

Preterm milk
Milk produced by mothers of premature infants.

preterm milk might also be higher in its concentration of calcium, IgA, sodium, potassium, chloride, phosphorus, magnesium, medium chain and polyunsaturated long-chain fatty acids, and total lipids, but lower in its lactose level than term milk. Thus the opinion developed that premature infants who are fed their mother's milk might demonstrate superior growth and development to that observed in premature infants fed banked human milk. In general this suspicion has proved to be true for very low-birth-weight infants as reported by researchers who have completed appropriate comparisons. It appears, however, that commercial infant formulas designed for low-birth-weight infants may also be superior to banked human milk in supporting growth of these babies.

The controversy surrounding the nutritional adequacy of human milk for very low-birth-weight infants still exists. Although recent observations suggest that premature infants can thrive on milk from their own mothers, it is known that protein and sodium concentrations are marginal and calcium and phosphate levels are too low to support optimum development of the skeleton. In the face of immature gastrointestinal and renal function and poor nutrient stores, the very low-birth-weight infant who is provided human milk will often profit from an organized supplementation program.

It is even possible to supplement human milk with a powdered or liquid product designed to improve nutritional adequacy for very low-birth-weight infants.* The powdered fortifier contains protein and carbohydrate and increases the caloric density of breast milk to about 24 kilocalories per ounce. The product is sold in premeasured packets; one packet is designed for addition to 25 ml of human milk. The liquid fortifier is similar in composition and is designed to be mixed with human milk or fed alternately with human milk.

COMPOSITION OF MATURE HUMAN MILK
Protein

Amount and types of protein. It is well known that different animals show different rates of growth. This fact appears to be related to their milk. The slowest rate of growth is found in humans and human milk contains the least protein. The major proteins found in breast milk are caseins and whey proteins. Caseins are phosphorus-containing proteins that occur only in milk. The **whey** proteins, like lactalbumin and lactoferrin, are synthesized in the mammary gland. Other proteins, including protein hormones and serum albumin, are transported to the milk from the plasma. The concentration of protein found in human milk is lower than the previously accepted value of 1.5 g/100 ml that was calculated from analyzed nitrogen content. Since human milk has been found to contain 25% of its nitrogen in nonprotein compounds, the lower protein concentration (0.8 to 0.9 g/100 ml) is now accepted as the true amount.

Initial changes. The protein content of human milk, like that of other mammals, falls rapidly over the first few days of lactation and reflects a relatively higher loss of those proteins important in immune functions. Colostrum averages about 2% protein; transitional and mature milk average 1.5% and 1.0%, respectively.

Relation to maternal diet. Observations of many women in a variety of countries have shown that protein content of human milk is not reduced in mothers consuming a diet low in protein or poor in protein quality. A study in Pakistan supports this idea.[7] Here the protein quality and quantity of milk collected from women of a very low socioeconomic group in Karachi were similar to those of well-nourished women there and in other parts of the world. Of interest, however, was the observation that the concentration of lysine and

Whey
The thin liquid of milk remaining after the curd, containing the mild protein casein, and the cream have been removed; contains other milk proteins lactalbumin and lactoferrin.

---

*Human Milk Fortifier, Mead Johnson Laboratories (powdered); Similac Natural Care, Ross Laboratories (liquid).

TABLE 5-3   *Significant Features About the Amino Acid Composition of Human Milk*

Characteristic	Explanation
Lower in methionine and rich in cystine	An enzyme, cystathionase, is late to develop in the fetus; this impairs optimum conversion of methionine to cystine, which is needed for growth and development; methionine may increase in the bloodstream of an infant fed cow's milk but not one fed human milk; hypermethioninemia may damage the central nervous system
Lower in phenylalanine and tyrosine	The enzymes tyrosine aminotransferase and parahydroxyphenyl pyruvate oxidase are late in developing: cow's milk-fed babies may develop hyperphenylalaninemia and hypertyrosinemia, which may adversely affect development of the central nervous system, especially in the premature; breast milk offers much less problem
Rich in taurine	Breast milk provides taurine for bile acid conjugation, and it *may* also be a neurotransmitter or neuromodulator in the brain and retina; humans cannot synthesize taurine well; cow's milk contains little taurine; the requirement for taurine in the developing neonate is uncertain

methionine in the free amino acid content of milk samples from malnourished women was reduced when compared with milk from healthy, well-nourished mothers. The investigators suggest that this finding could imply a reduction in nutritional *quality* of the protein in these samples. It is important to recognize, however, that dietary amino acid deficits may be readily subsidized from maternal tissues as long as reserves are available from which to draw in order to maintain protein homeostasis. Temporary fluctuations in free amino acid levels may be apparent, but alterations in quantity or quality of intact milk proteins are much less likely to occur until maternal protein stores are severely depleted.

Effect of chronic maternal protein deficit. With chronic protein undernutrition, breast milk composition may change. One study was carried out to assess the effects of prolonged lactation on the quantity of protein and patterns of amino acids in breast milk obtained from Thai women at various times during lactation.[8] Protein levels decreased from 1.56% during the first week to a low of about 0.6% from 180 to 270 days and then rose to about 0.7%. Using these data, one can calculate that a 3-month-old infant in the 50th percentile for weight would require about 1250 ml of milk per day to meet protein needs. Since few infants in developing countries would receive this volume of milk daily and since supplemental sources of protein are scarce, the protein status of such infants could be significantly compromised.

Amino acids. The amino acid content of human milk is recognized as ideal for the human infant. It is relatively low in several amino acids that are known to be detrimental if found in the blood at high levels, for example, in the genetic disease phenylalanine; on the other hand it is high in other amino acids that the infant cannot synthesize well, such as cystine and taurine. Some of the positive features of amino acid composition of human milk are summarized in Table 5-3. These characteristics are especially useful to infants whose biochemical capabilities are underdeveloped at birth.

Nonprotein nitrogen. The total amount of nonprotein nitrogen in human milk averages nearly 25% of all nitrogen and is significantly higher than that found in cow's milk (about 5%). The importance of this to infant nutrition and health is unknown. Nonprotein nitrogen sources consist of a variety of organic, and trace amounts of inorganic, compounds shed into the milk supply. Among these compounds are peptides and free amino acids, the latter of which may provide a nutritional advantage to the infant. Nonprotein nitrogen sources also include urea, creatinine, and sugar amines. Scientists have speculated that it is of nutritional significance that each species of mammal seems to carry a characteristic pattern of free amino acids in its nonprotein nitrogen pool.

Taurine. Much recent discussion has centered on the amino acid taurine. Since taurine is found in particularly high levels in fetal brain tissue, it has been proposed that it may play a role in the development of the brain. In addition, taurine is associated with bile acid and thus plays an important role in digestion and may function in the management of cholesterol in the body. Since human milk contains much more taurine than does cow's milk, it has been speculated that the breastfed infant might profit significantly from the higher taurine intake. Interestingly, however, observations have shown that breastfed babies maintain plasma taurine levels that are similar to those of formula-fed infants. It would therefore appear that taurine is not an essential amino acid for infants. However, the general consensus is that taurine is a conditionally essential nutrient for human infants and children, especially those born prematurely.[9]

Lipids

Amount. The total lipid content of human milk varies considerably from one woman to another and is even affected by parity and season of the year. Separate observations by different investigators around the world give the following average levels of fat in human milk: 2.02%, 3.1%, 3.2%, 3.27%, 3.95%, 4.5%, and 5.3%. Sampling methods may affect fat content, since the first milk (fore-milk) is low in fat and the last milk (hind-milk) shows about a threefold increase in the fat content.

Types. Nearly 90% of the lipid in human milk is present in the form of triglycerides. But small amounts of phospholipids, cholesterol, diglycerides, monoglycerides, glycolipids, sterol esters, and free fatty acids are also found. The fatty acid composition of human milk differs greatly from that of cow's milk. The content of the essential fatty acid linoleic acid is considerably greater in human milk than in cow's milk. The content of short-chain saturated fatty acids (C4 to C8) is greater in cow's milk. Of equal interest is the observation that human milk contains more cholesterol than cow's milk and much more cholesterol than commercial infant formulas. A beneficial effect of this higher cholesterol level has been suggested on grounds that (1) it is needed by the rapidly growing central nervous system for **myelin** synthesis, and (2) in early life it stimulates the development of enzymes necessary for cholesterol degradation.

Recent research has demonstrated that human milk contains not only linoleic acid and linolenic acid but also **eicosapentanoic acid (EPA)** and **docosahexanoic acid (DHA).** Interestingly, infant formula does not contain the longer-chain forms EPA and DHA. Since animal experiments have provided evidence that these **omega-3 fatty acids** may be essential for the normal prenatal and postnatal development of the brain and retina, the contribution that human milk makes to this developmental process is receiving much attention.[10]

Maternal diet effect on composition. The composition of the fat in human milk varies significantly with the diet of the mother. Lactating women fed a diet rich in polyunsaturated fats, such as corn and cottonseed oils, produce milk with an increased content of polyunsaturated fats. This is best seen by comparing total vegetarians with nonvegetarian, as seen in Table 5-4. Over the years, as dietary unsaturated fat intake has increased in the United States, the fatty acid composition of breast milk samples has reflected this change (Table 5-5).

When maternal energy intake is severely restricted, fatty acid composition of human

Myelin
The fatty coating of nerve fibers.

Eicosapentanoic acid (EPA)
(Gr *eicosa,* twenty; *penta,* five) Long-chain polyunsaturated fatty acid composed of a chain of 20 carbon atoms with 5 double (unsaturated) bonds; one of the omega-3 fatty acids found in fatty fish and fish oils.

Docasahexanoic acid (DHA)
(Gr *docosa,* twenty-two; *hexa,* six) Long-chain polyunsaturated omega-3 fatty acid having a 22 carbon chain with 6 double (unsaturated) bonds; metabolic product of omega-3 EPA, found in fatty fish and fish oils. The body synthesizes both EPA and DHA from the essential fatty acids linoleic and linolenic acids.

Omega-3 fatty acids
Group of long-chain polyunsaturated fatty acids having important precursor roles in producing highly active hormone-like substances, the *eicosanoids,* involved in critcal metabolic activities such as vascular muscle tone and blood clotting.

TABLE 5-4 *Mean Breast Milk Fatty Acid Concentration in Vegetarians (Vegans) and Nonvegetarians (Controls)*

Methyl Esters	Vegans*	Controls*
Lauric ($C_{12:0}$)	39	33
Myristic ($C_{14:0}$)	68	80
Palmitic ($C_{16:0}$)	166	276
Stearic ($C_{18:0}$)	52	108
Palmitoleic ($C_{16:1}$)	12	36
Oleic ($C_{18:1}$)	313	353
Linoleic ($C_{18:2}$)	317	69
Linolenic ($C_{18:3}$)	15	8

*Mean values expressed as milligrams per gram total methyl esters detected for four vegans and four controls (nonvegetarians).
Modified from Sanders TAB et al: *Am J Clin Nutr* 31:805, 1978.

TABLE 5-5 *Reports of Fatty Acid Composition of Human Milk*

Fatty Acid	Breast Milk Content (Percent of Total Fatty Acid)	
	1953*	1977†
Lauric ($C_{12:0}$)	5.5	3.8
Myrisitic ($C_{14:0}$)	8.5	5.2
Palmitic ($C_{16:0}$)	23.2	22.5
Palmitoleic ($C_{16:1}$)	3.0	4.1
Stearic ($C_{18:0}$)	6.9	8.7
Oleic ($C_{18:1}$)	36.5	39.5
Linoleic ($C_{18:2}$)	7.8	14.4
Linolenic ($C_{18:3}$)	—	2.0

*Based on data from Macy IG et al: *The composition of milks,* Pub No 254, Washington, DC, 1958, National Research Council.
†Based on data from Guthrie HA, Picciano ME, Sheehe D: *J Pediatr* 90:39, 1977.

milk resembles that of **depot fat.** This effect is to be expected; it represents fat mobilization in response to the reduction in energy intake. A substantial increase in the proportion of dietary kilocalories from carbohydrate will result in an increase in milk content of fatty acids with carbon chain lengths less than 16. The significance of this latter observation is unknown.

As far as cholesterol is concerned, there is no evidence that its concentration in human milk is altered by the maternal diet. In fact, milk cholesterol level stays between 100 and 150 mg/L even in hypercholesterolemic women and increases only in severe cases of pathologic hypercholesterolemia.

Fat-digesting enzymes. Human milk contains several lipases. One is a serum-stimulated lipase (lipoprotein lipase) that may appear in the milk as a result of leakage from the mammary tissue. Another fat-digesting milk enzyme has a similar activity to that of pancreatic lipase, breaking down triglycerides to free fatty acids and glycerol. This enzyme

Depot fat
Body fat stored in adipose tissue

Lipolysis

(Gr *lipos*, fat; *lysis*, dissolution) Fat digestion or break-down.

Carnitine

A naturally occurring amino acid ($C_7H_{15}NO_3$) formed from methionine and lysine, required for transport of long-chain fatty acids across the mitochondrial membrane where they are oxidized as fuel substrate for metabolic energy.

Mitochondrion

(Gr *mitos*, thread; *chondrion*, granule) Cell's "powerhouse," small elongated organelle located in the cell cytoplasm; principal site of energy generation (ATP synthesis); contains enzymes of the final energy cycle (citric acid cycle) and cell respiratory chains, as well as ribonucleic acid (RNA) and deoxyribonucleic acid (DNA) for some synthesis of protein.

Nanomole (nmol)

(Gr *nanos*, dwarf; *molekul*, molecule) Metric system unit for measuring extremely small amounts. Prefix *nano-* used in naming units of measurement to indicate one-billionth of the unit with which it is combined. Mole is the chemical term for the molecular weight of a substance expressed in grams-gram molecular weight.

Polymer

(Gr *poly-*, many; *meros*, part) Large compound formed by chains of simple repeating molecules, e.g., glucose polymer oligosaccharide.

is present in the fat fraction and appears to be inhibited by bile salts. It probably is responsible for **lipolysis** of milk refrigerated or frozen for later use. Additional lipases in the skim milk fraction are inactive until they encounter bile. These lipases, the bile salt-stimulated lipases, are believed to be present only in the milk of primates and are thought to serve some useful purpose for this species. Since the bile salt-stimulated lipases have been clearly shown to be stable and active in the intestine of infants, they can contribute significantly to the hydrolysis of milk triglycerides and partly account for the greater ease in fat digestion that is commonly demonstrated by breastfed babies.

Carnitine. Both human milk and cow's milk contain **carnitine,** which plays an important role in the oxidation of long-chain fatty acids by facilitating their transport across the **mitochondrial** membrane. The body's supply of carnitine is derived in part by ingestion of dietary carnitine and in part by ingestion of dietary carnitine and in part by endogenous synthesis from the essential amino acids lysine and methionine. Newborns are especially in need of carnitine since fat provides a major source of energy. It has been suggested that carnitine may be an essential nutrient for the newborn since infants may have a limited synthetic capacity, especially those born prematurely.[11] Human milk contains about 50 to 100 **nmol** of carnitine per milliliter; formula products based on milk or beef contain 50 to 656 nmol/ml. Those formulas prepared from soy isolate, and specialized formulations from egg white and casein, carry an amount equal to or less than 4 nmol/ml. For this reason most manufacturers of soy-based infant formulas now add carnitine to their products. Whether or not infants using any of these formulas or provided human milk require additional carnitine has been the subject of much debate. At this point, it appears that supplemental carnitine is unnecessary for the vast majority of neonates.

Carbohydrate

Lactose. Lactose, a disaccharide composed of glucose and galactose, is the main carbohydrate in human milk. In all species of mammals studied, milk is isotonic with plasma, which helps keep the cost of milk secretion low. Lactose exerts 60% to 70% of the total osmotic pressure of milk. The concentrations of lactose in human milk are remarkably similar among women and there is no good evidence that they can be influenced by maternal dietary factors.

Lactose is relatively insoluble and is slowly digested and absorbed in the small intestine. The presence of lactose in the gut of the infant stimulates the growth of microorganisms that produce organic acids and synthesize many of the B vitamins. It is believed that the acid milieu that is created helps to check the growth of undesirable bacteria in the infant's gut and to improve the absorption of calcium, phosphorus, magnesium, and other minerals. Since human milk contains much more lactose than cow's milk (7% and 4.8%, respectively), these gut-associated benefits of lactose are more significant in the breastfed than in the bottle-fed infant.

Other carbohydrates. Chromatographic processing of human milk samples has revealed trace amounts of glucose, galactose, and an array of moderate chain length carbohydrates (oligosaccharides). Some of these appear to be protective even though they are present in low concentrations. Nitrogen-containing sugars promote the growth of lactobacilli, the dominant acid-producing bacteria in the lower intestinal tract of breastfed infants. Specialized oligosaccharides inhibit the binding of selected bacterial pathogens or their toxins to epithelial cells by acting as "trapping receptors."

Amylase. Although human milk does not contain much complex carbohydrate, it does contain a starch-splitting enzyme, amylase, which is quite stable at pH levels found in the stomach and small bowel.[12] This enzyme may provide an alternative pathway for digestion of glucose **polymers** and starches in early infancy when pancreatic amylase is low or absent in duodenal fluid. The physiologic importance of mammary amylase may be analogous to that of the bile salt-stimulated lipase found in human milk.

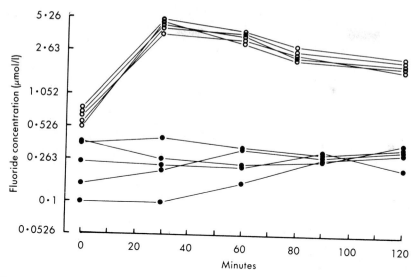

FIG. 5-7 Plasma *(open symbols)* and breast milk *(closed symbols)* fluoride concentrations in mothers after oral dose of 1.5 mg fluoride as sodium fluoride solution. (Conversion: fluoride – 1 mol/L $\approx$ 19 ng/ml.)

From Ekstrand J: No evidence of transfer of fluoride from plasma to breast milk, *Br Med J* 283:761, 1981.

Minerals

Comparison with cow's milk. One of the most striking differences between human and cow's milk lies in the mineral composition. As with protein, it is believed that this difference may be related to the rate of growth of the species for which the milk was intended. According to typical estimates, there is six times more phosphorus, four times more calcium, three times more total ash, and three times more protein in cow's milk than in human milk. The high mineral and protein composition of cow's milk distinctly affects the amount of mineral and protein waste products provided to the kidney. One might speculate that the kidney of the newborn infant is prepared to handle the "waste" derived from breast milk but is stressed unduly by the requirements placed on it when cow's milk, especially nonfat milk, is selected as an alternate.

Major and trace minerals. The major minerals found in mature human milk are potassium, calcium, phosphorus, chlorine, and sodium. Iron, copper, and manganese are found in only trace amounts, and since these elements are required for normal red blood cell synthesis, infants fed too long on milk alone become anemic. Minute amounts of zinc, magnesium, aluminum, iodine, chromium, selenium, and fluoride are also found in breast milk. Infants who are not provided with fluoridated water in addition to breast milk may benefit from a daily oral fluoride supplement of regulated dosage predetermined by the physician or pharmacist. Providing the lactating woman with a fluoride supplement does not significantly alter her milk output of fluoride (Fig. 5-7).

Varying mineral composition. The total mineral content of human milk is fairly constant, but the specific amounts of individual minerals may vary with the status of the mother and the stage of lactation. Observations from a number of laboratories have shown declining concentrations of several minerals over the weeks and months following the onset of lactation (Fig. 5-8). Of substantial interest are other reports in which dietary intake and supplementation habits of mothers have been compared with mineral composition of milk. In most situations little relationship has been found between maternal mineral intake and

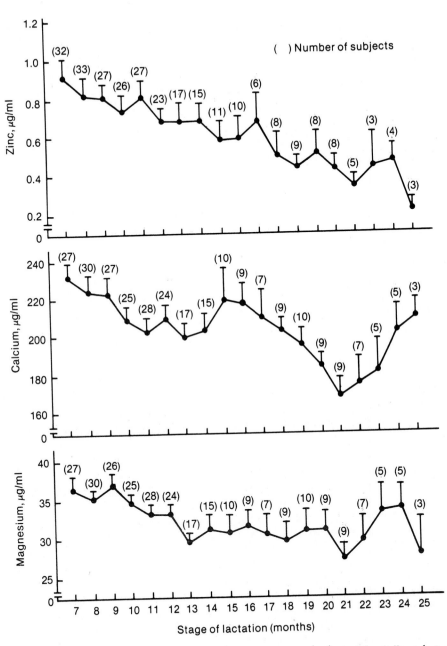

FIG. 5-8   Concentrations of zinc, calcium, and magnesium in milk samples collected at a morning feeding from 7 to 25 months of lactation. *Vertical bars* represent SEM.

Based on data from Karra MV et al: *Am J Clin Nutr* 43:495, 1986.

mineral content of milk. However, since the adequacy of maternal intake of some minerals has been questioned, this may place the mother at risk.

Iron and zinc bioavailability. Some minerals are more easily absorbed from breast milk than from cow's milk or commercial formulas. McMillan and others reported that nearly 50% of the iron in human milk is absorbed, whereas availability of iron from cow's milk and iron-fortified formulas is only 10% and 4%, respectively.[13,14] More recently Garry and

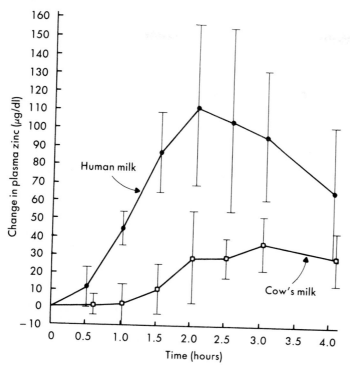

FIG. 5-9   Changes in plasma zinc concentration after ingestion of 25 mg of zinc with human milk (five subjects) and cow's milk (seven subjects). Points represent means ± SD variation from baseline value.

From Casey CE, Walravens PA, Hambidge KM: Availability of zinc: loading tests with human milk, cow's milk, and infant formulas, *Pediatrics* 68:394, 1981.

associates found that iron absorption from human milk may be much higher than 50% during the first 3 months of life.[15] An explanation for this improved absorption has not been found.

Iron supplementation. Whether or not breastfed infants should receive iron supplements is still the subject of much debate.[15,16] Several studies suggest that infants who are breastfed during the first 6 months of life and receive little or no dietary iron other than that in human milk appear to be iron sufficient at age 6 months. However, based on changes in total body iron determined by body weights and hemoglobin and ferritin concentrations, Owen and others concluded that some nonsupplemented breastfed infants are in negative iron balance between ages 3 and 6 months.[16] One might suggest that human milk alone cannot provide sufficient iron for optimum infant nutrition after 5 or 6 months of life.

Like iron, the **bioavailability** of zinc is substantially better from human milk than from other alternative preparations.[17] In one study the bioavailability of zinc fed to rats in various milk solutions was 59.2% for human milk, 42% for cow's milk, and 26.8% to 39% for commercial formulas. In other work human subjects demonstrated better absorption of zinc from human milk than from cow's milk or selected infant formulas (Fig. 5-9). An explanation for the better absorption of zinc from human milk is still being sought. It has been suggested, however, that the unique distribution and binding of zinc, and some other elements, to high and low molecular weight fractions of milk very likely are related to the differences in bioavailability that have now been demonstrated by a number of investigators.

Bioavailability
   Amount of a nutrient ingested in food that is absorbed and thus available to the body for metabolic use.

Fat-Soluble Vitamins

General vitamin content. All the vitamins, both fat- and water-soluble, required for good nutrition and health are supplied in breast milk, but the amounts vary markedly from one person to another. The major factor influencing the vitamin content of human milk is the mother's vitamin status. In general, when maternal intakes of a vitamin are chronically low, the levels of that vitamin in human milk are also low. As maternal intakes of the vitamin increase, levels in milk also increase. For many vitamins, however, a plateau develops that is not exceeded in the face of further augmentation in vitamin intake through diet or supplement. As a general rule, milk concentrations of water-soluble vitamins are more responsive to maternal dietary intake than are the concentrations of fat-soluble vitamins.

Vitamin D. The amount of biologically active vitamin D in human milk has been found to be low (0.5 to 1.5 μg/L). However, maternal sunshine exposure and dietary intake affect infant vitamin D status through their effects on breast milk vitamin D content. This is supported by the recent finding that a short course of oral vitamin D (60 μg/day) supplementation or exposure to ultraviolet phototherapy quickly raised the levels of **antirachitic** (vitamin D) sterols in the plasma and milk of lactating women.[18] There was a peak effect in 1 week with oral vitamin D supplementation and 2 to 3 days after ultraviolet irradiation. The levels then rapidly returned to baseline. Other reports show a direct relationship between maternal and infant levels of 25-hydroxyvitamin D, implying that maternal vitamin D intake directly affects the vitamin D concentration in breast milk.

A question remains regarding the need for vitamin D supplementation in the term infant who is exclusively breastfed. Although some clinicians do not believe it is necessary, the bulk of data support the practice. Greer and associates found low serum 25-hydroxyvitamin D concentrations and early decreases in bone mineral content in breastfed infants not receiving supplemental vitamin D.[19,20] Ozsoylu and Hasanoglu reported low serum 25-hydroxyvitamin D levels at 1 month of age in breastfed infants not supplemented with vitamin D.[21] In some of the sunniest parts of the world, such as the Middle East, rickets is common in certain breastfed infants because cultural practices keep the babies well clothed and indoors for the first year.[22] Even in the United States, reports of resurgence in rickets among breastfed infants provoke considerable concern.[23,24] Since no harm is associated with vitamin D supplementation at 10 μg/day and since expense and inconvenience are trivial, support of this practice seems justifiable. For light-skinned suburban populations in sunny regions and seasons, one may worry less about compliance with this recommendation.

Vitamin A. Milk is a good source of vitamin A and its precursors. Its concentration in human milk is influenced by the quality and quantity of the dietary elements consumed by the mother. The vitamin A content of breast milk is reportedly much lower in some developing countries than in the West. Maternal serum vitamin A levels in these same regions are also typically low. Vitamin A or carotene intake of some Western mothers is higher in the spring and summer months because of greater supplies of green leafy and yellow vegetables. Modern methods of preservation, however, have extended the length of seasons for many vegetables and fruits so that dietary differences from season to season may be minimal for many women with access to supermarkets, home freezers, and other such luxuries of modern society.

Vitamin E. Levels of vitamin E in human milk are substantially greater than those in cow's milk. As might be expected, serum levels of vitamin E rise quickly in breastfed infants and are maintained at normal levels without much fluctuation. Cow's milk-fed babies demonstrate depressed circulating levels of vitamin E unless supplemented. Fortunately manufacturers of infant formulas have increased their levels of vitamin E fortification to avoid potential deficiency.

Vitamin K. In mature human milk vitamin K is present at a level of 2 μg/L. Cow's milk contains much more than this amount with a typical reported value of 60 μg/L. Vitamin

Antirachitic
(Gr *anti-*, against; *rachitis*, a spinal disorder) Agent that is therapeutically effective against rickets, a nutritional deficiency disease affecting childhood bone development in which vitamin D is lacking.

CASE STUDY

Vitamin K Deficiency in Breastfed Infants
Case 1

A 5-week-old infant had seizures and apnea following 24 hours of increasing irritability and poor eating. Birth weight was 3.9 kg following a 42-week uncomplicated pregnancy; a self-trained midwife assisted at the home delivery. Neither vitamin K nor prophylaxis for eye infection was given. *Jaundice* was treated with a "grow light" and supplements of vitamins A and E. The infant was breastfed; there was no history of illness or trauma. His mother took no medications, ate a regular diet, and took vitamin supplements.

On physical examination, jaundice, a bulging fontanelle, right-sided seizures, and a discharge from the left eye were observed. Weight was 4.6 kg (75th percentile); length, 53 cm (25th percentile); and head circumference, 38.5 cm (75th percentile). Persistent bleeding was noted following **venipuncture** and **intubation.** Cerebrospinal fluid was grossly bloody. Laboratory results were consistent with internal bleeding; **prothrombin time (PT)** and **partial thromboplastin time (PTT)** were greater than 200 seconds. A **subdural hematoma,** with obliteration of the right ventricle, was shown by **computed tomography** of the head.

Treatment consisted of 5 mg phytonadione (vitamin K), antibiotics, plasma, and phenobarbital salt. Laboratory studies, repeated following transfer to a hospital, showed significant decreases in clotting time indexes; PT and PTT were reduced to 11.6/11.6 (subject/control) and 35.4 seconds, respectively.

Case 2

A 4-week-old, breastfed infant was seen following 3-days of vomiting. She was treated with 250 ml of normal saline in each thigh. When needles were removed, bleeding was noted at the injection site. Tests on hospitalization showed indexes consistent with hemorrhaging, including a PT of 37.4/11.8 (patient/control) and a PTT of 107.5 seconds. Blood factors VII and X were both significantly decreased. Treatment began with 2 mg phytonadione; bleeding ceased within 1 hour of vitamin K administration and before the fresh frozen plasma had been infused. Repeat studies showed normalization of both clotting times and blood factors.

The patient had been born at home after an uncomplicated gestation to a gravida 5, para 4 mother. She received no vitamin K or prophylaxis for eye infection at birth. Her mother ate a regular diet and took vitamin supplements; penicillin had been taken for a possible uterine infection for 2 weeks following delivery.

Venipuncture
A technique in which a vein is punctured through the skin by a sharp, rigid stylet or cannula carrying a flexible plastic catheter or by a steel needle attached to a syringe or catheter.

Intubation
Passage of a tube into a body hole, specifically the insertion of a breathing tube through the mouth or nose, or into the trachea to ensure a patent airway for the delivery of an anesthetic gas or oxygen.

Prothrombin time
A method of detecting specific coagulation defects.

Partial thromboplastin time
A more specific way of detecting coagulation defects.

Subdural hematoma
A collection of blood trapped under the outside layers of the skull, usually resulting from trauma.

Computed tomography
An x-ray technique that produces a film representing a detailed cross-section of tissue structure.

K is produced by the intestinal flora, but it takes several days for the sterile infant gut to establish an effective microbe population. Even then, onset of hemorrhagic disease with bleeding as late as 4 weeks after delivery has been associated with breastfeeding if no vitamin K had been given at birth. It is recommended, therefore, that all newborn infants receive vitamin K.

Water-Soluble Vitamins

Effect of maternal intake. The levels of water-soluble vitamins in human milk are more likely to reflect maternal diet or supplement intake more than most other ingested compounds. Maternal dietary supplements with most of these vitamins have been shown to increase their content in breast milk. This is especially true in women whose dietary patterns or nutritional status are suboptimum. It appears that with some of these vitamins a plateau may be reached where increased intake has no further impact on milk composition. This idea was nicely demonstrated when varying levels of supplemental ascorbic acid were provided to lactating women.[25] With comparable diets, women consuming either 90 mg or 250 mg per day of ascorbic acid produced milk with similar concentration of this vitamin. Women taking 1000 mg of ascorbic acid per day produced milk that was only slightly higher in its ascorbic acid content.

Vitamin B_6. Felice and Kirksey have provided evidence that milk concentration of vitamin B_6 may be a sensitive indicator of vitamin B_6 status of the mother.[26] They further suggest that the majority of lactating women produce milk with a vitamin B_6 content that is substantially less than that recommended for good health and growth of infants. These researchers observed that mothers receiving 2.5 mg/day of supplemental vitamin B_6 failed to supply their breastfeeding infants with 0.3 mg of vitamin B_6 per day, which is the RDA for young infants.[27]

Vitamin B_{12}. The vitamin B_{12} content of human milk has been found to range from 0.33 to 3.2 **ng**/ml (mean 0.97 ng/ml), and ingestion of supplemental B_{12} does not significantly affect milk content.[28] Human milk from well-fed mothers was found to contain adequate amounts of B_{12}. Its bioavailability, however, depends on the sufficiency of **proteolytic enzymes** to release it from its bound form. Infantile neurologic disorders related to vitamin B_{12} deficiency have been reported in breastfed infants of strict vegetarian women.[29,30]

Resistance Factors

A thorough discussion of the composition of breast milk must include mention of the beneficial components of human milk that are not classified as nutrients (Table 5-6).

Bifidus factor. One of the earliest resistance factors to be described in human milk was the bifidus factor, which may be a nitrogen-containing polysaccharide that favors the growth of **Lactobacillus bifidus**. Its uniqueness to human milk has recently been confirmed.[31] *L. bifidus* confers a protective effect against invasive enteropathogenic organisms.

Immunoglobulins. Various **immunoglobulins** are present in human milk, including IgA, IgG, IgD, and IgE. Although IgG appears to migrate from maternal serum into milk, evidence suggests that IgA, IgD, and IgE are produced locally in mammary tissue. A variety of studies support the idea of migration of **lymphoblasts** from maternal gut-associated lymphoid tissue to the mammary glands followed by local production of immunoglobulins at this site and secretion of them into the milk. This mechanism allows for maternal lymphoblasts to obtain antigenic exposure from distant sites and carry this experience to the mammary tissue where synthesis of appropriate antibodies can occur for protection of the suckling infant.

Secretory IgA (sIgA) is the predominant immunoglobulin in human milk. It is found in large amounts in colostrum and in smaller, but still significant, levels in mature breast milk. Secretory immunoglobulins have been shown to be a major host resistance factor against organisms that infect the gastrointestinal tract, in particular *E. coli* and the enteroviruses. Also, a protective effect against other organisms has been demonstrated. Human milk clearly exhibits a prophylactic effect against septicemia of the newborn.

Other host resistance factors. Some of the other host resistance factors in breast milk are also worthy of mention. Lysozyme, an antimicrobial enzyme, occurs in breast milk at 300 times the concentration found in cow's milk. **Lactoferrin** has been described recently as a compound with a "monilia-static" effect against **Candida albicans**. It inhibits the growth of staphylococci and *E. coli* by binding iron, which the bacteria require to proliferate. **Lactoperoxidase,** which has been shown in vitro to act with other substances

TABLE 5-6   *Antiinfectious Factors in Human Milk*

Factor	Function
Bifidus factor	Stimulates growth of bifidobacteria, which antagonizes the survival of enterobacteria
Secretory IgA (sIgA), IgM, IgE, IgD, and IgG	Act against bacterial invasion of the mucosa and/or colonization of the gut (show bacterial and viral neutralizing capacity; activate alternative complement pathway)
Antistaphylococcus factor	Inhibits systemic staphylococcal infection
Lactoferrin	Binds iron and inhibits bacterial multiplication
Lactoperoxidase	Kills streptococci and enteric bacteria
Complement (C_3, C_1)	Promotes opsonization (the rendering of bacteria and other cells susceptible to phagocytosis)
Interferon	Inhibits intracellular viral replication
Lysozyme	Lyses bacteria through destruction of the cell wall
B_{12}-binding protein	Renders vitamin B_{12} unavailable for bacterial growth
Lymphocytes	Synthesize secretory IgA; may have other roles
Macrophages	Synthesize complement, lactoferrin, lysozyme, and other factors; carry out phagocytosis and probably other functions

in combatting streptococci, is also found in human milk. Specific **prostaglandins** have also been defined, and these may protect the integrity of the gastrointestinal tract epithelium against noxious substances.[32]

Lymphocyte-macrophage activities. Of additional interest is the discovery that the **lymphocytes** in human milk produce the antiviral substance interferon. **Macrophages** are also found in colostrum and mature milk; 21,000/mm³ reportedly are present in a typical colostrum specimen. Macrophages are motile and phagocytic and have been shown to produce **complement**, lactoferrin, lysozyme, and other factors. The full role of the macrophages is still under investigation, but they undoubtedly have a protective function, both within the mammary lacteals and subsequently within the baby. A number of investigators have studied the activities of lymphocytes in human milk. Milk samples from lactating mothers have been collected at various times postpartum and examined for cell types present and in vitro activities of the various identified cells. The greatest number of cells appear in colostrum with numbers dropping significantly during the following 8 weeks.

Effect of maternal malnutrition. As one might expect, maternal malnutrition adversely affects not only the nutritional composition of human milk but also its content of immunologic substances. Observations of malnourished Colombian women showed that colostrum contained only one third the normal concentration of IgG and less than half the normal level of albumin. Significant reductions in colostrum levels of IgA and the fourth component of complement (C4) were also observed.[33] These differences tended to disappear in mature milk, accompanied by improvement in the nutritional status of the malnourished mothers during the first several weeks postpartum. Therefore, the protective qualities of colostrum and milk may be significantly influenced by maternal nutritional status.

Contaminants

The lactating woman is often exposed to a variety of nonnutritional substances that may be transferred to her milk. Such substances include drugs, environmental pollutants,

Prostaglandins
Potent hormone-like unsaturated fatty acids that act in extremely low concentrations on local target organs.

Lymphocytes
Mature leukocytes, special lymphoid white blood cells, T cells and B cells, forming major components of the body's immune system; also found in human milk.

Macrophage
(Fr *makros*, large; *phagein*, to eat) Large phagocytes, cells of the immune system that engulf and consume microorganisms, other cells, or foreign particles, and interact with T cells and B cells to produce inflammatory process and antibodies.

Complement
Series of enxymatic serum proteins that interact with an antigen-antibody complex to promote phagocyte activity or destroy other cells.

TABLE 5-7 *Abbreviated Guide to Drug Therapy in Nursing Mothers*

Drugs That Are Contraindicated During Breastfeeding

Drug	Reported Sign or Symptom in Infant or Effect on Lactation
Bromocriptine	Suppresses lactation
Cyclophosphamide	Possible immune suppression; unknown effect on growth or association with carcinogenesis; neutropenia
Cyclosporine	Possible immune suppression; unknown effect on growth or association with carcinogenesis
Doxorubicin	Possible immune suppression; unknown effect on growth or association with carcinogenesis
Ergotamine	Vomiting, diarrhea, convulsions (doses used in migraine medications)
Lithium	$\frac{1}{3}$ to $\frac{1}{2}$ therapeutic blood concentration in infants
Methotrexate	Possible immune suppression; unknown effect on growth or association with carcinogenesis; neutropenia
Phenindione	Anticoagulant; increased prothrombin and partial thromboplastin time in one infant (not used in USA)

Drugs of Abuse That Are Contraindicated During Breastfeeding

Drug	Effect
Amphetamine	Irritability, poor sleep pattern
Cocaine	Cocaine intoxication
Heroin	Withdrawal symptoms (i.e., shakiness)
Marijuana	Only one report in literature; no effect mentioned
Nicotine (smoking)	Shock, vomiting, diarrhea, rapid heart rate, restlessness; decreased milk production
Phencyclidine (PCP)	Potent hallucinogen

*Radiopharmaceuticals That Require Temporary Cessation of Breastfeeding**

Drug	Recommended Alteration in Breastfeeding Pattern
Gallium-67 (^{67}Ga)	Radioactivity in milk present for 2 wks
Indium-111 (^{111}In)	Small amount present at 20 hr
Iodine-125 (^{125}I)	Risk of thyroid cancer; radioactivity in milk present for 12 days
Iodine-131 (^{131}I)	Radioactivity in milk present 2 to 14 days depending on study
Radioactive sodium	Radioactivity in milk present 96 hr
Technetium-99m (^{99m}Tc), ^{99m}Tc macroaggregates, ^{99m}TcO$_4$	Radioactivity in milk present 15 hr to 3 days

Continued.

viruses, caffeine, alcohol, and food allergens. Although moderate amounts of many of these agents are believed to pose no risk to nursing infants, some substances provoke concern because of known or suspected adverse reactions.

Drugs. Much research has focused on the release of drugs into the milk of lactating women. Whether the mother drinks it, eats it, sniffs it, inserts it as an anal or vaginal

TABLE 5-7 *Abbreviated Guide to Drug Therapy in Nursing Mothers—cont'd*

Drugs That Have Caused Significant Effects on Some Nursing Infants and Should Be Given to Nursing Mothers With Caution†

Drug	Effect
Aspirin (salicylates)	Metabolic acidosis (dose related); may affect platelet function; rash
Clemastine	Drowsiness, irritability, refusal to feed, high-pitched cry, neck stiffness (one case)
Phenobarbital	Sedation; infantile spasms after weaning from milk containing phenobarbital, methemoglobinemia (one case)
Primidone	Sedation, feeding problems
Salicylazosulfapyridine (sulfasalazine)	Bloody diarrhea in one infant

*Consult nuclear medicine physician before performing diagnostic study so that a radionuclide with the shortest excretion time in breast milk can be used. Before study, the mother should pump her breast and store enough milk in freezer for feeding the infant; after study, the mother should pump her breast to maintain milk production but discard all milk pumped for the required time that radioactivity is present in milk.

†Measure blood concentration in the infant when possible.

Adapted from American Academy of Pediatrics, Committee on Drugs: Transfer of drugs and other chemicals into human milk, *Pediatrics* 84:924, 1989. Reproduced by permission of Pediatrics.

suppository, or injects it, some level of the active agents in the drug enters the maternal tissues and blood and finally migrates to the breast milk. The difference in method of administration determines the amount of drug that finally enters the blood and the speed with which it reaches the capillaries of the breast. In general the amount of a drug excreted in milk is not more than 1% to 2% of the maternal dose. Although concern exists about the amount of a given drug in the breast milk, of greater concern is the amount that actually reaches the infant's bloodstream. Unfortunately, there is no accurate way to measure this because other factors also affect the level in the infant's bloodstream. The tolerance of the chemical to the pH of the stomach and the enzymatic activity of the intestinal tract is significant. The volume of milk consumed by the infant is a factor as well.

Some drugs appear in human milk in sufficient quantities to be harmful to the infant (Table 5-7).[34] Sedatives used to relieve tension may produce drowsiness in the baby as well as the mother. Lithium and reserpine produce a bluish tint to the skin along with other disorders. Valium residuals in mother's milk induce lethargy in breastfed babies. Lithium carbonate, a drug prescribed for relief of manic depression, may induce lowered body temperature, loss of muscle tone, and bluish skin in the nursing infant. Both cyclophosphamide and methotrexate cause bone marrow depression when ingested by infants. A variety of disorders follow intake by infants of breast milk contaminated with antimicrobial agents of one kind or another. Penicillin in breast milk may produce an allergic reaction in a sensitive infant. Other antibiotics may produce similar reactions, as well as sleepiness, vomiting, and refusal to eat. Radioactive thyroid medications may damage the thyroid gland. Bowel problems in infants may result from maternal consumption of some laxatives, such as anthraquinone, aloes, cascara, emodin, and rheum (rhubarb). Safe laxatives include magnesia, castor oil, mineral oil, bisacodyl (Ducolax), senna phenophthalein or nonprescription Ex-Lax, and fecal softeners. Heroin or the painkiller dextropropoxyphene (Darvon) can lead to infant addiction. Treatment of the heroin-addicted mother with methadone is problematic, since one infant death has been

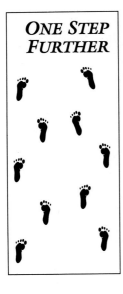

ONE STEP FURTHER

Barriers to Postpartum Treatment for Drug and Alcohol Addiction

Negative attitudes toward this population may generate resistance to treating the women.

The trend toward legal intervention in the pregnancies of women with alcohol and other drug problems discourages many from seeking care. Women fear criminal prosecution or loss of their children to foster care.

Nationwide, substance abuse treatment services are insufficient and inadequate to meet the needs of pregnant women and women who need child care while they're in treatment.

Cultural insensitivity exists in treatment programs.

Transportation to treatment is lacking or difficult to arrange.

Lack of residential programs that accept women and their children.

Long intervals between locating and being admitted to a program.

Community outreach providing information about programs is not available.

Alcohol and other drug problems often are not diagnosed because physicians and other clinicians lack adequate training in the identification of substance abuse and the consequences of drug use during pregnancy.

reported during maternal methadone therapy. Barriers to postpartum treatment for drug and alcohol addiction are discussed in the box above.

If a mother needs a specific medication and the hazards to the infant are believed to be minimal, the following important adjustments can be made to minimize the effects.

1. **Action time.** Do not use the long-acting form of the drug because the infant has even more difficulty in excreting the agent, which usually requires detoxification in the liver. Accumulation in the infant is then a genuine concern.
2. **Dose schedule.** Schedule the doses so the least amount of the drug gets into the milk. Given the usual absorption rates and peak blood levels of most drugs, having the mother take the medication immediately after breastfeeding is the safest time for the infant.
3. **Observations.** Watch the infant for any unusual signs or symptoms such as change in feeding pattern or sleeping habits, fussiness, or rash.
4. **Drug amount in milk.** When possible, choose the drug that produces the least amount in the milk.

One of the best sources of information on drugs in relation to human milk and infant health is the family pharmacist. It is also wise to read the product label to evaluate product composition and precautionary statements. Effective December 26, 1979, all drug manufacturers in the United States were required to provide relevant information on the labels of new drugs developed and marketed since that date. Whatever is known about excretion of the drug into milk and whatever is known of the effect on the infant will be indicated on the label. If nothing is known, the label will state that fact. In such a case, and in all use of drugs, the prudent mother will exercise due caution.

Environmental contaminants. The current concern over pesticide residues, industrial wastes, and other environmental contaminants is not without cause. Many of these compounds have accidentally contaminated food and water supplies around the world. In general the chemical contaminants that appear in breast milk have high lipid solubility, resistance to physical degradation or biologic metabolism, wide distribution in the environment, and slow or absent excretion rates. Of greatest concern among such chemicals are the **organohalides** such as polychlorinated biphenyls (PCBs) and dichlorodiphenyl

Organohalides
(Gr *organon*, organ; Chem *halides,* compounds of fluorine, chlorine, bromine, or iodine) Chemical compounds used as pesticides or in industrial processes, e.g., DDT and PCBs.

TABLE 5-8 *"Typical" Levels, FDA Action Levels, Allowable Daily Intake, and Calculated Daily Intake of Representative Breastfed Infants*

Substance	Typical Levels* (ppb)	FDA Action Levels for Cow's Milk† (ppb)	Allowable Daily Intake (µg/kg)	Daily Intake of Breastfed Infants‡ (µg/kg)
Dieldrin	1-6	7.5	0.1	0.8
Heptachlor epoxide	8-30	7.5	0.5	4
PCBs	40-100	62.5	1	14
DDT (including metabolites)	50-200	50	5	28

*Levels considered typical in whole milk in the United States.
†Assuming 2.5% fat. FDA action levels represent the limit at or above which the FDA will take legal action against a product to remove it from the market.
‡Intake of a 5 kg infant drinking 700 ml of milk per day; levels are based on high values given under typical levels.
Modified from Rogan WJ, Bagniewska A, Damstra T: *N Engl J Med* 302:1450, 1980.

trichloroethane (DDT).[35] Long-term low-level exposure to the organohalides results in a gradual accumulation of residues in fat, including the fat of breast milk. Lactation is the only way in which large amounts of such residues can be excreted.

Savage and associates conducted a study of environmental contaminants that focused on levels of chlorinated hydrocarbon insecticide residues in nearly 1500 human milk samples around the United States.[36] The majority of samples showed low but detectable levels of most of these insecticides or their metabolites, but significant differences were found among the five geographic regions. The southeastern United States had the highest mean residue levels, whereas the northwest had the lowest levels. Although nursing infants around the United States would generally receive low levels of some of these residues, a small number could be exposed to fairly high amounts.

It is clear that human milk is a variable source of contaminants, but it is difficult to define a "safe" level of exposure to these compounds. However, both the World Health Organization and the U.S. Food and Drug Administration have set "regulatory" or "allowable" levels for daily intake of several organohalides (Table 5-8). These standards provide a large margin of safety, so the fact that a given infant exceeds the level does not mean that such exposure is toxic. Much remains to be learned about the chemical contamination of human milk. Meanwhile, it is heartening to know that very few cases of illness caused by transmission of environmental chemicals through breast milk have appeared.

Heavy metals. Lead and mercury, both heavy metals, are transferred placentally to the fetus and also to the infant via maternal milk. Rat studies have shown that lactation increases lead absorption from the gut, which leads ultimately to an increased level of lead excretion via the milk. The exact mechanism for this phenomenon is not known. However, lactose may play a dominant role, since it is known to facilitate the absorption of calcium, other trace elements, and lead.

Nicotine. Nicotine enters human milk and can cause nicotine "poisoning" of the breastfed infant. Infants 3 to 4 days of age whose mothers smoked 6 to 16 cigarettes a day were reported to refuse to suckle, to become apathetic, vomit, and retain urine and feces. In a chain-smoking mother the nicotine content of milk may reach 75 µg/L. In the case of mothers who smoke very little it is likely that the amount of nicotine the infant would get

> ### SMOKING DURING PREGNANCY AND LACTATION AND ITS EFFECTS ON BREAST MILK VOLUME
>
> Ten smoking and ten nonsmoking mothers were studied with regard to volume of milk production and growth of their infants. Nonsmoking mothers had significantly greater breast milk production (961 g per day) than smoking mothers (693 g per day). Babies of smoking mothers showed significantly reduced rates of growth. These results indicate that cigarette smoking has a negative influence on breast milk volume; the lower growth rates of the infants of smokers suggest also that their breast milk output was insufficient to support the energy requirements of their infants.

Ethanol
Chemical name for beverage alcohol.

Cushing's syndrome
Condition first described by Boston surgeon Harvey Cushing (1869-1939), due to hypersecretion of adrenal corticotropic hormone (ACTH) or excessive intake of glucocorticoids, with rapidly developing fat deposits of face, neck, and trunk, giving a characteristic cushing-old "moon face" appearance.

from breathing cigarette smoke in the immediate environment would be more significant than that obtained from milk. The long-term impact of such exposure is unknown.

Caffeine. Caffeine passes from the maternal bloodstream into breast milk. Although a small dose of caffeine comparable to that obtained from a cup of coffee is transported at low levels from the mother to her milk (1%), caffeine does reach the infant where it can accumulate over time.[37] Wakeful, hyperactive infants sometimes are victims of caffeine stimulation. A mother who drinks more than six to eight cups of any caffeine-containing beverage in a day's time might expect her infant to demonstrate "coffee nerves." Such an infant does not require hospitalization, and verification of blood caffeine levels is not mandatory, although it might be helpful. An elimination trial should suffice to evaluate the role of maternal caffeine ingestion, and subsequent elimination, on infant behavior.

Alcohol. Beverage alcohol also passes from the mother's bloodstream into her breast milk. **Ethanol** has been shown to reach human milk in a similar concentration to that in maternal blood. Interestingly, however, the major breakdown product of ethanol, acetaldehyde, does not appear in human milk even though significant amounts may have been measured in maternal blood.

The role of the mammary gland in eliminating acetaldehyde may be similar to that of the placenta. If human milk contains large amounts of ethanol, the nursing infant may develop a pseudo-**Cushing's syndrome,** as described by Binkiewica, Robinaon, and Senior.[38] The 4 month-old infant they describe (Fig. 5-10) was breastfed by a mother who consumed at least fifty 12-oz cans of beer weekly, plus generous amounts of other more concentrated alcoholic drinks. When the mother stopped drinking but continued to nurse, the infant's growth rate promptly increased and her appearance gradually returned to normal. The mother also noted that she did not sleep as much as she did before.

Observations of lactating women consuming various levels of alcohol suggest that regular consumption of several drinks per day is associated with delayed psychomotor development at 1 year of age.[39] Whether this adverse result indicates permanent damage is unknown. Until more information is available, lactating women are well advised to limit consumption of alcoholic beverages.

The AIDS virus. Evidence suggests that the AIDS virus can be transmitted from mother to infant through breast milk. This recent finding has provoked much concern from the standpoint of providing appropriate advice about infant feeding to high-risk women. Should one encourage or discourage breastfeeding for such women? The current thinking in the United States is that breastfeeding should be discouraged when a woman is known to carry this virus. The World Health Organization, however, supports the concept that infants in many developing countries run greater risks of dying of diarrheal disease if they are not breastfed than of developing AIDS from the breast milk exposure (see the box on

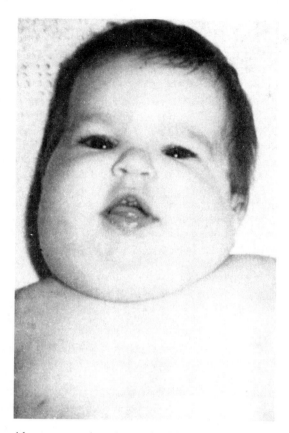

FIG. 5-10 Cushingoid appearance in a 4-month-old infant whose mother consumed at least 50 cans of beer weekly plus generous portions of other, more concentrated alcoholic beverages.

From Binkiewiez A, Robinson MJ, Senior B: Pseudo-Cushing syndrome caused by alcohol in breast milk. *J Pediatr* 93:965, 1978.

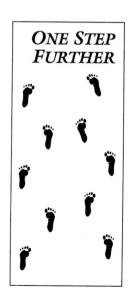

ONE STEP FURTHER

Recommendations About Breastfeeding When Carrying the AIDS Virus

- *Centers for Disease Control and Prevention (CDC) (United States)* Infected women should be advised against breastfeeding to avoid postnatal transmission to a child who may not be infected.
- *World Health Organization (WHO)* This group contends that there is insufficient evidence to conclude that breastfeeding is an *important* mode of HIV transmission. It is noted that breastfeeding is of special importance in the Third World, where safe, effective substitutes are not accessible to most women. It also notes that more uninfected than infected breastfed babies of HIV-positive mothers have been reported. And it points out that women who become infected via postpartum transfusions seem to be a special subset of infected mothers; the more common situation seems to involve women who are infected before or during pregnancy. WHO therefore recommends continued promotion, support, and protection of breastfeeding in both developed and developing countries and in the case of women known to be HIV-infected, that careful consideration be given to the availability of safe, effective use of alternatives before advising against breastfeeding.

CASE STUDY

Aids and Breast Milk

In 1986, Ziegler et al reported a case in which a newborn infant apparently contracted the acquired immunodeficiency syndrome (AIDS) virus through breast milk from his mother. The child was delivered by cesarean section and the mother contracted the AIDS virus after blood transfusion given in conjunction with her cesarean section. In this case, the blood transfusion was given after delivery and the baby was breastfed for 6 weeks. Thirteen months later, AIDS developed in the donor of one of the units of blood used for transfusion, resulting in testing of the mother and the child. Both the mother and the child were found to be positive for the virus. The mother had AIDS-related complex. The baby had a transient episode of failure to thrive and then developed lymphadenopathy and eczema but was otherwise well. The spouse and siblings were seronegative.

A subsequent study conducted in Kigali, Rwanda, involved observation of 212 mother-infant pairs who were negative for human immunodeficiency virus Type I (HIV-1) at delivery. All of the infants were breastfed. Mothers were followed for 3 months; those who became positive for HIV-1 were compared with those who did not; comparisons were completed after 16.6 months of further evaluation. Results indicated that HIV-1 infection can be transmitted from mother to infants during the postnatal period. Colostrum and breast milk were considered to be efficient routes for the transmission of HIV-1 from recently infected mothers to their infants.

From Wasserberger J, Ordog GJ, Stroh JJ: AIDS in breast milk, *JAMA* 255:464, 1986; and Van de Perre P et al: Postnatal transmission of human immunodeficiency virus Type I from mother to infant, *N Engl J Med* 325:593, 1991.

p. 194). Debate on this issue continues around the world. In the meantime, breast milk banks are taking special precautions to screen out donors who potentially could contribute virus-contaminated specimens. Samples are also pasteurized sufficiently to destroy viruses that might be present.[40-43]

DIET FOR THE NURSING MOTHER
General Recommendations

The committee on Recommended Dietary Allowances (RDA) of the Food and Nutrition Board considers the optimum diet for the lactating woman to be one that supplies somewhat more of each nutrient than that recommended for the nonpregnant female (Table 5-8).[44] Obviously, the needs of specific women relate directly to the volume of milk produced daily.

Energy

Prenatal storage. During pregnancy most women store approximately 2 to 4 kg of body fat, which can be mobilized to supply a portion of the additional energy for lactation. It is estimated that stored fat will provide 200 to 300 kcal per day during a lactation period of 3 months. This amount of energy represents only part of the energy needed to produce milk. The remainder of the energy needs should derive from the daily diet the first 3 months of lactation. During this time lactation can be successfully supported and readjustment of maternal fat stores can take place. If lactation continues beyond the initial 3 months or if maternal weight falls below the ideal weight for height, the daily extra energy allowance may need to be increased accordingly. If more than one infant is being nursed during the first few months of life, maternal kilocalorie stores will be more quickly used, and daily supplemental energy needs may double when maternal stores are depleted.

Efficiency of milk production. The efficiency of milk production has been estimated by several researchers by the observation of energy intake and energy utilization of breastfeeding and nonbreastfeeding mothers. English and Hitchcock compared the energy intake of 16 nursing mothers and 10 nonnursing mothers and found that the energy intake of breastfeeders in the sixth and eighth postpartum week was 2460 kcal/day.[45] The energy intake of nonnursing mothers during the same postpartum period was 1800 kcal/day—a difference of 580 kcal. In a later study lactating women were found to take in 2716 kcal/day and nonnursing mothers 2125 kcal/day—a difference of 590 kcal. By adding the assumed energy equivalents of body weight being lost, total energy available to the two groups was about 2977 and 2364 kcal/day, respectively. If one assumes that the energy requirements for basal metabolism and activity are equivalent for the two groups, the energy needed for daily milk production is close to 560 kcal. The production efficiency of human milk is therefore about 90%.

Energy needs. Recent observations of lactating women have led some researchers to propose that energy needs have been overestimated. Butte and others found that typical women who were producing about 750 ml of milk per day had a mean daily energy intake of 2171 plus 545 kcal per day.[46] Observations of postpartum weight loss patterns and subsequent calculations of energy balance led them to an estimation of 80% efficiency in energy utilization for milk production. When energy available from the diet (2171 kcal/day) was added to the energy derived from tissue mobilization (315 kcal/day) and the caloric equivalent of the milk was subtracted (597 kcal/day), a net balance of 1889 kcal/day was left for maintenance and activity. These findings suggest that successful lactation is compatible with gradual weight reduction and attainable with energy intakes less than current recommendations.

Similarly, Manning-Dalton and Allen evaluated postpartum weight loss patterns, breastfeeding completeness, and daily kilocalorie intakes of well-nourished North American women.[47] In spite of low mean kilocalorie intakes (2178 kcal/day), breastfeeding was successful, and weight loss during the 12 to 90 days postpartum averaged only 2.0 kg for the entire sample and 1.6 kg for the solely breastfeeding women. These authors emphasize that almost every aspect of maternal energy balance in lactation needs further investigation. In the meantime it should be recognized that the U.S. Recommended Dietary Allowance for energy in lactation is probably higher than necessary, especially for the well-nourished woman with a sedentary lifestyle. It is also apparent that the commonly held belief that breastfeeding helps the mother lose weight cannot be substantiated.[48]

Postpartum maternal weight concerns. For many women the usual slow rate of weight loss after childbirth may not satisfy their desires for immediate return to prepregnancy body weight. It is therefore likely that dietary restriction may be self-imposed, even though it is discouraged by health professionals. Suggested measures for improving nutrient intake of women with restrictive eating patterns can be found in the box on p. 196. It is important to recognize that moderate to severe restriction of caloric intake during lactation will compromise the woman's ability to synthesize milk. This is especially significant in the early weeks of lactation initiation before the process is firmly established. As a result of this effect of caloric restriction on milk production, lactating women should be advised to accept a gradual rate of weight loss in the first 6 months after childbirth. Otherwise, lactation success may be limited and the infant may suffer from insufficient milk supply to meet growth needs.

❖

SUGGESTED MEASURES FOR IMPROVING NUTRIENT INTAKE OF WOMEN WITH RESTRICTIVE EATING PATTERNS

- **Type of restrictive eating pattern**
  Excessive restriction of food intake, i.e., ingestion of < 1800 kcal of energy per day, which ordinarily leads to unsatisfactory intake of nutrients compared with the amounts needed by lactating women

- **Corrective measures**
  Encourage increased intake of nutrient-rich foods to achieve an energy intake of at least 1800 kcal per day; if the mother insists on curbing food intake sharply, promote substitution of foods rich in vitamins, minerals and protein for those lower in nutritive value; in individual cases, it may be advisable to recommend a balanced multivitamin-mineral supplement; discourage use of liquid weight loss diets and appetite suppressants

  Complete vegetarianism, i.e., avoidance of all animal foods, including meat, fish, dairy products, and eggs

  Advise intake of a regular source of vitamin B_{12}, such as special vitamin B_{12}-containing plant food products or a 2.6-μg vitamin B_{12} supplement daily

  Avoidance of milk, cheese, or other calcium-rich dairy products

  Encourage increased intake of other culturally appropriate dietary calcium sources, such as collard greens for blacks from the southeastern United States; provide information on the appropriate use of low-lactose dairy products if milk is being avoided because of lactose intolerance; if correction by diet cannot be achieved, it may be advisable to recommend 600 mg of elemental calcium per day taken with meals

  Avoidance of vitamin D-fortified foods, such as fortified milk or cereal, combined with limited exposure to ultraviolet light

  Recommend 10 μg of supplemental vitamin D per day

From Institute of Medicine: *Nutrition during lactation,* Washington, DC, 1991, National Academy of Sciences.

Protein

Along with the recommended energy increment, a 15 to 20 g increase in daily protein intake is advised for lactating women. The extra protein is believed to be necessary to cover the requirement for milk production with an allowance of 70% efficiency of protein utilization.

The increased needs for protein, as well as energy, can be met easily by consumption of about three to four extra cups of milk per day. Although this will provide the needed protein and energy, it will not cover the increased recommendations for other nutrients—ascorbic acid, vitamin E, and folic acid. Thus other foods such as citrus fruits, vegetable oils, and leafy green vegetables will also need to be added to the daily diet to supply these nutrients. The Daily Food Guide for Women, discussed in Chapter 3, provides a helpful food pattern for the reproductive years, including increases needed for pregnancy and lactation.

Vegetarian Diets

Maintenance of lactation while consuming a vegetarian diet can be managed well, providing all the basic principles of sensible vegetarian eating are followed carefully. The nutritional needs of the lactating vegetarian woman are the same as those of the lactating woman with a more traditional diet. Appropriate extra sources of kilocalories and protein must be clearly defined. If dairy products are acceptable in the chosen dietary regimen, extra milk can be used as indicated. If dairy products are not included in the accepted list of foods, extra energy and high quality protein must be obtained from appropriately combined vegetables, legumes, grains, nuts, and other such food sources in larger amounts. Calcium needs can be met by eating large quantities of some green leafy vegetables (for example, kale), calcium-fortified foods, and other significant sources of vegetable calcium. Dietary supplements may be unacceptable. Thus, intelligent daily diet planning is essential for maintenance of successful lactation and health of the vegetarian mother.

The Question of Supplementation

Although lactation increases a woman's requirement for nearly all nutrients, these increased needs can be provided by a well-balanced diet as outlined. For this reason nutritional supplements are generally unnecessary except when there is a deficient intake of one or more nutrients. It is true, for example, if the lactating woman does not tolerate milk, calcium supplementation as well as alternative energy and protein sources are needed to help prevent unnecessary calcium withdrawal from bones.

Although there is no evidence that calcium composition of human milk can be influenced by dietary intake of calcium, it is clear that dietary calcium deficiency promotes mobilization of calcium from bones to maintain milk calcium levels during lactation. Older clinical literature documents cases of **osteomalacia** in mothers who nursed their infants for long periods of time while on inadequate diets. Also, it has been proposed that the relatively high incidence of osteomalacia and **osteoporosis** in the United States is partially related to the waning intake of dairy products by adult women. Whether or not this is the case is still unknown. It stands to reason, however, that prolonged lactation accompanied by poor calcium intake may significantly compromise the calcium status of the skeletal system and increase its susceptibility to fractures and other forms of trauma.

Cost of Nutritional Support for Lactation

The cost of providing adequate nutritional support for the lactating mother depends heavily upon what foods she selects to meet her nutritional needs. Some older studies suggest that human milk costs more than bottle-feeding because of the extra nutrients the mother must consume. It is clear, however, in examining the costs of appropriate extra foods for the lactating mother that human milk is cheaper than proprietary cow's milk formulas if economical food choices are made (Tables 5-9, 5-10, and 5-11). The present difference between the costs of commercially prepared cow's milk formulas and human milk undoubtedly will continue to increase in coming years, since the price of "double cycle" animal food products, including cow's milk, continues to escalate. Beyond the price consideration, however, it is hard to justify "wastage" of human milk and the resultant unnecessary draw on the precious supply of other animal protein available to the world's population. Human milk represents a vital national resource that, if utilized to its fullest extent, could markedly improve not only the health and nutritional status of today's children but also the "natural resource base" of many underdeveloped countries.

ADVANTAGES OF BREASTFEEDING
Basic Values

Human milk was designed for human infants. The process of lactation is normal for mammals. It is therefore not surprising that a number of advantages have been defined for mothers and infants who participate in the breastfeeding experience (see box on p. 200). The degree of advantage varies among mother-infant pairs, since availability of alternative

Osteomalacia
(Gr *osteon*, bone; *lakia*, softness) Condition marked by softening of the bones due to impaired mineralization with excess accumulation of osteoid tissue (immature young bone matrix that has not had mineralization to harden); results from deficiency of vitamin D and calcium.

Osteoporosis
(Gr *osteon*, bone; *poros*, pore) Abnormal thinning of bone, producing a porous, fragile, lattice-like bone tissue of enlarged spaces, prone to fracture or deformity.

TABLE 5-9 *Recommended Daily Dietary Allowances for Lactation*

	First 6 Months	Second 6 Months
Energy (kcal)	+500	+500
Protein (g)	65	62
Vitamin A (RE*)	1300	1200
Vitamin D (μg)	10	10
Vitamin E activity (mg αTE)†	12	11
Ascorbic acid (mg)	95	90
Folacin (μg)	280	260
Niacin (mg‡)	20	20
Riboflavin (mg)	1.8	1.7
Thiamin (mg)	1.6	1.6
Vitamin B_6 (mg)	2.1	2.1
Vitamin B_{12} (μg)	2.6	2.6
Calcium (mg)	1200	1200
Phosphorus (mg)	1200	1200
Iodine (μg)	200	200
Iron (mg)	15	15
Magnesium (mg)	355	340
Zinc (mg)	19	16

*RE, Retinol equivalents.
†α-Tocopherol equivalents; 1 mg d-α-tocopherol = 1 αTE.
‡Although allowances are expressed as niacin, it is recognized that on the average, 1 mg of niacin is derived from each 60 mg of dietary tryptophan.
Modified from Food and Nutrition Board, National Research Council, National Academy of Sciences: *Recommended dietary allowances,* ed 10, Washington, DC, 1989, US Government Printing Office.

foods, environmental conditions, and lifestyle characteristics are markedly different from one setting to another. Reviewing the issue with an open mind, however, leaves no doubt that in the majority of situations breastfeeding provides distinct benefits for both child and family.

Antiinfective Properties

Around the turn of the century there was little knowledge of microbiology or of immunology, and bottle-fed infants suffered from a much higher incidence of diarrhea and acute gastrointestinal tract infection. They also experienced higher mortality rates than breastfed infants. Throughout much of the United States and the industrialized West, techniques for microbial control of the artificial diet have lessened the differences in mortality between bottle-fed and breastfed infants. However, small differences are still apparent in the number and severity of illnesses contracted by bottle-fed and breastfed infants.

Although the protective effect of breast milk is fully appreciated, not all studies show that breastfed babies demonstrate reduced morbidity. It is also true that the reported morbidity among breastfed infants may have nothing to do with the antiinfectious properties of human milk but might instead relate to different parenting strategies or lifestyle characteristics of mothers who choose to breastfeed instead of bottle-feed. Whatever the case, substantial data suggest that breastfeeding reduces infant morbidity, especially in the early months of life.[49]

TABLE 5-10   *Nutrients, Amounts, and Estimated Cost of Foods Needed to Meet Additional Nutritional Requirements of a Lactating Woman: Standard (Nonbudget) Plan*

Suggested Foods	Amounts	Cost*	Calories	Protein	A	C	B_1	B_2	B_3	Calcium	Iron
Milk, fresh, 2%	2 cups	.36	290	18	700		0.14	0.82	0.4	576	
Meat (round steak)	2 oz	.87	150	13	35		0.04	0.11	2.8	6	1.7
Vegetable, dark green or yellow (broccoli, cooked)	¾ cup	.25	20	2.5	1990	70	0.07	0.15	0.6	68	0.6
Other vegetable or fruit (grapefruit)	½ fruit	.15	45	1	10	44	0.05	0.02	0.2	19	0.5
Citrus fruit (orange juice)	½ cup	.14	60	1	275	60	0.11	0.01	0.5	12	0.1
Enriched (or whole grain) bread	1 slice	.16	65	3			0.09	0.03	0.8	24	0.8
TOTAL		1.93	630	38.5	3010	174	0.5	1.14	5.3	705	3.7

*Costs of May 1991, Seattle, Wash.

TABLE 5-11   *Nutrients, Amounts, and Estimated Cost of Foods Needed to Meet Additional Nutritional Requirements of a Lactating Woman: Budget Plan*

Suggested Foods	Amounts	Cost*	Calories	Protein	A	C	B_1	B_2	B_3	Calcium	Iron
Nonfat dry milk (prepared for drinking)	2 cups	.26	180	18	20		0.18	0.88	0.40	592	
Peanut butter	2 oz	.32	190	8			0.04	0.04	4.8	18	0.6
Vegetable, dark green or yellow (carrots, cooked)	¾ cup	.20	25	0.5	7610	4.5	0.04	0.03	0.04	24	0.45
Citrus fruit (tomato juice)	½ cup	.15	25	1	970	20	0.06	0.04	0.95	86	1.1
Enriched (or whole grain) bread	2 slices	.16	130	6			0.18	0.06	1.6	48	1.6
TOTAL		1.08	550	33.5	8600	24.5	0.5	1.05	7.79	768	3.75

*Costs of May 1991, Seattle, Wash.

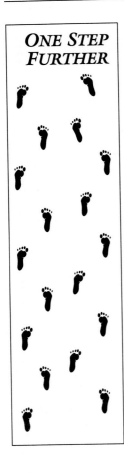

ONE STEP FURTHER

Benefits of Breastfeeding

Best for Baby
- Designed exclusively for human infants
- Nutritionally superior to any alternative
- Bacteriologically safe and always fresh
- Provides immunity to viral and bacterial diseases
- Stimulates the infant's own immunologic defenses
- Decreases risk of respiratory and diarrheal diseases
- Prevents or reduces the risk of allergy
- Promotes correct development of jaws, teeth, and speech patterns
- Decreases tendency toward childhood obesity
- Promotes frequent tender physical contact with mother
- Facilitates maternal-infant attachment

Best for Mother
- Promotes physiologic recovery from pregnancy:
    - Promotes uterine involution
    - Decreases risk of postpartum hemorrhage
    - Increases period of postpartum anovulation
- Promotes psychological attachment
- Facilitates positive self-esteem in maternal role
- Allows for daily rest periods
- Eliminates need to mix, prepare, use, and wash feeding equipment
- Saves money not spent on formula and equipment
- Decreases risk of breast cancer and ovarian cancer

Optimum Nutrition

A main advantage of breastfeeding is freedom from "formulogenic disease." The complications of improper dilutions, such as incorrect caloric density and excessive renal solute load, are not concerns for breastfed babies. Colostrum and breast milk contain factors whose functions are unclear, as well as micronutrients whose value to the newborn only become apparent when they are omitted from infant formulas. Human milk appears to have a fat composition and protein content ideally suited to the growth rate of the human infant; it is the standard by which formulas are measured.

Appropriate Growth and Development

Bottle-fed and breastfed infants follow similar growth curves from birth until the third or fourth month of age. From the fourth month on, the bottle-fed infant gains weight at a faster rate, especially beyond the sixth month of life. A sizable number of pediatric specialists feel that the slower rate of growth among older breastfed infants represents the ideal pattern for optimum health. It has even been suggested that the National Center for Health Statistics standards are not appropriate for evaluating the growth performance of breastfed infants and that growth curves based exclusively on breastfed infants should be used for that purpose. Thus far such curves are not available, and agreement about what represents optimum growth in infancy has not yet been reached.

Butte and others have demonstrated recently, however, the efficiency with which human milk is utilized by the young infant for maintenance and growth.[50] Forty-five healthy full-term infants who were exclusively breastfed were observed for the first 4 months of life. The amount of breast milk ingested over a 24-hour period was determined by test weighing using automatic electronic scales. At each feeding over a subsequent 24-hour period, milk samples were expressed from alternate breasts for analysis. Although adequate growth was demonstrated by the infants, this was accomplished with energy and protein intakes substantially less than that currently recommended. In the case of energy the following observations were recorded:

	Energy intake (kcal/day)	Energy intake (kcal/kg/day)
1 month	520 + 131	110 + 24
2 months	468 + 115	83 + 19
3 months	458 + 124	74 + 20
4 months	477 + 111	71 + 17

Reduced Risk of Allergy

Development of food allergy has been associated with the penetration into the body of intact proteins or large peptide fragments with antigenic determinants. Under ordinary circumstances, secretory antibodies, efficient intraluminal digestion, and impermeable intestinal epithelial cells and intercellular junctions combine to form a "mucosal barrier" in the healthy intestine. Intestinal absorption of whole protein macromolecules is thought to be maximum in the newborn period and to decrease with age. Formula feeding, as opposed to breastfeeding, has been associated with increased susceptibility to food allergies. Whether this is more directly related to exposure to "foreign" **antigens** in commercial formulas, to differences in intestinal morphology with different food sources, to a protective action of breast milk, or to a combination of these mechanisms has not been determined. Recent studies suggest that breast milk may promote early closure of the mucosal barrier. In other studies **antibodies** directed toward milk components have been found in human milk, and these may be involved in the prevention of allergies by hindering the intestinal absorption of intact immunogenic food proteins by the neonate.

Although arguments against the value of breastfeeding for allergy prevention have been presented in the literature with some vigor, these contributions clearly represent the minority viewpoint. It seems appropriate, therefore, that families with a history of allergy should be counseled about the desirability of breastfeeding combined with an allergen-avoidance diet for the baby during the majority of the first year of life.

Allergy to breast milk is uncommon, and some researchers question whether it exists at all. It has been shown, however, that allergens from foods that a mother consumes may enter her breast milk and occasionally promote an allergic reaction in a sensitive infant.[51] Sometimes alteration of maternal diet may be useful.[52] Gerard proposes that if food allergies are present on both sides of the family, the lactating mother should vary her diet and avoid large intake of any one specific food, particularly of cow's milk and egg products.[53] If the baby later develops symptoms suggestive of allergy, the mother should modify her diet rather than place her baby on a cow's milk or soy formula.

Normal Psychologic Development

Breastfeeding has been referred to as the period of "exterior gestation" because it provides continuity with the intrauterine environment while providing security and nourishment. Some workers have suggested that prolactin, coupled with sensory input from the baby, produces "mothering" responses in most women. Many women who have raised both breastfed and bottle-fed infants state that they feel a special closeness to the breastfed child that persists into adult life. Much attention has been focused on what might

Antigens

(*antibody* + Gr *genan*, to produce) Any disease agents, such as toxins, bacteria, viruses, and other foreign substances, that stimulate the production of *antibodies* to combat and destroy them.

Antibodies

Immune system components, specific immunobglobins, especially secretory IgA in the bowel and upper respiratory mucosa, that destroy invading antigens.

TABLE 5-12 *Cost per Day of the Most Commonly Used Prepared Formulas, Basic Equipment, and Fuel* *

Formula Products and Other Expenses	Cost per Day with Bottles and Nipples			Cost per Day with Disposable Holders and Liners		
Dry, powdered (52 scoops per can)	$1.87			$1.87		
Double-strength liquid (13 oz. can)		2.10			2.10	
Ready-to-feed liquid (32 oz can)			2.49			2.49
Unbreakable bottles with nipples ($10.68/dozen)	.12	.12	.12			
Extra nipples ($3.32/dozen)	.03	.03	.03			
Electricity (to clean and sterilize water/bottles)	.04	.04	.04			
or						
Disposable holders				.11	.11	.11
Liners (one used per feed)				.30	.30	.30
TOTAL	2.06	2.29	2.68	2.28	2.51	2.90

*Costs of May 1991, Seattle, Wash.

be termed *maternal-infant bonding.* Breastfeeding promotes strong emotional ties while meeting the infant's most basic physical need.

Reduced Risk of Obesity

Attempts have been made to assess the value of breastfeeding as protection against the development of obesity. But present data do not allow for satisfactory assessment of the merits of these statements. Published reports have yielded conflicting findings. For the time being it therefore seems inappropriate to advocate breastfeeding as a means of protection against infantile obesity.

Other Infant Benefits

An array of other advantages for babies have been proposed as being associated with breastfeeding. Many clinicians have suggested that low-birth-weight infants who are provided human milk are less likely to develop **necrotizing enterocolitis.**[54] Several researchers have proposed that breastfeeding protects against the development of clinical symptoms of **celiac disease, Crohn's disease,** and insulin-dependent diabetes mellitus (IDDM).[55-56] Support for these and other hypotheses are limited, but future observations may confirm their validity.

Maternal Benefits

Involution of uterus. One of the earliest documented maternal benefits of breastfeeding is the effect of oxytocin on the **involution** of the uterus. Early breastfeeding, even on the delivery table, stimulates contractions of the uterus that help to control blood loss.

Suppression of ovulation. The stimulation of the nipples and resultant secretion of prolactin suppress ovulation in many women, particularly when supplements and solids are not offered to the baby. This is believed to be of major significance in promoting short-term child spacing in the developing countries. When solid foods become a major source of nourishment for the child, nipple stimulation and prolactin levels decrease in the lactating

Necrotizing enterocolitis (Gr *nekrosis*, deadness; *enteron*, intestine) Infectious tissue-destroying intestinal disease; acute inflammation of intestinal mucosa.

Celiac disease An inborn error of metabolism characterized by the inability to hydrolyze peptides contained in the protein gluten.

Crohn's disease A chronic inflammatory bowel disease of unknown origin usually affecting the lower bowel. Diarrhea and severe abdominal pain are symptoms.

Involution (L *involutio: in*, into, *volvere*, to roll) Process of rolling or turning inward, shrinking an organ to its normal size, as the uterus after childbirth.

mother, and ovulation and menstruation usually begin again.

Ease of feeding. One of the prime benefits expressed by most women who breastfeed is the ease with which feeding is managed, particularly at night. The actual time spent nursing the infant may be greater during the first 2 weeks for the breastfeeding mother, since the infant eats more frequently to build up the mother's milk supply. More total time is spent in "nursing" by the bottle-feeding mother, however, since she must make the formula, clean the bottles, and heat the feedings before serving them.

Economy. Economy can no longer be used as a *major* reason for breastfeeding in the United States, but for some women it may be a relevant factor. Although the "old" evaporated milk formula costs about the same as the additional food required by the lactating woman, **proprietary formulas,** especially ready-to-feed ones (the only type that rivals breastfeeding in convenience), may be more expensive than breastfeeding. For some people, both in the United States and elsewhere, the expense of a commercial formula is prohibitive (Table 5-12).

Proprietary
(L *proprietarius,* owner) Referring to commercial products, such as infant formulas and medicinal items, which are designed, manufactured, and sold only by the owner of the patent, formula, brand name, or trademark associated with the product.

INCIDENCE OF BREASTFEEDING
General Background

In spite of the recognized benefits of breastfeeding for the child and the mother, the number of babies in the United States who were formula-fed climbed to an estimated 82% in the 2 decades before 1970. Comparable statistics were reported from England and France in the period following World War II.

Current Trends

Increased practice. More recent reports indicate that this prior trend reversed in the early 1970s and reached a peak in the early 1980s (Fig. 5-11).[3] More mothers are not only breastfeeding but also continuing to do so for a longer period of time throughout the months of their infants' most rapid growth and high nutritional demands. It is also

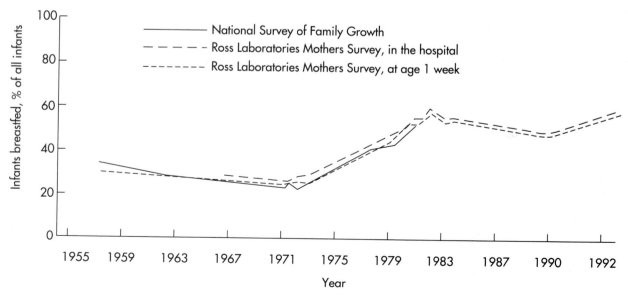

FIG. 5-11 Percentage of infants breastfed, by survey and year.

From Institute of Medicine, National Academy of Sciences: *Nutrition during lactation,* Washington, DC, 1991, National Academy Press and Ross Mothers Survey, preliminary 1992 report.

TABLE 5-13 *Percentage of Mothers Breastfeeding Newborn Infants in the Hospital and Infants at 5 or 6 Months of Age in the United States in 1989,* by Ethnic Background and Selected Demographic Variables*

Category	Total		White	
	Newborns	5-6 Month Infants	Newborns	5-6 Month Infants
All mothers	52.2	19.6	58.5	22.7
Parity				
Primiparous	52.6	16.6	58.3	18.9
Multiparous	51.7	22.7	58.7	26.8
Marital status				
Married	59.8	24.0	61.9	25.3
Unmarried	30.8	7.7	40.3	9.8
Maternal age				
< 20 years	30.2	6.2	36.8	7.2
20-24 years	45.2	12.7	50.8	14.5
25-29 years	58.8	22.9	63.1	25.0
30-34 years	65.5	31.4	70.1	34.8
≥ 35 years	66.5	36.2	71.9	40.5
Maternal education				
No college	42.1	13.4	48.3	15.6
College‡	70.7	31.1	74.7	34.1
Family income				
< $7,000	28.8	7.9	36.7	9.4
$7,000-$14,999	44.0	13.5	49.0	15.2
$15,000-$24,999	54.7	20.4	57.7	22.3
≥ $25,000	66.3	27.6	67.8	28.7
Maternal employment				
Full time	50.8	10.2	54.8	10.8
Part time	59.4	23.0	63.8	25.5
Not employed	51.0	23.1	58.7	27.5
U.S. census region				
New England	52.2	20.3	53.2	21.4
Middle Atlantic	47.4	18.4	52.4	21.8
East North Central	47.6	18.1	53.2	20.7
West North Central	55.9	19.9	58.2	20.7
South Atlantic	43.8	14.8	53.8	18.7
East South Central	37.9	12.4	45.1	15.0
West South Central	46.0	14.7	56.2	18.4
Mountain	70.2	30.4	74.9	33.0
Pacific	70.3	28.7	76.7	33.4

*Mothers were surveyed when their infants were 6 months of age. They were asked to recall the method of feeding the infant when in the hospital, at age 1 week, at months 1 through 5, and on the day preceding completion of the survey. Numbers in the columns labeled "5-6 Month Infants" are an average of the 5-month and previous day responses.

†Hispanic is not exclusive of white or black.

‡College includes all women who reported completing at least 1 year of college.

Data from A. Ryan, Ross Laboratories, personal communication, 1990, as presented in Institute of Medicine, National Academy of Sciences: *Nutrition during lactation,* Washington, DC, 1991, National Academy Press.

| Black | | Hispanic† | |
Newborns	5-6 Month Infants	Newborns	5-6 Month Infants
23.0	7.0	48.4	15.0
23.1	5.9	49.9	13.2
23.0	7.9	47.2	16.5
35.8	12.3	55.3	18.8
17.2	4.6	37.5	8.6
13.5	3.6	35.3	6.9
19.4	4.7	46.9	12.6
29.9	9.4	56.2	19.5
35.4	13.6	57.6	23.4
35.6	14.3	53.9	24.4
17.6	5.5	42.6	12.2
41.1	12.2	66.5	23.4
14.5	4.3	35.3	10.3
23.5	7.3	47.2	13.0
31.7	8.7	52.6	16.5
42.8	14.5	65.4	23.0
30.6	6.9	50.4	9.5
26.0	6.6	59.4	17.7
19.3	7.2	46.0	16.7
35.6	5.0	47.6	14.9
30.6	9.7	41.4	10.8
21.0	7.2	46.2	12.6
27.7	7.9	50.8	22.8
19.6	5.7	48.0	13.8
14.2	3.7	23.5	5.0
14.5	3.8	39.2	11.4
31.5	11.0	53.9	18.2
43.9	15.0	58.5	19.7

apparent that the increased incidence of breastfeeding has not been limited to higher income, better-educated mothers. From 1971 to 1981 the incidence at 2 months postpartum more than tripled among mothers in lower income families. The incidence of breastfeeding increased five times among mothers whose education did not extend beyond elementary or high school. Incidence of breastfeeding among mothers on the WIC program has increased. As might be expected, breastfeeding in any 1 year, especially long term, is much more common among mothers who have successfully breastfed a previous child. Even mothers of preterm infants, however, may nurse for long periods of time. Current trends in breastfeeding are summarized in Table 5-13.

Maternal employment. Recent surveys have considered the employment status of the mother as it relates to choices about infant feeding.[57,58] One report involved a large population of women in the Baltimore area.[57] These women were interviewed twice during the first 3 months postpartum. Planning to be employed during the first 6 months of the postpartum period did not affect the choice to initiate breastfeeding. However, actually being employed was significantly associated with cessation of breastfeeding as early as 2 or 3 months postpartum. Less than one half of mothers who were employed were still breastfeeding at the second postpartum interview, whereas two thirds of those who were not employed were still breastfeeding. Among employed mothers, working no more than 20 hours/week appeared to be associated with continued breastfeeding.

Regional differences. Regional differences have been reported in the current incidence of breastfeeding.[3] The highest rates of initiating breastfeeding in the hospital (Fig. 5-12) and at 5 or 6 months postpartum (Fig. 5-13) are found in the Mountain and Pacific regions. Rates in the East South Central region are the lowest. Ethnic differences within census regions are the same as those seen in national data.

Influence of change in medical attitude. One of the greatest influences on the current trend toward breastfeeding is the change in medical attitude. Today the American Academy of Pediatrics (AAP) actively recommends breastfeeding, as indicated by its Committee on Nutrition.

Beginning with its 1978 report, the AAP has recommended that all physicians encourage mothers to breastfeed their infants.[59,60] The AAP Committee on Nutrition declared:

1. Despite technologic advances in infant formulas, breast milk is "the best food for every newborn infant."
2. All physicians need to become "much more knowledgeable" about infant nutrition in general and breastfeeding in particular.
3. Attitudes, practices, and instruction in prenatal clinics and maternity wards should be changed to encourage breastfeeding.
4. In hospitals, mothers and infants should be kept together after birth so babies can be fed on demand.
5. Not only should information about breastfeeding be supplied to all school children, but nursing should also be portrayed as natural on television and other media.
6. To prevent conflict between breastfeeding and employment, legislation should mandate 3 to 4 months postdelivery leaves so that working mothers can breastfeed.

This hearty endorsement was followed in 1982 by a critical evaluation of how and why breastfeeding should be encouraged.[60] The AAP again voiced its support for the promotion of breastfeeding but made note of the maternal characteristics and family circumstances that may need attention when deciding on infant feeding strategies.

To reinforce the needed changes in health care practices, the AAP provided specific guidelines for activities to support breastfeeding. The final recommendations of the AAP include the following practices[60]:

- Education about breastfeeding in school for boys as well as girls since later support

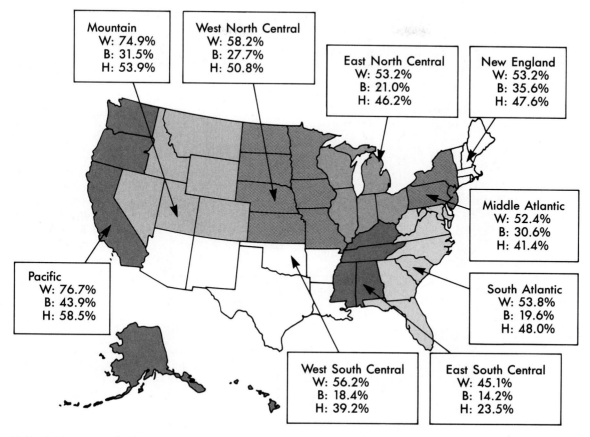

FIG. 5-12 Breastfeeding initiation rates, by census region and ethnic background. *W,* white; *B,* black; *H,* Hispanic.

Data from the 1989 Ross Mothers Survey (A. Ryan, Ross Laboratories, personal communication, 1990). Institute of Medicine, National Academy of Sciences: *Nutrition during lactation,* Washington, DC, 1991, National Academy Press.

by the father helps breastfeeding succeed
- Public education through television, newspapers, magazines, and radio to enhance the acceptability of breastfeeding
- Improved education about breastfeeding techniques in medical and nursing schools, and residency programs in obstetrics, pediatrics, and family practice
- Factual educational material designed to present advantages of breastfeeding
- Encouragement not to use breastfeeding alternatives for relief, vacation, or night feeding until nursing is well established
- Breastfeeding information provided in prenatal classes and at any prenatal contact
- Decreased sedation of the mother for labor and birth
- Extended contact between mother and infant in the first 24 hours
- Rooming in encouraged except when specifically contraindicated
- Avoidance of routine supplemental feeding
- Lactation suppressants not given unless requested by the mother
- Discharge packs of formula given only at the discretion of the physician or at the request of the mother, not as a routine hospital practice

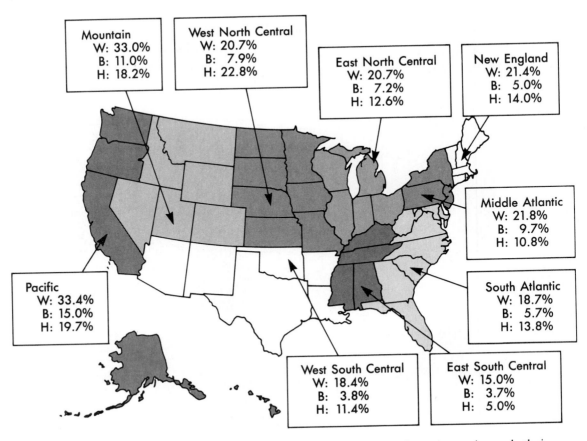

FIG. 5-13 Breastfeeding rates at 5 to 6 months postpartum, by census region and ethnic background. *W,* white; *B,* black; *H,* Hispanic.

Data from the 1989 Ross Mothers Survey (A. Ryan, Ross Laboratories, personal communication, 1990). Institute of Medicine, National Academy of Sciences: *Nutrition during lactation,* Washington, DC, 1991, National Academy Press.

- Development of day nurseries adjacent to school or work places to encourage and support working and school-aged mothers to breastfeed
- Utilization of lay support groups such as La Leche League
- Encouragement of continued breastfeeding of the hospitalized child
- Relactation instruction when necessary

PRENATAL AND POSTPARTUM COUNSELING
The Decision to Breastfeed

The decision to breastfeed is a significant one for the parents and is usually made relatively early in the pregnancy. The factors that influence this decision are complex and interrelated.

Where parents have not yet made a decision or have not been exposed to the advantages of breastfeeding, it is the responsibility of the health care professionals to support lactation as the optimum method of infant feeding. Although health professionals must support the parents' ultimate decision regarding feeding method, they too often fail to take a positive stand in support of lactation early enough in the prenatal period to influence the decision-making process. It has long been recognized that physicians who support lactation have higher percentages of breastfeeding mothers.

Involving other family members often is a good promotional tool. A study of 1525 women showed that if the woman is married, her husband's opinion is a strong influence on her decision to breastfeed. There also was a strong association between the child's grandmother's method of feeding. Outside influence can be subtle, too. Encouraging staff to wear pro-breastfeeding buttons, use bookmarks and note pads and breastfeeding slogans, and integrating such convenience as a private breastfeeding or pumping room into the regular scheme of things sends a powerful message: WE SUPPORT THE BREASTFEEDING FAMILY.

Historically, health professionals have been taught to be neutral in discussions of infant feeding. The notion here was that if health care workers supported breastfeeding, it might make bottle-feeding mothers feel guilty. However, some lactation advocates feel that bottle-feeding mothers aren't feeling guilty, but rather very angry with health professionals for not having disclosed the facts which would have given them a stronger motivation to begin or to continue breastfeeding. An opinion held by many is that women fail to breastfeed because professional personnel have failed to take this major physiological process seriously, and so frequently provide inaccurate diagnosis and inappropriate advice.

There are a few breastfeeding concerns that most prospective mothers have; by treating them seriously, honestly and respectfully, we can go a long way toward promoting breastfeeding. These concerns include:

1. How does it feel?
2. Does it hurt?
3. How long should I breastfeed?
4. What if the baby gets hungry in public?
5. What happens when I return to work?
6. What about sex?

There are some concepts that apply to all mother-baby couples; these can be shared with prospective parents so that they are prepared to breastfeed. These concepts lay the foundation upon which individual differences between mother-baby couples can be built. Techniques that work for one mother may not work for another; the same can be said for differences between siblings which were breastfed. What worked for the first or second baby may not work with the third. Sticking with the basics in the prenatal period is therefore important. These include the following:

1. Benefits of breastfeeding to mother and baby
2. Prenatal assessment and preparation of nipple
3. How breastfeeding works
4. Assessing a "Baby Friendly" hospital (see box on p. 211)

Experienced breastfeeding educators maintain that preparation for breastfeeding takes place 99% in the head and 1% in the nipples. Every prenatal contact is an opportunity to reinforce the choice to breastfeed.

When the decision has been made to breastfeed, an individual or small group instruction session is indicated. Simply handing out pamphlets is not very effective. These sessions may be held early in the second trimester. Both parents should be included in the instruction session if possible. Fathers tend to be more supportive if they know what to expect and understand possible difficulties they may encounter. The prenatal visit provides the opportunity to get to know the parents, to find out how much they know about breastfeeding, what fears and apprehensions they may have, and to estimate how much help and support the mother is likely to need in the early weeks of breastfeeding. It is important to remember that there is a typical breastfeeding personality. Women who appear to be

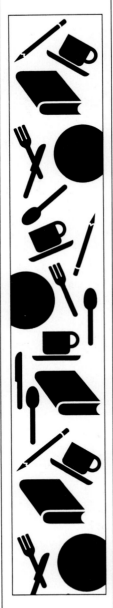

STRATEGIES FOR NUTRITION EDUCATION

Initiation and Duration of Breastfeeding: Benefits of Home Support Visits

Public health nutritionists and dietitians agree that breastfeeding is best for both mother and baby. Healthy People 2000: National Health Promotion and Disease Prevention Objectives has set the goal that 75% of all mothers will breastfeed and 50% will continue breastfeeding for at least 5 to 6 months. Current practices fall well below those goals and breastfeeding is lowest among low income, less well educated, and African-American and Hispanic mothers. Many new mothers do not have a relative or other support person nearby to answer questions about breastfeeding or to help with problems that may arise after they have left the hospital. This lack of support after returning home appears to be critical to the decision to discontinue breastfeeding. Intervention programs that provide home support by trained lactation counselors have resulted in about a two-fold increase in the number of mothers who are continuing to breastfeed after two months.

Schedule for Visits

It is important to visit the nursing mother within 1 to 2 days after she leaves the hospital and as often as needed during the first two weeks until breastfeeding is established. At that time it can be determined if further visits are necessary or if the process is moving along smoothly. Mothers should be provided with the telephone number of their counselors so they may obtain answers to questions as they arise.

Activities for Visits

Information provided in early visits might include the frequency of feeding, relaxation techniques, and how to determine if intake is adequate in the breastfed infant. The lactation counselor might also observe the breastfeeding process and make suggestions regarding the positioning of the infant and nipple care to avoid the development of sore nipples. Concerns relating to the adequacy of breast milk and the development of sore, cracked nipples are major factors leading to the discontinuation of breastfeeding.

Selection and Training of Lactation Counselors

Lactation counselors providing home support might include public health nutritionists, dietitians, or nurses sponsored by a local hospital, visiting nurse association or WIC (Supplemental Food Program for Women, Infants, and Children). To reduce the costs of a home support program trained paraprofessionals supervised by a home health agency or the Expanded Food and Nutrition Education Program (EFNEP) might provide lactation counseling.

Factors to be considered in the recruiting and training of lactation counselors include:
- workshops to develop a strong knowledge base on lactation
- hands-on experience with breastfeeding mothers in a supervised clinic situation
- at ease when observing breastfeeding and offering assistance
- nonjudgmental approach to the attitudes and decisions of others

Serafino-Cross P, Donovan PR: Effectiveness of professional breastfeeding home support, *J Nutr Educ* 24:117, 1992. US Department of Health and Human Services: *Healthy People 2000: National Health Promotion and Disease Prevention Objectives*, DHHS Pub No (PHS) 91-50213, Washington, DC, 1991, US Government Printing Office.

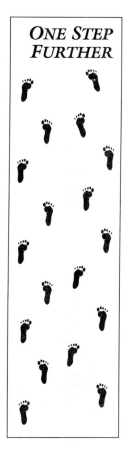

ONE STEP FURTHER

Is Your Hospital "Baby Friendly?"

WHO/UNICEF has jointly launched a new initiative aimed at promoting breastfeeding through the creation of "baby friendly" hospitals.

Institutions that adopt and apply the "10 steps to successful breastfeeding" will be designated as "Baby Friendly" and will receive a plaque or other award of public recognition.

Every health facility providing maternity services and care for newborn infants should:

1. Have a written breastfeeding policy that is routinely communicated to all health care staff
2. Train all health care staff in skills necessary to implement this policy
3. Inform all pregnant women about the benefits and management of breastfeeding
4. Help mothers initiate breastfeeding within a half-hour of birth
5. Show mothers how to breastfeed, and how to maintain lactation even if they should be separated from their infants
6. Give newborn infants no food or drink other than breast milk, unless medically indicated
7. Practice rooming-in—allow mothers and infants to remain together 24 hours a day
8. Encourage breastfeeding on demand
9. Give no artificial teats or pacifiers (also called dummies or soothers) to breastfeeding infants
10. Foster the establishment of breastfeeding support groups and refer mothers to them on discharge from the hospital or clinic

Representatives of the International Pediatric Association, at whose meeting the "Baby Friendly" compaign was introduced, ask for the assistance of all health professionals as partners in this initiative. The UNICEF resolution also calls on "manufacturers and distributors of breast milk substitutes to end free and low-cost supplies of infant formula to maternity wards and hospitals by December 1992," to reduce their detrimental effect on breastfeeding.

"nervous" can learn to breastfeed successfully if they cultivate a relaxed and confident attitude. This is best accomplished by adequate instruction along with professional and family support.

Lactation Education Program

In the beginning of the lactation education program, the health professional should discuss the advantages of breastfeeding as outlined earlier here. She should listen and respond to any concerns that the parents may have. Then the physiology of lactation and the mother's diet should be discussed.

The general physiology of lactation should be covered, explaining briefly the structure of the breast and hormonal controls of the process. A good understanding of mammary gland physiology is a great aid in promoting confidence in the ability to lactate. Women should realize that breast size is not a factor in the success of lactation. They should be informed that the glandular structure is adequately developed in virtually all women during pregnancy and differences in breast size are mainly the result of variation in the content of adipose tissue. Simplified diagrams and explanations such as those provided in this chapter may be useful for breastfeeding education.

A brief discussion of the dietary requirements for lactation should be included in the prenatal visits. It is usually sufficient to stress that additional amounts of the same types of foods that belong in any well-balanced diet, with special attention to good sources of calcium and vitamin C, will adequately provide the additional nutrition. Although fluid is an essential component of breast milk and its consumption should be encouraged, thirst dictates fluid requirements in most women. The body's ability to conserve fluid by concentrating urine allows women to succeed in lactation with wide variations in levels of fluid intake.

Nipple Conditioning

Although several studies suggest that prenatal nipple conditioning does not prevent nipple soreness during early lactation, it may be useful for some women. In societies where the breast is uncovered or where clothing is loosely worn, nipple soreness is much less a problem. The woman who plans to breastfeed should purchase a nursing brassiere that will suffice for the increased size required for the last few months of pregnancy, as well as for lactation. If her breasts are very heavy, or if the woman feels uncomfortable with the weight unsupported, the brassiere can be worn day and night. One of the easiest ways to get the nipples used to tactile stimulation is to leave the flaps on the brassiere open as much as possible during the day and night. This allows the nipples to rub against clothing, gradually desensitizing them.

Lanolin
(L *lana*, wool) Fatty substance extracted from wool, used in ointments and salves.

No special ointments or preparations are generally required for nipple conditioning. Pure **lanolin,** a component of many of the breast creams on the market, appears to be harmless (unless an allergy to wool exists), but products containing alcohol or petroleum-based products are to be avoided, since they remove natural lubricants from the nipple and areola. Since soap is drying, it is advisable to wash the nipple area with water only.

Inverted Nipples

Inverted nipples occasionally occur. They can be diagnosed by pressing the areola between the thumb and forefinger. A flat or normal nipple will protrude; a truly inverted nipple will retract. Truly inverted nipples are rare. When they do occur, they can usually be treated by massage.

Not only may exercises be helpful in the prenatal period to prepare flat or inverted nipples for lactation, but also use of a nipple shield, or breast shield, may be even more effective (Fig. 5-14). The rubber nipple tip of the shield should be removed and only the plastic base with the hole in the center applied over the areola inside a well-fitting brassiere. The constant, even pressure will cause the nipple to evert through the hole. The shield can be worn daily for the last weeks or months of pregnancy.

If inverted nipples are discovered at the first feeding in the hospital, the mother should use the electric pump to pull the nipples out, then place the infant quickly on the breast. If an electric pump is not available, a manual cylinder-type pump can be used. Between feedings, the mother should wear a breast shield and supportive brassiere.

Effect of Anesthetics

Another major consideration to be discussed during prenatal visits is the effect of anesthetics and analgesics given during labor and delivery on early feedings. Research indicates that even the nerve conduction anesthetics affect the newborn's reflexes and may impair ability to suck well. The baby may be lethargic and disinterested in feeding or may take the breast and suck only weakly until the effects of the anesthesia have worn off. This information may be useful to the mother in selecting an anesthetic, if it is to be used. The baby who is uncooperative because of sedation can still breastfeed successfully. It will probably take just a few days longer to establish a let-down reflex and to produce an

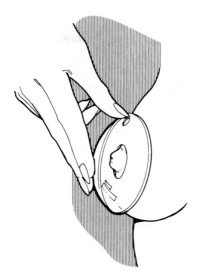

FIG. 5-14   Breast shield in place.

adequate milk supply. The baby who is severely affected may not suck well until after the third or fourth day of life. With the current trend toward early hospital discharges, it might be beneficial to keep mother and baby in the hospital for an extra day or to provide good follow-up care at home to ensure that lactation gets off to a good start.

Resources

The mother should be encouraged to jot down questions that arise. Several excellent books on breastfeeding are referenced at the end of this chapter. Most are available in paperback and from public libraries. Some large clinics have established their own lending libraries. Clients will benefit from talking with mothers who are already successfully breastfeeding. If no suitable candidates can be found from office files, local chapters of La Leche League, an international organization of mothers and professionals dedicated to spreading information about breastfeeding, will usually be able to assist the parents.

In-Hospital Postpartum Support

Breastfeeding will often be a new experience for the mother, as well as for the baby. The new mother may be apprehensive and unsure of herself, and need help and guidance in handling the infant. The clinician who is to instruct the mother at the first feeding should try to make her feel as much at ease as possible. The father should be encouraged to be present at feedings and during instruction if the hospital permits it and if the mother is comfortable with his presence. The father's support, knowledge, and understanding will be valuable later on. He may remember techniques and advice the mother has forgotten.

Positions for feeding. There are two basic breastfeeding positions, each of which is subject to a wide variety of individual adaptations. The chief requirements are (1) the comfort of the mother throughout the feeding, and (2) the positioning of the baby so that the process of swallowing is not impaired.

If the mother has had an **episiotomy** or operative delivery (cesarean section), she may be more comfortable breastfeeding lying down. She should position herself comfortably on her side, using pillows for additional support as required. The baby should be placed on his side with his mouth parallel to the nipple. A roll of receiving blankets makes a good

Episiotomy
(Gr *epision*, pubic region; *tome*, a cutting) Surgical incision into the peritoneum and vagina for obstetric purposes.

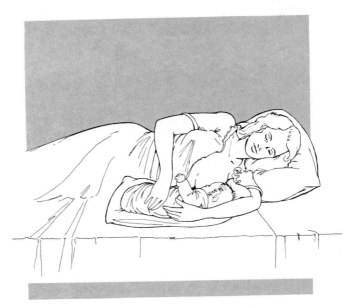

FIG. 5-15   Recommended recumbent position for breastfeeding.

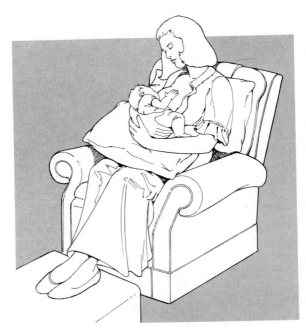

FIG. 5-16   Recommended positioning for breastfeeding while sitting in a comfortable chair.

support for the baby's back. This position is illustrated in Fig. 5-15. The baby can then feed comfortably from the lower breast without undue nipple traction or unnecessary distortion of the infant's alimentary tract. Both baby and mother will probably need help in repositioning to feed from the other breast.

The second common position for breastfeeding is that in which the mother sits in a comfortable chair that provides good back support, arm rests, and, if possible, foot and leg

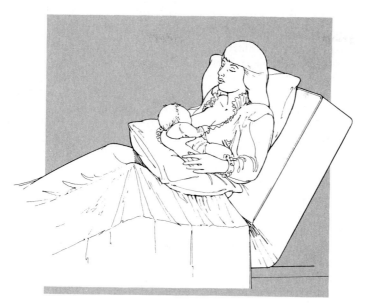

FIG. 5-17 Modified positioning for breastfeeding while sitting in a hospital bed.

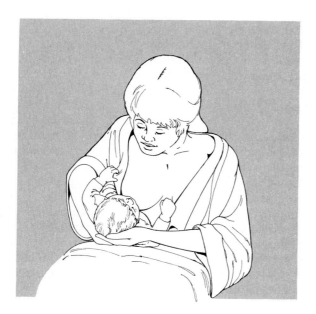

FIG. 5-18 Baby is tucked under right arm like a football and is nursing on right breast.

support. She cradles the baby in her arm, placing his head over her elbow so that his mouth is adjacent to the nipple. A pillow may be required on her lap to support the baby's body and under her elbow to prevent her arm from becoming too tired while holding the baby's head in the proper position for feeding. This position is illustrated in Fig. 5-16 and must be reversed for feeding on the opposite breast. This position can be modified for use in the hospital bed (Fig. 5-17). If this is to be successful, the head of the bed should be raised fully and the foot adjusted to provide leg support. Pillows will be required to support the arm holding the baby's head. An additional blanket roll or pillow under the mother's knees may make the position more comfortable. After feeding has begun, the position should be checked to make sure that nipple traction and distortion of the infant's alimentary tract are at a minimum.

Another popular position, especially with small babies or twins, is the "football hold". The baby's head is held in the palm of the hand while the forearm is used to support the baby's torso (Fig. 5-18). This allows the mother to move the baby easily until the proper position of the baby's mouth relative to the nipple is achieved. The "football hold" can be used while "tailor" sitting in bed with the mother's back supported. It is especially comfortable for mothers who have had cesarean deliveries.

TYPICAL CONCERNS OF THE BREASTFEEDING MOTHER

Even though the prenatal and early postnatal assistance with lactation may have been of high quality, mothers will likely have additional problems and questions during the first few weeks. A variety of concerns often develop and attention to these concerns may well determine the duration of breastfeeding for some distraught mothers.

Anxiety Over Quantity and Quality of Milk Supply

Sufficient quantity. Milk is produced to equal demand in almost all women. If the let-down reflex is functioning adequately, insufficient quantity is rarely a problem. The mother's concern may come from a well-meaning friend or relative who has casually remarked, "Mrs. X didn't have enough milk for her baby so she had to bottle-feed." Nurses and other helpers should try to impress on the new breastfeeding mother that in many societies of the world *all* women breastfeed their babies and virtually *all* women in our society who really want to breastfeed can do so, too. If feeding sessions have been frequent and of adequate duration, milk supply is probably ample. Pediatricians suggest careful monitoring of the infant's growth by weighing every week during the first month of life. A gain of about one third to one half pound per week is suggested. This can be reassuring to the mother and can help the clinician detect growth problems early on.

Baby's responses. Mothers may need to be reminded that babies do not always cry from hunger. Sometimes they may need to be "burped" or have diapers changed. Often they may merely require companionship and sometimes a baby cries for no apparent reason. If the baby is growing well and has at least six wet diapers a day, assuming he is receiving no additional water or formula, the mother should be comforted by knowing that the milk supply is adequate and that this fussy baby might be even fussier if he were being bottle-fed.

Milk quality. Too many well-meaning "advisors" are quick to volunteer that "your milk obviously doesn't agree with him" or "he's got gas (or colic); it must be something you ate." Such comments immediately give the mother a sense of guilt. Although the protein and fat content of human milk varies slightly according to time of day, stage of lactation, and the individual woman, evidence indicates that maternal nutrient stores "subsidize" the requirements of lactation if occasionally dietary intake is inadequate. Breast milk is therefore seldom "too rich" or "too thin" if the maternal diet is adequate and the let-down reflex functions.

Mother's diet and rest. Adverse reaction to foods in the maternal diet has been known to occur. From 4 to 6 hours are required for components of metabolites of a specific food to appear in breast milk. The food producing a reaction can often be identified and omitted from the mother's diet. Most foods that could be tolerated during pregnancy will be well tolerated by the mother and the infant during lactation. If a food consistently seems to bother mother or child, it can be omitted to see if relief, real or imagined, occurs.

Adequate rest, diet, and fluids are essential, especially if the milk supply needs to be increased. Mothers do not "lose" their milk. However, sometimes a busy schedule and lack of food or rest interfere with milk production. When this happens it is wise to take a day off to "make more milk." With rest, fluids, good diet, and of course more frequent feedings, milk supply usually parallels demand within 24 to 48 hours. Growth spurts, and thus increasing demand, are common at about 6 to 12 weeks of age.

Other general anxieties. Other causes for anxiety are the softening of the breast that occurs once lactation has become established, the presence (or absence) of milk leaking, changes in infant stool patterns, and lack of sleeping through the night. All of these are normal and do not indicate lack of breast milk. Growth failure is the only true indication of inadequate nutrition in the normal breastfed infant. When this occurs it is most frequently observed after the baby is 6 months of age. About this time some women find that their breast milk alone does not provide sufficient nutrition to maintain optimum growth. In fact, however, research has demonstrated that exclusive breastfeeding can be adequate for periods varying from 2 to 15 months and that there is no specific age at which breastfeeding becomes inadequate.

Excess milk flow. Sometimes the mother's concern is actually an oversupply of milk. She should be encouraged to use manual expression to slow the flow of milk before a feeding and to express to a comfort level between feedings. This expressed milk may be frozen for supplements or donated to milk banks for premature or critically ill infants. The mother should continue to offer both breasts at each feeding but decrease time to 5 to 10 minutes per side. The use of a pacifier for increased sucking time may be desirable.

Nipple Soreness

Normal reaction versus true problem. Many women who breastfeed experience varying degrees of general nipple discomfort when feeding. The discomfort associated with the first few seconds of feeding and alleviated by the feeding is normal. It is caused by the stimulation of the breast tissue by oxytocin during let-down. True nipple soreness, which is accompanied by tenderness and redness of the areola, is evidence of tissue breakdown and is better prevented than treated.

Treatment. Some women, particularly those with fair skin, seem more susceptible to this problem. If nipples must be treated, they should be treated promptly rather than allowing the condition to progress to cracked and fissured nipples open to infection. In addition to the techniques already discussed for nipple conditioning and prevention of soreness, the following suggestions may be useful:

1. Check for proper tongue position below nipple and make sure the baby's grasp includes some of the areola. Express milk if necessary to allow proper grasp of nipple.
2. Feed the baby on demand. If he gets too hungry he may suck harder, causing further soreness.
3. Vary the position with each feeding, allowing the baby to suck on slightly different areas of the areola with each feeding.
4. Begin each feeding on the breast that is least tender. Allow the baby to suck until the let-down reflex has occurred, then switch to the tender side and allow the baby to empty the breast. Promptly return to the less tender side to finish the feeding.
5. Promptly terminate feedings when completed. Allowing an infant to suck on an empty breast causes increased tissue damage. From 7 to 10 minutes on each side should be sufficient if nipples are tender. Offer a pacifier if necessary.
6. Let nipples dry well before replacing brassiere flaps, allowing air to circulate on them as freely as possible. Air drying for 10 minutes after a feeding and before using any breast cream is a good procedure.
7. Avoid soaps, alcohol, and especially petroleum-based compounds on the nipple area, as they cause further irritation. Lanolin or a commercial breast cream may be applied

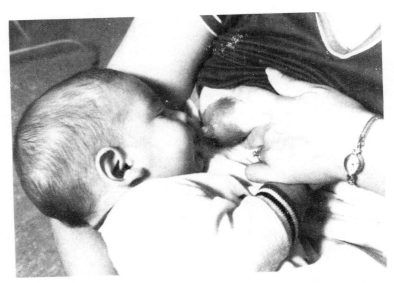

FIG. 5-19 When breast is offered to infant, areola is gently compressed between two fingers and breast is supported to ensure that infant is able to grasp areola adequately.

From Lawrence R: *Breastfeeding: a guide for the medical profession,* ed 3, St Louis, 1989, Mosby.

Tannic acid
Compound of certain plants such as tea leaves, giving an astringent taste and having astringent properties that promote local tissue healing; an herbal remedy.

after the areola has dried. **Tannic acid** has long been recognized for its role in promoting healing. Thus some mothers have found that a used tea bag, thoroughly cooled and applied to the nipple area two or three times a day, helps to promote healing.

Engorgement

Causes. Engorged breasts are hot, heavy, and hard with milk. Many physicians and nurses see this as basically a hospital-acquired condition caused by infrequent feeding. This is at least partly true, and the consequences may be a hungry, frustrated baby and a mother suffering from pain and stress. However, in some women a general increase in circulation to the mammary tissue and edema in the tissues are thought to combine with the newly produced milk to cause mild to extreme discomfort, regardless of feeding frequency. The only component of this situation that can be remedied is the milk. There is no more effective "breast pump" than a hungry baby.

Edema
(Gr *oidema,* swelling) Unusual increase of fluid in the intercellular tissue spaces, local or generalized.

Treatment. During engorgement the baby should be put to breast at least every 3 hours. The mother should compress the areola between two fingers to make it easier for the infant to grasp (Fig. 5-19). If the milk supply greatly exceeds demand, the baby should be allowed to suck only to relieve the sensation of fullness (about 5 minutes) at each breast. Some milk may be manually expressed before offering the breast to the baby if the nipple is difficult for the baby to grasp. If the baby is uncooperative (for example, sleepy), manual expression will have to be used to relieve the pressure of accumulating milk. A firmly-fitting brassiere may make engorgement less painful.

Venous stasis
(L *venosus,* vein; Gr *stasis,* standing still) A stoppage, or decreased flow, of blood draining an organ, causing engorgement of the affected tissue.

Many women find relief from discomfort by the application of moist heat to the breast. This may be done with wet towels, a warm shower or bath, or steam from a sink or basin of water. For the ambulatory mother suffering from engorgement, face cloths wet with warm water and folded into plastic bags can be held in place by the brassiere. Since much of the discomfort is caused by **edema** resulting from **venous stasis,** moist heat to increase the circulation would seem a more beneficial prescription than ice packs. However, some women have found that ice or cold packs make them feel better, possibly because cold merely dulls the sensation of discomfort. Massage is also useful to help soften the breast and assist the baby in draining the ducts. If the mother is really uncomfortable, a mild analgesic can be recommended. Typical engorgement occurs only on the first full day of milk production and is of short duration, usually about 24 hours.

Leaking

A number of women experience leaking from their breasts during the first few weeks of breastfeeding. Usually it is caused by fullness in the breast or the milk letting down and is part of the normal breastfeeding experience. It may occur during a nursing from the opposite breast, just before a nursing when the breasts are full, or when nursings are missed altogether. Sometimes it is caused by psychologic conditioning. For example, a woman may leak in response to hearing a baby cry, picking up her own baby to nurse, or simply thinking about breastfeeding her baby. Some mothers may be reassured by leaking, since it is a sign of a plentiful milk supply and a functioning let-down. Often the mother and baby only need time to adjust to one another, and leaking will subside as harmony develops between supply and demand.

Supplemental Feedings

Occasional bottle-feeding. Rare is the mother who does not want—indeed, need—to be away from her infant for a brief period that will undoubtedly include a feeding. For this reason it is a good idea to introduce the baby to an occasional bottle at least by the end of the first month and about once a week or so thereafter. Many infants do not accept a bottle from their mothers but will take it from their father or a sitter. The breastfeeding infant will often swallow more air with a bottle-feeding and may need to be "burped" more frequently, particularly if he seems to take the milk very quickly.

Preparation of single feeding. Powdered formula offers advantages for use as a single feeding supplement when human milk is not available. The proper number of measures of powder can be placed in the bottle and the nipple and cap put in place. Then if the bottle is needed, about half of the required amount of cold water can be added. The bottle should be shaken thoroughly to dissolve the powder, and then the remainder of the liquid should be added as very warm water. With this method, formula dilutions are less likely, the bottle is at serving temperature, and the cost is considerably less than ready-to-feed formula—a real advantage if the baby only takes 1 or 2 ounces and the remainder has to be discarded. Any unmixed, unneeded bottle can safely be left in the diaper bag for the next time. If refrigerated, a can of formula powder will last at least 6 months.

Expression of Milk

Manual technique. Manual expression of milk is a useful technique for the breastfeeding mother to learn. Although some women may find it a laborious procedure, there is often no substitute. Actually, the procedure is simple. First apply moist heat to the breast and massage gently for 5 to 10 minutes before expression or until a let-down reflex can be obtained. Then place the thumb on top and the forefinger under the areolar margin, gently pushing the finger and thumb back toward the chest wall to grasp behind the milk sinuses (Fig. 5-20). Squeeze gently in a "pumping" motion toward the nipple to remove the milk that has collected in the milk sinuses. Repeat the procedure, rotating the position of the grasp on the nipple occasionally so that all the sinuses are drained. Some women will find that the milk flows freely once a let-down occurs. Others will only be able to express a few drops at a time.

Breast pump. Mothers who need to express milk for a period of a day or weeks, such as in the case of a working mother or the mother of a hospitalized infant, might find it

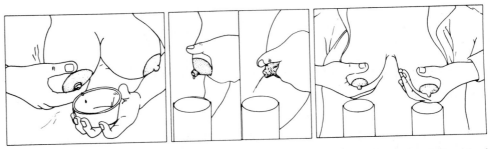

FIG. 5-20 Manual expression of breast milk. Front view, side view, and two-handed method.

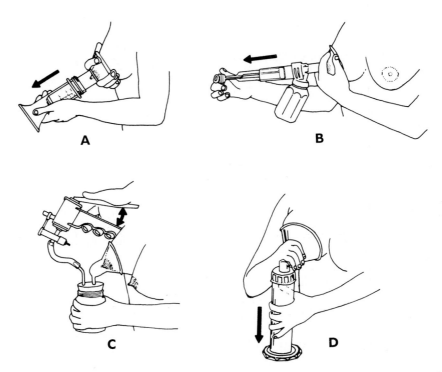

FIG. 5-21 Several popular varieties of manual breast pumps. **A,** Marshal or Kaneson. **B,** Medela. **C,** Lloyd-B. **D,** Egnell hand-operated pump.

From Worthington-Roberts BS, Williams SR: *Nutrition in pregnancy and lactation,* ed 5, St Louis, 1993, Mosby.

considerably easier and more comfortable to use a breast pump. Some very good manual pumps are now on the market (Fig. 5-21), and several high-quality electric breast pumps (Fig. 5-22) are also available. Each one simulates the nursing experience by providing alternating periods of negative and positive pressure. Many cities have rental sources of breast pumps. La Leche League maintains a rental supply of electric breast pumps in some cities. Manual breast pumps frequently do not work well and can cause considerable discomfort and even nipple damage because of the tremendous uninterrupted negative pressure used to extract the milk.

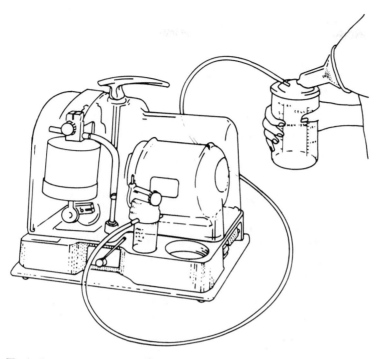

FIG. 5-22   Typical electric breast pump.

From Worthington-Roberts BS, Williams SR: *Nutrition in pregnancy and lactation,* ed 5, St Louis, 1993, Mosby.

Storage of Milk

If expressed human milk is to be saved for future feeding, care must be taken to assure that it is safe from microbes with minimal loss of its nutritional or protective characteristics. Fresh human milk is bacteriologically safe for up to, but no longer than, 6 hours after expression.[61] Freezing not only protects milk from contamination but also promotes minimal change in milk composition.[62] Membranes of milk cells are destroyed by this process and some hydrolysis of triglycerides occurs.[63] However, immunoglobulin levels, antibody titers, and nutritional properties are virtually unchanged. Heat treatment and **lyophilization** promote additional losses.[64,65] Fat and protein digestibility are reduced and milk cells damaged. Levels of many of the protective factors are also substantially reduced. Recent data suggest, however, that rapid high-temperature treatment allows for retention of nutritional and immunologic qualities.[66]

Several efforts have been made to determine if the type of storage container influences the quality of the milk. Paxson and Cress reported that the placement of human milk into glass containers markedly reduces retrieval of the white cells even though **phagocytosis** is unaffected.[67] These workers recommended that human milk be collected in plastic containers. However, Goldblum and associates reported that the type of container made little difference in the number of identifiable cells after 4 hours of storage.[68] They also found that levels of some of the protective factors declined with storage during the 4-hour period, but no one type of container proved to be superior for the storage of all of the measured immunologic factors. These investigators concluded that because of the

Lyophilization
(Gr *lyein,* to dissolve; *philein,* to love, having an affinity for a stable solution) Process of rapid freezing and dehydration of the frozen product under high vacuum to stabilize or preserve a biologic substance.

Phagocytosis
(Gr *phagein,* to eat; *cyte,* hollow vessel, anything that contains or covers) Engulfing of microorganisms, other cells, or foreign particles by phagocytes.

profound loss of sIgA antibodies in polyethylene bags, the difficulty in handling the flexible bags, and the potential breakage of the Pyrex glass containers, polypropylene containers were best for future work.

Duration of Breastfeeding

The tradition in most parts of the world is to breastfeed for 2 to 3 years. Weaning is rather natural at this age, since the child can now feed himself and eat a full adult diet. He also has teeth and can walk and talk a little and thus express wishes and disagreements. The mother, too, may again become pregnant at this time so that her attention will need to be directed toward the new infant.

Spontaneous termination. Many young children spontaneously give up breastfeeding at about 1 year of age or soon thereafter, especially if they are receiving adequate supplementary foods. Some mothers feel much relief, and others feel sad or rejected. Some children cling to the breast for years, and again maternal response to this behavior is mixed. There are also a few children who cling to the breast and refuse to eat solid foods. These are usually children a year of age who have had solids introduced too late. It is essential that these children be trained to eat solid food, and the sooner the training takes place, the easier it will be for the parent.

The individual mother-child couple must determine their own ideal duration of breastfeeding. Factors to consider include the following:

1. Convenience of the mother
2. Needs of the child, both psychologic and physiologic
3. Availability of satisfactory alternative or supplemental feeds
4. Custom in the community

Whether a mother breastfeeds her child for 2 months or 2 years, the main concern of the health care provider is to support the mother in her decision, and to help her avoid cessation of breastfeeding against her wishes.

SPECIAL PROBLEMS
Maternal and Infant Conditions

Contraindications to lactation. Although each case must be evaluated on its own merit, there are very few conditions that automatically preclude breastfeeding. The genetic disease **galactosemia** is one *absolute* contraindication to breastfeeding. Breast milk is a rich source of lactose, and the very survival of infants with galactosemia depends on their receiving a non-lactose-containing formula. Galactosemia is a rare disorder, occurring in approximately 1 in every 60,000 births. Another genetic disease **phenylketonuria (PKU)** is also often mentioned as a contraindication to breastfeeding. However, breast milk has relatively low levels of phenylalanine. In fact, infants who are exclusively breastfed may receive a phenylalanine intake near the amount recommended for treating PKU. Total or partial nursing can therefore be used, although close monitoring of the infant's blood phenylalanine levels is required.

Mothers with a known transmissible viral disease, such as acquired immunodeficiency syndrome (AIDS) should probably not breastfeed. Breastfeeding is also inappropriate in cases of alcoholism, heroin addiction, malaria, or severe chronic disease resulting in maternal malnutrition. Patients with active tuberculosis should not breastfeed. However, if the mother is being treated with an antituberculosis drug and is culture negative, breastfeeding is allowed. In such cases, careful checks of mother and infant are necessary because an accumulation of the antituberculin drug, Isoniazid, can cause liver damage. Women with diagnosed breast cancer are usually advised not to breastfeed so that the needed treatment can be given immediately.

Galactosemia

Rare inherited disease in newborns caused by a missing enzyme (galactose-1-phosphate uridyl transferase—G-1-PUT), required for conversion of galactose (from lactose) to glucose. Untreated galactose accumulation in the blood causes extensive tissue damage and potential death. Normal growth and development now follows newborn screening and immediate initiation of a galactose-free diet with a special soy-base formula.

Phenylketonuria (PKU)

A genetic disease caused by a missing enzyme, phenylalanine hydroxylase, required for the metabolic conversion of the essential amino acid phenylalanine to the amino acid tyrosine. Untreated, profound mental retardation occurs. Normal growth and development now follows current mandatory newborn screening and immediate initiation of a low phenylalanine diet with special "low-phe" formula such as Lofenalac.

Mothers requiring drug therapy for management of chronic medical conditions may not be able to breastfeed if the only drug of choice is contraindicated during lactation. Recommendations of the American Academy of Pediatrics related to lactation and drug use are periodically updated (Table 5-7).

Cesarean birth. Mothers who have had operative deliveries ("C-sections") usually find that they can breastfeed successfully after the effects of the anesthesia have worn off for both the mother and child. In fact the mother can minimize the effects of pain medication on her baby by taking it 15 to 30 minutes directly before nursing. It may be possible for the mother to avoid some discomfort by requesting that the intravenous line be placed in a position that allows her maximum ability to handle her baby. Use of plenty of pillows will allow her to reduce the discomfort of pressure on her incision. If she can be comfortable in more than one position, she may be able to increase the number of nursing positions and reduce the severity of nipple soreness. Despite the few potential problems, the rate of successful breastfeeding among cesarean mothers is no different from that of mothers who deliver vaginally.

Poor let-down function. Some women seem to have more trouble than others in establishing a satisfactory let-down reflex. The extent to which the mother's emotional state contributes to the problem must be assessed. Anxiety and stress are known separately to decrease milk output since adrenalin inhibits oxytocin release. Anything that encourages relaxation should enhance let-down. A warm bath, moist heat to the breasts, gentle massage, and tactile stimulation, as well as soft lights and soft music, have been known to help. A moderate amount of alcohol seems to be beneficial as a relaxant for the mother and seems to enhance the let-down. Excessive amounts of alcohol and caffeine, however, have both been reported to interfere with the let-down reflex. The mother who habitually smokes to relax should avoid doing so during nursing and use other means, such as mental exercises. Failing that she should at least wait until the infant is sucking vigorously and the ejection is well established, then in the meanwhile continue her efforts to quit smoking entirely. Marijuana contains a psychoactive chemical (9-tetrahydrocannabinol) that acts on the hypothalamus and eventually disrupts pituitary production of prolactin as well as other hormones.

Colds and influenza. The presence of colds or other mild viral infections such as influenza is usually no reason to discontinue lactation as long as the mother feels able to breastfeed. The infant has usually been exposed to the infection by the time the mother realizes that she is affected. There is good evidence that the infant has some immunity through maternal antibodies. If the infant is infected, it is often a very mild form. When the infant has a cold, congestion makes breathing difficult during nursing. Use of a nasal aspirator to remove mucus and aid breathing may be of some help.

Clogged milk ducts. This condition is caused by incomplete emptying of one or more ducts. This sometimes occurs when the infant's feeding position does not allow for equal drawing on all of the milk sinuses, causing stasis. Milk or cast-off cells accumulate within a duct and form a localized plug or blockage. Milk then builds up behind the plug. Tenderness may develop in the area of the plug, and a lump may be felt at the point of blockage. Under these circumstances of simple obstruction, no fever, flulike symptoms, or systematic reactions typically occur. The remedy is (1) more frequent feeding, especially on the affected side; (2) rest; (3) analgesics, if necessary; and (4) application of moist heat. If the mother can lie down and allow the infant to nurse on the affected breast for half an hour or longer, the improvement is often dramatic. If treatment is prompt, recovery should be nearly complete within 24 hours.

It is highly desirable that the plug be removed quickly, since plugged ducts can develop into larger blocked-off areas called a "caked breast." This may be followed by a breast infection and considerable discomfort. If the plug can be released, however, improvement can be rapid. Sometimes plugs dissolve or are reabsorbed by maternal tissues. If the plug is released and comes out with the milk, it may be brownish or greenish and thick and stringy. This is no danger for the baby, but he may temporarily reject the milk.

Mastitis. The symptoms of **mastitis**, breast infection, are similar to those of engorgement. The breast is tender, distended with milk, and may feel hot to touch. Fever may be present. Treatment consists of prompt medical attention, antibiotic therapy, bed rest, and continued breastfeeding. Discontinued feeding causes increased stasis and further pain. Frequently the source of the infection is an untreated infection in the infant. Recurrent breast infections may require culturing of the milk or the baby's mouth to determine which antibiotics to prescribe. Infrequently the cause of the infection may be exposure to bacteria carried by other family members. If all other treatments prove ineffective, cultures should be taken from the rest of the family to determine the source of bacteria and prescribe simultaneous treatment for all involved. In any case, weaning should not be attempted until the infection has cleared up.

Abscess. When breast infections are not successfully treated, they may develop into a serious and painful condition called an abscess, in which there is localized pus and swelling of tissue. An abscess should be viewed as a serious problem requiring immediate medical attention. Diagnosis is made by culturing the secretions from the breast. Usual treatment includes antibiotics along with massage, pumping, and sometimes surgical drainage. It may be necessary to discontinue nursing on the affected side, but usually it can continue on the unaffected breast.

Maternal Disease

Chronic disease. Heart disease, diabetes, hepatitis, nephrosis, and most other chronic medical conditions are not themselves a contraindication to breastfeeding. Usually if the condition can be managed well enough to allow successful maintenance of pregnancy, breastfeeding may be the feeding method of choice because it is less tiring for the mother.

Diabetes. Since management of the diabetic woman in pregnancy has become increasingly more successful, many diabetic mothers are now choosing to breastfeed. In fact some mothers with diabetes enjoy a postpartum remission of their diabetes, which may last through lactation and in some cases several years longer. The remission has been attributed to the hormone interactions that affect the hypothalamus and pituitary gland during pregnancy, labor, delivery, and lactation.

Since persons with diabetes are known to be prone to infection, mastitis may pose a significant threat, and vaginitis may be more common. Infection of the nipples may also occur because of *Candida albicans.* Careful anticipatory care, avoidance of fatigue, and early antibiotic management of developing problems are wise.

Thyroid disease. When hypothyroidism is diagnosed in the mother, it is generally treated with full replacement therapy of desiccated thyroid. Under such circumstances breastfeeding is not contraindicated. If the mother is truly hypothyroid, care should be taken to rule out hypothyroidism in the infant. Diagnosis is made by evaluating blood values and is not a hazard to the nursing infant.

Unlike hypothyroidism, the diagnostic procedures and therapeutic management of the mother with hyperthyroidism present some hazards to the breastfed infant. Treatment includes antithyroid medication, which inhibits the synthesis of thyroid hormones. Compounds in this medication may appear in breast milk and may build up in the infant's circulation. With careful monitoring and thyroid medication, nursing may proceed successfully. However, care must be taken to watch for **bradycardia** and other signs of hypothyroidism, including goiter.

Cancer. A mother with a diagnosis of breast cancer should not nurse her infant in order to have definitive treatment immediately for herself. However, not all lumps in the lactating

Mastitis
(Gr *mastos,* breast; *itis,* inflammation) Breast infection; inflammation of the mammary gland.

Bradycardia
(Gr *bradys,* slow; *kardia,* heart) A slow heart beat, evidenced by slowing of the pulse rate to less than 60 beats/min.

breast are cancer, or even benign tumors. The lactating breast is lumpy by nature, and the lumps shift day by day. If a mass is located and the physician thinks it should be biopsied, it can be done under local anesthesia without weaning the infant. Usually such a lump is diagnosed as a benign mass. Immediate surgery to remove the mass may relieve tremendous anxiety without necessarily sacrificing breastfeeding.

Infectious disease. Infectious diseases that require isolation of the mother from other adults, as well as from children, may be a contraindication to breastfeeding.

Family and Social Situations

Multiple births. It is entirely possible to nurse more than one infant and many case reports support this fact. Historical observations of wet nurses indicate that support of six babies simultaneously is within the realm of physiologic capability. The key deterrent to nursing twins or triplets is not usually the milk supply but the time. Nursing two infants at the same time is clearly more efficient. A number of tricks have been proposed to accommodate more than one infant, but as they become larger and more active, it may be a real challenge to keep them simultaneously nursing without assistance from the father or a friend. The nursing mother of more than one infant needs to conscientiously attend to her own rest and nourishment.

Working during lactation. Many women believe that breastfeeding conflicts with working outside the home. This is a myth, since the two can go nicely together. The reduced incidence and severity of illness in the breastfeeding infant may actually reduce the days the mother misses from work. It is desirable for the working mother to have a minimum of 4 to 6 weeks at home with her nursing infant before returning to a full-time job. This time will allow for the successful establishment of lactation and the development of a close mother-child relationship. This strong foundation will provide the mother with substantial motivation to continue breastfeeding as her work commitments increase and her time with the infant decreases. The dedicated working mother will want to learn to express her milk so that she can provide it to her infant and maintain her lactation capacity for the days she has to work.

Pregnancy during lactation. Occasionally a mother may wish to nurse an infant after she becomes pregnant again. This circumstance is physiologically possible, but the nutritional and psychologic demands on the mother are substantial. Some women may even experience uterine contractions while nursing and in some cases may need to consider weaning to avoid the possibility of spontaneous abortion. The child may become discouraged from nursing because of the changing composition and taste of the milk produced as the pregnancy proceeds. The mother's milk supply may also decrease, and this may cause her child to lose interest in nursing.

Nursing siblings—tandem nursing. With sufficient sucking stimulus, most mothers can produce enough milk to successfully nurse a young infant, as well as an older child. It is important, however, to consider the emotional needs of the older sibling and the physical well-being of the mother. If the mother feels that the older child may satisfy his sucking needs and benefit emotionally from the breastfeeding experience, she may decide to continue nursing both children. However, if she feels that this undertaking is too demanding or she resents the older child nursing, she is well advised to wean the older child as soon as possible.

If the mother decides to wean the toddler, she should go about it gradually. It may be rather difficult while she is nursing the young baby, since the older one may want to nurse when he sees the younger sibling at the breast. An obvious solution is to nurse the baby at the times when the older child is not around or is happily occupied with other things. The mother will need to decide on some alternative activities and snacks to take the place of breastfeeding so that the transition from nursing to total weaning will go smoothly.

Relactation. Relactation is the resumption of lactation after it has been stopped some time beyond the immediate postpartum period. This process may be attempted by women who have for various reasons not nursed their infant for a while or by women who change their minds about lactation after weaning has taken place. To reactivate the lactation process requires that appropriate stimuli are provided to the breasts. The baby's sucking or manual stimulation may be accompanied by use of medications or hormones. Success generally depends on the mother's determination and the baby's willingness to suckle at the less than satisfying breast. The longer the interlude between initial lactation and relactation, the more likely the effort is to fail.

A mother needs to decide if she really wishes to attempt relactation. Considerable motivation is required, and initially the effort may be very time consuming. It should be clear to the mother that she may not be able to produce an adequate milk supply to meet all the infant's nutritional requirements. In fact such a goal may be unrealistic and undesirable. The majority of mothers who express great pleasure in their relactation experience indicate that the mother-infant relationship is of far greater short- and long-term importance than the act of the breastfeeding alone. They emphasize that breastfeeding is as much *nurturing at* the breast as it is *nutrition from* the breast. In many instances undue emphasis on a complete milk supply actually hinders the mother's ability to achieve it.

The mother who is attempting relactation needs to build up her milk supply by making sure that she receives satisfactory rest and nutrition along with frequent sucking stimulus. She may encourage the infant to suckle by simply cuddling and stroking, but in addition may apply a sweet-tasting substance to the end of the nipple. She may effectively offer the baby a supplement and avoid nipple confusion between the bottle and the breast by use of a nursing supplementer, the Lact-Aid. The Lact-Aid Nursing Trainer is a plastic bag that can be filled with formula and affixed to the mother's clothing near the breast during a feeding. A similar product called the Lactation Supplementer has recently been developed by Medela. While the baby nurses at the mother's breast, he receives formula through a small tube attached to the bag at one end and taped to the mother's nipple at the other (Fig. 5-23). Gradual weaning from the Lact-Aid or the Lactation Supplementer can be provided by putting less and less in the bag, in response to cues indicating an increase in maternal lactation, that is, excess supplement left in bag after nursing, very wet diapers, soft stools, spitting up after feedings, and increased time between feedings.

Nursing the adopted infant. It is extremely time consuming, and sometimes impossible, to induce lactation without having been pregnant. Even when a pregnancy has been carried out in the past, great motivation is required to nurse an adopted infant. Chances increase if the mother has given birth or nursed another baby. If she is currently nursing another baby or has recently weaned one, her chances for success are good. A mother embarking on this nursing experience should have realistic motives and goals. She should not expect to provide all the infant's nutrition through lactation but should look forward to a satisfying emotional experience.

The nipple preparation and relactation techniques described above apply also to the adoptive mother. In addition, it is useful for the mother to pump her breasts to stimulate milk production. She can gradually increase the frequency and duration of this activity until it reaches a level of about 20 minutes every 2 hours when the baby's arrival is near. The mother should realize that it may be quite a while before she sees any results from her pumping and that even a small amount of milk means success. The milk supply will increase rapidly when the baby begins suckling. If the mother is not able to obtain her baby soon after birth, however, her chances of success may decline, since the baby will have been bottle-fed and may suffer from nipple confusion.

The fact that some women have succeeded in nursing their adoptive infants does not mean that all adoptive mothers can nurse or should attempt to do so. This point was well

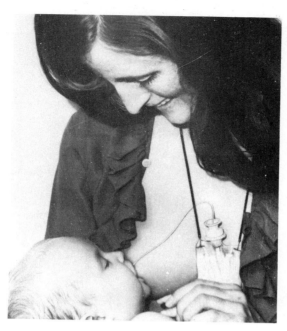

FIG. 5-23 Lact-Aid nursing trainer in use.
Courtesy of Lact-Aid International, Inc, PO Box 1066, Athens, TN 80206.

made by a physician whose family had recently adopted a young infant.[69] He pointed out that adoptive parents often have decided to adopt a child after a long period of reproductive failure and a trying experience with an adoptive agency. When the adopted infant finally arrives, the parents have to cope with a considerable role handicap. In view of the substantial time commitment of induced lactation and the stress and frustration that can be associated with it, one must really ask whether the advantages outweigh the disadvantages. Attempting lactation may set the mother up for another failure of physical function and loss of self-esteem, and in addition it requires much time and energy that could be devoted to more significant areas of social adjustment. *No pressure should ever be put on the adoptive mother to breastfeed.* If she wishes to try, she should have support and guidance. However, if she finds that she and her family are frustrated and exhausted, she should immediately reevaluate her intentions and not be encouraged to continue.

Teenage mothers. Most teenage mothers elect to keep their babies even when their home environments are neither supportive nor conducive to successful lactation. The self-image of the teenager may be poor, and she may have much doubt about her self-worth. She frequently feels uncomfortable in her new role as a mother. If the young mother expresses some interest in breastfeeding, effort should be made to determine her motives, and advantages and disadvantages should be discussed. It should be determined whether or not breastfeeding would significantly compromise her ability to continue in school or provide for the infant's other needs. Physiologically, teenagers are entirely capable of breastfeeding, although some will have less functional breast tissue than adult women. Teenage mothers are capable of satisfactory milk production and experience the same difficulties as other women. When problems arise, however, teenagers are less likely to overcome them and continue breastfeeding. They obviously require much support. Those with good support systems often breastfeed for the same amount of time as older mothers.

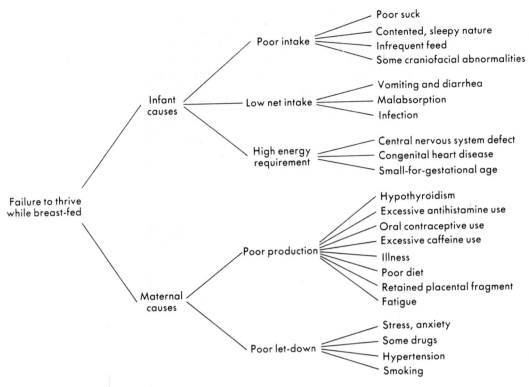

FIG. 5-24   Diagnostic flowchart for failure to thrive.
Modified from Lawrence R: *Breastfeeding: a guide for the medical profession,* ed 3, St Louis, 1989, Mosby.

Failure to Thrive

Causes. Failure of some breastfed infants to thrive has been reported for several decades and in many respects is no less puzzling today than when it was first described. A flow chart summarizing possible maternal and infant causes of the problem is provided in Fig. 5-24. In some cases there may be no history of excessive crying or dissatisfaction. The infant takes the breast well, nurses for a sufficient length of time, and sleeps well. There may be nothing to indicate abnormal nutrition, or whether the infant is getting enough to eat (see box on p. 229), until marked signs of dehydration and even marasmus appear.

Suckling process. According to Frantz and Fleiss, a major cause of failure to thrive in the totally breastfed infant is a weak or ineffective suck.[70] As these clinicians have repeatedly observed, the baby who is gaining weight poorly often has a rapid flutter-type chewing suckle that does not seem to have any drawing pause between the jaw motions, and swallowing occurs only every 3 to 15 suckles. On the other hand, they have noted that the babies who gain weight well also have a chew action to their jaw motions but display a slight pause in their cheeks between each suckle, and they appear to swallow with every suckle. The quality of the suckle often improved when an effort was made to hold the tongue down at the start of the feed and the tongue position was periodically checked. It also helped to have the mother switch breasts frequently, switching when inappropriate suckling began to develop. In some cases the Lact-Aid Nursing Trainer was found to be useful. Since minimum effort is required by infants to fill their mouths with milk, they have to create a chain reaction of suckle, swallow, suckle, and swallow.

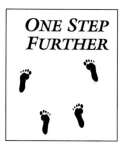

ONE STEP FURTHER

How to Tell If the Infant Is Getting Enough to Eat

1. Urination six or eight times a day. Most breastfed infants will have at least one or two stools a day during the first few weeks and may have as many as one every feeding
2. Adequate weight gain
3. Good color and skin tone
4. Feeding every 1½ to 3 hours, after which baby seems content

 ## CASE STUDY

A Breastfeeding Infant's Early Growth Pattern

A young mother and her 3-month-old infant appear in the clinic for routine well-baby care. The infant appears to be healthy but small. The body measurements reveal that weight falls on the 5th percentile and height plots on the 40th percentile. The mother reports that she is breastfeeding her baby, that things are going well although she is very tired, and that the baby is well behaved and rarely cries.

Questions for analysis
1. Define appropriate questions for the mother
2. Outline a strategy to determine if the infant is receiving sufficient nutritional support through breast milk
3. Propose an acceptable monitoring protocol
4. Suggest solutions to the various problems that might be identified

Evaluation of growth rate. The breastfed infant should be evaluated regularly to determine if growth is proceeding normally. If the infant fails to thrive, even after techniques to enhance let-down and improve milk supply, and then improves when placed on a formula, breastfeeding should either be abandoned or a regular program of supplementary feeding established. The important point is to monitor growth closely enough that a life threatening emergency and panic-weaning to bottle can be avoided. In some cases of failure to thrive at the breast, the mother should receive additional support to allay feelings of guilt and failure that will inevitably arise. Breastfeeding of a subsequent child is not necessarily contraindicated.

COMMON REASONS FOR FAILURE OF LACTATION
Poor Maternal Attitude

Probably the chief reason for failure of breastfeeding is a poor maternal attitude toward lactation in the first place. The mother who does not sincerely want to breastfeed her infant but agrees to do so to placate her family, friends, or nurse will have a very difficult time. Fear, worry, distraction, anger, and other such emotions have a potent effect on the let-down reflex. When this reflex functions poorly, the infant receives only a portion of the milk supply because the bulk of the milk stored in the alveoli is not released. The infant cries from hunger and eventually fails to gain weight. This provides negative feedback to the mother and a vicious cycle begins.

Inadequate Milk Supply

Failure to establish adequate milk supply by frequent feeding on demand is a great deterrent to successful lactation. Before breastfeeding is abandoned, the clinician should check to see if caloric intake has been adequate to support lactation. Are there anxieties and distractions to nursing that can be eliminated? Is the mother getting enough rest? Is she taking oral contraceptives or other medication that suppresses lactation? The problem may be inhibition of the let-down reflex rather than failure of milk production. Is the hospital routine nonsupportive? Other problems can stem from use of supplements too soon and too frequently, and from early introduction of solid foods.

Lack of Information and Support

Another common reason for failure of lactation is lack of information and support for the mother. Many women do not have the support of friends or relatives who have successfully breastfed infants. These women are often poorly informed about the physiology of lactation and about the virtually fool-proof method of meeting the infant's nutritional needs. New breastfeeding mothers may have fears of the milk supply being too low in quality or quantity to support the infant's growth requirements. They may become discouraged when the infant does not feed well because he has been sedated during labor and delivery. They may be discouraged by nipple discomfort or engorgement, common complaints during the first few days of breastfeeding. Often a new mother feels mildly depressed around the fourth or fifth day postpartum, and any initial lactation problems will be magnified out of proportion. This is particularly true if the mother does not see these occurrences as normal. If the parents have had adequate prenatal instruction and good counseling during the hospital stay, the chances of weathering these storms are greatly increased. If the breastfeeding mother has the support of her partner and understanding professionals who can provide kind words to bolster her confidence even when things are going fine, she will feel she has a place to turn for help and advice when things go badly. Under these circumstances problems that cannot be avoided can be more easily overcome.

Summary

From many standpoints evidence supports the suitability of breast milk for the human infant. The important role of the health professional in counseling breastfeeding mothers is now recognized. Effective functioning as a breastfeeding counselor demands a thorough understanding of the process of lactation and a sincere desire to help inexperienced mothers decide for themselves about the best approaches to infant feeding in their own circumstances.

In-depth knowledge about the problems women experience with lactation needs recognition. Workable management strategies need to be devised. Because support for breastfeeding has been voiced by an array of health care disciplines and lay groups, and because breastfeeding counseling is now of high quality, breastfeeding should remain popular in the future. Continued attention should be given, however, to early childhood exposure to lactation along with effective educational programs for both boys and girls.

1. Diagram the structural components of the female mammary gland and define the process of human milk synthesis and movement through the system.
2. Describe the basic physiology of lactation referring to appropriate anatomic sites, hormonal contributions, and other significant details.
3. Outline the advantages and disadvantages of breastfeeding.
4. Define the significant characteristics of human milk that make it particularly suitable for human infants.
5. Outline a dozen concerns expressed by breastfeeding mothers and describe appropriate approaches to counseling women about these concerns.

References

1. Worthington-Roberts BS, Williams SR: *Nutrition in pregnancy and lactation*, ed 5, St Louis, 1993, Mosby.
2. Shaul DMB: The composition of milk from wild animals, *Int Year Zoo Book* 4:333, 1962.
3. Institute of Medicine, National Academy of Sciences: *Nutrition during lactation*, Washington, DC, 1991, National Academy Press.
4. Hartmann PE et al: Studies on breastfeeding and reproduction in women in Western Australia—a review, *Birth Fam J* 8:215, 1982.
5. Lovelady CA et al: Lactation performance of exercising women, *Am J Clin Nutr* 52:103, 1990.
6. Lawrence RA: *Breastfeeding: a guide for the medical profession*, ed 3, St Louis, 1989, Mosby.
7. Lindblad BS, Rahimtoola RJ: A pilot study of the quality of human milk in a lower socioeconomic group in Karachi, Pakistan, *Acta Paediatr Scand* 63:125, 1974.
8. Chavalittamrong B et al: Protein and amino acids of breast milk from Thai mothers, *Am J Clin Nutr* 34:1126, 1981.
9. Sturman JA: Taurine in development, *J Nutr* 118:1169, 1988.
10. Simopoulos AP: α-3 Fatty acids in growth and development and in health and disease, *Nutr Today* 23:10, 1988.
11. Carroll JE et al: Carnitine deficiency revisited, *J Nutr* 117:1501, 1987.
12. Heitlinger LA et al: Mammary amylase: a possible alternate pathway of carbohydrate digestion in infancy, *Pediatr Res* 17:15, 1983.
13. McMillan JA et al: Iron sufficiency in breast-fed infants and the availability of iron from human milk, *Pediatrics* 58:686, 1976.
14. McMillan JA et al: Iron absorption from human milk, simulated human milk and properietary formulas, *Pediatrics* 60:896, 1977.
15. Garry PJ et al: Iron absorption from human milk and formula with and without iron supplementation, *Pediatr Res* 15:822, 1981.
16. Owen GM et al: Iron nutriture of infants exclusively breastfed the first five months, *J Pediatr* 99:237, 1981.
17. Casey CE et al: Availability of zinc: loading tests with human milk, cow's milk and infant formulas, *Pediatrics* 68:394, 1981.
18. Hollis BW et al: *The effects of oral vitamin D supplementation and ultraviolet phototherapy on the antirachitic sterol content of human milk*, American Society of Bone and Mineral Research Annual Meeting, 1982 (abstract).
19. Greer FR et al: Bone mineral content and serum 25-hydroxyvitamin D concentration in breastfed infants with and without supplemental vitamin D, *J Pediatr* 98:696, 1981.
20. Greer FR et al: Bone mineral content and serum 25-hydroxyvitamin D concentrations in breastfed infants with and without supplemental vitamin D: one year follow-up, *J Pediatr* 100:919, 1982.
21. Ozsoylu S, Hasanoglu A: Vitamin D supplementation in breast-fed infants, *J Pediatr* 100:1000, 1982.

22. Finberg L: Human milk feeding and vitamin D supplementation—1981, *J Pediatr* 99:228, 1981.

23. Bachrach S et al: An outbreak of vitamin D deficiency rickets in a susceptible population, *Pediatrics* 64:871, 1979.

24. Edidin DV et al: Resurgence of nutritional rickets associated with breastfeeding and special dietary practices, *Pediatrics* 65:232, 1980.

25. Byerly LO, Kirksey A: Effects of different levels of vitamin C intake on the vitamin C concentration in human milk and the vitamin C intakes of breast-fed infants, *Am J Clin Nutr* 41:665, 1985.

26. Felice JH, Kirksey A: Effects of vitamin B_6 deficiency during lactation on the vitamin B_6 content of milk, liver, and muscle of rats, *J Nutr* 111:610, 1981.

27. Borschel MW, Kirksey A: Relationship of plasma pyridoxal phosphate levels to vitamin B_6 intakes during the first six months, *Fed Proc* 42:1331, 1983.

28. Sandberg DP et al: The content, binding, and forms of vitamin B_{12} in milk, *Am J Clin Nutr* 34:1717, 1981.

29. Specker BL et al: Vitamin B_{12}: low milk concentrations are related to low serum concentrations in vegetarian women and to methylmalonic aciduria in their infants, *Am J Clin Nutr* 52:1073, 1990.

30. Kuhn T et al: Maternal vegan diet causing a serious infantile neurological disorder due to vitamin B_{12} deficiency, *Eur J Pediatr* 150:205, 1991.

31. Beerens H et al: Influence of breastfeeding on the bifid flora of the newborn intestine, *Am J Clin Nutr* 33:2434, 1980.

32. Reid B et al: Prostaglandins in human milk, *Pediatrics* 66:870, 1980.

33. Miranda R et al: Effect of maternal nutritional status on immunological substances in human colostrum and milk, *Am J Clin Nutr* 37:632, 1983.

34. American Academy of Pediatrics, Committee on Drugs: The transfer of drugs and other chemicals into human milk, *Pediatrics* 84:924, 1989.

35. Jacobson JL: Determinants of polychlorinated biphenyls (PBBs), polybrominated biphenyls (PBBs), and dichlorodiphenyl trichloroethane (DDT) levels in the sera of young children, *Am J Public Health* 79:1401, 1989.

36. Savage EP et al: National study of chlorinated hydrocarbon insecticide residues in human milk, USA, *Am J Epidemiol* 113:413, 1981.

37. Le Guennec JC, Billon B: Delay in caffeine elimination in breast-fed infants, *Pediatrics* 79:264, 1987.

38. Binkiewicz A et al: Pseudo-Cushing syndrome caused by alcohol in breast milk, *J Pediatr* 93:965, 1978.

39. Little RE et al: Maternal alcohol use during breastfeeding and infant mental and motor development at one year, *N Engl J Med* 321:425, 1989.

40. Seitzer V, Benjamin F: Breastfeeding and the potential for human immunodeficiency virus transmission, *Obstet Gynecol* 75:713, 1990.

41. Belec L et al: Antibodies of human immunodeficiency virus in breast milk of healthy, sero-positive women, *Pediatrics* 85:1022, 1990.

42. Davis MK: *The role of human milk in human immunodeficiency virus infection.* In Atkinson SA et al, editors: *Breastfeeding, nutrition, infection and infant growth in developed and emerging countries,* St Johns, Newfoundland, Canada, 1990, ARTS Biomedical Publishing and Distributing.

43. Mehta NR, Subramanian KNS: Human milk banking: current concepts, *Indian J Pediatr* 57:361, 1990.

44. Food and Nutrition Board, National Research Council: *Recommended dietary allowances,* ed 10, Washington, DC, 1989, National Academy Press.

45. English RM, Hitchcock NE: Nutrient intakes during pregnancy, lactation, and after the cessation of lactation in a group of Australian women, *Br J Nutr* 22:615, 1968.

46. Butte NF et al: Maternal energy balance during lactation, *Fed Proc* 42:922, 1983.

47. Manning-Dalton C, Allen LH: The effects of lactation on energy and protein consumption, postpartum weight change and body composition of well nourished North American women, *Nutr Res* 32:293, 1983.

48. Potter S et al: Does infant feeding method influence maternal postpartum weight loss? *J Am Diet Assoc* 91(4):441, 1991.

49. Popkin BM et al: Breast-feeding and diarrheal morbidity, *Pediatrics* 86:874, 1990.

50. Butte NF et al: Human milk intake and growth of exclusively breastfed infants, *J Pediatr* 104:187, 1984.

51. Perkin JE: Maternal influences on the development of food allergy in the infant, *Top Clin Nutr* 5:6, 1990.

52. Zeiger RS et al: Effect of combined maternal and infant food-allergen avoidance on development of atopy in early infancy: a randomized study, *J Allergy Clin Immunol* 84:72, 1989.

53. Gerrard JW: Allergy in breast-fed babies to ingredients in breast milk, *Ann Allergy* 42:69, 1979.

54. Lucas A, Cole TJ: Breast milk and neonatal necrotizing entero-colitis, *Lancet* 336:1519, 1990.

55. Auricchio S et al: Does breastfeeding protect against the development of clinical symptoms of celiac disease in children? *J Pediatr Gastroenterol Nutr* 2:428, 1983.

56. Riccardi G, Rivellese AA: Can diabetes mellitus be prevented by diet? *Diab Nutr Metab* 2:259, 1989.

57. Gielen AC et al: Maternal employment during early postpartum period: effects on initiation and continuance of breast-feeding, *Pediatrics* 87:298, 1991.

58. Kurinu N et al: Does maternal employment affect breast-feeding? *Am J Public Health* 79:1247, 1989.

59. American Academy of Pediatrics, Committee on Nutrition: Nutrition and lactation, *Pediatrics* 68:435, 1981.

60. American Academy of Pediatrics: The promotion of breast-feeding, *Pediatrics* 69:654, 1982.

61. Pittard WB et al: Bacteriostatic qualities of human milk, *J Pediatr* 107:240, 1985.

62. Friend BA et al: The effect of processing and storage on key enzymes, B vitamins, and lipids of mature human milk. I. Evaluation of fresh samples and effects of freezing and frozen storage, *Pediatr Res* 17:61, 1983.

63. Bitman J et al: Lipolysis of triglycerides of human milk during storage at low temperature: a note of caution, *J Pediatr Gastroenterol Nutr* 2:521, 1983.

64. Bjorksten B et al: Collecting and banking human milk: to heat or not to heat? *Br Med J* 281:765, 1980.

65. Goldsmith SJ et al: IgA, IgG, IgM and lactoferrin contents of human milk during early lactation and the effect of processing and storage, *J Food Protection* 46:4, 1983.

66. Goldblum RM et al: Rapid high-temperature treatment of human milk, *J Pediatr* 104:380, 1984.

67. Paxson CL and Cress CC: Survival of human milk leukocytes, *J Pediatr* 94:61, 1979.

68. Goldblum RM et al: Human milk banking. I. Effects of container upon immunologic factors in mature milk, *Nutr Res* 1:449, 1981.

69. Carey WB: *Am J Dis Child* 135:973, 1981.

70. Frantz KB, Fleiss PM: *Ineffective suckling as a frequent cause of failure to thrive in the totally breast-fed infant.* In Freier S, Eidelman AI, editors: *Human milk: its biological and social value,* Amsterdam, 1980, Excerpta Medica.

Further Reading

Lawrence RA: Breast-feeding: a guide for the medical profession, ed 4, St Louis, 1994, Mosby. This manual provides a thorough review of the process of lactation, the composition of human milk, and counseling recommendations for breast-feeding women. The manual is especially aimed at physicians and other health care professionals.

Neville, MC, Neifert MR, editors: *Lactation: physiology, nutrition, and breast-feeding,* New York, 1983, Plenum Press.

This book provides a complete review of research related to lactation, human milk, and the breast-feeding experience.

Report of the Task Force on the Assessment of the Scientific Evidence Relating to Infant-feeding Practice and Infant Health: *Pediatrics* 4(suppl), October, 1984.
This task force report gives a comprehensive overview of infant feeding practices around the world and their relationship to infant health.

US Department of Health and Human Services: *Report of the Surgeon General's workshop on breast-feeding and human lactation,* Washington, DC, 1984, US Government Printing Office.
This report provides a summary of the recommendations of the expert committee that developed the policy of the US Surgeon General's office about breastfeeding.

US Department of Health and Human Services: *Follow-up report of the Surgeon General's workshop on breast-feeding and human lactation,* Washington, DC, 1986, US Government Printing Office.
This follow-up report defines the impact of the Surgeon General's recommendations (1984) regarding breast-feeding.

Additional New Readings

Auerbach KG: Assisting the employed breast-feeding mother, *J Nurs Midwifery* 35:26-34, 1990.

Dewey KG et al: Breast-fed infants are leaner than formula-fed infants at 1 year of age: The Darling Study, *Am J Clin Nutr* 57:140, 1993.

Ellis LA and Picciano MF: Milk-borne hormones: regulators of development in neonates, *Nutrition Today* p. 6, Sept./Oct. 1992.

Frank JW, Newman J: Breastfeeding in a polluted world: uncertain risks, clear benefits, *Can Med Assoc J* 149:33, 1993.

Gielen AC et al: Maternal employment during the early postpartum period: effects on initiation and continuation of breast-feeding, *Pediatrics* 87:298-304, 1991.

Goldberg GR et al: Longitudinal assessment of the components of energy balance in well-nourished lactating women, *Am J Clin Nutr* 54:788, 1991.

Institute of Medicine: *Nutrition services in perinatal care,* 2e, National Academy of Sciences, Washington DC, 1992.

Institute of Medicine: *Nutrition during pregnancy and lactation: an implementation guide,* National Academy Press, Washington DC, 1992.

Kang-Yoon SA et al: Vitamin B_6 status of breast-fed neonates: influence of pyridoxine supplementation of mothers and neonates, *Am J Clin Nutr* 56:548, 1992.

Michaelsen KF et al: The Copenhagen Study on infant nutrition and growth: breast milk intake, human milk macronutrient content and influencing factors, *Am J Clin Nutr* 59:600, 1994.

Frank JW, Newman J: Breastfeeding in a polluted world: uncertain risks, clear benefits, *Can Med Assoc J* 149:33, 1993.

Gielen AC et al: Maternal employment during the early postpartum period: effects on initiation and continuation of breast-feeding, *Pediatrics* 87:298-304, 1991.

Goldberg GR et al: Longitudinal assessment of the components of energy balance in well-nourished lactating women, *Am J Clin Nutr* 54:788, 1991.

Institute of Medicine: *Nutrition services in perinatal care,* 2e, National Academy of Sciences, Washington DC, 1992.

Institute of Medicine: *Nutrition during pregnancy and lactation: an implementation guide,* National Academy Press, Washington DC, 1992.

Kang-Yoon SA et al: Vitamin B_6 status of breast-fed neonates: influence of pyridoxine supplementation of mothers and neonates, *Am J Clin Nutr* 56:548, 1992.

Michaelsen KF et al: The Copenhagen Study on infant nutrition and growth: breast milk intake, human milk macronutrient content and influencing factors, *Am J Clin Nutr* 59:600, 1994.

Potter S et al: Does infant feeding method influence maternal postpartum weight loss?, *J Am Diet Assoc* 91:441, 1991.

Sowers MF et al: Changes in bone density with lactation, *JAMA* 269:3130, 1993.

Spake J, Harris MB: Reasons for continuing and ceasing breastfeeding in low income Hispanics and whites, *J Nutr Educ* p. 37, Jan/Feb 1993.

Specker BL et al: Calcium kinetics in lactating women with low and high calcium intakes, *Am J Clin Nutr* 59:593, 1994.

6

Nutrition During Infancy

Peggy Pipes

Basic Concepts

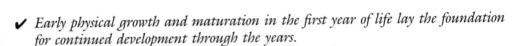

✔ *Early physical growth and maturation in the first year of life lay the foundation for continued development through the years.*

✔ *Individual energy and nutrient needs reflect rapid growth demands for fuel, building materials, and basal metabolism.*

✔ *An appropriate milk source, breast milk or alternate formulas, with gradual solid food additions, supply both nutritional and developmental needs.*

✔ *Maturing oral structures and function determine developing infant eating skills and appropriate textures of food.*

✔ *Infant feeding behavior follows a defined developmental sequence.*

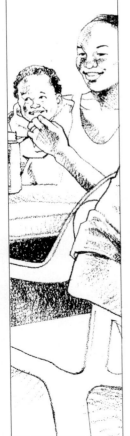

*T*he first year after birth is one of dramatic change for normal human infants. The torso grows longer and subcutaneous fat accumulates. Infants progress from being newborns with no head control to being babies who pull themselves up to a standing position and begin to take steps. They change from securing their nourishment with a reflexive suck to picking up finger foods with a precise pincer grasp. They develop voluntary and independent movements of the tongue, lip, and jaw and begin rotary chewing. At 1 year they are beginning self-feeding and can drink from a cup if help is provided.

This chapter stresses the importance of an adequate energy and nutrient intake consumed in a loving and supportive environment. Milk and other foods supply the materials necessary for rapid linear growth and weight gain. Foods also support developmental progress. Adding appropriate textures and varieties of food when infants are developmentally ready provides the stimulus for learning new skills, while feeding infants in a loving and nurturing environment helps them develop a sense of security and trust.

Human milk, or alternate formula if needed, is the baby's source of nutrients and energy for the first 4 to 6 months. The addition of semisolid foods progressing to "table foods" in the latter part of the first year provide important growth nutrients and support oral and fine motor development. Normal full-term infants fed on demand regulate their intake to in the latter part of the first year provide important growth nutrients and support oral and fine motor development. Normal full-term infants fed on demand regulate their intake to consume precisely the amount they need to grow appropriately and soon establish their own schedule.

Parents have a number of options in the selections of food to offer infants in developed countries. In developing areas of the world there are fewer reasonable approaches to infant feeding. Sanitation, economics, and maldistribution of food mandate breastfeeding as the only safe and economically feasible approach. Malnutrition in infancy in a number of developing countries results from ignorance, poverty, and corporate greed. The discussions in this chapter are directed at the feeding of infants in developed areas of the world.

GROWTH AND MATURATION

From birth to 1 year of age, normal human infants triple their weight and increase their length by 50%. They progress from sucking a nipple reflexively to obtain food to beginning voluntary self-feeding in a sitting position. They change from a diet composed solely of milk to one that includes many finger and table foods, as well as beverages, that they will consume as adults. They bond with their parents and acquire a sense of trust, and each infant develops an ego identity as a unique person. Growth and maturation can be compromised or accelerated by undernutrition or overnutrition. Also, the stage of maturation determines the developmental readiness to progress in the acceptance of foods, texture, and self-feeding, for example, readiness to receive spoon foods and to self-feed with finger-foods. Throughout this important first year of life, infant feeding and nutrition influence both physical and psychosocial growth and development.

Physical Growth

In the 24 hours after birth infants' adaptation to the out-of-placenta environment is critical. They begin to breathe, to receive oxygen for themselves and remove carbon dioxide from their tissues. They assume responsibility for their own circulation, temperature regulation, and metabolic support. Digestion and absorption begin when they consume food.

Weight. Birth weight is determined by the mother's prepregnancy weight and her weight gain during pregnancy. After parturition, genetics, environment, and nutrition determine rates of gains in weight and height. Immediately after birth there is a weight loss due to a loss of fluid and some catabolism of tissue. This loss averages 6% of body weight but occasionally exceeds 10%. Birth weight is usually regained by the tenth day. Thereafter, weight gain during infancy proceeds at a rapid but decelerating rate. Average weight gains for the first 4 months are 20 to 25 g per day, and during the next 8 months are 15 g per day. By 4 months of age, most infants weigh twice their birth weights, and by 12 months they usually weigh three times what they weighed at birth. Males increase in weight to twice their birth weights earlier than do females, and smaller newborns increase in weight to twice their birth weight sooner than do heavier neonates.

Length. Infants usually increase their lengths by 50% the first year, the average length being 25 to 30 cm (10 to 12 inches). But a period of "catch-up" or "lag-down" growth

Growth velocity
(L *velocitas,* speed) Rapidity of motion or movement; rate of childhood growth over normal periods of development, as compared with a population standard.

Growth acceleration
Period of increased speed of growth at different points of childhood development.

Growth deceleration
Period of decreased speed of growth at different points of childhood development.

Extracellular water
Alternate term for collective body water or fluids outside of cells.

Intracellular water
Collective body water or fluids inside of cells; in body composition measures a large proportion assigned to total lean body mass, a vital component in cell metabolism.

Adipose tissue
(L *adipis,* fat, lard) Loose connective tissue in which fat cells (adipocytes) accumulate and are stored.

Lean body mass
Collective fat-free mass of body composition; most metabolically active portion of body tissues.

may occur. The majority of infants who are born small but are genetically determined to be longer shift **percentiles** on **growth grids** during the first 3 to 6 months. However, larger infants at birth whose genotypes are for smaller size tend to grow at their fetal rates for several months before the lag-down in growth becomes evident. During this lagdown period their length drops from a higher to a lower percentile rating on the growth chart. Often a new percentile rating is not apparent until the child is 13 months of age.[1] Figs. 6-1 and 6-2 depict catch-up and lag-down growth in the first year. Racial differences have been noted in rates of growth. American black males and females are smaller than Caucasians at birth, but they grow more rapidly during the first 2 years.

Growth Charts

It is important that one concerned with infants' nutrient and energy intake be aware of how their growth is progressing. Height and weight data plotted on growth charts show how growth is proceeding. Measurements must be taken accurately, then weight and height values recorded on growth charts so that **growth velocity** as well as **acceleration** or **deceleration** can be monitored.

The most commonly used growth grids in North America are those prepared by an expert committee of the National Center for Health Statistics (NCHS).[2] Data collected by the Fels Research Institute from large numbers of a nationally representative sample of children were used to determine standards for children from birth to 36 months of age. The grids are prepared so that age values lie along the **axis** and height or weight values are plotted along the abscissa. Measurements at one age rank the baby's height or weight in relation to 100 other infants of the same age. Weight-height percentiles rank the baby's weight in relation to 100 other babies of the same length. Then sequential measurements plotted on the growth grid indicate if the baby is maintaining, reducing, or increasing the percentile rating as growth proceeds.

Changes in Body Composition

Changes during growth occur not only in height and weight but also in the components of the tissue. Increases in height and weight and skeletal maturation are accompanied by changes in body composition—water, lean body mass, and fat.

Body water. Total body water as a percentage of body weight decreases throughout infancy from approximately 70% at birth to 60% at 1 year of age. Reduction of body water is almost entirely extracellular. **Extracellular water** decreases from about 42% of body weight at birth to 32% at 1 year of age. At the same time **intracellular water** increases with the rapid growth of tissue. This change results from decreases in the water content of **adipose tissue** as well as increases in adipose tissue, but largely from relative increases in lean body mass with its higher water content.

Lean body mass. The fat-free mass of the body matures, the percentage of protein increasing as the percentage of total body water decreases. Fomon estimates that the protein content of the fat-free **lean body mass** gained increases from 12.5% at 1 month to 17% at 1 year in males and to 16.7% at 1 year in females.[3]

Body fat. The fat content of the body develops slowly during fetal life. Fat accounts for 0.5% of body weight at the fifth month of fetal growth and 16% at term. After birth, fat accumulates rapidly until approximately 9 months of age. Between 2 and 6 months of age the increase in adipose tissue is more than twice as great as the increase in the volume of muscle. Sex-related differences appear in infancy, the female depositing a greater percentage of weight as fat than the male.

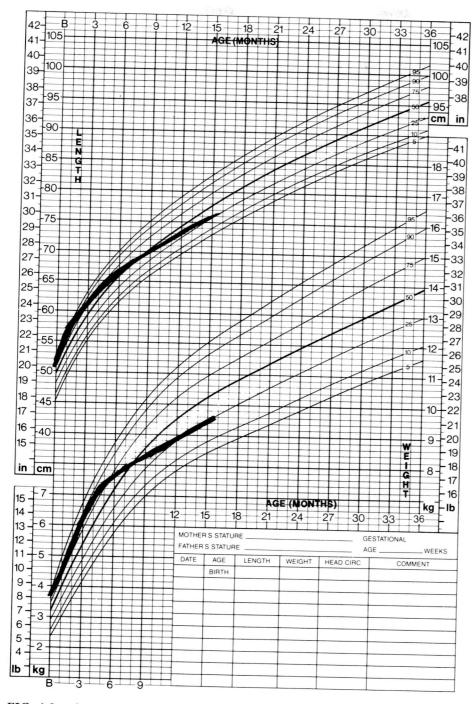

FIG. 6-1 Growth grid of a large infant who "lagged down" to her genetic potential. (Courtesy Ross Laboratories.)

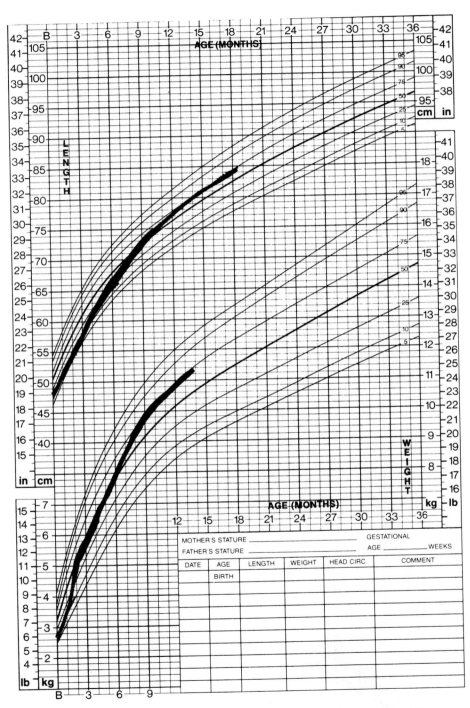

FIG. 6-2 Growth grid of a small infant who "caught up" to his genetic potential. (Courtesy Ross Laboratories.)

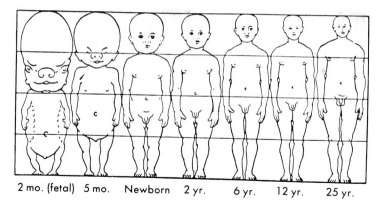

FIG. 6-3 Changes in body proportions from second fetal month to adulthood.
From Robbins WJ et al: *Growth,* New Haven, Conn, 1928, Yale University Press.

Changes in Body Proportions

Increases in height and weight are accompanied by dramatic changes in body proportions. The head proportion decreases as the torso and leg proportion increases (Fig. 6-3). At birth, the head accounts for approximately one fourth of the total body weight. When growth has ceased, the head accounts for one eighth of the total body length. Between birth and adulthood, leg length increases from approximately three eighths of the newborn's birth length to one half of the adult's total body height.

Psychosocial Development

Feeding is the fundamental interaction from which the relationship between parents and infants evolves and the infant's psychosocial development proceeds. A parent's responsiveness to the infant's cues of hunger and satiation, and the close physical contact during a feeding facilitate a healthy psychosocial development. During the first year feeding when hungry teaches the baby a sense of trust and well-being, that his needs will be met. For optimal development in early infancy babies need to be fed as soon as they express hunger. As they grow older and learn to trust that their needs will be met they can wait longer for the initiation of the meal. **Tactile** stimulation is important. Babies need to be held and cuddled while they are fed. Some individuals feel this skin-to-skin contact facilitates bonding. Propping the bottle needs to be discouraged. In the early months attachments are indiscriminate; after six months attachments are formed to the parenting figure.

Identification of the infant's cues of hunger and satiation are basic to developing a sense of trust and to learning to regulate appetite. Cues change rapidly as development proceeds during the early years. The observant parent will recognize the changes and respond appropriately as the baby grows and develops. Table 6-1 lists some of the cues of hunger and satiation in the first year.

Parents' ability to interpret cues and negotiate the feeding experience with their babies fosters healthy parent-child interactions.

Tactile
(L *tactio,* to touch)
Sense of touching, perception by the touch.

Digestion and Absorption

The digestive capacity of the infant matures and increases during the first year of life. The developing stomach and intestine provide an increasing ability to handle various nutrients and textures provided by the food. The full-term newborn is, however, prepared

TABLE 6-1   *Hunger and Satiety Behaviors of Infants*

Age	Hunger	Satiety
Early infancy	Fusses and cries Mouths the nipple	Draws away from nipple Falls asleep
16-24 weeks	Actively approaches breast or bottle Leans forward to spoon	Releases nipple and withdraws head Fusses or cries Bites nipple Increases attention to surroundings
28-36 weeks	Vocalizes eagerness for bottle or food	Changes position Shakes head Keeps mouth tightly closed Hands become more active
40-52 weeks	Points or touches spoon or feeder's hand	Behaviors as above Sputters with tongue and lips Hands bottle or cup to feeder

Gastric pH

(Gr *gaster*, stomach; *pH*, power of the hydrogen ion — H⁺) Chemical symbol relating to H⁺ concentration or activity in a solution; expressed numerically as the negative logarithm of H⁺ concentration: pH 7.0 is neutral — above it alkalinity increases, and below it acidity increases. The hydrochloric acid (HCl) gastric secretions make gastric pH about 2.0.

Trypsin

(Gr *tryein*, to rub; *pepsis*, digestion) Protein-splitting enzyme formed in the intestine by action of enterokinase on inactive precursor trypsinogen.

Chymotrypsin

(Gr *chymos*, chyme, creamy gruel-like material produced by gastric digestion of food) One of the protein-splitting and milk-curdling pancreatic enzymes, activated in the intestine from precursor chymotrypsinogen; breaks peptide linkages of the amino acids phenylalanine and tyrosine.

to digest and absorb an adequate supply of nutrients for normal growth and development. Table 6-2 indicates the percentage of adult-level factors needed for digestion that are present at birth.

Stomach actions. The stomach capacity at birth, 10 to 12 ml, increases to 200 ml by 12 months. The **gastric pH** is slightly alkaline at birth but within 24 hours acid secretion reaches a peak comparable to that of a 3-year-old child. It then declines to a low level, remaining lower than that of the adult for the first few months.[4] The stomach at birth empties in about 2 ½ to 3 hours. Newborns require small, frequent feeds. As the infant matures the emptying rate depends on the amount and composition of food consumed. Fat is the last of the macronutrients to leave the stomach, contributing to the satiety of the feed.

Intestinal actions. The intestines of newborns are larger in relation to body size than the adult and therefore have a larger surface area for absorption. **Reverse peristalsis** is common.

Enzymatic secretions provide the capacity for infants to digest and absorb the milk and food consumed.

Proteins. The newborn's concentrations of **trypsin** are near adult levels. Concentrations of **chymotrypsin** and **carboxypeptidase** in the duodenum are only 10% to 60% of the adult levels. Babies can digest adequate protein even though the quantity is limited. Newborns can completely digest about 1.95 g/kg/day of protein, 4-month-old babies about 3.75 g/kg/day.[4] In other words, a 3.5 kg newborn would be expected to digest 6.75 g of protein. An intake of 12.5 oz (369.6 ml) of human milk will meet the suggested energy intake and provide approximately 4.0 g protein. A formula-fed infant who consumes the same quantity will receive 5.54 g protein; either protein intake is adequately digested by the infant.

Fats. Pancreatic **lipase** activity is low in the newborn, especially in the premature infant. The bile acid pool, although present, is reduced. When compared to the adult on the basis of body surface area, the newborn, although able to synthesize **bile,** has a bile acid pool one half that of the adult. Lingual and gastric lipase and milk lipases also contribute to the

TABLE 6-2   *Factors Necessary for Digestion Present at Birth*

Factors	% of Adult
H$^+$	< 30
Pepsin	< 10
Chymotrypsinogen	10 to 60
Procarboxypeptidase	10 to 60
Enterokinase	10
Peptidases	> 100
Fat	
Lingual lipase	> 100
Pancreatic lipase	5 to 10
Pancreatic colipase	?
Bile acids	50
Carbohydrate	
Alpha amylases	
Pancreatic	0
Salivary	10
Lactase	> 100
Sucrase-insomaltase	100
Glucoamylase	< 100 (?)

From Lebenthal E: Impact of development of the gastrointestinal tract on infant feeding, *J Pediatr* 102:1, 1983.

infant's ability to digest **lipids.** The fatty acid composition of the dietary fat influences how much of it will be digested and absorbed by the infant. **Triclycerides** with saturated fatty acids are not as well utilized as those with unsaturated fatty acids. Also, the position of a fatty acid on the fat's glycerol base affects absorption. Stearic acid is poorly absorbed in any position. Free palmitic acid **hydrolized** from positions 1 and 3 is poorly absorbed, whereas palmitic acid on position 2 of the glycerol base remains with the glycerol as a monoglyceride that appears to be well absorbed. Fatty acids in human milk are better absorbed than those in cow's milk. Newborns absorb approximately 85% to 90% of the fat provided by human milk. Many infants absorb less than 70% of cow's milk fat.[3] Plant oils are more efficiently absorbed than animal fats. Mixtures of vegetable oils in commercially prepared infant formulas are well absorbed.

Carbohydrates. Sugars are well utilized. **Maltase, isomaltase,** and **sucrase** activity reach adult levels by 28 to 32 weeks gestation. Lactase, present in low levels at 28 weeks gestation, increases near term and reaches adult levels at birth. Pancreatic **amylases** are low or absent up to 4 months of age. Salivary amylase, present at birth, rises to adult concentrations between 6 months and 1 year of age. Even though a large percentage of the salivary amylase is suspected of being inactivated by hydrochloric acid in the stomach, young infants do digest some starch. This is thought to be due to the presence of glycosidase and glucoamylase present in the **brush border** of the small intestines. These enzymes hydrolyze starch to glucose.

Renal Function

The newborn has an immature kidney. The functional development of the **nephron** is not complete until 1 month of age. The tubules are short and narrow and do not reach mature proportions until approximately 5 months. In addition, the pituitary gland

Carboxypeptidase
(L *carbo,* coal, carbon, fundamental element in all organic compounds) The chemical group *carboxyl*—COOH—at the end of the carbon chain identifies the compound as an organic acid. The end of the word, *peptidase,* indicates a protein-splitting enzyme, which together with the first part means that this is an enzyme that acts on the peptide bond of the terminal amino acid having a free-end carboxyl group.

produces only limited quantities of the antidiuretic hormone (ADH) vasopressin, which normally inhibits diuresis. These factors limit the newborn's ability to concentrate urine and to cope with fluid and **electrolyte** stress, i.e., electrolyte-dense formula, limited fluid intake, and diarrhea. By 1 month of age, the normal infant can maintain water balance as efficiently as the adult.

Renal solute load. The major percentage of **solutes** presented to the kidney for excretion are the nitrogenous end products of protein metabolism, sodium, potassium, phosphorus, and chloride. If none of these elements were utilized in new body mass or lost by nonrenal routes, such as perspiration, they would need to be excreted in the urine. They are therefore referred to as the potential **renal solute load.** The potential renal solute load can be calculated by assuming all nitrogen is excreted, dividing dietary nitrogen by 28 and adding sodium, potassium, chloride, and phosphorus in the feed expressed as **milliosmoles,** abbreviated **mOsm.**[5]

These solutes must be concentrated in water derived from that preformed in the diet and formed from the oxidation of protein and carbohydrates. Each milk for normal infants yields approximately 95 ml of water per 100 ml consumed. Some is utilized in new tissue, and some is lost in the feces or by evaporation. The solutes are dissolved in the remainder.

The concentrating capacity of some neonates has been reported to be as limited as 700 mOsm/L; of others as great as that of older children and adults, 1200 to 1400 mOsm/L. Human milk has a potential renal solute load of 93 mOsm/L, commercially available cow milk-based formula of 133 mOsm/L, and soy formula of 177 mOsm/L.[5]

Difficulties with the renal solute load are unlikely in normal infants fed human milk or a correctly prepared formula. Problems may occur when elevated environmental temperature or fever increase evaporative loss, when diarrhea occurs, and/or when infants reduce the volume of fluids they consume.

NUTRIENT NEEDS OF INFANTS

Individual differences of infants in nutrient reserves, body composition, growth rates, and activity patterns make defining actual nutrient requirements impossible. Estimates have been made from intakes of infants growing normally and from the nutrient content of human milk. Nitrogen balance studies have been conducted to establish amino acid requirements. Fat and calcium absorption have been examined. The Recommended Dietary Allowances (RDAs) are planned to provide a margin of safety to allow for maximum protection. Because of the declining growth rates during the latter part of the first year, recommended intakes have been set for two 6-month periods, from birth to 6 months and from 6 months to 1 year.[6]

Energy

The energy requirement in infancy is determined primarily by body size, physical activity, and rates of growth. Since large variations in these variables are seen among infants at any age and in any one infant from month to month, ranges of energy needs are large. Total energy needs (kcal/day) rise during the first year, but energy needs per unit of body size decline in response to changes in rates of growth. The recommended **energy intake** (Table 6-3) falls from 108 kcal/kg in the first 6 months to 98 kcal/kg for 6 months to 1 year.[6] These figures were derived from estimates made by the World Health Organization (WHO) based on studies of intakes of healthy thriving infants in developed countries. They are about 15% higher than estimated energy expenditures, which indicate a requirement of 95 kcal/kg/day during the first 6 months and 84 kcal/kg/day in the last half of the first year.

Renal solute load
Collective number and concentration of solute particles in solution, carried by the blood to the kidney nephrons for excretion in the urine, usually nitrogenous products from protein metabolism, and the electrolytes Na$^+$, K$^+$, Cl$^-$, and HPO$_4$.

Milliosmoles (mOsm/L)
Osmole (Gr *osme,* small), standard unit of osmotic pressure; equal to the gram molecular weight of solute divided by the number of particles (ions) into which a substance dissociates in solution. Thus milliosmole would be a much smaller unit of measure of osmotic pressure — $1/1000$ of an osmole, equal to $1/1000$ gram molecular weight of a substance divided by the number of ions into which a substance dissociates in 1 liter (L) of solution. The term *osmolality* refers to this concentration of solutes per unit of solvent.

Energy intake
Energy value of carbohydrate, fat, and protein in food, measured in kilocalories.

TABLE 6-3 *Recommended Energy Intake for Infants*

Age	Energy (kcal)
≤6 months	kg × 108
6 months–1 year	kg × 98

From National Academy of Sciences: *Recommended dietary allowances,* ed 10, Washington, DC, 1989, National Academy Press.

It has been estimated that approximately 50% of the energy expenditure is due to the basal metabolic rate. Energy expended for growth declines from approximately 32.8% of intake during the first 4 months to 7.4% of intake from 4 to 12 months.[3] The contribution of physical activity to total energy expenditure is quite variable but can be expected to increase with age as motor skills develop. Some infants are quiet and cuddly while others spend a considerable amount of time crying, kicking, or just exploring with motor skills they have acquired. The most appropriate way to judge the adequacy of babies' energy intake is to monitor the adequacy of their linear growth and weight gain.

Protein and Amino Acids

Protein needs. Infants require protein for synthesis of new body tissue during growth, increases in the protein content of the body, as well as synthesis of enzymes, hormones, and other physiologically important compounds. Increases in body protein are estimated to average about 3.5 g/day for the first 4 months, and 3.1 g/day for the next 8 months.[3] The body content of protein increases from about 11.0% to 15.0% over the first year. The recommended intake is 2.2 g/kg for the first 6 months and 1.6 g/kg from 6 to 12 months. Fomon and associates have suggested that during infancy, amino acid and protein requirements expressed per unit of kilocalories consumed, reflecting both size and rate of growth, would be more meaningful than expressions of requirements on the basis of body weight alone.[3] They estimate the protein requirement to be 1.6 g/100 kcal for children 1 to 4 months of age, and 1.4 g/100 kcal for children 8 to 12 months of age. Protein intake of breastfed infants growing and gaining normally ranges from 2.43 g/kg/day in the first month to 1.51 g/kg/day in the fourth month.[7] The American Academy of Pediatrics has set minimum protein standards for infant formula of 1.8 g/100 kcal with a protein efficiency ratio equal to that of casein.[8]

Amino acid needs. Nine amino acids are dietary essentials in infancy. Amino acid requirements have been estimated by Holt and Snyderman from studies in which pure amino acids were supplied in proportions of amino acids in human milk.[9] The requirement of an amino acid was defined as the least amount required to maintain satisfactory nitrogen retention and weight gain when nitrogen levels and other amino acids were held constant. Fomon and Filer have estimated amino acid requirements from intakes of infants between the ages of 8 and 112 days who were fed whole protein in cow's milk formulas and soy formulas.[10] Satisfactory linear growth and weight gain, nitrogen balance, and serum concentrations of albumin equivalent to those of normal breastfed infants were used as criteria of adequacy.

Requirement standards. The FAO/WHO expert committee has suggested that a composite of the lower estimates of the data from the studies of Holt and Snyderman and from Fomon and Filer would provide estimates of the upper range of **essential amino acid** requirements of infants age 0 to 6 months.[9-11] The National Research Council has accepted these estimates as shown in Table 6-4.

TABLE 6-4   Estimated Amino Acid Requirements of Infants 3-4 Months of Age

Amino Acid	mg/kg/dy
Histidine	28
Isoleucine	70
Leucine	161
Lysine	103
Methionine plus cystine	58
Phenylalanine plus tyrosine	125
Threonine	87
Tryptophan	17
Valine	93

From Energy and Protein Requirements, Report of a Joint FAO/WHO Ad Hoc Committee, World Health Organization technical report series No 522, *FAO Nutr Meet Rep No 52,* Geneva, 1973, World Health Organization.

Under certain conditions, other amino acids become essential. For example, the infant who has phenylketonuria cannot metabolize phenylalanine to tyrosine and tyrosine becomes essential. Premature infants require an external source of tyrosine and cystine.

Fat and Essential Fatty Acid

Fat needs. Fat, the most calorically concentrated energy nutrient, supplies between 40% and 50% of the energy consumed in infancy. The energy provided by fat spares protein for tissue synthesis. Its caloric concentration is an asset during periods of rapid growth when energy demands are great. Fat provides 45% to 50% of the energy content of commercial formula and 55% of the energy content of human milk. Commercial infant semisolid foods other than egg yolks are relatively low in fat.

Essential fatty acid. Although polyunsaturated linoleic and linolenic acids are both classified as essential, the importance of linolenic acid is not firmly established.

One of the earliest manifestations of fatty acid deficiency recognized in animals was an increased basal metabolic rate. Infants deficient in **linoleic acid** have an eczema-like dermatitis. Also, infants who are fed formulas low in this essential fatty acid consume greater numbers of kilocalories than do those who receive adequate amounts of linoleic acid to maintain normal growth. Caloric utilization has been reported to vary with intakes of linoleic acid up to 4% and 5% of the total kilocalories.

The requirement for linoleic acid is estimated to be 0.6% of energy intake; the recommended intake is 1.2%. A requirement of only a few milligrams/day and a suggested intake of 0.5 gm/day of linolenic acid has been made.

Approximately 5% of the total kilocalories in human milk and 1% of the kilocalories in cow's milk are provided by linoleic acid. Commercially available infant formulas contain blends of vegetable oils and contribute greater amounts of linoleic acid.

Water

Infants require more water per unit of body size than do adults. A larger percentage of water is located in the extracellular and **vascular spaces.** As noted before, young infants have an immature kidney. These two factors make the infant vulnerable to water imbalance. The water requirement is determined by water loss, water required for growth, and solutes derived from the diet.

Linoleic acid
The ultimate essential amino acid for humans.

18:2 fatty acid
Naming system for fatty acids according to structure: carbon chain length and number of double (unsaturated) bonds. Thus, an 18:2 fatty acid would have a long chain of 18 carbon atoms with two double bonds. This is the chemical shorthand for linoleic acid.

Vascular spaces
Spaces within fluid vessels in the body, blood vessels and lymph vessels; contain body fluids in transit, greater amount in blood and remainder in the interconnecting lymphatic system.

TABLE 6-5 *Range of Average Water Requirements of Infants and Children Under Ordinary Circumstances*

Age	Amount of Water (ml/kg/day)
3 days	80-100
10 days	125-150
3 mo	140-160
6 mo	130-155
9 mo	125-145
1 yr	120-135
2 yr	115-125

Modified from Behrman RE, Kliegman RM, editors: *Nelson textbook of pediatrics,* ed 14, Philadelphia, 1992, WB Saunders.

Water is lost by evaporation through the skin and respiratory tract (**insensible water loss**), through perspiration when the environmental temperature is elevated, and by elimination in urine and feces. During growth additional water is necessary since water is needed as a constituent of tissue and for increases in the volume of body fluids. The amount of water required for growth, however, is very small. The body requirement for water is the sum of the above demands.

Water lost by evaporation in infancy and early childhood accounts for more than 60% of that needed to maintain homeostasis, as compared to 40% to 50% in the adult. At all ages approximately 24% of the basal heat loss is by evaporation of water through the skin and respiratory tract. This amounts to 45 ml of insensible water loss per 100 kcal expended. Fomon estimates evaporative water loss at 1 month of age to average 210 ml/day and at age 1 year, 500 ml/day.[3] Evaporative losses increase with fever and increased environmental temperature. Increases in humidity decrease respiratory loss. Loss of water in the feces averages 10 ml/kg/day in infancy.

The range of water requirements is shown in Table 6-5. The National Research Council recommends an intake of 1.5 ml/kcal of energy expenditure for infants.[6] Water intoxication resulting in **hyponatremia,** irritability, and coma can result if infants are fed too much water. Reported cases include infants fed 8 oz of water after each feeding or fed water instead of formula because of financial inability of parents to buy formula.[12] Under normal conditions, infants fed breast milk or infant formulas do not need additional water.

Minerals and Vitamins

Demands for minerals and vitamins are influenced by growth rates, mineralization of bone, increases in bone length and blood volume, and by energy, protein, and fat intakes. RDAs have been established for three major and four trace minerals and for 11 vitamins, as shown in Table 6-6. Ranges of safe intakes have been suggested for five trace minerals and two vitamins. Although all of these nutrients are essential, the discussion here focuses on those that are most commonly of concern during infancy.

Calcium. The recommended intake of calcium is planned to meet the needs of formula-fed infants who retain less than half of the calcium they consume. Breastfed infants retain two thirds of their calcium intake. The allowances are easily met by infants consuming commercially available formulas. The allowances are not applicable to breastfed

Insensible water loss
Daily water loss through the skin and respiration, so-named because a person is not aware of it. An additional smaller amount is lost in normal perspiration, the amount varying with the surrounding temperature.

Hyponatremia
Abnormally low levels of sodium (Na^+) in the blood; can be easily caused by excess water intake to point of water intoxication, with resulting dilution of the major electrolyte (Na^+) in extracellular circulating fluids.

TABLE 6-6 *Recommended Dietary Allowances for Minerals and Vitamins for Infants*

Age (yrs)	Calcium (mg)	Phosphorus (mg)	Iodine (μg)	Iron (mg)	Magnesium (mg)	Zinc (mg)	Selenium (μg)
0.0-0.5	400	300	40	6	40	5	10
0.5-1.0	600	500	50	10	60	5	15

	Fat-Soluble Vitamins			
	Vitamin A (μg RE)	Vitamin D (μg)	Vitamin E (mg α-TE)	Vitamin K (μg)
0.0-0.5	375	7.5	3	5
0.5-1.0	375	10	4	10

	Water-Soluble Vitamins						
	Thiamin (mg)	Riboflavin (mg)	Niacin (mg NE)	Vitamin B_6 (mg)	Folate (μg)	Vitamin B_{12} (μg)	Vitamin C (mg)
0.0-0.5	0.3	0.4	5	0.3	25	0.3	30
0.5-1.0	0.4	0.5	6	0.6	35	0.5	35

RE, retinol equivalent; α-TE, α-tocopherol equivalent; NE, niacin equivalent.
Reprinted with permission from *Recommended dietary allowances,* ed 10. © 1989 by the National Academy of Sciences. Published by National Academy Press, Washington, DC.

Erythropoiesis
Synthesis of new red blood cells.

Ferrous sulfate
Iron fortification compound in infant formulas used as needed to prevent anemia.

Iron absorption
Degree of iron absorption, relatively small at best, depends upon its acid reduction, either by accompanying food such as orange juice or by the gastric HCl secretions, from the ferric form (Fe^{+++}) in foods to the ferrous form (Fe^{++}) required for absorption. After absorption it is oxidized back to the ferric form required for incorporation in body metabolism.

infants. The calcium-phosphorus ratio, previously thought to be a factor in calcium absorption, is no longer a concern.

Iron. Infant iron needs are supplied from two different sources, prenatal reserves and food sources.

Prenatal reserves. Before birth, the fetus accumulates iron in proportion to body size. Premature and low-birth-weight infants have limited reserves that are quickly depleted. Even with the advantage of full-term iron stores, the rapidly growing infant is at risk for iron deficiency because of the increase in blood volume as the baby grows larger. The concentration of hemoglobin at birth averages 17 to 19 g/100 ml of blood. During the first 6 to 8 weeks of life it decreases to approximately 10 to 11 g/100 ml because of a shortened life span of the fetal cell and decreased **erythropoiesis.** After this age there is a gradual increase in hemoglobin concentration to 13 g/100 ml at 2 years of age.

Food sources. Forty-nine percent of the iron in human milk, 10% of the iron in cow's milk, and 4% of the iron in iron-fortified formulas is absorbed.[13] Commercially available formulas are prepared both with and without the inclusion of **ferrous sulfate.** Iron-fortified commercial infant cereals are fortified with electrolytically reduced iron. Absorption of this iron averages 5%. Many have recommended mixing this cereal with a fruit juice containing vitamin C to enhance the **iron absorption.** Normal full-term breastfed infants can maintain satisfactory hemoglobin levels without supplemental iron in early infancy.

However, if they continue to be fed only breast milk after 4 to 6 months they are at risk of negative iron balance and may deplete reserves by 6 to 9 months.[14]

After 3 to 4 months, the addition of iron-fortified cereals or an iron supplement becomes important. If the infant is to be formula-fed, it is advisable to select a formula with iron.[15]

Zinc. The infant's zinc needs are met by a limited tissue supply at birth and early food sources.

Body stores. The infant is born without zinc body stores. Tissue concentrations at birth are similar to those of adults. Therefore, infants rapidly become dependent on a dietary source. Variations in concentrations of plasma zinc during growth reflect the continued utilization and depletion of body stores of zinc. Although there are not enough data to state a requirement, the RDA standard has been set for 5 mg during the first year. One study comparing hair zinc concentration of breastfed and bottle-fed babies during the first 6 months of life found that only male bottle-fed infants experienced a significant decline in hair zinc concentration, suggesting that males had a higher requirement for zinc during the period studied.[16]

Food sources. Colostrum contains 20 mg/L of zinc, three to five times as much as later milk. Human milk contains 4 mg/L of zinc in the first month declining to 0.6 mg/L at 6 months.[17] Cow's milk contains 3 to 5 mg/L of zinc. Formulas are supplemented and contain 5 mg/L. Animal studies suggest that the bioavailability of zinc is 59.2% in human milk, 43% to 53.9% in cow's milk, and 26.8% to 39.5% in infant formula.[18] The recommended intake of 5 mg/day is applicable for formula-fed infants.

Fluoride. The importance of fluoride in the prevention of dental caries has been well documented. It is also recognized that flouride can cause dental fluorosis (ranging from fine white lint to entirely chalky teeth) with intakes that range from 4-100 μg/kg/day in infancy.

Breast milk has a very low fluoride content. Powdered formula has higher concentrations than concentrated formula. Commercially prepared infant cereals, wet pack cereals, poultry-containing products, and fruit juice produced with fluoridated water are significant sources of fluoride in infancy.

There is evidence that the previously recommended supplementation with fluoride may place children at risk for fluorosis. Fomon currently recommends no fluoride supplements for infants. After tooth eruption he recommends that fluoridated water be offered several times a day to breastfed infants, to those who receive cow's milk, and when formulas are made with water providing less than 0.3 mg of fluoride/liter.[3]

Vitamins. The specific functions of vitamins in metabolic processes make the requirement for each vitamin dependent upon the related intakes of energy, protein, carbohydrates, and fats. Exact needs are difficult to define. Most vitamins cross the placenta and accumulate in the fetus at greater concentrations than in the mother. Maternal hypovitaminemia will be reflected in the fetus. Vitamins A, E, and beta-carotene (vitamin A precursor) concentrations are lower in the newborn infant's blood than in the mother's. The concentration of water-soluble vitamins in the blood of the neonate is higher than in that of the mother.

Fat-soluble vitamins in excess of need are not excreted but are stored. Reserves can be accumulated. The toxicity of excessive intakes of vitamins A and D is well documented. In contrast to vitamins A, D, E, and K, the water-soluble vitamins are "stored" only in the sense of small degrees of tissue saturation that turn over rapidly so deficiencies can occur in a relatively short period if the nutrient is absent from dietary intake.

Fat-soluble vitamins. The infant's needs for the fat-soluble vitamins A, D, E, and K are met by food sources and in some instances added supplementation.

Vitamin A. The milk of well-nourished women contains 40 to 70 μg/dl **retinol** and 20 to 40 μg/dl of **carotenoids**. The recommended intake of 375 μg/retinol equivalents (RE) per day in the first year reflects the RE intake of an infant consuming 750 ml per day with a margin for the **coefficient of variation** between women.

Vitamin D. Although 2.5 micrograms (μg) (100 international units [IU]) of vitamin D prevents rickets and ensures adequate absorption of calcium and normal mineralization of bone in the infant, better calcium absorption and some increase in growth has been

Retinol
Chemical name for vitamin A derived from its function relating to the retina of the eye and light-dark adaptation. Daily RDA standards are stated in retinol equivalents (RE) to account for sources of the preformed vitamin and its precursor provitamin A beta-carotene.

noted with intakes of 10 μg (400 IU)/day. Vitamin D can be formed by the action of sunlight on the skin. The amount formed depends on several variables, and amounts formed cannot be readily measured. To assure an adequate intake, the recommended intake as **cholecalciferol** is 7.5 μg (300 IU)/day for the first 6 months and 10 μg (400 IU)/day for the remainder of the first year. Breastfed infants who are not exposed to sunlight should receive a supplement of 5.0 to 7.5 μg (200 to 300 IU) daily. The U.S. RDA standards, as well as those of the international community, no longer use the former concept of *International Unit*, which was based on the biologic activity (in the case of vitamin D, 1 IU equals 0.025 μg) of a given amount of the vitamin to achieve its function, but now express RDAs in direct amounts needed for health.

Vitamin E. Defining appropriate intakes for vitamin E is complicated by large variations in the susceptibility to peroxidation of fatty acids in the diet and tissues. The recommended intake during infancy reflects the **tocopherol** concentration of human milk in which 6% of the kilocalories are provided by polyunsaturated fatty acid.

Vitamin K. Vitamin K, essential for the formation of **prothrombin** and other factors involved in blood clotting, is of particular concern for the breastfed infant. The newborn has low plasma prothrombin levels. The intestinal flora is very limited and human milk provides low levels of vitamin K (2 μg/L). If the breastfed infant does not receive supplements, the infant is at risk for intracranial hemorrhage. A **prophylactic** intramuscular dose of 0.5 to 1 mg of vitamin K or an oral dose of 1 to 2.1 mg of vitamin K is usually given to infants at birth in the hospital. Home-delivered infants who are to be breastfed need the same supplement.

Water-soluble vitamins. The current RDAs set standards for six of the B vitamins— thiamin, riboflavin, niacin, B_6, B_{12}, and folate—and for vitamin C. Only safe and adequate estimates for two additional B vitamins, biotin and pantothenic acid, are possible at this time.

Thiamin. Requirements for thiamin are related to energy intake since it functions as a vital coenzyme factor in energy metabolism. One study, based on the consumption of 1 L of human milk, suggests that the minimum requirement for thiamin during infancy is 1.7 mg/day. The Academy of Pediatrics estimates the allowance of thiamin for infants as 0.4 mg/1000 kcal consumed.

Riboflavin. Requirements for riboflavin are also related to energy intake, reflecting its coenzyme role in energy metabolism. An intake of 0.4 mg of riboflavin per day has been noted to maintain blood and urine levels in infants weighing 5.9 to 9.0 kg. The average breastfed infant who consumes 750 ml/day of breast milk receives 0.26 mg of riboflavin, or 0.48 mg/1000 kcal.

Niacin. The fact that the amino acid tryptophan can be converted to niacin makes basic requirements for niacin difficult to determine. Human milk contains 1.5 mg of niacin and 210 mg of tryptophan per liter. Minimum requirements for niacin appear to be 4.4 mg/1000 kcal. The allowance for infants before 6 months of age is 8 **niacin equivalents (NE)**/1000 kcal. For infants older than 6 months, allowances are based on the same standard as that for adults, 6.6 NE/1000 kcal.

Vitamin B_6. Vitamin B_6 (**pyridoxine**) functions as an essential coenzyme factor in the metabolism of amino acids and lipids, as well as nucleic acid, a key component of the genetic structure in the cell nucleus deoxyribonucleic acid (DNA). The requirement for this vitamin increases as the protein intake increases. The recommended intake, 0.3 mg/day during the first 6 months of life and 0.6 mg/day the last half of the first year, is based on experience with commercial infant formulas.

Vitamin B_{12}. Vitamin B_{12} (**cobalamin**) functions as a co-enzyme in the degradation of certain amino acids and of fatty acids with **odd-numbered carbon chains**. It is essential, along with folate, in metabolic processes that transfer single carbon fragments from one

Tocopherol
(Gr *tokos*, childbirth; *pherein*, to carry) Chemical name for vitamin E, so-named by early investigators because their initial work with rats indicated a reproductive function, which did not turn out later to be the case with humans, in whom it functions as a strong anti-oxidant to preserve structural membranes such as cell walls.

Prothrombin
(Gr *pro-*, before; *thrombos*, clot) Bloodclotting factor (number II), synthesized in the liver from glutamic acid and CO_2, catalyzed by vitamin K.

Niacin equivalent (NE)
Current international measure for recommended amounts of the B-vitamin niacin that accounts for the preformed vitamin and the amino acid precursor tryptophan, from which the vitamin can be synthesized. Thus, 1 NE equals 1 g niacin or 60 mg of dietary tryptophan.

Pyridoxine
Chemical name for vitamin B_6, derived from its ring-like structure. In its active form, pyridoxal phosphate, it acts as a coenzyme in many types of transamination and decarboxylation reactions in amino acid metabolism.

compound to another in amino acid metabolism and nucleic acid synthesis. Deficiency of either vitamin results in growth retardation. The allowances for vitamin B_{12} are based on 0.3 μg/day for the young infant and 0.5 μg/day for the infant over 6 months of age. Symptoms of B_{12} deficiency have been found in a few breastfed infants whose mothers had followed a strict vegan diet or who had **pernicious anemia.**

Folate. Body stores of folate at birth are small and rapidly depleted. Serum and **erythrocyte** levels fall below adult levels by two weeks of age and remain there during the first year of life. The allowance for folate is 3.6 mg/kg per day for the first year. The folate needs of infants are adequately met by both human and cow's milk. Goat's milk is folate deficient for the human infant.

Vitamin C. Newborn infants consuming 7 to 12 mg/day of vitamin C (**ascorbic acid**) have been protected from scurvy. An intake of 30 mg/day, based on the amount provided by human milk, is recommended during the first 6 months of life, and 35 mg/day for the next 6 months. Infants who are fed human milk or commercial infant formula will receive adequate vitamin C.

Vitamin and mineral supplements. Full-term infants who receive milk from a well-nourished lactating mother will receive all the vitamins they need, with the exception of vitamin D. Breastfed infants should receive vitamin D supplements by 2 months of age. Infants who receive a commercially available formula that is properly prepared will be adequately nourished with vitamins.

The need for supplemental iron depends on the composition of the diet consumed. Solely breastfed infants should receive a supplement by 4 to 6 months of age. Those who receive iron-fortified cereals will probably not need supplements. Infants receiving iron-fortified formula will need no supplemental iron.

MILK FOR INFANTS
Human Milk and Formula

The advantages of human milk for feeding human infants are numerous and breastfeeding is encouraged by most health professionals. Many mothers breastfeed their infants for a few months and then offer them a formula. Most normal full-term infants who are not breastfed receive a cow's milk-based formula. Infants who do not tolerate cow's milk may receive a soy or hydrolyzed casein formula.

Differences in human and cow's milk were discussed in Chapter 5. From such comparisons it soon becomes apparent that if cow's milk is offered to infants it must be modified. Products prepared for infant feeding do indeed modify cow's milk. In fact, many attempt to simulate human milk.

Nutrient Composition Regulations

Guidelines for energy and minimum and maximum levels of nutrients in formulas have been established by a number of groups including the Committee on Nutrition of the American Academy of Pediatrics,[8] the European Society of Paediatric Gastroenterology and Nutrition,[19-22] a joint WHO/FAO commission,[23] and the Food and Drug Directorate in Canada. In the United States regulations regarding the composition of infant formula are established by the Food and Drug Administration.[25] Minimum levels for most nutrients and maximum levels for some have been established. It has been suggested that upper limits need to be established for all nutrients.[3]

Modified Cow's Milk Formulas

Commercially manufactured formulas prepared from nonfat milk are available and generously used for feeding in infancy. Three formulas are casein-based, utilizing fat-free

Cobalamin
Chemical name for vitamin B_{12}, from its structure as a complex red crystalline compound of high molecular weight, with a single cobalt atom at its core. Its food sources are of animal origin, but the ultimate source is from the colonies of synthesizing microorganisms inhabiting the gastrointestinal tract of herbivorous animals.

Erythrocyte
(Gr *erythro-*, red; *cyte*, hollow vessel) Red blood cell.

milk as the protein source; three others are whey predominant (Table 6-7). Combinations of vegetable oils, a high percentage of which are absorbed by infants, are added. Also, oleo oil is added to one whey-based formula. Lactose is added to increase the caloric concentration to approximately that of human and cow's milk. Vitamins and minerals are added. Formulas are marketed both with and without ferrous sulfate in amounts that provide 12 mg per quart. Pediatricians encourage the use of formulas with iron.

Hypoallergenic Formulas

Soy formulas. The most commonly used products for infants who have conditions that contraindicate the use of cow's milk are the soy milks. These formulas are constructed of protein isolated from soy meal fortified with methionine, corn syrup or sucrose, and soy or other vegetable oils to which vitamins and minerals have been added. The **trypsin inhibitor** in raw soybean meal is inactivated during heat processing. The **goitrogenic** effect of soy is diminished by heating and the addition of iodine.

Casein hydrolysate formulas. Three other formulas are marketed for infants who do not tolerate either soy or cow's milk. Nutramigen, prepared from a **casein hydrolysate** and corn oil; Progestimil, which contains a casein hydrolysate and medium-chain triglycerides; and Alimentum which contains free amino acids, **elemental formula** components. All three formulas have an unpleasant odor and taste and are rarely accepted by infants if not introduced before 8 to 9 months of age. The composition of non-cow's milk–based formulas is given in Table 6-8.

Preparations for Toddlers

Three manufacturers market formula for children over one year for whom cow's milk is inappropriate. One soy-based formula that includes corn syrup solids and sugar as carbohydrate and vegetable oils as fat is fortified with iron. There are also two elemental formulas for oral feeding of children over one year. These formulas are milk, lactose, and gluten free.

Formula and Milk for Older Infants

One cow's milk-based formula is marketed for older babies. This formula, designed to accompany the feeding of semisolid foods, is higher in protein and lower in fat than formula for the younger infant. However, examination of the nutrient intakes of infants from 6 months to 1 year reveals that their intakes are completely adequate without the additional protein. Pediatricians feel there is no justification for the use of these milks.

The use of whole, 2%, 1%, or nonfat cow's milk in the first year is strongly discouraged. It has been noted to contribute to the incidence of anemia. Not only is there no iron in this milk, it may cause a very tiny blood loss from the intestinal tract. If a test of the baby's feces is done with paper impregnated with guaiac solution and/or a fecal hemoglobin test is performed, small amounts of blood may be found. Over time, this may lead to anemia.[26]

Formulas prepared for younger infants are perfectly adequate for the first year.

Substitute and Imitation Milks

Feeding infants formulas made from recipes that have not been proven to support adequate nutrition should be strongly discouraged. Malnutrition was observed in infants fed a barley water, corn syrup, and whole milk formula suggested in a magazine for mothers.[27] Kwashiorkor, an advanced protein-deficiency state of malnutrition, has been reported in infants fed a nondairy creamer as a substitute for milk.[28]

Substitute or imitation milks should not be offered to infants. Substitute milk is defined by the Food and Drug Administration as nutritionally equivalent to whole or nonfat milk based on their content of only 14 or 15 nutrients. It does not include all nutrients

---

Trypsin inhibitor

A natural substance in raw soybeans that is responsible for a toxin in the bean. Fortunately this substance is destroyed by heat and rendered inactive.

Goitrogens

Natural substance in certain foods such as soybeans that cause hypothyroidism and a compensatory enlargement of the thyroid gland, producing symptoms of iodine-deficiency goiter; effect diminished by adequate heating of the soy meal and adding iodine supplementation.

Casein hydrolysate formula

Infant formula with base of hydrolyzed casein, major milk protein, produced by partially breaking down the casein into smaller peptide fragments, making a product that is more easily digested.

Elemental formula

Infant formula produced with elemental, ready to be absorbed, components of free amino acids and carbohydrate as simple sugars.

TABLE 6-7 *Nutrient Content of Commercially Available Cow's Milk-Based Formula*

Nutrient Source	Similac	Gerber	Bonamil	Enfamil	S.M.A.	Good Start
Protein	Casein	Casein	Casein	Reduced mineral whey, casein	Demineralized whey, casein	Reduced-mineral whey
Fat	Soy oil, coconut oil, corn oil	Soy oil, coconut oil, soy lecithin	Soy oil, coconut oil	Soy oil, coconut oil, palm oil	Oleo; soybean, safflower, and coconut oils	Palm, safflower, soy, and coconut oil
Carbohydrate	Lactose, hydrolyzed cornstarch	Lactose	Lactose	Lactose	Lactose	Lactose

Nutrients per 100 ML – normal dilution

	Similac	Gerber	Bonamil	Enfamil	S.M.A.	Good Start
Energy (kcal)	67	67	67	67	67	67
Protein (g)	1.5	1.5	1.5	1.5	1.5	1.6
Fat (g)	3.6	3.6	3.8	3.3	3.6	3.4
Carbohydrate (g)	7.2	7.2	7.1	6.9	7.2	7.4
Vitamin A (IU)	200	200	200	209	200	300
Vitamin D (IU)	40	40	40	43	40	60
Vitamin E (IU)	2	2	2	1.3	1	1
Vitamin C (mg)	6	6.0	5.5	5.5	5.5	8
Thiamin (µg)	67	67	67	53	67	60
Riboflavin (µg)	100	100	100	102	110	130
Niacin (mg) (equiv.)	0.7	0.7	.5	0.85	.5	.75
Pyridoxine (µg)	40	40	42	43	42	15
Vitamin B$_{12}$ (µg)	.17	0.16	.13	.15	.13	.2
Folate (µg)	10	10	5	10.6	5	9
Calcium (mg)	49	50	46	53	42	43
Phosphorus (mg)	39	39	36	36	28	24
Magnesium (mg)	3.4	4	4	5.3	4.5	4.5
Iron (mg)	Trace	Trace	Trace	Trace	Trace	Trace
Zinc (mg)	0.5	0.5	0.5	0.5	0.5	0.5
Copper (µg)	60.0	60	47	64	47	53
Iodine (µg)	6	5.4	3.3	4.1	6	5.6

TABLE 6-8 *Nutrient Content of Soy Formulas and Other Milk Substitutes for Infants*

Nutrient Source	Prosobee	Isomil	Nutramigen	Progestimil
Protein	Soy protein	Soy protein	Casein hydrolysate	Casein hydrolysate
Fat	Soy oil	Coconut oil, soy oil	Soy, coconut and palm oils	Corn oil, medium-chain triglycerides, soy oil
Carbohydrate	Corn syrup solids	Corn syrup solids, sucrose	Modified tapioca starch, sucrose	Corn syrup solids, modified tapioca starch
Nutrients per 100 ML—normal dilution				
Energy (kcal)	68	68	67	68
Protein (g)	2.0	1.8	1.9	1.9
Fat (g)	3.6	3.7	2.7	3.8
Carbohydrate (g)	6.8	6.9	9.1	7.0
Vitamin A (IU)	210	203	210	256
Vitamin D (IU)	42.0	41.0	42.0	51.0
Vitamin E (IU)	1.4	2.0	2.1	2.5
Vitamin C (mg)	5.5	6.0	5.5	7.9
Thiamin (μg)	52.0	41.0	52.0	52.0
Riboflavin (μg)	63.0	61.0	63.0	63.0
Niacin (mg) (equiv.)	0.8	0.9	0.8	0.8
Pyridoxine (μg)	42.0	41.0	42.0	42.0
Vitamin B_{12} (μg)	0.2	0.3	0.2	0.2
Folic acid (μg)	11.0	10.0	10.6	10.6
Calcium (mg)	63.0	71.0	63.0	63.0
Phosphorus (mg)	50.0	51.0	42.0	42.0
Magnesium (mg)	7.4	5.1	7.4	7.4
Iron (mg)	1.3	1.2	1.3	1.3
Zinc (mg)	0.5	0.5	0.5	0.5
Copper (μg)	63.0	51.0	63.0	63.0
Iodine (μg)	7.0	10.0	4.8	4.8

recommended as components of infant formulas. Imitation milk simulates milk but does not meet the standard of identity for substitute milk.[29]

Formula Preparation

Types of formula available. Manufacturers market three basic types of formulas, each of which is prepared according to its form: (1) *liquid concentrates* prepared for feeding by mixing equal amounts of the liquid and water; (2) *ready-to-feed* formulas that require no preparation are available in an assortment of sizes (4-, 6-, and 8-oz bottles and 32-oz containers); and (3) *powdered* formulas that are prepared by mixing 1 level tablespoon of powder for each 2 oz of water. All of these formulas, when properly prepared and adequately supplemented, provide the nutrients important for the infant in an appropriate caloric concentration and present a solute load reasonable for the full-term infant. Errors in dilution caused by lack of understanding of the proper method of preparation, improper

Nutrient Source	Alimentum	Gerber Soy	Next Step Toddler
Protein	Cystine, tyrosine, tryptophan	Soy protein	Soy protein
Fat	Medium-chain triglycerides, safflower and soy oils	Soy, coconut oils, soy lecithin	Coconut oil, soy oil, palm oil, sunflower oil
Carbohydrate	Sucrose, modified tapioca starch	Corn syrup	Corn syrup solids

Nutrients per 100 ML — normal dilution

	Alimentum	Gerber Soy	Next Step Toddler
Energy (kcal)	68	67	67
Protein (g)	1.9	2.0	2.2
Fat (g)	3.7	3.6	3.0
Carbohydrate (g)	6.9	6.7	8.0
Vitamin A (IU)	304	203	203
Vitamin D (IU)	30.4	40	40
Vitamin E (IU)	2.0	2	1.4
Vitamin C (mg)	6.0	6	8
Thiamin (μg)	41.0	40	54
Riboflavin (μg)	61.0	61.0	61.0
Niacin (mg) (equiv.)	0.9	0.7	0.7
Pyridoxine (μg)	41.0	40	60
Vitamin B$_{12}$ (μg)		.3	.2
Folic acid (μg)	10.0	10	11
Calcium (mg)	71.0	64	78
Phosphorus (mg)	51.0	50.0	61.0
Magnesium (mg)	5.1	5.4	5.4
Iron (mg)	1.2	1.2	1.2
Zinc (mg)	0.5	0.5	0.8
Copper (μg)	50.7	50.7	50.7
Iodine (μg)	6.0	10	10.1

measurements, adding extra water to make the formula last longer, or the belief of the parents that their child should have greater amounts of nutritious food can lead to problems.

Results of errors in formula preparation. Failure to gain appropriately in height and weight has been observed as a result of dilution of ready-to-eat formulas in the manner that concentrated formulas are prepared. Mothers have been known to add extra water in the belief that more dilute formula might reduce spitting up by their infants.

Feeding dilute formula over time can lead to undernutrition and water intoxication with symptoms of hyponatremia, irritability, and in severe cases, coma.

Feeding undiluted concentrated formula increases kilocalories, protein, and solutes presented to the kidneys for excretion and may predispose the young infant to hypernatremia, dehydration, and **tetany** as well as obesity. Problems of improper formula preparation have most frequently been reported with the use of powdered formula and occur most often when an increased need for water caused by a fever or infection is superimposed on consumption of an already high-solute formula. Infants fed concentrated formula during such illnesses may become thirsty, demand more to drink, or refuse to consume more liquid because of anorexia secondary to the illness. When presented with more milk concentrated in the protein and solutes, the **osmolality** of the blood increases and **hypernatremic dehydration** may result. Cases of cerebral damage and gangrene of the extremities have been reported to be the result of hypernatremic dehydration and **metabolic acidosis**.[30]

Anticipatory guidance of parents of young infants should include information on the variety of formulas available, differences in methods of preparation of each product, and the dangers of overdiluted formula and excessive water intake.

Sterilization of formulas. Because commercially prepared liquid formulas are sterile before they are opened and powdered formulas are free of viable microorganisms of public health significance sterilization is no longer recommended. Most parents prepare formula for one bottle at each feeding and immediately feed the infant.

To prepare formula by clean technique, the hands of the person preparing the formula should be washed carefully. All equipment to be used during preparation, including the cans that contain the milk, the bottles, and the nipples, must be thoroughly washed and rinsed. Once opened, cans of formula must be covered and refrigerated. The formula is prepared immediately before each feeding as described above. After the formula has been heated and the infant has been fed, any remaining milk should be discarded. Warm milk is an excellent medium for bacterial growth.

SEMISOLID FOODS IN THE INFANT'S DIET

In spite of the fact that no nutritional or developmental advantage can be expected from the early introduction of semisolid foods, many families feed them in the first month of infant life. Some parents add semisolid foods hoping that the added foods will encourage their infants to sleep through the night, a commonly held belief that has proved to be untrue. Other parents feed semisolid foods because they think that their infants are hungry or because they consider the acceptance of these foods a developmental landmark.

Many infants receive foods with texture such as baked potato or drained tuna fish by the time they can sustain a sitting posture. When they reach out and secure foods with a pincer grasp, finger foods such as zwieback and arrowroot cookies can be offered.

Age of introduction. The age of introduction of semisolid foods to infants in the United States declined between 1920, when these foods were seldom offered before 1 year of age, and the period between 1960 and 1970 when they were frequently offered in the first weeks and months of life. Concern that this early introduction of semisolid foods predisposed infants to obesity and allergic reactions caused many healthcare professionals in the pediatric community to reexamine the appropriate age to introduce these foods. It is currently recommended that the feeding of semisolid foods be delayed until the consumption of food is no longer a reflex process and the infant has fine, gross, and oral motor skills appropriate to consume them, that is, at approximately 4 to 6 months of age.

FEEDING BEHAVIORS
Developmental Readiness

Illingworth and Lister have defined a "critical or sensitive" period of development in relation to eating.[31] This is a time at which a specific stimulus, solid food, must be applied to the organism to learn a particular action, accepting and eating table foods. They point out that infants learn to chew at about 6 or 7 months of age, thus at this point they are

---

Osmolality
(Gr *osmos*, impulsion through a membrane) Property of a solution that depends on the concentration of the particles (solutes) in solution per unit of solvent base; measured as milliosmoles per liter (mOsm/L).

Hypernatremic dehydration
An abnormally high sodium ion concentration in the extracellular fluid, due to water loss or restriction, drawing cell water to restore osmotic balance, causing dangerous cell dehydration.

Metabolic acidosis
Abnormal rise in acid partner of the carbonic acid-base bicarbonate buffer system by excess of organic acids, which displace part of the base bicarbonate in the buffer system and cause the H^+ concentration to rise.

developmentally ready to consume food. If solid foods are withheld until a later age, the child will have considerably more difficulty in accepting them.

In 1937 Gesell and Ilg published their now classic observations made during extensive studies of the feeding behavior of infants.[32] Their observations are as valid today as they were then. **Cineradiographic** techniques developed since then have permitted more detailed descriptions of the actions involved in sucking, suckling, and swallowing.

Development of Oral Structures and Functions

It is important to recognize that even though the normal neonate is well prepared to suck and swallow at birth, the physical and motor maturation during the first year alter both the form of the oral structures and the methods by which the infant extracts milk from a nipple. Each of these changes influences the infant's eating skills. At birth the tongue is disproportionately large in comparison with the lower jaw and essentially fills the oral cavity. The lower jaw is moved back relative to the upper jaw, which protrudes over the lower by approximately 2 mm.[33] When the mouth is closed, the jaws do not rest on top of each other; the tip of the tongue lies between the upper and lower jaws. There is a "fat pad" in each of the cheeks. It is thought that these pads serve as a prop for the muscles in the cheek, maintaining rigidity of the cheeks during suckling. The lips of the neonate are also instrumental in suckling and have characteristics appropriate for their function at this age. A mucosal fold disappears by the third or fourth month, when the lips have developed muscular control to seal the oral cavity. The newborn infant sucks reflexively, the young infant beginning at 2 or 3 weeks of age suckles, and as infants grow older they learn mature sucking. Some description of these two processes therefore seems important.

Suckling

The processes of breast and bottle suckling are similar. The nipple of the breast becomes rigid and elongated during breastfeeding so that it resembles a rubber nipple in shape, and both assume a similar position in the infant's mouth. The infant grasps the nipple in the mouth. The oral cavity is sealed off by pressure from the middle portions of the lips assisted by the mucosal folds of the jaws. The nipple is held in the infant's mouth with the tip located close to the junction of the hard and soft **palate.**

During the first stage of suckling, the lower jaw and tongue are lowered while the mouth is closed, thus creating a negative pressure. The tip of the tongue moves forward. The lower jaw and tongue are next raised, compressing the beginning base of the nipple. The compression is moved from the beginning base to the tip of the nipple as the tip of the tongue withdraws, thus stroking or milking the liquid from the nipple. The moved-back position of the lower jaw maximizes the efficiency of the stroking action. As the tongue moves back, it comes in contact with the tensed soft palate, thus causing liquid to squirt into the side food channels. The location of the **larynx** is further elevated by the muscular contractions during swallowing. As the liquid is squirted back in the mouth, the epiglottis is positioned so that it parts the stream of liquid, passing it to the sides of the larynx instead of over it. Thus liquid does not pass over the laryngeal entrance during early infancy because of the relatively higher position of the larynx and the parting of the stream of liquid by the epiglottis.

Sucking

Mature sucking is an acquired feature of the **orofacial muscles.** It is not a continuous process. Upon accumulation of sufficient fluid in the mouth, sucking and breathing are interrupted by a swallowing movement. The closure of the nasopharyngeal and laryngeal sphincters in response to the presence of food in the **pharynx** is responsible for the interruption of the nasal breathing.

Cineradiographs
(Gr *cine-, kinesis,* movement; L *radius,* ray; Gr *graphein,* to write) Fluoroscopic motion film records of internal structures and their functions.

Palate
(L *palatum,* palate) The partition separating the nasal and oral cavities, with a hard bony front section and a soft fleshy back section.

Larynx
(Gr *larynx,* upper part of windpipe) Structure of muscle and cartilage lined with mucous membrane, connected to top part of the trachea and to the pharynx; essential sphincter muscle guarding the entrance to the trachea and functioning secondarily as the organ of the voice.

Orofacial muscles
(L *os, oris,* mouth) Adjoining muscles of the mouth and face.

Pharynx
(Gr *pharynx,* throat) The muscular membranous passage between the mouth and the posterior nasal passages and the larynx and esophagus.

Adenoidal pad
(Gr *adenos*, gland; *ei-dos*, form) Normal lymphoid tissue in the nasopharynx of children.

Epipharynx
(Gr *epi*, on; *pharynx*, throat) Nasopharynx; the part of the pharynx that lies above the level of the soft palate.

Lymphoid tissue
(L *lympha*, water) Tissues related to the body system of lymphatic fluids.

During swallowing the food lies in the swallow preparation position on the groove of the tongue. The farther back portion of the soft palate is raised toward the **adenoidal pad** in the roof of the **epipharynx.** The tongue presses upward against the nipple so that the swallow of milk follows gravity down the sloping tongue and reaches the pharynx. As the milk in the mouth moves downward, the rear wall of the pharynx comes forward to displace the soft palate toward the back surface of the tongue and the larynx is elevated and arched backward. The accumulated milk is expressed from the pharynx by peristaltic movements of the pharyngeal wall toward the back of the tongue and the larynx. The milk spills over the joining folds of the pharynx and epiglottis folds into the side food channels and then into the esophagus.

The tonsils and **lymphoid tissue** play an important role as infants swallow. They help keep the airway open and the food away from the rear pharyngeal wall as the infant is held in a reclining position, thus delaying nasopharyngeal closure until food has reached the pharynx.

As the infant grows older the oral cavity enlarges so that the tongue no longer fills the mouth. The tongue grows differentially at the tip and attains motility in the larger oral cavity. The elongated tongue can be protruded to receive and pass solids between the gum pads and erupting teeth for mastication. Mature feeding is characterized by separate movements of the lip, tongue, and gum pads or teeth.

Sequence of Development of Feeding Behavior

The sequence of development of feeding behavior is related to the individual maturation of the infant.

Newborns. The "rooting reflex" caused by stroking of the perioral skin including the cheeks and lips causes an infant to turn toward the stimulus, so that the mouth comes in contact with it. Stimulus placed on the lips causes involuntary movements toward it, closure, and pouting in preparation for sucking. These reflexes thus enable the infant to suck and receive nourishment. Both rooting and suckling can be elicited when the infant is hungry but are absent when the infant is satiated. During feeding the neonate assumes a tonic position, the head rotated to one side and the arm on that side fisted. The infant seeks the nipple by touch and obtains milk from the nipple with a rhythmic suckle.[32] Semisolid foods, introduced by spoon at an early age into the diets of many infants, are secured in the same manner as milk, by stroking movements of the tongue with the tongue projecting as the spoon is withdrawn. Frequently, the food is expelled from the mouth.

Age 16 to 24 weeks. By 16 weeks of age the more mature suckling pattern becomes evident, with the tongue moving back and forth as opposed to the earlier up-and-down motions. Spoon feeding is easier because the infant can draw in the lower lip as the spoon is removed. The tonic neck position has faded, and the infant assumes a more symmetric position with the head at midline. The hands close over the bottle. By 20 weeks of age the infant can grasp on tactile contact with a palmar squeeze. By 24 weeks of age the infant can reach for and grasp an object on sight. In almost every instance the object goes into the mouth.

Age 24 to 28 weeks. Between 24 and 28 weeks of age chewing movement, an up-and-down movement of the jaws, begins. This movement, coupled with the ability to grasp and the hand-to-mouth route of grasped objects, as well as sitting posture, indicates a readiness of the infant to finger feed. Infants at this age grasp with a **palmar grasp.** Therefore, the shape of the food presented to the child to finger feed is important. Cookies, melba toast, crackers, and teething biscuits are frequently introduced at this stage.

Age 28 to 32 weeks. Between 28 and 32 weeks of age the infant gains control of the trunk and can sit alone without support. The sitting infant has greater mobility of the shoulders and arms and is better able to reach and grasp. The grasp is more digital than the earlier palmar grasp. The infant is able to transfer items from one hand to the other

Palmar grasp
Early grasp of the young infant, clasping an object in the palm and wrapping whole hand around it.

and learns to release and resecure objects voluntarily. The beginning of chewing patterns, up-and-down movements of the jaws, is demonstrated. The tongue shows more maturity in regard to spoon feeding than in drinking. Food is received from the spoon by pressing the lips against the spoon, drawing the head away, and drawing in the lower lip. The infant is aware of a cup and can suck from it. Milk leaks frequently from the corners of the mouth as the tongue is projected before swallowing.[32]

Age 6 to 12 months. The introduction of soft mashed, but not strained, foods is appropriate at this stage of development. In fact, it is at this stage of development that Illingworth and Lister believe it is critical to introduce the infant to harder-to-chew foods. Between 6 and 12 months of age the infant gradually receives greater amounts of food from the family menu and less and less of the pureed and strained items. Foods should be carefully selected and modified so that they are presented in a form that can be manipulated in the mouth without the potential of choking and aspirating, as may occur with small grains of rice or corn. Many parents mash well-cooked ground meat dishes, such as ground

TABLE 6-9 *Sequence of Development of Feeding Behavior*

Age	Reflexes	Oral, Fine, Gross Motor Development
1-3 months	Rooting and suck and swallow reflexes are present at birth Tonic neck reflex present	Head control is poor Secures milk with suckling pattern, the tongue projecting during a swallow By the end of the third month, head control is developed
4-6 months	Rooting reflex fades Bite reflex fades Tonic neck reflex fades by 16 weeks	Changes from a suckling pattern to a mature suck with liquids Sucking strength increases Munching pattern begins Grasps with a palmar grasp Grasps, brings objects to mouth and bites them
7-9 months	Gag reflex is less strong as chewing of solids begins and normal gag is developing Choking reflex can be inhibited	Munching movements begin when solid foods are eaten Rotary chewing begins Sits alone Has power of voluntary release and resecural Holds bottle alone
10-12 months		Develops an inferior pincer grasp Reaches for a spoon Bites nipples, spoons, and crunchy foods Grasps bottle and foods and brings them to the mouth Can drink from a cup that is held Tongue is used to lick food morsels off the lower lip Finger feeds with a refined pincer grasp

Modified from Gessell A, Ilg FL: *Feeding behavior of infants,* Philadelphia, 1937, JB Lippincott.

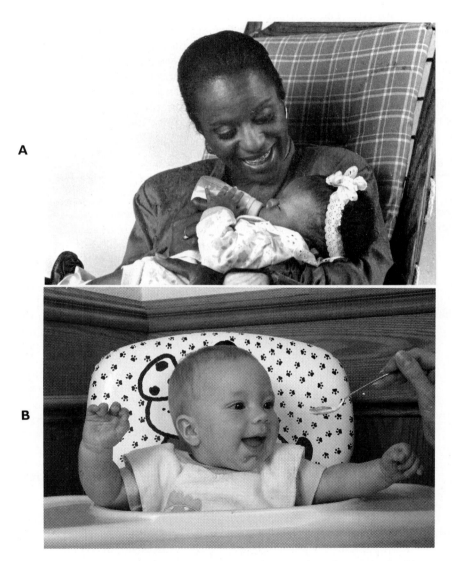

FIG. 6-4 Sequence of development of feeding behaviors. **A,** Infant sucks liquids. **B,** 8-month-old infant is fed table food.

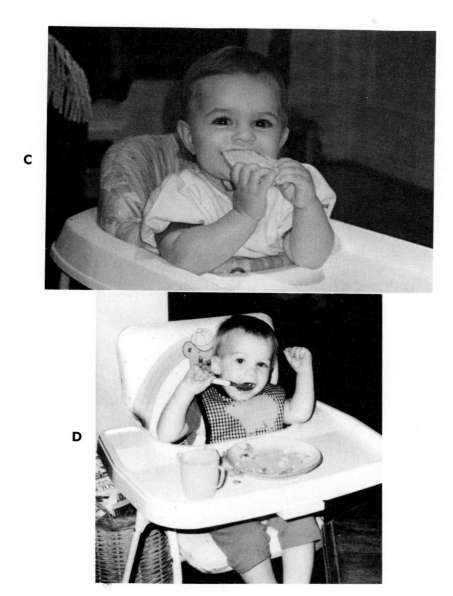

FIG. 6-4, cont'd   **C,** 10-month-old infant finger feeds with both hands. **D,** 11-month-old infant begins to feed himself.   *Continued.*

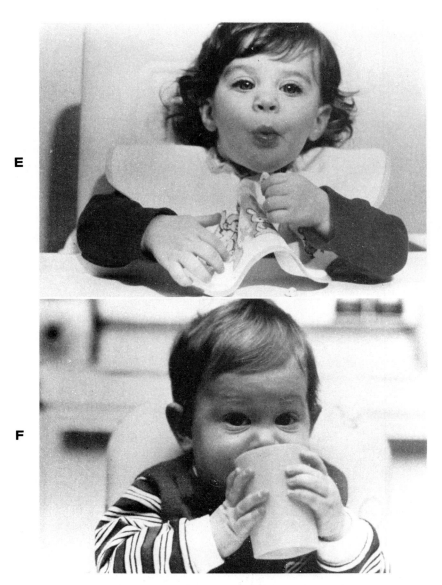

FIG. 6-4, cont'd **E,** 10-month-old infant purses her lips. **F,** 12-month-old infant drinks from a cup.

meat in gravies or sauces, which appear to be easily accepted, as are liverwurst, minced chicken livers, and drained tuna fish. Custards, puddings, and ice cream soon become favorites.

By 28 weeks of age infants are able to help themselves to their bottle in sitting postures, although they will not be able to tip the bottle adaptively as it empties until about 32 weeks of age. By the end of the first year they can completely manage bottle-feeding alone.

By 32 weeks of age infants bring their heads forward to receive the spoon as it is presented to them. The tongue shows increased motility and allows for considerable increased manipulation of food in the mouth before swallowing. At the end of the first year, infants are able to manipulate food in the mouth with definite chewing movements.

During the fourth quarter of the first year, the child develops an increasingly precise **pincer grasp.** The bottle can be managed alone and can be rescued if it is lost. The child can drink from a cup only if help is provided. Infants at this age are increasingly conscious of what others do and often imitate the models set for them.[32] By 1 year of age the patterns of eating have changed from sucking to beginning rotary chewing movements. Children understand the concept of the container and the contained, have voluntary hand-to-mouth movements and a precise pincer grasp, and can voluntarily release and rescue objects. They are thus prepared to learn to feed themselves, a behavior they learn and refine in the second year.

This development of feeding behavior is summarized in Table 6-9 and is shown in the sequence of illustrations in Fig. 6-4.

FOOD CHOICES
Commercially Available Infant Foods

A vast number of commercially prepared foods are marketed for feeding the infant. The new mother may select organically grown products or products prepared from farms and

Pincer grasp
Later digital grasp of the older infant, usually picking up smaller objects with a precise grip between thumb and fore-finger.

Directions for Home Preparation of Infant Foods

1. Select fresh, high-quality fruits, vegetables, or meats.
2. Be sure all utensils, including cutting boards, grinders, knives, etc., are thoroughly clean.
3. Wash your hands before preparing the food.
4. Clean, wash, and trim the foods in as little water as possible.
5. Cook the foods until tender in as little water as possible. Avoid overcooking, which may destroy heat-sensitive nutrients.
6. Do not add salt. Add sugar sparingly. Do not add honey to foods for infants less than 1 year of age.*
7. Add enough water so that the food has a consistency that is easily pureed.
8. Strain or puree the food using an electric blender, a food mill, a baby food grinder, or a kitchen strainer.
9. Pour puree into ice cube tray and freeze.
10. When food is frozen hard, remove the cubes and store in freezer bags.
11. Thaw and heat in serving container the amount of food that will be consumed at a single feeding (in water bath or microwave oven).

---

*Botulism spores have been reported in honey, and young infants do not have the immune capacity to resist this infection.

From Pipes PL: *Nutrition in infancy.* In Krause MV, Mahan LK, editors: *Food, nutrition, and diet therapy,* ed 7, Philadelphia, 1984, Saunders.

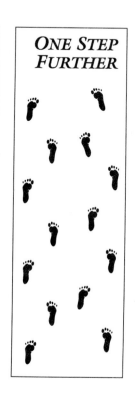

ONE STEP FURTHER

vineyards that probably use fertilizers and insecticides. She will find jarred single foods and juices and dinners of vegetables mixed with meat, several juices mixed together, and can choose from 2½ oz, 4 oz, or 6 oz jars (first foods, second foods, third foods). Some may find toddler meals interesting. Juices are marketed in 4 oz, 8 oz, and 25.3 oz bottles, some prepared from fresh fruit, others from concentrates. This wide range of choice among current products in the U.S. baby food market may at first appear confusing to the new mother and she may choose to prepare some of the basic foods herself from fresh produce (see the box on p. 263).

Foods as Sources of Nutrients

The range of nutrients found in any group of foods for infants is quite wide, as indicated in Table 6-10. Ready-to-serve dry infant cereals are fortified with electrically reduced iron. Three level tablespoons of cereal will provide about 5 mg of iron, or from one half to one third of what the infant requires. Therefore, cereal is usually the first food added to the infant's diet. Cereal and fruit mixtures in jars are fortified with ferrous sulfate to provide 7 to 9 mg of iron per 4.5 oz jar.

Strained and junior vegetables and fruits provide carbohydrate and variable amounts of vitamins A and C. Vitamin C is added to a number of the fruits and all of the fruit juices. Several fruits, including apricots, have sugar added and are marketed as fruit desserts. Tapioca is added to a number of the fruits. Milk is added to creamed vegetables and wheat is incorporated into mixed vegetables.

Strained and junior meats are prepared with only water, except for lamb which has lemon juice added. Strained meats, which have the highest caloric density of any of the commercial baby foods are an excellent source of high-quality protein and **heme iron.** Water is the most abundant ingredient in meat and vegetable combinations and high-meat dinners. The introduction of these products should be delayed until it has been determined that the infant has no allergic reactions to any of the wide variety of ingredients they contain.

Heme iron
Dietary iron from animal sources, from heme portion of hemoglobin in red blood cells. More easily absorbed and transported in the body than nonheme iron from plant sources, but supplying the smaller portion of the body's total dietary iron.

TABLE 6-10   *Ranges of Selected Nutrients Per Ounce in Commercially Prepared Infant Foods*

Food	Energy (kcal)	Protein (gm)	Iron (mg)	Vitamin A (RE)	Vitamin C (mg)
Dry cereal	120	2.0-10.0	14.3	*	*
1st Foods, 2nd Foods, & 3rd Foods fruits	12-29	0.0-0.3	0.0-0.1	0.3-34	*-6.3
1st Foods, 2nd Foods & 3rd Foods vegetables	9-20	0.2-0.9	0.0-0.3	0.3-440	0.0-2.2
2nd Foods & 3rd Foods meats	28-37	3.8-4.4	0.2-0.4	*	*
2nd Foods & 3rd Foods dinners	12-22.4	0.5-1.1	0.1-0.2	0.3-341	*-5.3
2nd Foods & 3rd Foods desserts	19-25	0.0-0.5	0.0-0.1	*-10.5	*-4.0

*Quantity insignificant.
© 1995 Gerber Products Company: Nutrient Values, Fremont, MI, Rev1294. 1st Foods, 2nd Foods, and 3rd Foods are trademarks of Gerber Products Company.

A number of dessert items are also available, including puddings and fruit desserts. The nutrient composition of these products varies, but all contain sugar and modified corn or tapioca starch.

Home Preparation of Infant Foods

In spite of the fact that the manufacturers of infant foods no longer add salt or sugar to most of their commercially prepared products, many parents prefer to make their own infant foods at home with a food grinder, blender, or strainer. The foods should be carefully selected from high-quality fresh, frozen, or canned fruits, vegetables, and meats, and prepared so that nutrients are retained. The preparation area and all utensils used must be meticulously cleaned. Salt and sugar should be used sparingly, if at all. When the food has been cooked, then pureed or strained, it should be packaged in individual portions and refrigerated or frozen so that a single portion can be heated and fed without compromsing the quality and bacterial content of the entire batch (Fig. 6-5). The box on p. 263 provides directions for the home preparation of infant foods. Care must be taken not to use additional seasoning, as home-prepared infant foods usually have a greater caloric content than the commercial products do, and many have a higher salt content.

Table Food

Cultural influence. Food from the family menu is introduced at an early age in the diets of many infants. The age of introduction and type of food offered will reflect cultural practice. For example, crumbled cornbread mixed with pot liquor (the liquid from cooked vegetables) may be fed to infants in the southern states by 3 months of age, "sticky" rice may be fed to Oriental infants in the Pacific Northwest by 6 to 7 months of age, mashed beans with some of the cooking liquid are often given to Hispanic-American infants at 2 to 4 months of age, and mashed potatoes are offered to many infants by 3 to 4 months of age. Examples of nutrient content of some selected table foods commonly fed to older infants are given in Table 6-11.

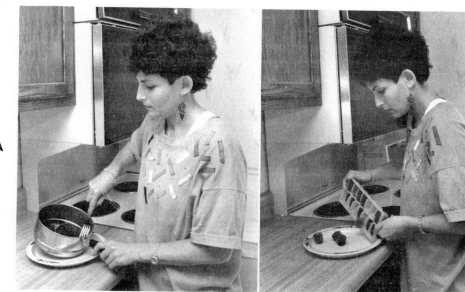

FIG. 6-5 **A,** Mother prepares food for her infant. **B,** After the food is frozen in ice-cube trays, she removes the cubes and stores them in individual portions for later use.

TABLE 6-11 *Nutrient Content of Selected Table Foods Commonly Fed to Infants*

Food	Portion Size	Energy (kcal)	Protein (g)	Iron (mg)	Vitamin A (IU)	Vitamin C (mg)
Cooked cereal (farina)	¼ cup	26	0.8	Dependent on level of fortification		
Mashed potato	¼ cup	34	1.1	0.2	10	5
French fried potato	3, 1 to 2 inches	29	0.4	0.2		
Spaghetti	2 tbsp	19	0.6	0.2		
Macaroni and cheese	2 tbsp	54	2.1	0.2	107	
Liverwurst	½ oz	45	2.1	0.8	925	
Hamburger	½ oz	41	3.4	0.5	5	
Eggs	1 medium	72	5.7	1.0	520	
Cottage cheese	1 tbsp	5	1.9		23.7	
Green beans	1 tbsp	3	0.15	0.2	43	1
Cooked carrots	1 tbsp	2.81			952	
Banana	½ small	40	0.5	0.35	90	5
Pudding	¼ cup	70	2.2	Trace	102	
Lollipop	1 oz hard candy	109				
Saltine crackers	1	12	0.2			
Vanilla wafer	¼ inch thick, 1¾ inch diameter	18	0.2			
Cheese strips	¼ oz	28	1.78		92	

From Adams CF: *Nutritive value in American foods in common units,* Agriculture Handbook no 456, Washington, DC, 1975, US Department of Agriculture.

Botulism
A serious, often fatal, form of food poisoning from ingesting food contaminated with the powerful toxins of the bacteria *Clostridium botulinum*. The toxin blocks transmission of neural impulses at the nerve terminals, causing gradual paralysis and death when affecting respiratory muscles. Most cases result from eating carelessly home-canned food, so all such food should be boiled at least 10 minutes before eating. Cases reported in infants have been related to eating spore-containing honey, so it should not be used.

Form and texture. Solid foods offered to infants should be in a form easily masticated and not given in small pieces. Choking and aspiration can occur if small pieces of hot dogs, grapes, hard candy, nuts, and other food in small, hard pieces are consumed.

Honey. Sometimes honey is used as a sweetener for home-prepared infant foods and formulas. Honey is also recommended for use on pacifiers to promote sucking in hypotonic infants. However, honey has been implicated as the only food source of spores of *Clostridium botulinum* during infancy. These spores are extremely resistant to heat and are not destroyed by present methods of processing honey. **Botulism** in infancy is caused by ingestion of the spores, which germinate into the toxin in the lumen of the bowel. Honey should not be fed to infants less than 1 year of age.[34]

Feeding the Infant

Presented with the breast of an adequately fed lactating mother, or the nipple on a bottle of properly prepared formula, the hungry infant receives both biochemical and psychosocial nurturance.

Feeding schedule. The infant held in a semireclining position who is offered the nipple sucks and receives the major portion of nourishment in 20 minutes.

If they are initially fed on demand babies will have both the physical and psychosocial aspects of the care addressed and will soon establish their own schedule. Newborn infants

Feeding Infants: Safe Food Handling

As the number of mothers working outside the home continues to rise, increasing numbers of infants are being cared for in public or private day care centers. Babies are very susceptible to food-borne illness and unsafe food practices in day care centers can lead to serious infections, debilitating gastrointestinal disturbances and diarrhea, and even death. It is important to take extra care when handling infant food or formula to avoid bacterial contamination. Moreover, infectious disease can be spread from one infant to another through poor sanitation practices with bottles or other feeding utensils. Appropriate storage methods are essential to avoid food spoilage or the unwanted growth of harmful microorganisms. A nutritionist or dietitian supervising food and nutrition procedures in day care settings should implement staff training in sanitation practices, food and formula preparation, and safe food handling. Suggestions for training lessons are given below.

Sanitation Practices
- Importance of procedures for washing hands before preparing or handling food or formula, touching bottles or feeding utensils, and after changing an infant's diaper or clothing
- Procedures for washing and sterilizing bottles, nipples, and caps or other feeding utensils

Food Preparation
- Methods for mixing dry powdered infant formula or liquid concentrates carefully according to directions; underdiluted formula (containing too little water) puts an excessive burden on the baby's kidneys and digestive system and may lead to dehydration; overdiluted formula (containing too much water) does not contain adequate kilocalories and nutrients
- Methods for checking cans of formula carefully before using, discarding those with dents, bulges or rust spots; noting that the vacuum seal on a jar of baby food has not been broken before using—you should hear a pop when you open the jar
- Methods for serving to include not using the baby food jar as a serving dish, and placing the amount of food to be fed in a dish for serving (if the spoon is placed in the jar it will contaminate the remaining food making it unfit for later use or for feeding to another child); not putting any leftover food back in the jar

Food Storage
- Storing opened jars of baby food in the refrigerator and using within 2 to 3 days
- Refrigerating prepared bottles of formula for no more than 24 hours and expressed breast milk for no more than 48 hours
- Discarding breast milk or formula remaining in the bottle after feeding
- Warming bottles of formula or breast milk immediately before serving

Modified from US Department of Agriculture: *Feeding infants; A guide for use in the child care food programs,* FNS-258, Washington DC, 1989, US Government Printing Office.

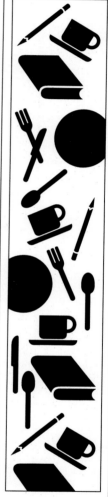

will initially feed six to eight times a day at intervals of 2 to 4 hours and will consume 2 to 3 oz at a feeding. By 2 weeks of age most infants will have increased the amount of milk consumed at a feeding and reduced the number of feedings to six. By 2 months of age most infants are fed five times a day and sleep through the night. By 6 months of age most babies consume three meals and four milk feedings a day.

Intakes of infants. Volume of intake and energy consumption is influenced not only by the infant's requirements for maintenance, growth, and activity, but also by the parents' sensitivity to and willingness to accept cues of hunger and satiety, eagerness for the infant to feed, and skill at feeding. Infants eat differently, and mothers vary in their sensitivity to the child's cues. Thoman found that mothers with their first baby spent more time stimulating their infants during feeding than did mothers who had several children, yet their infants spent less time sucking during breastfeeding and consumed less from bottles at feeding than did infants of multiparous mothers.[35] The stimulation prolonged the pauses between sucking and reduced the total consumption of food.

Growth Response to Feeding

Formula-fed newborn infants have been reported to regain to their birth weights more rapidly than breastfed infants. Thereafter, weight gains until 3 months appear similar in breastfed and bottle-fed babies, after which bottle-fed infants gain more rapidly.[36]

Energy intakes. Per unit of size, infants consume the greatest number of kilocalories between 14 and 28 days of age, a time referred to by many pediatricians as the "hungry period." After this time, although total quantity of energy intake increases, intakes per unit of size decrease. Infants consume greater amounts of food and nutrients as they grow older but less and less per unit of body size.

Wide ranges of volume of intake and energy consumption throughout the first year of life have been noted in formula-fed infants by several researchers. Formula-fed infants consume more calories per unit of body size than do breastfed infants during the first year. Gains in weight are greater in formula-fed infants as are increases in body mass per gram of protein intake. There is, however, no evidence of functional advantage to the more rapid growth.[37]

TABLE 6-12 *Suggested Ages for the Introduction of Semisolid Foods and Table Food*

	Age (months)		
Food	4 to 6	6 to 8	9 to 12
Iron-fortified cereals for infants	Add		
Vegetables		Add strained	Gradually delete strained foods, introduce table foods
Fruits		Add strained	Gradually delete strained foods, introduce chopped well-cooked or canned foods
Meats		Add strained or finely chopped table meats	Decrease the use of strained meats, increase the varieties of table meats
Finger foods such as arrow-root biscuits, oven-dried toast		Add those that can be secured with a palmar grasp	Increase the use of small-sized finger foods as the pincer grasp develops
Well-cooked mashed or chopped table foods, prepared without added salt or sugar			Add
Juice by cup			Add

Texture progress. Stages of development of feeding behavior indicate readiness for the addition of semisolid and table foods. Ages at which these stages occur and when foods other than milk are offered are shown in Table 6-12.

Food Selection

Because of the great variability in energy and nutrients provided by foods offered to infants, selection of foods and the amounts offered should be based on the infant's rate of gain in height and weight as well as on nutrient needs. Iron-fortified infant cereals are usually the first foods added to the infant's diet. It makes little difference whether fruits or vegetables are introduced next. New foods should be added singly, no more than one new food every 3 days. The introduction of vegetables containing nitrates—for example, carrots, beets, and spinach—is usually delayed until the infant is at least 4 months of age, because nitrate can be converted to nitrite in the stomach of the young infant, resulting in methemoglobinemia.

Infants gradually increase their acceptance of new foods by slowly increasing the quantity they accept. Breastfed infants appear to accept greater quantities than do formula-fed infants.[38]

It is generally recommended that the introduction of fruit juice be delayed until it can be consumed by cup. Also, it is important that intakes of fruit juice not negate their intake of more calorically dense foods. If excessive amounts of juice are consumed the infants may fail to thrive. Examples of foods and milks that might be consumed by infants at various ages are shown in Table 6-13.

During feeding both the mother and the infant receive satisfaction and pleasure. The infant is pleased because hunger is satiated. The mother is pleased because she has fulfilled the needs of her infant. Successful feeding provides the basis for the warm, trusting relationship that develops between infants and their mothers. Infants swallow air as well as milk during feeding. Holding the child in an upright position and gently patting the back encourages expulsion of swallowed air and prevents distension and discomfort.

Feeding-Related Concerns

Colic. Parents of colicky babies—those who are otherwise healthy and well-fed but who cry constantly for several hours, draw their legs onto their abdomens, and pass large amounts of gas—often request changes in their infants' formulas. This rarely resolves colic and frequent change in formulas should be discouraged. It has been suggested that colic in some breastfed babies may be resolved by eliminating milk from the mother's diet. A casein hydrolysate formula may alleviate symptoms in some but not all bottlefed infants.[40]

Spitting up food. Spitting up can occur in infants and usually causes concern for parents.

✣ *SYMPTOMS THAT REQUIRE FURTHER INVESTIGATION*

Poor nippling and/or suck
Stiffening during a feed
Reflux
Very slow linear growth
Slow or no weight gain
Delayed acquisition of feeding behaviors
Refusing spoon foods when developmentally ready
Refusing textured foods when developmentally ready (textural aversion)

TABLE 6-13 *Sample Menus for Infants at Various Ages*

Age	Weight (kg)	Energy Needs (kcal/kg)	Menu
2 months	5	540	26-28 oz human milk or infant formula
6 months	7.75	775	3 oz human milk or infant formula
			4 tbsp strained applesauce
			½ cup iron-fortified infant cereal
			4 tbsp strained pears
			1 piece zwieback
10 months	9.5	925	24 oz formula or human milk
			½ cup iron-fortified cereal
			½ cup applesauce
			1 piece melba toast
			1 oz finely chopped chicken
			½ mashed baked potato + ½ tsp oleo
			3 oz junior vegetable
			1 arrowroot cookie
			¼ oz cheese strip
			1 6-oz beef noodle dinner
			2 tbsp well-cooked broccoli
			¼ cup vanilla pudding
			2 saltine crackers

During the early months of life, some otherwise healthy infants spit up a small amount of any milk or food digested at each feeding. Although the infants do not fail to thrive, parents may seek help in resolving the situation. There is no therapy. The problem usually resolves itself by the time the infant can sustain a sitting position.

Screening for Infants With Special Health Care Needs

During observations of feeding and assessment of physical growth infants with problems may be identified. A poor suck and poor weight gain may be indicative of abnormalities of muscle tone which may later be diagnosed as cerebral palsy. Stiffening and arching during a feed may precede the diagnosis of spasticity. Delays in achieving the developmental landmarks identified in table may be indicative of generalized developmental delays. Short stature and poor weight gain may result from physical or neurological difficulties. The box on p. 269 identifies physical parameters that may be observed during feeding that should be reported for further investigation. Assessment and intervention for babies who have these symptoms will require an interdisciplinary team that will include physicians, therapists skilled in oral motor intervention, nurses, and dietitians.

Nursing bottle syndrome. A characteristic pattern of tooth decay in infants and younger children of all the upper and sometimes the lower posterior teeth, known as nursing bottle syndrome, is often observed in children who are given sweetened liquid by bottle at bedtime or who are breastfed frequently when they sleep with their mothers. As children suck, the tongue protrudes slightly from the mouth, covering the lower front teeth. Liquids are spread over the upper teeth and the lower posterior teeth. Sucking stimulates the flow of saliva, which washes the debris from the teeth and promotes the secretion of compounds that buffer the acids in the plaque. When children are awake they swallow the liquid quickly. However, if they fall asleep, sucking stops and the salivary flow and buffering are reduced. The sweetened liquid pools around the teeth not protected by the extended tongue, and the bacterial plaque has contact with the carbohydrates during the hours of sleep.

Infant formulas, fruit juice, human milk, and cow's milk consumed when infants are falling asleep may cause this decay. To prevent this dental destruction it has been suggested that infants be held when feeding and burped and put to bed as soon as they fall asleep.

Infant obesity. In the past, there has been speculation that formula feeding and the early introduction of semisolid foods might be factors in excessive intakes of energy and the development of infant obesity, and that obese infants very often become obese adults. However, a number of studies have shown that neither breastfeeding nor bottle-feeding nor the age of introduction of semisolid foods are causes of obesity in infancy. Obesity in infancy has not been found to be predictive of obesity in later life. One study found measures of fatness at 8 years of age no greater in children who had been bottle-fed as compared to those who had been breastfed.[41] A longitudinal study of children found that infants who were obese at 6 months and 1 year of age became progressively thinner as they grew older. Weight gain in infancy was not found to be predictive of obesity at 9 years of age.[42]

CASE STUDY

Case 1

Danny's Grandmother Wonders About His Weight

Danny is 6 months old, a happy and healthy baby. However, his grandmother seems worried about his weight. At the well-child clinic today, his mother says she feels that Danny is doing well, but she asks for some answers to questions raised by her mother-in-law. Danny's chart shows his weight/height record:

	2 weeks	2 months	4 months	6 months
Weight (kg)	5.34	7.60	9.59	10.60
Height (cm)	57.10	62.50	67.10	72.60

Danny was solely breastfed until 4 months of age. At that time semisolid foods were added to his diet and he was given a cow's milk-based formula. Now, at 6 months of age, his usual intake is:

Formula, commercially prepared (20 kcal/oz)	32-40 oz
Rice or oatmeal baby cereal	8 tablespoons dry
Strained pears or applesauce	½ cup
Strained squash or carrots	½ cup

Questions for analysis
1. In what percentile do his height, weight, and weight-height plot on his growth chart?
2. Is there any reason for concern about Danny's rate of weight gain?
3. Is this diet appropriate for him? How would you counsel his mother?

CASE STUDY

Case 2

Scott's Mother is Concerned Her Baby is Obese

Baby Scott weighed 7 lb 6 oz and measured 21 ¼ inches at birth. He was solely breastfed for 3 months. At that age he seemed to be very hungry, wanting to eat every hour. A soy-based formula was introduced and breastfeeding was discontinued; the soy formula was chosen because of the mother's lactose intolerance during infancy rather than an indication that baby Scott could not tolerate cow's milk-based formula. The infant's parents introduced commercially prepared dry infant cereal, mixing 1 to 2 ounces of formula with ¼ cup cereal. He suckled the cereal as he had the milk. His stools became hard and difficult to expel. At 4 months fruit and fruit juice were introduced once a day.

Baby Scott is currently fed in a high chair. He has good head control and will remain sitting if placed in that position. He leans toward and opens his mouth for the spoon. His parents notice that his tongue seems to move without his jaw. He swallows by pushing his tongue to the roof of his mouth but continues to have a thrust swallow.

Lengths and weights recorded at the pediatrician's office are:

	Length	Weight
1 month	23 in	10 lb 7 ½ oz
2 months	24 in	13 lb 5 oz
3 months	25 ½ in	14 lb
4 months	27 in	16 lb 4 oz
5 months	28 in	17 lb 9 oz

His current diet includes the following:

6 a.m	8 oz soy-based formula
9 a.m.	¼ cup infant oatmeal or barley cereal mixed with 1 oz formula
Noon	8 oz soy-based formula
4 p.m.	2 ½ oz strained fruit
5 p.m.	8 oz soy-based formula
8:30 p.m.	¼ cup cereal as offered at 9 a.m.

Questions for analysis

1. After plotting baby Scott's growth on an NCHS chart (see Appendix A), describe changes in growth parameters at 3 months. How did these patterns affect the baby's appetite and ultimately the decision to cease breastfeeding?
2. Describe the adequacy of the baby's current energy intake per unit of body weight.
3. What developmental landmarks can be expected next? How will they affect the foods offered and Scott's participation in his feeding? What anticipatory guidance would you offer this family in relation to Scott's feeding?
4. How would you expect the addition of new foods to Scott's diet to affect Scott's energy intake?

CASE STUDY

Case 3

Mother Wonders Why John Isn't Gaining Weight

Baby John is seen in a pediatrics clinic where he has been followed since shortly after birth. At 6 ½ months his mother does not want to feed John an iron-containing formula, is concerned about his constipation, and has questions about how to introduce semisolids into his diet. She has tried to introduce rice and oatmeal cereals, and fruits and vegetables without success.

Baby John, a male with trisomy 21 Down syndrome, was adopted at birth. He is mildly hypotonic. His father is currently unemployed. His mother has had previous experience with children who are delayed. She helped raise her brother who also was born with Down syndrome and currently lives with the family.

At three months baby John was hospitalized with tachypnea (an abnormally rapid rate of breathing). During that time his cardiac status was found to be normal. An upper GI series and video fluoroscopic swallowing study indicated no abnormalities and normal swallow.

The baby receives occupational/physical therapy during home visits twice a week.

He has had intermittent problems with constipation since birth. He currently produces slightly hard, dry stools every 2 to 3 days. His mother feels that iron-containing formula increases these problems and uses a low-iron formula. He consumes six 5 oz bottles of formula a day at intervals of 2 to 3 hours. He sleeps through the night. He has four to eight wet diapers a day.

Baby John's weights and lengths recorded in his chart are:

Age	Height	Weight
3 months	55.3 cm	4.8 kg
4 months	58.4	5.33
5 months	60.0	5.7
6 months	61.0	5.9

This 6-month-old hypotonic baby needs to be held when fed. His head control is poor. He consumes his food with a suckle using tongue thrust swallow.

Questions for analysis

1. Compare baby John's physical growth on an NCHS (Appendix A) and a Down growth chart (on p. 274).
2. What would you suggest be done about the mother's reluctance to use an iron-containing formula?
3. Is John's energy intake adequate?
4. Is it developmentally appropriate for John to be offered semisolid foods? How would you council his mother about adding new food to his diet?

Boys with Down Syndrome:
Physical Growth: 1 to 36 Months

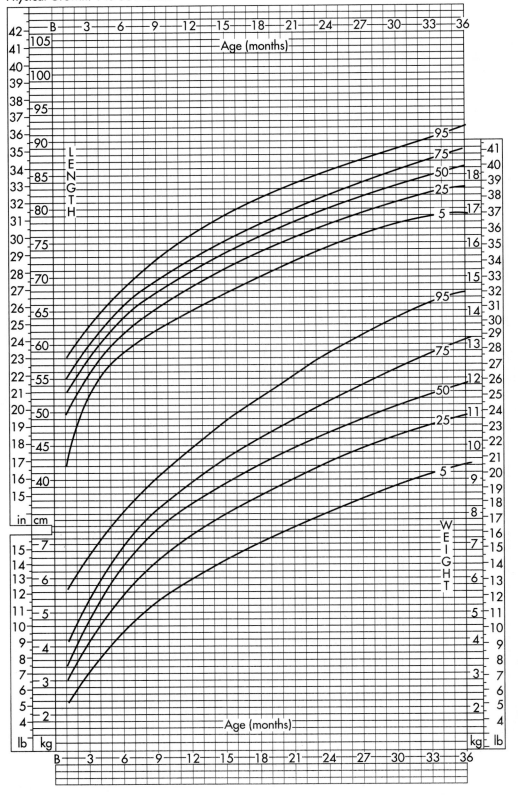

FIG. 6-6   Growth chart for boys with Down Syndrome, 1 to 36 months.

Summary

Adequate nourishment for infants can be achieved through consumption of a variety of combinations of milks, supplements, and semisolid foods. Maturation of the oral and fine motor skills indicates appropriate stages for the introduction of semisolid and solid foods. Current recommendations include breastfeeding by an adequately nourished mother and the introduction of semisolid foods at 4 to 6 months of age, and of finger foods when the infant reaches out, grasps, and brings items to his mouth.

If the mother is unable or unwilling to breastfeed her child, a variety of properly constructed infant formulas are marketed that have been proven to support normal growth and development in infants. It is to the formula-fed baby's advantage to receive a formula with iron.

Infants should be permitted to establish their own feeding schedule and be fed to satiety. When they develop a voluntary mature sucking pattern, the introduction of semisolid foods is appropriate. When munching and rotary chewing begin, the use of soft-cooked table foods is appropriate. Infants can begin to drink from a cup with help between 9 and 12 months of age.

Review Questions

1. Why is there such a wide range of acceptable intakes of energy during infancy?
2. Under what circumstances should the infant's water intake be carefully monitored?
3. What is the difference in fat absorption of human and cow's milk?
4. What supplements should be given to a solely breastfed 3-month-old male infant?
5. Describe the difference between sucking and suckling.
6. What developmental landmarks indicate a readiness for semisolid foods to be added to the infant's diet?
7. At what age is it reasonable to feed whole cow's milk?
8. Why is it important for a baby to go to sleep without a bottle?
9. At what age is it important to add iron to the breastfed infant's diet?
10. Explain how growth charts are used to assess the adequacy of a baby's energy and nutrient intake.

References

1. Smith D et al: Shifting linear growth during infancy, *J Pediatr* 89:225, 1976.
2. National Center for Health Statistics: NCHS growth charts, 1976, *Monthly vital statistics report,* vol 25, no 3, suppl (HRA) 76-1120, Rockville, Md, 1976, Health Resources Administration.
3. Fomon SJ: *Nutrition of normal infants,* St Louis, 1993, Mosby.
4. Lebenthal EL, Lee PIC, Heitlinger LA: Impact of development of the gastrointestinal tract on infant feeding, *J Pediatr* 102:1, 1983.
5. Ziegler E, Fomon J: Potential renal solute load of infant formulas, *J Nutr* 119:1785, 1989.
6. Food and Nutrition Board, National Research Council, National Academy of Sciences: *Recommended Dietary Allowances,* ed 10, Washington, DC, 1989, National Academy Press.
7. WHO (World Health Organization): *Energy and protein requirements, Report of a joint FAO/WHO/UNU Expert Consultation,* Technical Series 724, 1985, World Health Organization.
8. Committee on Nutrition, American Academy of Pediatrics: Commentary on breast-feeding and infant formulas, including proposed standards for formulas, *Pediatrics* 57:279, 1976.
9. Holt LE Jr, Snyderman SE: The amino acid requirements of infants, *J Am Nurs Assoc* 175:100, 1961.
10. Fomon SJ, Filer LJ: *Amino acid requirements for normal growth.* In Nyhan WL, editor: *Amino acid metabolism and genetic variation,* New York, 1967, McGraw-Hill.
11. Report of a Joint FAO/WHO Ad Hoc Expert Committee: *Energy and protein requirements,* World Health Organization Technical Series No 522, FAO Nutr Meet Ser No 52, Geneva, 1973, World Health Organization.

12. Partridge JC et al: Water intoxication secondary to feeding mismanagement, *Am J Dis Child* 135:38, 1981.

13. McMillan MA, Landau SA, Oski FA: Iron sufficiency in breast milk and the availability of iron from human milk, *Pediatrics* 58:686, 1976.

14. Calvo EB, Galindo AC, Aspres NB: Iron status in exclusively breast fed infants, *Pediatrics* 90:375-379, 1992.

15. Committee on Nutrition, American Academy of Pediatrics: Iron-fortified infant formulas, *Pediatrics* 84:114, 1989.

16. MacDonald LD, Gibson RS, Miles JE: Changes in hair zinc and copper concentrations of breast-fed and bottle-fed infants during the first six months, *Acta Paediatr Scand* 71:758, 1982.

17. Cavell PA, Widdowson EM: Intakes and excretion of iron, copper, and zinc in the neonatal period, *Arch Dis Child* 39:496, 1964.

18. Johnson PE, Evans GW: Relative zinc availability in human breast milk, infant formulas, and cow's milk, *Am J Clin Nutr* 31:416, 1978.

19. ESPGAN (European Society of Paediatric Gastroenterology and Nutrition), Committee on Nutrition: Guidelines on infant nutrition. I. Recommendations for the composition of an adapted formula, *Acta Paediatr Scand* Suppl. 287:1, 1981.

20. ESPGAN (European Society of Paediatric Gastroenterology and Nutrition) Committee on Nutrition: Guidelines on infant nutrition. II. Recommendations for the composition of follow-up formula and beikost, *Acta Paediatr Scand* Suppl 287:1, 1981.

21. ESPGAN (European Society of Paediatric Gastroenterology and Nutrition) Committee on Nutrition: Comments on the composition of cow's milk based follow-up formulas, *Acta Paediatr Scand* 79:250, 1990.

22. ESPGAN (European Society of Paediatric Gastroenterology and Nutrition) Committee on Nutrition: Comments on the content and composition of lipids in infant formulas, *Acta Paediatr Scand* 80:887, 1991.

23. Joint FAO/WHO Codex standards for foods for special dietary uses including foods for infants and children and related code of hygienic practice, CAC/Vol. 9, ed 1, suppl 4, Rome, 1989, Food and Agriculture Organization of the United Nations/World Health Organization.

24. Food and Drug Directorate: Food and drug regulations, Division 25, *Canada Gazette*, 124:73E-73H, 1990.

25. Food and Drug Administration: Rules and regulations: Nutrient requirements for infant formulas (21 CFR Part 107), *Fed Reg* 50:45106, 1985.

26. Ziegler EE et al: Cow's milk feeding in infancy: further observations on blood loss from the gastrointestinal tract, *J Pediatr* 116:11, 1990.

27. Fabius RJ et al: Malnutrition associated with a formula of barley water, corn syrup, and whole milk, *Am J Dis Child* 135:615, 1981.

28. Sinatra FR, Merritt RJ: Iatrogenic kwashiorkor in infants, *Am J Dis Child* 135:21, 1981.

29. Committee on Nutrition, American Academy of Pediatrics: Imitation and substitute milks, *Pediatrics* 73:876, 1984.

30. Comay SC, Karabus CD: Peripheral gangrene in hypernatremic dehydration of infancy, *Arch Dis Child* 50:616, 1975.

31. Illingworth RS, Lister J: The critical or sensitive period with special reference to certain feeding problems in infants and children, *J Pediatr* 65:839, 1964.

32. Gesell A, Ilg FL: *Feeding behavior of infants,* Philadelphia, 1937, JB Lippincott.

33. Subtelny JD: Examination of current philosophies associated with swallowing behavior, *Am J Orthod* 51:135, 1965.

34. Arnon SS et al: Honey and other environmental risk factors for infant botulism, *Pediatrics* 94:331, 1979.

35. Thoman EB: Development of synchrony in mother-infant interaction in feeding and other situations, *Fed Proc* 34:1587, 1975.

36. Butte NF, Smith EO, Garza C: Energy utilization of breast-fed and formula-fed infants, *Am J Clin Nutr* 51:350, 1990.

37. Henig MJ et al: Energy and protein intakes of breast-fed and formula-fed infants during the first year of life and their association with growth velocity: The Darling Study, *Am J Clin Nutr* 58: 152, 1993.

38. Sullivan SA, Birch LL: Infant dietary experience and acceptance of solid foods, *Pediatrics* 93:271, 1994.

39. Smith MM, Litshitz F: Excess fruit juice consumption as a contributing factor in nonorganic failure to thrive, *Pediatrics* 93: 438, 1994.

40. Lothe L, Lindberg T, Jakobsson I: Cow's milk formula as a cause of infantile colic, *Pediatrics* 70: 7, 1982.

41. Fomon SJ et al: Indices of fatness and serum cholesterol at eight years in relation to feeding and growth during infancy, *Pediatr Res* 18: 1223, 1984.

42. Shapiro LR et al: Obesity prognosis: a longitudinal study of children from the age of 6 months to 9 years, *Am J Public Health* 74: 968, 1984.

Further Reading

Fuchs GJ et al: Iron status and intake of older infants fed formula vs. cow's milk with cereal, *Am J Clin Nutr* 58:343, 1993.

104 infants who entered this study at 4 to 6 months were randomly assigned to one of four feeding groups; a ready-to-feed iron-fortified formula, one of two follow-up formulas, or whole cow's milk and cereal. At 12 months significantly more infants who had had whole milk and cereal had lower serum ferritin and corpuscular volume than those who had consumed the iron-fortified formula and significantly more had serum ferritin concentrations less than 12/L.

Duncan B et al: Exclusive breast-feeding for at least 4 months protects against otitis media, *Pediatrics* 91: 867, 1993.

A study designed to assess the relation of exclusive breastfeeding to the incidence of otitis media for the first year found that infants exclusively breastfed for 4 or more months had half the number of episodes of acute otitis media of infants not breastfed and 40% less than those whose diets were supplemented with other foods prior to 4 months.

Johnson CE et al: Selenium status of term infants fed human milk or selenite-supplemented soy formula, *J Pediatr* 122:739, 1993.

Infants fed human milk had plasma and erythrocyte selenium values higher than those fed a soy formula with selenite although plasma and glutathione peroxidase activities were normal in both groups indicating that functional requirements were met. The lower plasma and erothrocyte from soy formula indicated selenite is not accumulating in the body and was thought to be beneficial considering the potential toxicity of selenium.

Zeghound F et al: Vitamin D prophylaxis during infancy: comparison of the long-term effects of three intermittent doses (15, 5, or 2.5 mg) on 25-hydroxyvitamin D concentrations, *Am J Clin Nutr* 60:393, 1994.

This study tested the effectiveness and potential toxicity of three doses of vitamin D (15 mg given one time, 5 mg at intervals of 6 months, or 2.5 mg given every 3 months) in infants from birth to 6-9 months. Oral doses of 2.5 mg every three months seem to provide the best protection against Vitamin D deficiency and toxicity in high-risk infant populations.

Michaelsen KF et al: The Copenhagen cohort study on infant nutrition and growth: breast milk intake, human milk macronutrient content, and influencing factors, *Am J Clin Nutr* 59:600, 1994.

Breast milk intakes were measured in healthy term infants at 2, 4, and 9 months; macronutrient content of the milk was analyzed. Intakes at 2 and 4 months averaged 781 and 855 ml/day, respectively. Intake was correlated with the weight of the infant. Median protein intake was 1.3, and 1.0 g/kg at the same ages.

Graham SM, Arvela OM, Wise GA: Long-term neurologic consequences of nutritional vitamin B_{12} deficiency in infants, *J Pediatr* 121:710, 1992.

A review of six infants who had experienced Vitamin B_{12} deficiency during the first year found irritability, anorexia, failure to thrive, developmental regression, and poor brain growth to be consistent symptoms. During follow-up two of four of children were reported to have borderline intelligence at ages 4 and 5 years.

7

Nutrition in Childhood

Peggy Pipes
Cristine M. Trahms

Basic Concepts

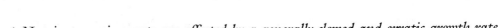

✔ *Nutrient requirements are affected by a generally slowed and erratic growth rate between infancy and adolescence and a child's individual needs.*

✔ *A child's food choices are determined by numerous family and community factors.*

✔ *Nutrient intake and developing food patterns in young children are governed by food availability and food choices.*

✔ *Considerations in feeding young children are guided by meeting physical and psychosocial needs.*

✔ *Nutrition concerns during childhood relate to growth and development needs for positive health.*

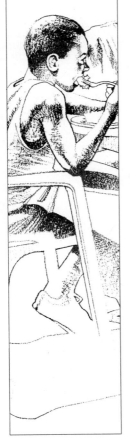

After the infant's first year of rapid growth, the interval between infancy and adolescence is a period of slower growth. This interval is a time for the acquisition of skills that permit independence in eating and feeding and the development of individual food preferences. The development of gross motor skills makes increased activity possible. Preschool children learn to control body functions, to interact with others, and to behave in a socially acceptable manner. School-age children attempt to develop personal independence and establish a scale of values. Individual variations in children become more noticeable in such areas as rates of growth, activity patterns, nutrient requirements, personality development, and food intakes.

There is a wide range of nutrient requirements of children at any age during this period. Body size and composition, activity patterns, and rates of growth influence basic needs. The foods available to and accepted by the child are determined not only by parental food selection but also by the mealtime environment, peer pressures, advertising, and the child's food experiences. If appropriate support is provided by parents, food patterns that support normal growth and weight, ensure good dental hygiene, and prevent nutritional deficiencies including iron-deficiency anemia can be established.

PHYSICAL GROWTH DURING CHILDHOOD
Growth Rate

The rapid rate of growth during infancy is followed by a deceleration during the preschool and school-age years. Weight gain approximates 4 to 6 lb (1.8 to 2.7 kg) per year. Length increases approximately 3 inches (7.6 cm) per year between 1 year and 7 to 8 years of age, then increases 2 inches (5.1 cm) per year until the pubertal growth spurt. Between 6 years of age and the adolescent growth spurt, gender differences can be noted. At age 6 boys are taller and heavier than girls. By age 9 the height of the average female is the same as that of the 9-year-old male and her weight is slightly more.

Racial differences have been noted in rates of growth. American black infants are smaller than American white infants at birth. However, they grow more rapidly during the first 2 years of life, and from 2 years of age through adolescence are taller than American white children of the same age. Asian children tend to be smaller than black children and white children.[1] Recent assessments of growth of specific populations of children indicate that Mexican-American children, regardless of family income, tend to be shorter and heavier than either African-American or white children of the same ages.[2] A longitudinal survey of Southeast Asian refugee children indicated a marked improvement in growth status of those children and eventual achievement of growth curves much like children of similar ethnic backgrounds.[3]

Body Composition

Muscle mass accounts for an increasingly greater percentage of body weight during the preschool years. Children become leaner as they grow older. Fatfold measurements decrease. Females, however, have more subcutaneous fat than males.

Brain growth is 75% complete by the end of the second year; by 6 to 10 years of age brain growth is complete. This results in a decrease in head size in relation to body size.

Body fluid proportion is similar to that of an adult by the time the child is 2 to 3 years of age. Rapid shifts in fluid between intracellular and extracellular compartments are less likely. The child is less vulnerable to dehydration than the infant. The extracellular fluid continues to decrease while intracellular fluid increases because of the growth of new cells. The approximate percentage of total body fluid is 59% in the toddler compared with 64% in the adult male.

Bone growth results in increased stature. Bone is not an inert tissue and is constantly being remodeled by destruction and renewal of collagen and the addition and loss of mineral. Increases in skeletal length are achieved by this process of dissolution and reshaping of bone. The school-age child with longer legs appears more graceful and slimmer than the preschooler.

Growth Charts

Normal differences in individual children become apparent in the percentile channel of growth followed by each child. Once the percentile ranking is established on the growth chart, children can be expected to maintain **growth channels** when sequential measurements over time are recorded. However, physicians will not predict later height from growth charts before a child is 2 years of age. It is more important to know that a child is maintaining his height and weight in relation to other children and in the weight-height percentile than it is to know that they are tall or short.

The infant growth charts, as described in Chapter 6 (p. 238), are constructed to 36 months of age and should be used until the child is at least 24 months old. The growth charts for children from 2 to 18 years of age were prepared from data from the National Health and Nutrition Examination Surveys (NHANES).[4] It should be noted that length

Growth channel
The progressive regular growth pattern of children, guided along individual genetically controlled channels, influenced by nutritional and health status.

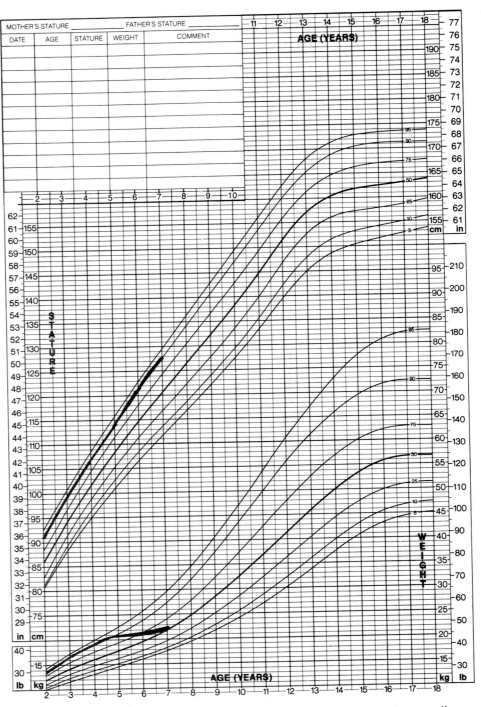

FIG. 7-1 The growth chart of a female whose weight remained in the 90th percentile over time but who became anorexic at 4½ years. She did not consume enough food to support an appropriate weight gain.

Courtesy Ross Laboratories.

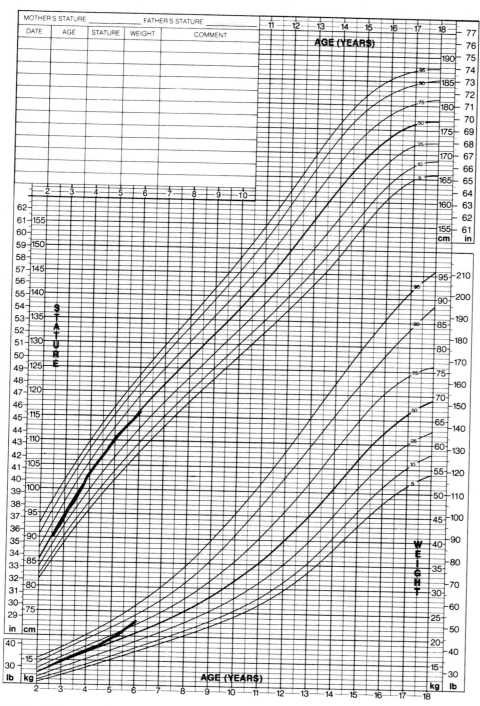

FIG. 7-2 The growth chart of a male who began eating excessive amounts of high calorie food at age 4½ years. His rate of weight gain increased.

Courtesy Ross Laboratories.

measurements on the infant chart are recumbent lengths and those on the children's chart are standing height measurements. Children should be weighed in stocking feet and standard examination clothing on a beam balance scale. Standing height is measured using a hard board while the heels, buttocks, and shoulders touch a flat wall (see Chapter 6). It is not unusual for small changes to occur in length percentile ratings on growth charts when changing from recumbent to upright measurement.

Excesses or inadequacies in energy and nutrient intakes as well as the genetic potential for growth will be reflected in patterns of growth. The child who is not eating sufficient food will show a decrease in channel of weight gain charts (Fig. 7-1). Changes in height or weight channel may also be a reflection of genetic potential for growth. If food deprivation is severe enough and lasts long enough, rates of linear growth will be reduced or growth will cease. Intakes of energy in excess of expenditure will be noted by increases in weight percentile (Fig. 7-2).[5-6]

Feeding Skills

The child's rate of physical growth will also be reflected in the development of self-feeding skills. Children learn to feed themselves independently during the second year of life. The 15-month-old child will have difficulty scooping food into the spoon and bringing food to the mouth without turning the spoon upside down and spilling its contents because of lack of wrist control. By 2 years of age spilling seldom occurs.

By 16 to 17 months of age a well-defined **ulnar deviation** of the wrist occurs and the contents of the spoon may be transferred more steadily to the mouth. By 18 months of age the child lifts the elbow as the spoon is raised and flexes the wrist as the spoon reaches the mouth so that only moderate spilling occurs, in contrast to earlier stages of self-feeding.

Handedness is not established at 1 year of age. Children may grasp the spoon with either hand and find when they try to fill the spoon that the bowl is upside down.

A refined pincer grasp will have been developed in the first year. Finger-feeding is easy and often preferred. Foods that provide opportunities for finger-feeding should be

Ulnar deviation

Turning and articulation of the *ulna* (inner and larger bone of the forearm on the side opposite the thumb) with the wrist joint to accomplish coordinated movement of the wrist and hand.

TABLE 7-1 *Appropriate Finger Foods for Young Children With a Refined Pincer Grasp*

Appropriate Foods (no skins or peeling)	Inappropriate Foods (may cause choking or gagging)
Dry cereal: Cheerios, Kix	
Banana slices	Dried fruits: raisins, coconut, dates
Soft cut-up fruit	Small fruit with skin or peel: grapes
Mealy apple	Raw vegetables
Canned or well-cooked vegetables (green beans, broccoli, carrots)	
Cheese sticks, hard cheese (cheddar, Monterey Jack)	Processed American cheese
Large curd cottage cheese	
Small pieces tender meats (small meatballs, chicken)	Hot dogs
Scrambled eggs	Nuts, including peanuts
Fish sticks (no bones)	Peanut butter
Oven-dried toast	Popcorn
Zwieback toast	Potato chips
Arrowroot biscuits	Corn chips
Graham crackers	Tortilla chips

provided at each meal (Table 7-1), avoiding inappropriate ones that may cause choking. Young children, especially preschoolers, are at risk of choking on food. Death from asphyxiation resulting from intakes of small pieces of food has been described primarily among children less than 2 years of age. Foods most often responsible include hot dogs, hard candy, nuts, and grapes. Children will often place food in the spoon with their fingers and may finger-feed foods that are commonly spoon-fed, such as vegetables and pudding.

By 15 months of age children can manage a cup, but will have difficulty in lifting, tilting, and lowering it. The cup is tilted, using the palm, often too rapidly. By 18 to 24 months of age the cup will be tilted by manipulation of the fingers.

Children refine the rotary chewing movements that began at 1 year of age. The ability to chew hard and fibrous foods will increase through the school years.

NUTRIENT NEEDS OF CHILDREN

Recommendations for energy intakes for children have been derived from intakes of normal healthy children growing satisfactorily. Recommendations for nutrient intakes are based on only a few balance studies, mostly extrapolated from requirements for infants and adults. It is important to remember that the range of adequate intakes is quite wide among groups of children. The Recommended Dietary Allowances (RDAs) provide guidelines for studying groups of children but not for evaluating diets of individual children.[7]

Energy

Individual needs. The energy requirements for individual children are determined by resting energy expenditure (REE), rate of growth, and activity. REE varies with the amount and composition of **metabolically active** tissue, which varies with age and gender. However, gender differences are relatively small until children reach 10 years of age and no gender differences have been made in recommended energy intakes before these ages. The average energy cost of growth after infancy is small, about 5 kcal/g of tissue gained. The energy needs of individual children of the same age, gender, and size vary. Reasons for these differences remain unexplained. Differences in physical activity, in the metabolic cost of minimal and excessive protein intakes at equivalent levels of energy intake, and in the efficiency with which individuals utilize energy have all been hypothesized to exert an influence. The RDA guidelines established by the Food and Nutrition Board of the National Research Council are given in Table 7-2.[7,8]

Physical activity. The contribution of physical activity to total energy expenditure is quite variable among children and in individual children from day to day. At all ages activity patterns among children show wide ranges both in the time spent in the various activities and in the intensity of the activities. Some children may engage in sedentary activities such

Metabolic activity
Sum of biochemical actions and reactions in the body that build and maintain tissue, regulate body functions, and require a constant energy source. The most metabolically active body tissue is the lean body mass.

TABLE 7-2   Recommended Energy Intakes for Children

Age (years)	Weight (kg)	Height (cm)	Energy Allowances/Day (kcal)	Energy Allowances/kg/Day (kcal)
1-3	13	90	1300	102
4-6	20	112	1800	90
7-10	28	132	2000	70

From National Academy of Sciences: *Recommended dietary allowances,* ed 10, Washington, DC, 1989, National Academy Press.

as looking at books or watching television, whereas their peers may be engaged in physical activities that demand running, jumping, and general body movements. The energy expenditure for physical activity of fourth- and fifth-grade school children, for example, was estimated to be 31.2% and 25.3% of total energy expenditure for males and females, respectively.[9]

Studies indicate that the actual energy intakes of children agree with the recommended intakes. However, wide-ranging intakes will be noted among individual children. The most appropriate evaluation of adequacy of a child's energy intake is based on observation of rates of growth as depicted on growth charts and on measurements of body fat.

Catch-up growth. During a period of catch-up growth, the requirements for energy and nutrients will be greatly increased. Daily intakes of 150 to 250 kcal/kg of body weight have been recommended for children of preschool age. An intake of 200 kcal/kg/day should produce a weight gain of 20 g/day.[10]

Protein

Basis of need. The protein needs of children include those for maintenance of tissue, changes in body composition, and synthesis of new tissue. During growth, the protein content of the body increases from 14.6% at 1 year of age to 18% to 19%, which are adult values, by 4 years of age. Estimates of protein needs for growth range from 1 to 4 g/kg of tissue gained. As the rate of growth falls, maintenance requirements gradually represent an increasing proportion of the total protein requirement.

Recommended intakes. The recommended protein intake, calculated on the maintenance requirements of the adult, growth rates, and body composition, gradually decreases from 1.3 g/kg at 1 year of age to 1.0 g/kg at 10 years of age (Table 7-3).[7,11] This intake approximates 4% to 5% of the total kilocalories, less than most children consume. Protein provided 13% to 15% of the energy intake in the average child's diet.

An evaluation of a child's protein intake must be based on the adequacy of growth rate, the quality of protein in the foods eaten, combinations of foods that provide **complementary amino acids** when consumed together, and the adequacy of those nutrients, vitamins and minerals, and energy that are necessary for protein synthesis to proceed.

Inadequate protein intakes are rarely noted in North America. Some children have such limited energy intakes that part of the protein consumed must be used for body fuel. Children who consume a **vegan diet** have been reported to be shorter and leaner than the average child.[12,13]

Minerals and Vitamins

Minerals and vitamins are necessary for normal growth and development. Inadequate intakes will be reflected in slow growth rates, inadequate mineralization of bones, insufficient iron stores, and anemia. The RDAs are shown in Tables 7-4 and 7-5.

Calcium. How much calcium does a child need to grow properly? Attempts to establish

Complementary amino acids

Combinations of amino acids from a variety of combined protein foods that complement one another according to their relative amounts of the individual amino acids; in order to meet growth requirements for the nine essential amino acids that the body does not sufficiently synthesize.

Vegan diet

Strict vegetarian diet that does not allow any animal protein; requires careful food combinations of incomplete plant proteins to complement one another and achieve an overall adequacy of essential amino acids for growth needs.

TABLE 7-3   Recommended Dietary Allowances of Protein

Age (years)	Protein (g/kg)	Protein (g/day)
1-3	1.2	16
4-6	1.1	24
7-10	1.0	28

From National Academy of Sciences: *Recommended dietary allowances,* ed 10, Washington, DC, 1989, National Academy Press.

recommended intakes of calcium have caused considerable controversy for many years. Calcium is essential for bone growth and mineralization. More than 98% of body calcium is bone. Absorption of calcium fluctuates from 30% to 60% of intake. Lactose increases absorption. Binders such as **phytic acid** and **oxalic acid** reduce absorption. The level of dietary protein affects the urinary excretion of calcium. As levels of protein intake increase, levels of urinary calcium increase.

It is estimated that daily calcium accretion rates must average 150-200 mg calcium/day with a peak of 400 mg/day during rapid growth. Recommendations for children are set at 800 mg/day since growing children may need two to four times as much calcium per unit of body weight as adults require. It is suggested that low calcium intake is a factor that limits linear growth and bone mineralization. There is also the likelihood that efficiency of absorption and conservation of calcium may, in fact, increase with low calcium intake and high biologic requirement.[14]

Milk and other dairy products are the primary sources of bioavailable calcium. Thus children who consume limited amounts of these products risk a deficient calcium intake. **Zinc.** The trace mineral zinc is essential for normal protein synthesis and growth. Variations in plasma zinc concentrations during growth reflect the continual use and

Phytic acid
A compound in certain grains, such as wheat, that binds calcium and hinders its absorption.

Oxalic acid
A compound in a variety of foods, including green leafy vegetables, corn, soy products such as tofu, and wheat germ, that binds calcium in the food mix and hinders its absorption.

TABLE 7-4 *Recommended Daily Dietary Allowances for Minerals*

Age (years)	Calcium (mg)	Phosphorus (mg)	Iodine (µg)	Iron (mg)	Magnesium (mg)	Zinc (mg)	Selenium (µg)
1-3	800	800	70	10	80	10	20
4-6	800	800	90	10	120	10	20
7-10	800	800	120	10	170	10	30

TABLE 7-5 *Recommended Dietary Allowances of Vitamins*

Vitamin	Age (years)		
	1-3	4-6	7-10
Fat-Soluble			
Vitamin A (µg RE)	400	500	700
Vitamin D (µg)	10	10	10
Vitamin E (mg α-TE)	6	7	7
Vitamin K (µg)	15	20	30
Water-Soluble			
Thiamin (mg)	0.7	0.9	1.0
Riboflavin (mg)	0.8	1.1	1.2
Niacin (mg)	9	12	13
Vitamin B$_6$ (mg)	1.0	1.1	1.4
Folate (µg)	50	75	100
Vitamin B$_{12}$ (µg)	0.7	1.0	1.4
Ascorbic acid (mg)	40	45	45

From National Academy of Sciences: *Recommended dietary allowances*, ed 10, Washington, DC, 1989, National Academy Press.

depletion of body stores of zinc. Zinc deficiency has serious consequences; most notable are growth retardation, hypogeusia, and diarrhea, as well as impaired wound healing and cell-mediated immunity. Zinc intakes of children 1 to 3 years of age have been estimated to average 5 mg/day; those of children 3 to 5 years of age average 5 to 7 mg/day.[15]

There is speculation that poor linear growth in early childhood in some low-income populations may result from a growth-limiting zinc deficiency state. A study of Hispanic-American children 2 to 6 years of age who consumed 5 to 6 mg of zinc per day and whose linear growth was below the 10th percentile found low hair and plasma zinc levels. Increasing their zinc intake to 10 mg/day increased rates of linear growth.[16]

Small amounts of zinc are more efficiently absorbed than large amounts. Children in poor zinc status absorb zinc more efficiently than those in good status. High intakes of phytate and fiber depress zinc absorption. The bioavailability of zinc varies with the food source. Meats are a good source of available zinc; cereal grains contain a less available form of zinc. The average toddler in the United States consumes 8.5 mg of zinc per day.

Iron. Iron deficiency is the most common nutritional deficiency. It occurs most frequently in children 4 to 24 months of age, in adolescent males, and in females in their childbearing years. It may result from inadequate iron intake, impaired absorption, a large hemorrhage, or repeated small blood losses. Iron deficiency anemia in preschool children causes delayed mental and physical development and decreased resistance to infection.

The RDA guidelines assume 10% iron absorption and are planned to meet variations of need in individuals.[7] Iron requirements of individual children vary with rates of growth and increasing total iron mass, iron stores, variations in menstrual losses of iron in adolescent females, and the timing of the growth spurt of adolescents. Larger, more rapidly growing children have the greatest requirements for iron because they are increasing their blood volumes more rapidly.

Prevention of anemia. Many younger preschoolers do not have the oral motor strength to masticate meat and prefer **nonheme** plant sources of iron. The consumption of foods or a supplement containing vitamin C along with the foods containing nonheme iron can help increase the amount of the iron absorbed. Absorption can also be increased by consuming meat when nonheme iron is ingested. Iron absorption is decreased by antacids, bran, and tea. Also, directing parents to use more foods containing heme iron that are easier to chew, such as ground beef, can increase iron intake. For children whose iron intake is limited, a supplemental maintenance dose of iron (10 mg/day) may be indicated. Children with diagnosed iron-deficiency anemia will receive therapeutic doses of iron, 3 mg/kg/day, for 3 months.

> **Nonheme iron**
> The larger portion of dietary iron, including all of the plant food sources and 60% of the animal food sources, that lacks the more easily absorbed and bioavailable heme iron in the remaining 40% of the animal food sources that contain hemoglobin residues of iron-containing heme.

It is increasingly clear that iron deficiency anemia causes long-term developmental effects. The iron status of a group of infants in Costa Rica was re-evaluated at age 5 years. The children all demonstrated reasonable growth and iron status at that time. Those children who had demonstrated moderately severe iron-deficiency anemia (hemoglobin <10 mg/l) in infancy had lower mental and motor-functioning scores at age 5.[17]

Children whose families had incomes adequate to provide day care appeared to have difficulty in acquiring an adequate intake of iron. These children demonstrated normal growth attainment, energy intakes at 70% of the RDA, and a nutrient intake of >75% of the RDA for all nutrients except iron and folic acid which were 50% of the RDA. The low iron intakes were reflected in low biochemical indices for iron stores.[18]

It has been suggested, based on a review of iron supplementation studies worldwide, that a weekly iron supplement to young children at risk for iron deficiency may improve weight gain, appetite, and psychomotor and mental development.[19]

Vitamins. The function of vitamins in metabolic processes means that their requirements are determined by intakes of energy, protein, and saturated fats. Exact needs are difficult

TABLE 7-6A   *Estimated Safe and Adequate Daily Dietary Intakes of Selected Trace Minerals for Children*

Age (years)	Copper (mg)	Manganese (mg)	Fluoride (mg)	Chromium (μg)	Molybdenum (μg)
1-3	0.7-1.0	1.0-1.5	0.5-1.5	20-80	25-50
4-6	1.0-1.5	1.5-2.0	1.0-2.5	30-120	30-75
7-10	1.0-2.0	2.0-3.0	1.5-2.5	50-200	50-150
11+	1.5-2.5	2.0-5.0	1.5-2.5	50-200	75-250

TABLE 7-6B   *Estimated Minimum Requirements of Electrolytes*

Age (years)	Sodium (mg)	Potassium (mg)	Chloride (mg)
2-5	300	1400	500
6-9	400	1600	600
10-18	500	2000	750

From National Academy of Sciences: *Recommended dietary allowances,* ed 10, Washington, DC, 1989, National Academy Press.

to define. The RDA guidelines for most vitamins and for some trace minerals (Table 7-6) are interpolated from infant and adult allowances or calculated on the basis of energy and protein allowances.

Ethnic, geographic, and situation variation in nutrient intake and subsequent concerns about nutritional status and deficiency have long been documented. Recent studies have documented the extent of hungry children in the United States. It is estimated that one out of three poor children (living in households at or below 50 percent of poverty level) does not obtain even two thirds of the RDA for energy.[20]

Mexican-American Children

Mexican-American children have been considered at high risk for inadequate nutrient intakes. Mexican-American preschool children in San Diego demonstrated worrisome intakes ($<\frac{2}{3}$ of the RDA) for iron, zinc, vitamin D, vitamin C, and niacin. Mexican-American girls also had a significantly lower calcium intake. The study participants were all lower income to lower-middle income families.[21] Another recent report suggests that these children consume vegetables less often than other groups of children. Twenty-five percent of the children consumed no vegetables.[22]

American Indian Children

Long-term concern has been demonstrated about the adequacy of nutrient intakes and growth for American Indian children. Height and weight status of school-aged American Indian children was assessed. The overall prevalence of overweight in this group was 40% compared with the NHANES II reference population and about 29% compared with the HHANES-MA Mexican-American population. Overweight is much more prevalent in American Indian children than among other children in the United States at all ages and in both sexes.[23]

Foster Care

There is little known of the nutritional intake of young children in foster care in the United States. These children are vulnerable for many reasons including the crises in their lives and a high incidence of health problems. The chaotic social situation is considered to be a precursor for negative feeding behaviors and poor nutritional intake.[24]

Homeless Children

Unfortunately, homelessness is an all too common occurrence in the United States. It has been estimated that each night there are about 100,000 homeless children and about half of these children are under 6 years of age. Efforts have been made to assess the nutrition and growth of young children without homes. Compared with children of similar ages and income level in homes, homeless children demonstrated a growth pattern compatible with moderate, chronic nutritional deprivation, that is, stunting without wasting. This indicates a dietary pattern that is not deficient in total energy but rather inadequate in some nutrients and composed primarily of cheaper carbohydrate-rich foods.[25]

Height-for-age and weight-for-age measurements of homeless children in Baltimore were generally comparable to other groups of low income children.[26] Intakes of all nutrients except calcium (77% of the RDA) and zinc (79% of the RDA) met or exceeded the RDAs for preschool children. Nutrient-fortified ready-to-eat cereals were credited with providing many of the nutrients consumed since fruits, vegetables, and dairy products were seldom available.

Calculated nutrient intakes of young children living in temporary shelters indicated very low iron and folic acid intakes, 40% and 30% of the RDA, respectively, and moderate intakes of all other nutrients (>60% RDA). The overall dietary adequacy score was low.[27]

Vitamin Supplementation

Dietary evaluation. Vitamin supplementation of children's diets should be recommended only after careful evaluation of the child's food intake. Diets of children who restrict their intake of milk because of documented or suspected allergies, lactose intolerance, or for psychosocial reasons should be monitored for adequate intakes of riboflavin and vitamin D. Diets of infants and children receiving goat's milk should be carefully monitored for food sources of folate. Diets of children who consume limited amounts of fruits and vegetables should be checked for sources of vitamins A and C.

Children at risk. The Committee on Nutrition of the American Academy of Pediatrics has defined six groups of children at particular risk and for whom vitamin supplementation may be appropriate.[28]

1. Children from deprived families, especially those who suffer from parental neglect or abuse
2. Children who have anorexia, poor and capricious appetites, poor eating habits, or those who consume fad diets
3. Children with chronic disease
4. Children on dietary regimens to manage obesity
5. Pregnant teenagers
6. Children who consume vegan diets

Those children needing supplements can be determined by a nutritional assessment, and in addition to the above, might include children with food allergies, limited food acceptance, or frequent or chronic illness. Any vitamin supplements, especially those that are colored and sugar coated, should be stored in places inaccessible to young children.

The importance of appropriate vitamin supplementation of breastfed infants is discussed in Chapter 6. After infancy, however, the percentage of toddlers who are given vitamin supplements declines. But over half of the preschool and school-age children receive multivitamin/mineral preparations.

Vitamin supplementation is often considered advisable. No significant differences have been noted in biochemical indices with the exception of red blood cell folate of children who used supplements compared with those who did not, even though mean intakes of vitamin B_6 of the nonsupplemented group were 30% below the RDA.[29] Many of the nonsupplemented children did not ingest two thirds of the RDA for folate. All blood values were in the range of accepted standards. In general, supplements are more often used by children from families who are better educated. Fewer children take iron supplements alone; supplemental iron is most often consumed as a part of a multiple vitamin/mineral supplement.[30]

FACTORS THAT INFLUENCE FOOD CHOICES

The adequacy of children's food intake depends not only on the foods available to them but also on cultural, environmental, interactional, and societal factors. Most investigators who have studied food choices have focused on preschoolers because it is at this stage of development that parents often become confused about the children's food selections and concerned that their children are not eating the kinds and amounts of foods they should. Food acceptance and factors that influence it assume increasing attention.

Food Acceptance

Acceptance of food is affected by factors that include nutritional status, degree of satiation, taste, previous experiences, and beliefs about specific foods. Infants have a preference for sweetened water, a preference that can be extinguished by offering only beverages that are not sweetened.[31] Young infants seem to have an aversion to bitter tastes and an indifference to salty tastes. Tastes for salt change from neutral to preferred at 4 months of age when the salt taste is combined with other tastes in food. Preschoolers reject salty beverages but prefer a higher level of salt in soup than do adults.[32]

Recently work has focused on genetic factors that influence food preferences.[33] Monozygotic twin pairs demonstrated a greater similarity in food preferences than dizygotic twin pairs. Foods with similar preferences were orange juice, broccoli, cottage cheese, chicken, sweetened cereal, and hamburger. A strong genetic influence was demonstrated for phenylthiocarbamide (PTC). Individuals sensitive to the bitter taste of compounds like PTC tended to have more food dislikes than those who were less sensitive. Foods identified as tasting bitter were turnips, broccoli, green beans, strawberries, bacon, grapefruit, orange, and apple, all of which contain some PTC. Sensitivity to bitter tastes, tested by sensitivity to 6-n-propylthiouracil (PROP), appears to have a genetic basis for influencing food preferences.[34]

Parental Influences

Parents have a profound influence on food-related behaviors of young children. Many research studies have documented that parents, with or without conscious effort, guide the food preferences of their young children and establish the style for where food is eaten, how it is eaten, with whom it is eaten, and the quantity of food eaten.

Nutrition knowledge. The nutrition knowledge of parents and other caregivers appears to be an important factor in children's food choices. The degree to which knowledge of nutrition is incorporated into family meal planning seems to be related to positive attitudes toward self, problem-solving skills, and family organization. This relationship held in spite of a professed concern by all mothers interviewed about the total diet offered to young children and the importance of mealtime with children.[35] The ordinal position of the preschool child in the family appears to influence choices of specific foods regardless of equivalent knowledge of nutrition between groups of mothers.[36] When a preschool child is the youngest child in the family, the mothers appear to be less susceptible to the child's requests for new products. Mothers are willing, however, to accommodate that preference when the preschooler is the oldest child in the family. In a recent study parents of 4- to 7-year-old children reported that types of foods made available and eaten for meals were influenced by the likes and dislikes of the children. However, snack food availability and portion sizes were controlled by the adult that was present.[37]

Young children influence how families spend their food dollars. Child-prompted purchases comprised about 14% of the family food budget. Over half of child-prompted food items were calorie dense.[38] Mothers reported feeling a sense of guilt because they realized that their families, including young children, ate foods they preferred rather than the foods she felt to be nutritious.[39]

Models. The models set for children by their families and other persons close to them exert a strong influence on their developing food patterns. Parental food preferences exert a definite influence. Food habits of siblings exert an influence equal to that of parents. Parents report that they know little about nutrition but think it is important.

Parent-child interactions. Children's interactions with their parents influence their acceptance of foods and the food patterns they develop. If parents casually accept transient strong food preferences preschoolers develop, these passing food behaviors are soon forgotten. However, parents who find these behaviors difficult to accept and give much attention to them by trying to bribe or encourage the child to eat, discussing the children's dislikes in front of them, or providing a preferred food when they refuse to eat may pattern that behavior into a permanent food habit. A child's social-emotional environment is directly related to the adequacy of the child's dietary intake. Companionship at mealtime, a positive home atmosphere, and appropriate food-related parenting behaviors are strongly associated with improved quality of diet.[40]

The parent-child interaction also has an important influence on the amount of food consumed. There appear to be differences between the interactions of thinner children and their mothers and fatter children and their mothers both in food and nonfood situations. Thinner children and their mothers talk more with each other and eat less food more slowly than fatter children and their mothers.[41] Preferences for foods are enhanced when foods are offered as a reward or with a brief positive social interaction with adults.[42]

Contingencies. It is also a common practice for parents to use rewards such as "Clean your plate and you can have dessert" to achieve a child's acceptance of foods. While this practice often achieves its immediate goal, the long-term effects are often negative. Children understand that external pressure is usually applied to get them to eat a less-preferred food. When the contingency is removed they eat less of the food.[43] The ability of the child to recognize hunger and satiation has also been studied by Birch.[44] Of all the children in the study, 95% ate less lunch after a high-caloric density preload than a low-caloric density preload. Only 60% of the adults followed the same pattern. Parental monitoring (or threat of parental monitoring) decreased the number of nonnutritious foods chosen and thus the total energy content of the meal.[45]

Quantities of food consumed. If normal well-nourished children are offered a variety of nutritionally appropriate foods and permitted to eat those foods they select in the amounts they wish, they will consume an appropriate energy intake. Studies conducted in the 1920s and early 1930s on 6-month-old to 4-year-old foundlings in a Chicago hospital presented the children with 10 unprocessed foods at each meal. The children were permitted to self-select the foods and amounts they ate at any meal. A more recent study by Birch with 15 children in a day care center used the same menu for 2 days each week for 3 weeks in the day care center and at home. Foods included in the menu would provide appropriate nutrient intake. In both studies there was considerable variability in the quantity of food each child consumed from one day to the next. However, the children self-selected an appropriate energy intake when the study days were averaged.[9,46] It is important to note that both researchers utilized a laboratory setting and controlled for a variety of parent-child interaction issues that influence food acceptance. These studies do, however, provide a model of an optimal method of achieving the acceptance of a nutritionally appropriate diet by children.

Influence of Television on Children

Sylvester et al[47] have summarized the research on children and television over the past 20 years. They state, "Children spend enough time in front of TV to warrant concern as to the content and effect of this medium." It would appear that hours of viewing television for young children have been fairly constant over the last two decades. Younger children continue to watch more Saturday morning television than older children.

Food attitudes and requests. In addition to the many familial, cultural, and psychosocial influences on children's food habits, mass media have an impact on children's attitudes toward food and their requests for particular products. Of all the forms of mass media, television has the greatest impact on children because it reaches many children before they are capable of verbal communication and because it engages much of their time. Children spend more time watching television than they do in any other activity except for sleeping. Children from low-income families watch more television than do children from moderate- to high-income families. It has been estimated that children watch television 22 to 25 hours per week.

Obesity. Extensive television viewing can be detrimental to growth and development by encouraging sedentary and passive activities, thus promoting a lifestyle that may lead to obesity. An association between obesity and time spent watching television has been documented in 6- to 11-year-old children and in adolescents.[48] "The amount of TV viewing may be a factor in development of obesity . . . insofar as it precludes other activities that require much greater energy expenditure." Sylvester goes on to state,[47] "The major impact of TV is not the behavior it produces, but the behavior it prevents."

Snacking. Television viewing by children is also correlated with between-meal snacking. Snacking is significantly related to the amount of time spent viewing television. The total amount of TV watched positively correlates with the act of snacking. Short-term consumption behaviors appear to be influenced by the content and amount of TV viewed.[47]

Advertisers attempt to use children to influence their parents' purchasing behavior. They present frequent cues for food and drink and often encourage consumption of a wide variety of sugared products. Television programs, as well as advertising, present models of behavior children may imitate.

Television advertising. Kindergarten children often are unable to separate commercials from the program and frequently explain them as part of the program. Younger school-age children 5 to 10 years of age watch commercials more closely than do older children 11 to 12 years of age. Older children are more conscious of the concept of commercials, the purpose of selling, and the concept of sponsorship and are less likely to accept advertisers' claims without question. They perceive that television commercials are designed to sell products rather than entertain or educate. Children in the second grade have been found to have a concrete distrust of commercials based on experience with advertised products. Children in the sixth grade have been found to have global mistrust of all commercials.

TV and food choices. On Saturday morning TV programming for children more than 56% of the advertisements were for food; of these, nearly 44% were for fats, oils, and sweet foods. The most frequently advertised foods were high-sugar cereals. Most preschool children can not distinguish between programs and commercials.[49]

Certain attributes of food are promoted by television advertising as being superior to others. The main characteristics presented positively are "sweetness," "chocolatey," and "richness." Many food manufacturers, in other words, deemphasize the physiologic need for nutrients and encourage selection on the basis of sweet flavor. Exposure to such messages may distort a child's natural curiosity toward other characteristics of food such as the fresh crispness of apples or celery.

There has been ongoing concern about the influence of television on the growth and health of young children. Dietz and Gortmaker outline aspects of television watching that are of concern: (1) the relationship between increased television watching and snacking, (2) the increased consumption of foods advertised on television as watching time increases, (3) the direct association of increased viewing time with the number of attempts of the young child to influence the supermarket purchases of the parent. The foods advertised on weekend children's programs are usually ones of high-caloric density, which if purchased and consumed without an increase in activity can lead to inappropriate weight gain and poor food habits. The larger intake of highly concentrated sweets and fat foods plus the decrease in activity that is associated with excess television watching has led to an increase of obesity among children in the United States.[48]

Parental response. Children are influenced by television commercials and attempt to influence their parents' buying practices. Commercials for food have the strongest influence and mothers are more likely to yield to requests for food than for other products. Parents have a greater tendency to respond to requests from older children, but certainly do not ignore those of younger children. Mothers of children aged 3 to 8 years were interviewed to assess children's viewing habits and parental response to children's requests for food advertised on television. Children requested the foods they saw advertised on TV. The number of hours a week that a child watched TV correlated significantly with the reported number of requests for foods that were advertised and energy intake.[50] Highly child-centered mothers are less likely to buy children's favorite cereals than are mothers who are not as child centered. The American Academy of Pediatrics has taken a strong stand on this issue with the recommendation that televised advertising aimed at children be eliminated. The position paper states, "Parents rather than children should determine what children should eat."[28]

PRESCHOOL CHILDREN

Although clinical signs of malnutrition are rarely found in preschool children in North America and many low-income families show good management of scarce economic resources for food, there is evidence that some children receive diets that are limited in some nutrients and in some cases energy. A study of low-income Mexican-American preschoolers in Colorado found that the children consumed an adequate nutrient intake.[51]

Both longitudinal and cross-sectional studies of nutrient and energy intakes of children have shown large differences in intakes between individual children of the same age and gender. Some children consume two to three times as much energy as others.[9,46,52] After a rapid rise in intake of all nutrients during the first nine months of life, reductions can be expected in the intakes of some of the nutrients as increases occur in intakes of others. Several researchers have noted gender differences in intakes of energy and nutrients. In all studies males consumed greater quantities of food, thus greater amounts of nutrients and energy.

The Preschool Years

During the preschool years there is a decrease in intake of calcium, phosphorus, riboflavin, iron, and vitamin A because of discontinued use of iron-fortified infant cereals in the diets of children, a reduction in milk intakes, and a disinterest in vegetables. During this period children increase their intake of carbohydrate and fat. Protein intakes may plateau or increase only slightly. Between 3 and 8 years of age there is a slow, steady, and relatively consistent increase in intake of all nutrients. Since intakes of vitamins A and C are unrelated to energy intakes, greater ranges of intakes of these nutrients have been noted.

Normal Food Behaviors of Preschool Children

Food rituals. Few children pass through the preschool years without creating concern about their food intake. Between 9 and 18 months of age children display a disinterest in food that lasts from a few months to a few years. Strong preferences for specific foods are common. Likes and dislikes may change from day to day and week to week. For example, a child may demand only boiled eggs for snacks for a week and completely reject them for the next 6 months. Rituals become a part of food preparation and service. Some children, for example, accept sandwiches only when they are cut in half, and when parents quarter the sandwich the children may throw tantrums. Others demand that food have a particular arrangement on the plate or that dishes be placed only in certain locations on the table.

Appetites. During this period appetites are usually erratic and unpredictable. The child may eat hungrily at one meal and completely refuse the next. The evening meal is generally the least well received and is one of the most concern to the majority of parents. It is possible that children who have consumed two meals and several snacks have already met their needs for energy and nutrients before dinner time.

Food preferences. Parents report that preschool children enjoy meat, cereal grains, baked products, fruit, and sweets. They frequently ask for dairy products, cereal, and snack items such as cookies, crackers, and fruit juice. Food preferences during the preschool years seem to be for the carbohydrate-rich foods that are easiest to masticate. Cereals, breads, and crackers are selected often in preference to meat and other protein-rich foods. The use of dry **fortified cereals** as a primary source of many nutrients is increasing. Yogurt and cheese appear to be increasing in popularity among young children.

Fortified cereal
Cereal food products enriched by addition of minerals such as iron and zinc, and vitamins such as thiamin, riboflavin, niacin, folate, B_6, and B_{12}.

Frequency of Eating

Nearly 60% of children 3 to 5 years of age eat more than 3 times a day. They consume food on an average of 5 to 7 times a day, although ranges of 3 to 14 times a day have been noted. The frequency of food intakes appears to be unrelated to nutrient intakes except when children consumed food less than four or more than six times a day.[53] Children who consumed food less than 4 times a day consumed fewer kilocalories and less calcium, protein, ascorbic acid, and iron than the average intakes of other children their age. Those who consumed food more than 6 times a day consumed more energy, calcium, and ascorbic acid than average intakes of children their age. Snacks contribute 33% of the daily energy, 20% of the protein, 33% of the fat, and 40% of the carbohydrate consumed each day by 10-year-old children.[54] School-age children eat less frequently than younger children, about 4 or 5 times a day on school days. They usually have a snack after school which they often prepare themselves. These snacks contribute about one third of their total energy intake.[55]

The Preschool Child

In spite of the reduction of appetite and erratic consumption of food, preschool children do enjoy well-prepared and attractively served food. If simply prepared foods are presented in a relaxed setting, children will consume an appropriate nutrient intake. Meals and snacks should be timed to foster appetite. Intervals necessary between meals and snacks may vary from one child to another. Rarely can the clock be depended on to know appropriate intervals and times when it may be important for a child to eat. However, indiscriminate snacking dulls the appetite and such patterns should be discouraged.

Foods for young children. Children accept simple unmixed dishes more willingly than casseroles, and prefer most of their food at room temperature, neither hot nor cold. Food preparation is important. Children recognize poorly prepared food and are likely to refuse it. Most children eat most easily those foods with which they are familiar. Small portions of new foods can be introduced with familiar and popular foods. Even if the child only looks at the new food or just feels or smells it at first, this is a part of learning about it and accepting it.

Dry foods are especially hard for preschool children to eat. In planning a menu always balance a dry food with one or two moist foods. For example, it is wise to put a slice of meat loaf, relatively dry, with mashed potatoes and peas in a little cream sauce. Also, combinations of sharp, rather acid-flavored foods with mild-flavored foods are popular with young children, and they are pleased to find colorful foods such as red tomatoes, green peppers, and carrot sticks included in their meals.

Ease of manipulation. Foods eaten easily with the unskilled and seemingly clumsy hands of a young child are very important. Many small pieces of foods such as cooked peas or beans are difficult for a child to spoon up. Foods can be prepared so that a child can eat them with the fingers. Hard-cooked eggs may be served in quarters, cooked meat can be cut in small strips, and cooked green beans can be served as finger foods. Children like oranges that have been cut in wedges, skin and all, much better than peeled and diced oranges. Mixed-up salads, when there are layers of food to be eaten, are much more difficult to eat than simple pieces of raw vegetables with no salad dressing. Cottage cheese or similar foods should be served separate from the lettuce leaf on the child's plate. Creamed foods served on tough toast are difficult for children to manage.

Relatively small pieces of food that can be handled with the child's eating tools are best for preschool children. The problem of handling silverware and conveying food to the mouth at this early age is a greater task than many adults realize. Pieces of carrots that slide across the plate and are too small to remain on the fork are frustrating. On the other hand, cubes of beets so large that they must be cut into smaller pieces before they can be eaten exhaust the patience of a 2- or 3-year-old child. Most foods for these children should be served in bite-size pieces. When the child is 4 years of age and older, the skills to cut up some foods may have been developed. If, however, difficulty in managing food is noticed, small pieces should be served, with occasional encouragement to cut up some easier to manage foods. Canned pears and other soft fruits, for example, are usually easy to cut into bite-size pieces.

In general, the aim is to support the young child's early efforts at self-feeding and many creative adaptations can be helpful. Stringy spinach or tomatoes, for example, are a trial for anyone to eat. Much can be done with food shears in the kitchen to make these foods easier to eat. Finger foods such as pieces of lettuce or toast can be used in meals where some of the foods are difficult to handle. Small sandwiches, that is, a large one cut into four small squares, are popular with young children. As the young child matures, self-help skills become more sophisticated. In general, a 2-year-old child uses arm muscles for tasks, a 3-year-old child uses hand muscles, and a 4-year-old child uses finger muscles. This maturation enables the child to wipe, scrub, pour, mix, and peel foods for eating.[56]

Food characteristics. Three general food characteristics affecting taste, acceptance, and self-feeding skills development are important considerations in early feeding of young children. These aspects are texture, flavor, and portion sizes.

Texture. It is wise to serve one soft food for easy chewing, one crisp food for easy chewing and enjoyment of the sounds in the mouth, and one chewy food for emerging chewing skills without having too much to chew in each meal for young children. Pieces of meat seem to be hard for a young child to eat, which explains why children often prefer hamburgers to frankfurters. Most children's meat can be served as ground meat. Ground meat should be cooked only long enough for the color to change to brown, and not be allowed to become dry and crusted, which makes it hard for a child to eat. Some children may prefer moderately rare meat, which is even more moist, but care must be taken that it is cooked sufficiently to be safe.

Flavor. In general, young children reject strong flavors. Many children, however, do seem to like pickles and some spicy sauces, which may seem to contradict this. In general, it has been found that children like food only mildly salted. Pepper and other sharp spices and acids such as vinegar should also be used sparingly on children's food.

Portion sizes. Children are easily discouraged by large portions of food. Offer less than the child usually eats and permit seconds, rather than discourage him with portions that are too large. Appropriate portion sizes are shown in Table 7-7.

Parental concerns. Occasionally anxious or concerned parents need help with food sources of nutrients usually supplied by food refused or in establishing limits to the preschooler's food intakes and feeding behavior. Of the commonly expressed concerns, limited intakes of milk, refusal of meat and vegetables, eating too many sweets, and limited intakes of food appear to cause the most problems.

Milk. It is important to recognize that 1 oz of milk supplies 36 mg of calcium, and many children receive 6 to 8 oz of milk on dry cereal daily. Although they consume only 1 to 2 oz at a time, their calcium intakes may be acceptable when they consume milk with meals and snacks. When abundant amounts of fruit juice or sweetened beverages are available, children may simply prefer to drink them instead of milk. Other dairy products can be offered when milk is rejected. Cheese and yogurt are usually accepted. Powdered milk can be used in recipes for soups, vegetables, and mixed dishes.

Meat. Parents' perceptions of children's dislike of meat may need to be clarified, or an easier to chew form used. If in fact preschoolers do consistently refuse all food sources of heme iron, their daily intake of iron should be carefully monitored.

Vegetables. When vegetables are consistently refused, wars between parents and children should not be permitted to erupt. Small portions of 1 or 2 teaspoons should continue to be served without comment and should be discarded if the child does not eat them. Preschool behavior modification programs that included token rewards when children consumed vegetables served at mealtime have been found to increase children's acceptance and intake of them.[52]

Sweets. Parents concerned about children's excessive intakes of sweets may need help in setting limits on amounts of sweet foods they make available to their children. It may be important also to help them convey their concern and the need to set limits on the

CASE STUDY

A Preschooler's View of Milk and Vegetables

During a well-child clinic visit the mother of a 3-year-old boy expresses concern about his nutrient intake. She tells the clinical nutritionist, "He doesn't like to drink milk and refuses vegetables."

Questions for analysis
1. How does his food behavior compare with that of other preschool children?
2. What nutrients should be assessed in the food that he does eat?
3. What nonfood parameters should be evaluated?

TABLE 7-7   A Feeding Guide for Children

This is a guide to a basic diet. Fats, desserts, and sauces will contribute additional kilocalories to meet the needs of the growing child.

| Food | 1 year old | | 2-3 years old | |
	Portion Sizes	No. of Servings	Portion Sizes	No. of Servings
Milk	½ cup	4-5	¼-¾ cup	4-5
Meat and meat equivalents	¼-1 oz 2-4 tbsp	1	1-2 oz	2
Fruit and vegetables		4-5		4-5
Vegetables				
Cooked	1-2 tbsp		2-3 tbsp	
Raw	1-2 tbsp		few pieces	
Fruit				
Canned	2-4 tbsp		2-4 tbsp	
Raw	2-4 tbsp (chopped)		½-1 small	
Juice	2-4 oz		3-4 oz	
Grains and grain products	½ slice	3	¼-1 slice	3

Modified from Lownberg ME: The development of food patterns in young children. In Pipes P, Trahms CM: *Nutrition in infancy and childhood,* ed 5, St Louis, 1993, Mosby.

This is a guide to a basic diet. Fats, desserts, and sauces will contribute additional kilocalories to meet the needs of the growing child.

4-6 years old		7 years to Puberty		
Portion Sizes	No. of Servings	Portion Sizes	No. of Servings	Comments
½-¾ cup	3-4	1 cup	3	The following may be substituted for ½ cup of liquid milk: ½-¾ oz cheese ¼-½ cup yogurt 2½ tbsp nonfat dry milk powder
1-2 oz	2	2-3 oz	3	The following may be substituted for 1 oz of meat, fish, or poultry: 4-5 tbsp cooked legumes 1 egg 2 tbsp peanut butter
	4-5		4-5	Include one green leafy or yellow vegetable, e.g., spinach, broccoli, carrots, winter squash
3-4 tbsp few pieces		½ cup ½ cup		
4-6 tbsp ½-1 small 4 oz 1 slice	4	½ cup 4 oz 1 slice	6	Include one vitamin C–rich fruit or juice per day The following may be substituted for one slice of bread: ½ cup cooked cereal ½ cup spaghetti or other pasta ½ cup rice 5 saltines Whole grain products provide additional bulk to the diet

availability of these foods. Other family members, day care providers, and teachers may need to be involved in the plan for change.

Food intake. If children's food intakes are so limited that their intakes of energy and nutrients are compromised, parents may need help in establishing guidelines so that the children develop appetites. They should provide food often enough so that children do not get so hungry that they lose their appetite, yet not so often that they are always satiated. Intervals of 3 to 4 hours are often successful. Very small portions of foods should be offered, and second portions permitted when children consume the foods already served. Attention should always be focused on children when they eat, never when food is refused.

Group Feeding

Increasing numbers of mothers of young children are working outside the home. Over half of the 3- to 5-year-old children in the United States are in child care settings at least part-time each week. This has been estimated at 5.1 million preschool-aged children in child care centers and 4 million children in family day care homes. Children whose mothers work full time are often in a child care facility for 9 to 10 hours 5 days a week and receive both meals and snacks in this setting. Kindergartens and preschools also offer snacks and meals along with food experiences that are often included as part of the learning activities.

Family day care homes and day care centers are licensed by state agencies that mandate the meal pattern and types of snacks to be provided for the children, as well as the percentage of the recommended daily allowances that must be included in the menus. In general, a child in day care for 8 hours should receive at least one third the RDA from food and snacks; a child in day care for more than 8 hours should receive one half to two thirds of the RDA.

Breakfast should be provided for children who receive none at home. Snacks should be planned to complement the daily food intakes. Small portions of food should be served, and children should be permitted second servings of those foods they enjoy. Disliked or unfamiliar foods may be offered by the teaspoonful, and the child's acceptance or rejection received without comment. Children who eat slowly will need to be served first and permitted to complete the meals without being rushed to other activities. Teachers and caretakers should eat with the children without imposing their attitudes about food.

A new setting provides an opportunity for children to have exposure to many new foods. Day care centers, kindergartens, and preschools can provide an important educational setting for both children and their parents. Children learn how to prepare food, how food grows, how it smells, and what nutrients it contains. Parents learn through participation, observation, and conversation with the staff. An organized approach to feeding children must include parents, teachers, and other staff who offer food to children. Teachers and day care workers can provide important information to parents about how children successfully consume food, the nutrients children need, and the foods that provide these nutrients. Parents offer important information to the centers about their children's food acceptance and needs. Each needs to be reinforced positively by the other for their efforts to provide food for the children to be successful.

SCHOOL-AGE CHILDREN

Studies of the school-age population have found that most children are adequately nourished. One will, however, find groups in which an inadequate food and nutrient intake is of concern. In a comparison of first grade children in areas of low- and high-poverty areas in Washington state, obesity was the most common growth deviance observed. Eighteen percent of children from low-poverty areas and 12% from high-poverty areas had a weight-height ratio greater than the 90th percentile on the NCHS growth charts.[57] There have been several reports of failure-to-thrive and delayed onset of puberty because very zealous parents' efforts to prevent obesity and cardiovascular disease caused them to allow their children inadequate energy intake that was insufficient for normal growth.[58,59] It is clear that children who eat regular meals in preference to only snacking do better nutritionally. Studies have also revealed that currently the amount of fat in children's diets is the same as in the diets of adults, and these amounts are lower than they were several years ago.[60]

School entrance provides an opportunity to identify children whose growth parameters may indicate nutrition concerns, such as growth failure, obesity, and underweight. Feeding programs such as the school lunch and breakfast programs contribute significantly to children's nutrient intake.

Patterns of Nutrient Intake

By school age most children have established a particular pattern of nutrient intake relative to their peers. Although wide ranges of food intake, and thus of energy and nutrients, continue to be observed, those who consume the greatest amount of food consistently do so, whereas those consuming smaller amounts maintain these lesser intakes relative to their peers. Differences in intake between males and females gradually increase to age 12 and then become marked. Boys consume greater quantities of food, thus energy and nutrients, than girls.

Physical and Social Development

The school-age period is one of few apparent feeding conflicts. A natural increase in appetite creates normal increases in food intake. Because children spend their days at school, they adjust to a more ordered routine. As they explore the environment of school and peers, children will be influenced by these experiences (Fig. 7-3). Often the credibility of parents is questioned, in the face of advice from teachers, peers, or peers' parents. The school-age child has more access to money, grocery stores, and vending machines, and therefore to foods with questionable nutrient value. Many school-age children have some responsibility for preparing their own breakfasts or sack lunches and arrive home from school looking for a snack.

Food Patterns

Although school-age children usually increase the amount they eat and the varieties of food they accept, many continue to reject vegetables and mixed dishes. The range of food they voluntarily accept may be small. Sugar contributes 24% to 25% of the total

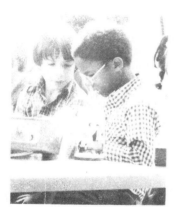

FIG. 7-3 Food habits are part of both physical and psychosocial development.
Steve Fritz.

kilocalories in the diets of many school-age children. Milk is the primary contributor. Sweetened beverages, fruits, fruit juice, cakes, cookies, and other dessert items are also significant contributors.

Food dislikes of older children consistently include cooked vegetables and mixed dishes. Children accept raw vegetables more readily than cooked ones but often take only a limited amount. Sweetness and familiarity are significant factors that influence food preferences in all children.

A common difficulty for parents is finding a time when school-age children are willing to sit down and eat a meal. Frequently they are so involved with other activities that it is difficult to get them to take time to eat. Often they satisfy their initial hunger and rush back to their activities and television programs, returning later for a snack. The food patterns of second and fifth graders were assessed. Forty percent of the children did not eat vegetables except for potatoes and tomato sauce; 20% did not eat fruit; 36% ate at least four different types of snack foods daily. Fifth graders ate significantly more snack foods than second graders and were also more likely to skip breakfast.[61]

Meal Patterns

Breakfast is an important meal. Even so, estimates of children who do not eat breakfast range from 8% to 29%. Children will have to rise earlier to eat an unhurried and balanced meal and may have to prepare it themselves. Early morning school activities may make preplanning necessary. Some may find a glass of milk and fruit juice important before early sports activities. Studies have shown that when breakfast is consumed, children have a better attitude and school record compared with when it is omitted. Pollitt, Leibel, and Greenfield found that 9- to 11-year-old well-nourished children who skipped breakfast showed a decrease in accuracy of response in problem-solving but an increase in immediate memory in short-term accuracy.[62] The effect was attributed to a heightened arousal level, which in turn had a qualitative effect on cognitive function.

Actually, most children do eat breakfasts that contribute at least one fourth of the RDA standard. A larger percentage of children in the lower grades eat breakfast than those in the middle and upper grades. Reasons for skipping breakfast included "not hungry," "no time," "on a diet," "no one to prepare food," "do not like food served for breakfast," and "foods are not available." Breakfast is noted as being an important contributor to overall dietary quality and adequacy in school-age children. Girls are more likely than boys to have breakfast at home (46%), and about 20% of all 10-year-old children skipped breakfast entirely.[63] The school-age child often participates in the National School Lunch Program administered by the Department of Agriculture, which provides cash reimbursement and supplemental foods to feeding programs that comply with federal regulations. Low-income children may receive reduced prices or free meals.

Children who do not participate in the school lunch program generally bring a packed lunch from home. Studies have indicated that, compared with the school lunch, these meals provide significantly fewer nutrients, but do supply energy. Little variety is seen in the lunches since favorite foods tend to be packed and lack of refrigeration limits the kinds of foods that can be carried.

The evening meal provides an opportunity for family interaction and socialization, as well as one of food and nutrient intake. Children should be expected to participate in both activities. It is important that parents not cater to children's food idiosyncrasies but offer them the family menu.

The emotional environment at the dinner table may influence nutrient intake. The evening meal is not the place for family battles or punitive action toward children. If eating is to be successful and enjoyable it must occur in a setting that is comfortable and free from stress and unreasonable demands.

School Meals

School feeding and nutrition education programs, when adequately implemented, provide not only important nutrients for children, but also an opportunity to learn to make responsible food choices. These feeding programs contribute significantly to the nutrient and energy intake of many low-income children. In fact, such feeding programs may provide motivation for children to go to school.

Since its inception in 1946, the National School Lunch Program has been administered by the U.S. Department of Agriculture. Federal regulations require that school lunches and

---

School Meal Initiative for Healthy Children: Improving Nutritional Health

STRATEGIES FOR NUTRITION EDUCATION

The National School Lunch Program was begun in 1946 and now serves about 25 million lunches every day. A school breakfast program was added in recent years to serve children who for socioeconomic or other reasons cannot eat breakfast at home. The National School Lunch Program has two important goals. First, this program strives to improve the dietary intake and nutritional health of the nation's children. Children who receive an appropriate supply of nutritious food and adequate kilocalories throughout the day are more physically, mentally, and emotionally prepared for learning. A second major goal of the National School Lunch Program is to promote nutrition education and teach children to make appropriate food choices for a lifetime. School meals should provide examples of healthy meal patterns based on the Food Guide Pyramid. Food habits are shaped early in life and the school nutrition program should introduce children to a wide variety of foods which they may or may not have eaten at home. To maximize this effort the food and nutrition education provided by the school breakfast and lunch program must be coordinated with education received in the classroom. Children must develop positive health attitudes and learn about the relationships of food, nutrition, and health. Some schools have developed a comprehensive curriculum in which food and nutrition concepts are introduced and reinforced from kindergarten through grade 12. Appropriate food and fitness behaviors can be integrated within all major subject areas in the school curriculum. Examples of appropriate learning activities are described below.

Social Studies: Foods consumed by different ethnic or cultural groups, foods grown in different parts of the world, nutrition labeling regulations, and functions of the Food and Drug Administration

Mathematics: Calculation of kilocalories or total nutrients consumed by the student per meal or per day; calculation of the kilocalories in a particular food based on the grams of fat, carbohydrate, and protein given on the label; calculation of the total cost of a meal and cost per person

Physical and Biological Sciences: Process by which food is digested; how nutrients are used for growth and regulation of body functions; food tests for protein, carbohydrate or starch; classification and origin of fruits and vegetables; energy and muscle function

Health and Physical Education: Exercise activities for lifelong enjoyment, exercise and weight management, components of a healthy diet, avoidance of addictive behaviors, and good food sources of particular nutrients

Communication Arts: Writing a story about a favorite food, writing and producing a class play about healthy food and activity behaviors, and making posters for the school lunch room about good food choices

From ADA supports USDA School Meals Initiative for Healthy Children but recommends more improvements for child nutrition, *J Am Diet Assoc* 94:841, 1994.

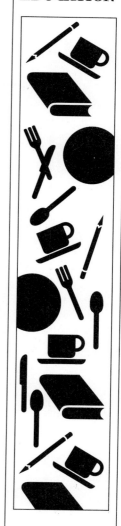

breakfasts be sold at reduced prices or be given free to children whose families cannot afford to buy them. The breakfast and lunch menus must be planned to meet the guidelines established for the National School Lunch Program. Tables 7-8 and 7-9 show minimum quantities of food required for the various age groups in a school breakfast and lunch.

To provide variety and to enlist participation and consumption, schools are encouraged to provide a selection of foods. About half of the schools participating in the lunch program also serve breakfast. Breakfast must include liquid milk, fruit or vegetable juice, and bread or cereal. Schools are encouraged to keep fat, sugar, and salt at moderate levels.

Current regulations require that schools involve students and parents in planning the school lunch program. They may be included in such activities as menu planning, enhancing the eating environment, program promotion, and related student community support activities.

Foods sold in competition with school lunch in snack bars or vending machines must provide at least 5% of the recommended dietary allowances for one or more of the following nutrients: protein, vitamin A, vitamin C, niacin, riboflavin, thiamin, calcium, and iron. This regulation eliminates the sale of soda water, water ices, chewing gum, and some candies until after the last lunch period. It should also encourage the offering of more fruits,

TABLE 7-8 *School Breakfast Pattern — School Breakfast Program*

Food Components		Minimum Quantities		
		Age 1-2	Age 3-5	Age 6 and Older
Milk	Beverage, on cereal, or both	½ c (4 fl oz)	¾ c (6 fl oz)	½ pt (8 fl oz)
Fruit/vegetable/juice*	Fruit or vegetable or both or full-strength fruit or vegetable juice	¼ c	½ c	½ c
Select *one* serving from each of the following components or *two* servings from one component				
Bread or bread alternate	Whole-grain or enriched bread	½ slice	½ slice	1 slice
	Whole-grain or enriched biscuit, roll, muffin	½ serving	½ serving	1 serving
	Whole-grain, enriched, or fortified cereal	¼ c or ⅓ oz	⅓ c or ½ oz	¾ c or 1 oz
Meat or meat alternate	Lean meat, poultry, or fish	½ oz	½ oz	1 oz
	Cheese	½ oz	½ oz	1 oz
	Large eggs	½	½	½
	Peanut butter	1 T	1 T	2 T
	Cooked dry beans or peas	2 T	2 T	4 T
	Nuts or seeds or both	½ oz	½ oz	1 oz

From Food and Nutrition Service, USDA: *Meal pattern requirements and offer versus serve manual,* FNS-265, 1990.
*A citrus fruit or juice or a vegetable that is a good source of vitamin C is recommended daily.

TABLE 7-9 *School Lunch Pattern – National School Lunch Program*

Components	Minimum Quantities				Recommended Quantities*
	Group I: Age 1-2; Preschool	Group II: Age 3-4; Preschool	Group III: Age 5-8; Gr. K-3	Group IV: Age 9 and Older; Gr. 4-12	Group V: Age 12 and Older; Gr. 7-12
Milk Whole and unflavored lowfat milk must be offered†	¾ c (6 fl oz)	¾ c (6 fl oz)	½ pt (8 fl oz)	½ pt (8 fl oz)	½ pt (8 fl oz)
Meat or meat alternate (quantity of the edible portion as served)					
Lean meat, poultry, or fish	1 oz	1½ oz	1½ oz	2 oz	3 oz
Cheese	1 oz	1½ oz	1½ oz	2 oz	3 oz
Large egg	½	¾	¾	1	1½
Cooked dry beans or peas	¼ c	⅜ c	⅜ c	½ c	¾ c
Peanut butter or an equivalent quantity of any combination of above	2 T	3 T	3 T	4 T	6 T
Vegetable or fruit 2 or more servings of vegetable or fruit or both to total	½ c	½ c	½ c	¾ c	¾ c
Bread or bread alternate (servings per week) Must be enriched or whole-grain—at least ½ serving‡ for group I or one serving‡ for groups II-V must be served daily	5	8	8	8	10

From Food and Nutrition Service, US Department of Agriculture: *Meal pattern requirements and offer versus serve manual*, FNS-265, 1990.
*The minimum portion sizes for these children are the portion sizes for group IV.
†This requirement does not prohibit offering other milk, such as flavored milk or skim milk, along with the above.
‡Serving, 1 slice of bread; or ½-cup of cooked rice, macaroni, noodles, other pasta products, other cereal products such as bulgur and corn grits; or 1 biscuit, roll, muffin, and similar products; or any combination of these.

vegetables, and fruit and vegetable juices in places that compete with the school lunch. Concentrated sources of sucrose have been a concern of many interested in dental health, the control of obesity, and the development of sound food habits for all children. Sufficient concern has been created in some school districts that only machines that provide fruit, milk, nuts, and seeds have been made available to students. Initially, sales have been found to decrease, but ultimately they increase. One school discovered that they made a greater profit on apples than on chocolate bars.

Many persons concerned about the prevention of atherosclerosis and obesity have made statements about the quantity and saturation of fats as well as the caloric density of foods in these school lunches. Indeed, some schools have responded to these concerns and provided low-fat menu options.

Although elementary school children are making more decisions regarding food selection, supervision and supportive guidelines may be necessary at lunchtime. Children may give priority to activities other than eating and rush through their meals. Some may refuse to eat the food on the menu. Children who need therapeutic diets will need guidance in the foods they should and should not eat. Model projects are underway to evaluate nutrient standard menu planning (NSMP), that is, using the nutrient content of foods to plan menus rather than the more traditional meal pattern components menu planning system. It is hoped that the new system will facilitate greater variety of foods of lower fat and sodium content in school lunch menus.[64]

PREVENTION OF NUTRITION AND HEALTH PROBLEMS

Nutrition concerns during childhood include iron-deficiency anemia, overweight and obesity, and dental caries. In addition some persons are worried about children's intakes of specific foods and food constituents such as artificial flavors and colors and sugar and their possible effect on behavior. Also, it is important to recognize that many risk factors for cardiovascular disease can be modified by changes in dietary patterns. Identification of children at risk and modifying fat and salt intakes as well as other contributing factors are important health promotion actions.

The prevention of iron-deficiency anemia has been discussed earlier in this chapter (p. 286). Any discussion on childhood nutrition should include attention to these other concerns as well.

Weight Management

An excessive rate of weight gain and deposition of fat occurs when energy intake exceeds energy expenditure. Over time this situation can lead to obesity. The possible influence of family factors in childhood on adult obesity has been debated for decades. A recent study in Denmark followed a cohort of school-aged children for 10 years, from mid-childhood to young adulthood. Parental neglect, that is, lack of emotional support and general hygiene, predicted a great risk of obesity in young adulthood, independent of age and body mass index in childhood, gender, and social background.[65] By monitoring rates of growth and deposition of adipose tissue, children who are accumulating more fat than would be anticipated can be identified, and measures to increase activity and decrease excessive caloric intake can be taken. Young children are increasingly concerned about their weight and are attempting to modify it. About 60% of fourth grade girls, compared to about 39% of boys, reported a desire to be thinner. Weight-related behaviors and concerns increased with increasing weight-for-age and body mass index. The most frequent weight-related behavior was increased consumption of diet soft drinks.[66]

Family attitudes. Adolescents make their own decisions about what and when they eat. Counseling must be directed to the teenagers themselves. But parents control the food available to younger children, create the environment that influences their acceptance of food, and can influence energy expenditure by the opportunities they create for physical activity for their children. It may be important to explore first with parents their reasons for encouraging their children to consume amounts of food that result in rapid weight gain. Some parents may not recognize that their expectations for the quantity of food they encourage their children to consume are excessive and that the "chubby" child is not necessarily the healthy child.

Parents may need help in developing appropriate parenting skills. They may need to learn how to respond to hunger and other needs of their infants and how to interact with their children. They may need help in identifying ways to help their children develop initiative and to cultivate friends and outlets in the community.[67]

Physical activity. The activity pattern of both the child and the family should be explored. It may be important to help parents find ways of increasing their child's level of activity. Parents who live in apartments often reinforce sedentary activities to reduce the noise level and complaints from neighbors. Those who live in one-family dwellings may have limited space for children's activities. City park departments, preschools, and schools frequently have programs that offer opportunities for increasing children's activities.

Appropriate energy intake. It is important to remember that at any age the range of appropriate energy intakes is large. Overweight children and children with familial trends to obesity may need fewer kilocalories than do their peers. Families of children with a familial tendency to obesity may require help in identifying the kinds and amounts of food that provide an energy intake that will support normal growth and weight gain.

Nutrition counseling. Programs of nutrition counseling should be family oriented and based on normal nutrition, emphasizing foods that provide a balance of nutrients as well as appropriate kilocalorie intakes. Families will need to realize that these efforts are directed at reduction in rates of weight gain and are not intended to effect weight loss. They must recognize that the food available and the models set for their child will determine the child's response to efforts to control weight gain. Family meals may need to be modified to include fewer fried foods, less gravy, and fewer rich desserts. Parents and siblings may have to modify their own eating practices to set appropriate examples. Teachers, babysitters, and day care providers should be alerted to and included in programs designed to control weight. Food experiences at school may need to be modified to exclude corn dripping with butter and chocolate cupcakes so frequently provided for special occasions. Low caloric snacks such as raw fruits and vegetables can be provided instead of cookies, candy, and hot dogs.

It is important to recognize that school-age children are very concerned about size. In fact, many are on self-imposed diets because they worry about becoming overweight. Weight control programs should be planned carefully so that they do not become the cause of an eating disorder in adolescence (see the box on p. 306).

Dental Caries

Dental caries, one of the most common nutritional diseases, affects children of all ages and family income levels. School children in the United States have an average of 3.07 decayed, missing, or filled permanent tooth surfaces (DMFS). This rate increases to 8.04 DMFS by age 17.[68] It has been documented that 61% of African-American and 55% of Mexican-American children exhibited tooth decay by age 8[69] and that 59% of all children aged 2 to 4 years old have never visited a dentist. As with other tissues, nutrition plays an important role during development in the acquisition of sound teeth and the surrounding

CASE STUDY

Wise Weight Management for a School-Age Girl

At the regular pediatric clinic visit of a 7-year-old girl, the pediatrician and pediatric nutritionist found that the girl's weight-for-height on the growth grid was above the 95th percentile. Her rate of weight gain had increased in the past year, crossing from the 50th to the 90th percentile.

Questions for analysis
1. What factors that influence her food intake and energy expenditure should be assessed?
2. What is a reasonable goal to correct her overweight status?
3. Outline a daily food plan to achieve this goal.

Buffering capacity
Function of the body's main buffer system of two balancing partners, an acid partner (carbonic acid) and a base partner (sodium bicarbonate), that act together to buffer or neutralize any incoming acid or base to maintain the necessary degree of acidity and alkalinity in the body fluids that is compatible with life and health.

Desquamation
(L *de-*; *squama*, scale). The shedding of epithelial tissue, mainly the skin and oral mucosa, in scales or small sheets.

Hydroxyapatite
An inorganic compound of calcium and phosphorus found in the matrix of bones and teeth; gives rigidity and strength to the structure.

structures that hold them and in the later susceptibility of the teeth to caries. Once the tooth has erupted, the composition of the diet, the presence of acid-producing bacteria, and the **buffering capacity** of the saliva interact and result in control or development of dental caries. Calcified dental tissues, unlike the long bones, which are subject to constant remodeling and repair, do not have the ability to repair themselves. Tooth destruction by decay is permanent.

Etiology. Dental plaque, a prerequisite for dental caries, has been described as a sticky, gelatinous mixture that contains water, salivary protein, **desquamated cells,** and bacteria. The plaque bacteria, using energy derived from the catabolism of dietary carbohydrate, synthesize several toxic substances including enzymes that have the potential to degrade the **enamel** and **dentin** and are precursors of acidic fermentation products. *Streptococcus mutans* appears to be the primary bacteria. These acids and enzymes cause demineralization of the **hydroxyapatite** of the enamel followed by **proteolytic** degradation and demineralization of the enamel and dentin. It has been proposed that when the acidic environment falls below 5.5, cariogenic bacteria invade the tooth and caries results. The saliva, the **pH** of which is 6.5 to 7.0, acts as a buffer and provides mechanical cleansing of the teeth.

Sugar. It has been well documented that when intakes of sugar could be controlled, sucrose is the most cariogenic carbohydrate. The incidence of caries can be reduced when the intakes of sugar are reduced. Glucose is thought to be the next most cariogenic sugar, and maltose, lactose, and fructose have been found to have equal effect. Starch can also cause the production of large amounts of plaque acid because the carbohydrate, once attacked by salivary amylase, is broken down into sugar and attacked by plaque bacteria.

Frequency of eating. The presence of sucrose, or even the total amount of sucrose in the diet, may not be the determining factor in the incidence of dental caries. An often quoted study in an institution for the mentally handicapped in Sweden showed that the more important factors were the frequency with which the sugar is consumed and the adhesiveness of the food to the teeth.[70] The researchers who conducted this 5-year study showed that the consumption of sticky candy between meals produced a high increase in the incidence of dental caries, whereas the increase in incidence of caries from the addition of sugar-sweetened water at mealtime was small. When sucrose was fed in chocolate or bread, an intermediate increase in the incidence of caries was noted. Other studies have not

Nutritional Snacks for Dental Health

- *Protein foods**
Natural cheese (cheddar, jack, string)
Milk
Cooked turkey, chicken, beef, ham
Plain yogurt
Peanut butter
Cottage cheese
Unsalted nuts and seeds
Tuna
Hard-cooked egg
- *Breads and cereals†*
Whole-grain breads
Whole-grain cereals
Whole-grain, low-fat crackers
Tortillas
English muffins
Rice crackers
Pita bread
Popcorn
Bagels

- *Fruits†*
Apples
Bananas
Pears
Berries
Oranges, other citrus fruits
Melon
Grapes
Unsweetened canned fruit
Unsweetened fruit juices
- *Vegetables*
Carrots
Celery
Green pepper
Radishes
Cucumbers
Cabbage
Cauliflower
Broccoli
Tomatoes
Jicama
Vegetable juices

Examples: Apple wedges with peanut butter; egg salad sandwich; raw vegetables with yogurt or cottage cheese dip; plain yogurt with unsweetened applesauce and cinnamon; tortilla with melted cheese; pita bread with tuna; popcorn with parmesan cheese; frozen banana rolled in plain yogurt and chopped nuts; rice cracker with peanut butter or cheese.

---

*These foods may be protective against lowering plaque pH when eaten with foods that contain fermentable carbohydrate.
†Fruits, juices, and most cereal/bread products contain fermentable carbohydrate; limit to 1 serving in a snack.
From Pipes PL, Trahms CM: *Nutrition in Infancy and Childhood*, St. Louis, 1993, Mosby.

ONE STEP FURTHER

supported these findings. Many researchers have found no difference between meal eating habits of caries-free and caries-prone individuals.

Snacking at bedtime is especially effective in increasing dental caries. Reduction of the flow of saliva, which occurs during sleep, reduces the natural cleansing mechanism and permits greater fermentation of cariogenic material. The ingestion of foods that alter the buffering capacity of the saliva, for example, milk and fats, which form a protective oily film on the tooth surface, may offer some protection for the teeth.

Control. The less frequently sucrose-containing foods are consumed and the less ability the foods have to adhere to the teeth, the more positive will be the outlook for the control of dental caries.

Fluoride. It has definitely been proven that fluoride can reduce the incidence of dental caries. Fluoride suppresses sugar metabolism by bacteria, makes enamel more resistant to acid, and stimulates remineralization of the teeth. A fluoridated water supply is an important approach to the prevention of dental caries.

Diet: Foods and frequency. Dietary control continues to be a most important and effective approach to the control of dental caries. The frequency of eating breads, rolls, and cereals has not been associated with an increase in dental caries, whereas the frequency of eating candy and chewing gum has been shown to increase the number and incidence of dental caries. Cookies, cakes, pies, and candies have been shown to cause profound falls in pH levels of the plaque. It is interesting that the more acid-carbonated beverages depress the pH less than apple and orange juice.[71] A study of 147 junior high school students' snacking patterns in relation to caries production showed chocolate candy to be the most carious snack food selected. Children who consumed fruit drinks, cookies, or apples at bedtime and between meals had a significant caries increment during the year studied. No carious lesions developed in 47 children who had higher intakes of fruit juice and oranges and lesser use of sugar-sweetened chewing gum than the other children.[72]

Plaque control. Researchers have studied the cariogenicity of foods by noting changes in the plaque pH before and immediately after a food is eaten. Foods that cause the plaque pH to fall below 5.5 are considered to be cariogenic. Certain foods do not cause the plaque pH between the teeth to fall to levels at which demineralization will occur. These foods have a relatively high protein content with basic amino acids, a moderate fat content, a strong buffering capacity, a high mineral content including calcium and phosphorus, and a pH greater than 6.0. They also stimulate saliva flow. Meats, nuts, and cheese have been found to be noncariogenic. In fact, they have a beneficial effect when consumed with other foods. Cheddar cheese has been observed to block caries formation caused by sweet snacks when sweets and cheese have been eaten alternately. Nutritional snacks for dental health are shown on p. 307.

Nutrition education. Children should be taught to select foods that provide the essential nutrients and to limit their consumption of cariogenic foods. It is important that they learn to include noncariogenic protective foods in their snacking patterns, especially when sucrose-containing foods are included in the menu. The important between meal snacks can be carefully planned to contribute nutrients without creating an oral environment conducive to tooth decay. Sweet foods such as dessert items should be consumed as infrequently as possible within the framework of acceptability to the child and to the family.

Food and Behavior

There has been considerable speculation that certain additives and food constituents such as sugar and caffeine may play a part in the etiology of hyperactivity in childhood. This condition is characterized by inattention, excess motor activity, impulsiveness, and poor tolerance for frustration; the onset of hyperactivity occurs before 7 years of age. It affects 5% to 10% of school-age children.

Additives. In recent years the hypothesis that artificial flavors and colors and naturally occurring **salicylates** cause hyperactivity in as many as 50% of children so affected has been popular. Many persons have felt that a diet that eliminated these constituents was indicated. But research has not supported this hypothesis. A very small percentage of children, however, have been identified to be "responders" to the additives.

Open clinical trials have indicated behavioral improvements in as many as 50% of hyperactive children. They have also reported that diet improved behavior in nonhyperactive children, suggesting that behavioral changes may be due to changes in the parent-child interactions and family dynamics.[73] A recent study using a total dietary replacement design once again looked at dietary manipulations in 24 preschool hyperactive boys. All children received both the experimental and control diets. Food dyes, food flavorings, preservatives, monosodium glutamate, chocolate, and caffeine were eliminated from the diet. Specific foods that the family felt to be detrimental to the child's behavior

Salicylates
Compound salts of salicylic acid, found in certain plants and in drugs such as common aspirin (acetylsalicylic acid—ASA).

were also eliminated. Almost 50% of the boys showed some behavioral improvement using the accepted rating scales. Sleep patterns also were better.[74]

Double-blind studies suggest that food additives do not play a major role in the etiology of hyperactivity in the majority of cases. Interestingly, two different researchers found an order effect. In one study parents noted a slight effect if the additive-free diet had been given first, and in another study teachers noted the same effect when the **placebo** was given first.[73]

Sugar. Sugar has also been hypothesized to play a role in the etiology of behavioral difficulties in children. Most of the reports that have indicted sugar have been based on clinical assessment, with few on controlled studies.

Several double-blind challenge studies have not found sugar to contribute to hyperactivity even in children whose mothers felt they were responders. However, speculation that sugar is an offender in the etiologies of the disorder continues on the basis of observations of behavior and food intake. An association was suggested between destructive aggressive behavior and sugar intake of 4- to 7-year-old hyperkinetic but not normal children on the basis of 7-day food diaries kept by the mothers and videotaped observations of behavior by trained observers.[75] Another study noted an inverse relationship in the percentage of sugar in the children's diets suggested by a 1-day dietary recall and standardized measures of intelligence and school achievement.[76] It should be noted that none of the above studies has shown a cause and effect relation between sugar and behavior.

Definitive evidence that sugar causes behavioral problems in children has not been found. However, there may be some children who are sensitive to sugar, and further investigation using a double-blind crossover design is appropriate.

Prevention of Atherosclerosis

Risk factors. Major risk factors associated with **atherosclerosis** and its resulting cardiovascular disease include obesity, a strong family history of heart disease, a sedentary lifestyle, hypertension, and elevated blood lipids, especially low-density lipoprotein (LDL) cholesterol. These risk factors are independent and continuous variables. Studies of adults have shown a significant relation between elevated serum cholesterol, blood pressure, and the extent of **atherosclerotic lesions.** The extent of the raised lesion is associated with total fat, saturated fat, cholesterol, and animal protein intakes.

Evidence that the atherosclerotic process leading to adult coronary heart disease begins in childhood includes (1) observations at autopsy of children and young adults who died of noncoronary events, and (2) epidemiologic studies of adult relatives of children with elevated plasma cholesterol levels. Findings at autopsy have described fatty streaks in the **aortas** of preschool children and fibrous plaques in coronary arteries of 20- to 22-year-old American soldiers who died in the Korean and Vietnamese wars. Epidemiologic studies indicate that blood lipids and lipoproteins track from birth to the young adult years.[77-79] It is also known that food habits developed in childhood continue into the adult years.

Because of these findings, it is becoming increasingly clear that the origin of atherosclerosis, especially in genetically predisposed persons, is in early childhood. Several groups have recommended changing the diet of all children over 2 years of age. The recommendation includes reduction of total dietary fat to less than 30% of the day's total kilocalories, saturated fat reduced to less than 10% of the total kilocalories, and cholesterol limited to 300 mg/day.[80]

Many pediatricians disagree with this universal recommendation, feeling that such diets may not provide sufficient energy and essential nutrients for normal growth and development. In fact, children of some conscientious parents trying to implement the recommendations have been diagnosed with growth deficits and failure to thrive.[59,60] The

Placebo
(L "I will please") An inactive substance or preparation used in controlled drug or nutrient studies to determine the efficacy of an agent under study.

Atherosclerosis
(Gr *athere*, gruel; *skleros*, hard) Condition characterized by gradual formation, beginning in childhood in genetically predisposed individuals, of fatty cheeselike streaks then harder plaques in the intima or inner lining of major blood vessels such as coronary arteries, eventually in adulthood cutting off blood supply to the tissue served by the vessel; the underlying pathology of coronary heart disease.

Atherosclerotic lesions
Characteristic lesions, called *athromas,* the fatty raised streaks and plaques that signal atherosclerosis, the underlying cardiovascular disease associated with elevated levels of serum lipids, especially cholesterol, and related risk factors such as smoking, obesity, and hypertension.

Aorta
Main large trunk blood vessel from the heart, leading down the center of the body through the chest and into the abdomen, from which the systemic arterial blood system proceeds.

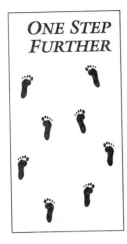

ONE STEP FURTHER

NCEP Report: Recommended Cholesterol Levels for Children and Adolescents				
	Total cholesterol		Low-density lipoprotein cholesterol	
	mmol/L	mg/dl	mmol/L	mg/dl
Acceptable	<4.4	<170	<2.8	<110
Borderline	4.4-5.1	170-199	2.8-3.3	110-129
High	≥5.2	≤200	≥3.4	≥130

The National Cholesterol Education Program, *Report of the Expert Panel on Blood Cholesterol Levels in Children and Adolescents*, Bethesda, Md, 1991, National Heart, Lung and Blood Institute.

Hyperlipidemia
(Gr *hyper*, above; *lipos*, fat; *haemia*, blood) General term for elevated concentrations of any or all of the lipids in the blood plasma.

American Academy of Pediatrics states that the recommendation should be followed with moderation.[28]

Panel report. A panel from the National Institutes of Health also recommends screening of high-risk children. Children, they indicate in their report, should be selected by their pediatricians for cholesterol screening if they have high-risk families, with parents or grandparents with diagnosed cardiovascular heart disease or a cardiac event before age 55, or if one or both parents have had elevated serum cholesterol levels over 240 mg/dl. The panel recommended dietary intervention for children with borderline low-density lipoprotein (LDL) cholesterol levels of 110 to 129 mg/dl, and drug therapy for children over 10 years of age who have very high serum cholesterol levels over 200 mg/dl or LDL cholesterol level above 130 mg/dl that does not respond to dietary intervention.[81]

The American Academy of Pediatrics recommends cholesterol testing only for children over age 2 who have a family history of **hyperlipidemia** or early **myocardial infarction.** If an elevated serum cholesterol is confirmed in the child, dietary counseling is advised. Drug therapy is advised only for children with serum cholesterol levels greater than 200 mg/dl and for those who do not respond to dietary intervention in a reasonable period of time.[82] The new guidelines in the National Cholesterol Education Program (NCEP) report for blood total cholesterol and LDL-cholesterol limits for children, shown in the box above, are consistent with the American Academy of Pediatrics recommendations, as well as national health guides and objectives of the American Heart Association, National Academy of Sciences, and the U.S. Surgeon General, and are supported by the American Dietetic Association.[83-87]

Summary

Children between 1 year and the onset of puberty grow at a steady rate. They acquire new skills, learn much about their environment, and test the limits of behavior the environment will accept. All of these factors influence the food they accept and the frequency with which they eat. As they grow older, children's food intakes become more influenced by peers, activities, and stimuli in their environment.

Prevention of nutrition problems is important during childhood. Of particular concern is the prevention of iron deficiency anemia, obesity, and dental caries, as well as reducing later adult risks for cardiovascular coronary heart disease in identified children of high-risk families.

1. Why do energy needs of children vary so widely at any age?
2. What independent feeding skills would you expect a normal 18-month-old child to have?
3. What factors influence food acceptance by children?
4. List food and feeding behavior concerns of most importance to mothers of preschool children.
5. List snack foods appropriate for children that are supportive of a program to prevent excessive weight gain and dental caries.
6. Describe the family history and blood lipid levels that would identify a child at risk for development of arteriosclerotic heart disease.

References

1. Smith DW: *Growth and its disorders,* Philadelphia, 1977, WB Saunders.
2. Ryan AS et al: An evaluation of the association between socioeconomic status and the growth of Mexican American children: data from the Hispanic Health and Nutrition Examination Survey (HHANES 1982-1984), *Am J Clin Nutr* 51:944S, 1990.
3. Yip R et al: Improving growth status of Asian refugee children in the United States, *JAMA* 267:937, 1992.
4. National Center for Health Statistics: NCHS growth charts, 1976, *Monthly Vital Statistics Report,* vol 25, no 3, suppl (HRA) 76-1120, Rockville, Md, 1976, Health Resources Administration.
5. Pipes PL, Trahms CM: *Nutrition in infancy and childhood,* St. Louis, 1993, Mosby.
6. Scott BJ et al: Growth assessment in children: a review, *Top Clin Nutr* 8:5, 1992.
7. Food and Nutrition Board, National Research Council: *Recommended dietary allowances,* ed 10, Washington, DC, 1989, National Academy of Sciences.
8. Pellet PL: Food energy requirements in humans, *Am J Clin Nutr* 51:711, 1990.
9. Birch LL et al: The variability of young children's energy intake, *N Engl J Med* 324:232, 1991.
10. Ashworth A, Millward DJ: Catch-up growth in children, *Nutr Rev* 44:157, 1986.
11. Pellet PL: Protein requirements in humans, *Am J Clin Nutr* 51:723, 1990.
12. Sabate J et al: Anthropometric parameters of school children with different lifestyles, *Am J Dis Child* 144:1159, 1990.
13. Pipes PL, Trahms CM: Nutrition in infancy and childhood, St. Louis, 1993, Mosby.
14. Prentice A: Calcium requirements of children, *Nutr Rev* 53:37, 1995.
15. Schlage C, Wortberg B: Zinc in the diet of healthy preschool and school children, *Acta Paediatr Scand* 61:421, 1972.
16. Walravens PA et al: Zinc supplementation in infants with a nutritional pattern of failure to thrive: a double-blind, controlled study, *Pediatrics* 83:1089, 1989.
17. Lozoff B et al: Long-term developmental outcome of infants and iron deficiency, *N Engl J Med* 325:687, 1991.
18. Drake MA: Anthropometry, biochemical iron indexes, and energy and nutrient intake of preschool children: comparison of intake at day care center and at home, *J Am Diet Assoc* 91:1587, 1991.
19. Stephenson L: Possible new developments in community control of iron-deficiency anemia, *Nutr Rev* 53:23, 1995.
20. Lobosco RM: A commentary on domestic hunger: a problem we can solve, *Top Clin Nutr* 9:8-12, 1994.
21. Zive MM et al: Vitamin and mineral intakes of Anglo-American and Mexican-American preschoolers, *J Am Diet Assoc* 95:329, 1995.
22. Murphy SP et al: An evaluation of food group intakes by Mexican-American children, *J Am Diet Assoc* 90:388, 1990.

23. Jackson MY: Height, weight and body mass index of American Indian school children 1990-91, *J Am Diet Assoc* 93:1136, 1993.

24. DuRousseau PC et al: Children in foster care: are they at nutritional risk? *J Am Diet Assoc* 91:83, 1991.

25. Fierman AH et al: Growth delay in homeless children, *Pediatrics* 88:918-1991.

26. Taylor ML, Koblinsky SA: Dietary intake and growth status of young homeless children, *J Am Diet Assoc* 93:464, 1993.

27. Drake MA: Dietary adequacy of children residing in temporary shelters, *J Am Diet Assoc* 91:A-77, 1991.

28. Barnes LA editor: *Pediatric nutrition handbook,* Committee on Nutrition, American Academy of Pediatrics, Elk Grove Village, Ill, 1993.

29. Breskin MW et al: Water soluble vitamins: intakes and indices in children, *J Am Diet Assoc* 85:49, 1985.

30. Terry RD, Oakland MJ: Parents' reasons for giving vitamin and mineral supplements to their preschoolers, *Top Clin Nutr* 5:67, 1990.

31. Beauchamp GK, Cowart BJ: Congenital and experimental factors in the development of human flavor preferences, *Appetite* 6:357, 1985.

32. Cowart BJ, Beauchamp GK: The importance of sensory content in young children's acceptance of salty tastes, *Child Dev* 57:1034, 1986.

33. Falciglia GE, Norton PA: Evidence for a genetic influence on preference for some foods, *J Am Diet Assoc* 4:154, 1994.

34. Anliker JA et al: Children's food preferences and genetic sensitivity to the bitter taste of 6-n-propylthiouracil (PROP), *Am J Clin Nutr* 54:16, 1991.

35. Swanson-Rudd J et al: Nutrition orientations of working mothers in the North Central Region, *J Nutr Educ* 14:132, 1982.

36. Phillips DE, Bass MA, Yetley E: Use of food and nutrition knowledge by mothers of preschool children, *J Nutr Educ* 10:73, 1980.

37. Burroughs ML, Terry RD: Parents' perspectives toward their children's eating behavior, *Top Clin Nutr* 8:45, 1992.

38. DeWalt KM: The use of itemized register tapes for analysis of household food acquisition patterns prompted by children, *J Am Diet Assoc* 90:559, 1990.

39. Kirk MC, Gillespie AH: Factors affecting food choices of working mothers with young families, *J Nutr Educ* 22:161, 1990.

40. Stanek K et al: Diet quality and the eating environment of preschool children, *J Am Diet Assoc* 90:1582, 1990.

41. Birch LL et al: Mother-child interaction patterns and the degree of fatness in children, *J Nutr Educ* 12:17, 1981.

42. Birch LL et al: The influence of social-affective context on the formation of children's food preferences, *J Nutr Educ* 13:115, 1981.

43. Birch LL et al: Eating as a "means" activity in contingency: effect on young children's food preferences, *Child Dev* 55:431, 1984.

44. Birch LL, Deysher M: Caloric compensation and sensory specific satiety: evidence for self regulation of food intake by young children, *Appetite* 7:323, 1986.

45. Klesges RC et al: Parental influence on food selection in young children and its relationship to childhood obesity, *Am J Clin Nutr* 53:859, 1991.

46. Story M, Brown JE: Do young children instinctively know what to eat? The studies of Clara Davis revisited, *N Engl J Med* 316:103, 1987.

47. Sylvester GP, others: Children's television and nutrition: friends or foes? *Nutr Today* 30:6, 1995.

48. Dietz WH, Gortmaker SL: Do we fatten our children at the television set? Obesity and television viewing in children and adolescents, *Pediatrics* 75:807, 1985.

49. Kotz K, Story M: Food advertisements during children's Saturday morning television programming: are they consistent with dietary recommendations? *J Am Diet Assoc* 94:1296, 1994.

50. Taras HL et al: Television's influence on children's diet and physical activity, *J Dev Behav Pediatr* 10:176, 1989.
51. Sanjur D et al: Dietary patterns and nutrient intake of toddlers from low-income families in Denver, *J Am Diet Assoc* 90:823, 1990.
52. Beal VA: Dietary intake of individuals followed through infancy and childhood, *Am J Public Health* 51:1107, 1961.
53. Eppright ES et al: The North Central Regional Study of diets of preschool children. III. Frequency of eating, *J Home Econ* 62:407, 1970.
54. Farris RP et al: Macronutrient intake of 10-year-old children, 1973 to 1982, *J Am Diet Assoc* 86:765, 1986.
55. Nicklas TA et al: Nutritional studies in children and implications for change: the Bogalusa Heart Study, *J Adv Med* 2:451, 1989.
56. Hertzler AA: Preschoolers' food handling skills-motor development, *J Nutr Educ* 21:100B, 1989.
57. Sherry B et al: Short, thin or obese? Comparing growth indexes of children from high- and low-poverty areas, *J Am Diet Assoc* 92:1092-5, 1992.
58. Pugliese MM et al: Parental health beliefs as a cause of non-organic failure to thrive, *Pediatrics* 80:175, 1987.
59. Lifshitz F, Moses N: Growth failure, *Am J Dis Child* 143:537, 1989.
60. McPherson RS et al: Intake and food sources of dietary fat among school children in the Woodlands, Texas, *Pediatrics* 86:520, 1990.
61. Wolfe WS, Campbell C: Food pattern, diet quality, and related characteristics of schoolchildren in New York state, *J Am Diet Assoc* 93:1280, 1993.
62. Pollitt EL et al: Brief fasting stress and cognition in children, *Am J Clin Nutr* 34:1526, 1981.
63. Nicklas TA et al: Breakfast consumption affects adequacy of total daily intake in children, *J Am Diet Assoc* 93:886-891, 1993.
64. Briggs M et al: Nutrient standard menu planning in child nutrition programs, *Top Clin Nutr* 9:37, 1994.
65. Lissau I, Sorensen TIA: Parental neglect during childhood and increased risk of obesity in young adulthood, *Lancet* 343:324, 1994.
66. Gustafson-Larson AM, Terry RD: Weight-related behaviors and concerns of fourth grade children, *J Am Diet Assoc* 92:818-822, 1992.
67. Hertzler AA: Obesity impact of the family, *J Am Diet Assoc* 75:525, 1981.
68. *Oral health of United States children: the national survey of dental caries in US school children (1986-1987),* NIH Pub No 89-2247, 1989, US Department of Health and Human Services, Bethesda, Md.
69. Tucker AW, Touger-Decker R: Improving nutrition and oral health of minority urban children: a model university/community program, *Top Clin Nutr* 9:49, 1994.
70. Gustafson BE et al: The Vipeholm dental caries study: the effect of different levels of carbohydrate intake on dental caries in 436 individuals observed for five years, *Acta Odontal Scand* 11:232, 1954.
71. White-Graves MV, Schiller MR: History of foods in the caries process, *J Am Diet Assoc* 86:241, 1986.
72. Clancy KL et al: Snack food intakes of adolescents and caries development, *J Dent Res* 56:568, 1977.
73. Levitsky DA, Strump BA: *Nutrition and the behavior of children.* In Walker WA, Watkins WF, editors: *Nutrition in pediatrics,* Boston, 1985, Little, Brown.
74. Kaplan BJ et al: Dietary replacement in preschool hyperactive boys, *Pediatrics* 83:7, 1989.
75. Printz RJ et al: Dietary correlates of hyperactive behavior in children, *J Consult Clin Psychol* 48:760, 1980.
76. Lester MB et al: Refined carbohydrate intake, hair cadmium levels, and cognitive function in children, *Nutrition and Behavior* 1:3, 1982.

77. Berenson GS et al: Serum high density lipoprotein and its relationship to cardiovascular disease risk factor variables in children—the Bogalusa Heart Study, *Lipids* 14:91, 1979.
78. Enos WF et al: Coronary disease among United States soldiers killed in action in Korea, *JAMA* 152:1090, 1952.
79. McNamara JJ et al: Coronary artery disease in combat casualties in Vietnam, *JAMA* 216:1185, 1971.
80. Department of Health and Human Services, National Heart, Lung, and Blood Institute, The National Cholesterol Education Program: *Report of the expert panel on population strategies for blood cholesterol reduction,* DHHS Pub No (NIH) 90-3046, Washington, DC, 1990, US Government Printing Office.
81. Department of Health and Human Services, National Heart, Lung, and Blood Institute, The National Cholesterol Education Program: *Report of the expert panel on blood cholesterol levels in children and adolescents,* NIH Pub No 91-2732, Bethesda, Md, 1991.
82. American Academy of Pediatrics, Committee on Nutrition: Indications for cholesterol testing in children, *Pediatrics* 83:141, 1989.
83. National Academy of Sciences, National Research Council, Food and Nutrition Board: *Diet and health, implications for reducing chronic disease risk,* Washington, DC, 1989, National Academy Press.
84. US Department of Health and Human Services, Public Health Services: *Healthy people 2000, national health promotion and disease prevention objectives,* DHHS Pub No (PHS) 91-50212, Washington, DC, 1990, US Government Printing Office.
85. ADA Reports: Timely statement on NCEP report on children and adolescents, *J Am Diet Assoc* 91(8):983, 1991.
86. National Cholesterol Education Program (NCEP): Report of the expert panel on blood cholesterol in children and adolescents, *Pediatrics* Supplement 89:575, 1992.
87. Statement on Cholesterol, Committee on Nutrition, American Academy of Pediatrics, *Pediatrics* 90:469, 1992.

Further Reading

Recently position papers and handbooks have been published to address the critical need for appropriate meal service in child care centers and educational programs. The components of nutrition education, appropriate food to provide needed nutrients, and a supportive physical and emotional environment are endorsed to protect and promote children's health and well-being.

Position paper of the American Dietetic Association: Child Nutrition Services: *J Am Diet Assoc* 93:334, 1993.

Position of ADA, SNE, and ASFSA: school-based nutrition programs and services, *J Am Diet Assoc* 95:367, 1995.

Nutrition standards in child care programs: technical support paper: *J Am Diet Assoc* 93:334, 1993.

Building for the future: nutrition guidance for the child nutrition programs, US Department of Agriculture, Food and Nutrition Service, FNS-279, 1992.

Edelstein S: *Nutrition and meal planning in child-care programs: a practical guide,* Chicago, Ill., 1992, The American Dietetic Association.

Several useful handbooks are available which address the complex issues of child health.

Sharbaugh CO editor: *Call to action: better nutrition for mothers, children and families,* 1991, National Center for Education in Maternal and Child Health.

Healthy children 2000: national health promotion and disease prevention objectives related to mothers, infants, children, adolescents and youth, Department of Health and Human Services, Public Health Service, Health Resources and Service Administration, Maternal and Child Health Bureau, 1991.

Eliades DC, Suitor CW: *Celebrating diversity: approaching families through their food,* Arlington, Va, 1994, National Center for Education in Maternal and Child Health.

Call to action: better nutrition for mothers, children, and families, Maternal and Child Health Bureau, Health Resources and Services Administration, Public Health Service, US Department of Health and Human Services.

Green M, editor: *Bright futures: guidelines for health supervision of infants, children, and adolescents,* Arlington, Va, 1994, National Center for Education in Maternal and Child Health.

Education programs now accommodate the special nutritional needs of children with developmental disabilities and chronic illnesses.

Yadrick K, Sneed J: Nutrition services for children with developmental disabilities and chronic illnesses in education programs, *J Am Diet Assoc* 94:1122, 1994.

An increasingly multi-cultural population requires that all health care providers have knowledge and skills in understanding the foodways of people in the United States.

Randall-David E: *Strategies for working with culturally diverse communities and clients,* Bethesda, Md, 1989, Association for the Care of Children's Health.

Lynch EW, Johnson MJ: *Developing cross-cultural competence: a guide for working with young children and their families,* Baltimore, 1994, Brookes Publishing.

Bronner Y: Cultural sensitivity and nutrition counseling, *Top Clin Nutr* 9:13-19, 1994.

Bronner Y et al: African-American/soul foodways and nutrition counseling, *Top Clin Nutr* 9:20-27, 1994.

Rodriguez J: Diet, nutrition, and the Hispanic client, *Top Clin Nutr* 9:28-39, 1994.

Wu-Jung CJ: Understanding food habits of Chinese Americans, *Top Clin Nutr* 9:40-44, 1994.

Eliades DC, Suitor CW: *Celebrating diversity: approaching families through their food,* Arlington, Va, 1994, National Center for Education in Maternal and Child Health.

8

Nutrition in Adolescence

Bonnie S. Worthington-Roberts
Jane M. Rees

Basic Concepts

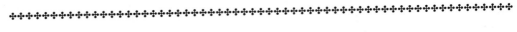

- ✔ *Adolescent growth and development include both rapid physical growth and dramatic psychosocial development with sexual maturing.*
- ✔ *Normal adolescent growth and development require increased nutritional support.*
- ✔ *Adolescent physical activities and health problems lead to specific nutritional needs.*
- ✔ *Personal needs guide approaches to adolescent nutrition assessment, counseling, and management.*

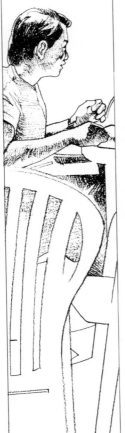

Adolescence is a phase of the life cycle that has long puzzled individuals and their parents as well as health professionals. An awareness of the characteristics and needs of this special group, however, can contribute to a greater appreciation for teenagers in general and for those who have special nutritional needs. Knowledge from other disciplines in the physical and social sciences must be integrated to provide a comprehensive basis for understanding nutritional issues. The unique characteristics of adolescent growth and development, both physical and psychologic, are relevant not only to theoretical discussions of the specific topics but also to clinical protocols, in which results from controlled studies are synthesized to derive solutions to long-term problems arising in uncontrolled real life situations.

In this chapter we see that typical eating habits of adolescents are affected by environment, lifestyle, and normal development. We also understand why counseling techniques useful in helping adolescents improve their nutritional practices include the most sophisticated ones available from the social sciences today. Specifically planned nutritional support for growth and development is required for such diverse circumstances as eating disorders, fitness activities and competitive sports, chronic disease, and pregnancy. Current research is beginning to shed light on the theories and myths that surround nutritional influence on adolescent behavior. While many questions related to adolescent nutrition remain unanswered, a body of sound, practical knowledge exists to guide adolescents in maintaining positive nutrition and health.

ADOLESCENT GROWTH AND DEVELOPMENT
Physiologic Growth

Puberty. The process of physically developing from a child to an adult is called puberty. Puberty, referring to maturation of the total body, is initiated by poorly understood physiologic factors. During late childhood slow growth begins to accelerate with pubescence until the rate is as rapid as that of early infancy. Fig. 8-1 shows that linear growth in centimeters per year during the teen years compares with that for the second year of life. The individual will gain about 20% of adult height and 50% of adult weight during pubertal growth.[1] Most of the body organs will double in size.

Initiation of puberty. What causes the upsurge in hormonal activity that initiates pubertal development? Current **radioimmunoassay** techniques allow the measurement of hormonal concentrations that previously were below the sensitivity limits of earlier assays. This advance allows the hormonal changes to be measured as they occur chronologically. However, even with the development of these refined laboratory techniques, the exact factor or combination of factors that triggers these changes is still unknown.[1] Many theories have been suggested. One popular theory proposes that there is a "gonadostat," an area in the brain that is extremely sensitive to the sex steroids estrogen, testosterone, and progesterone. This "gonadostat" governs the release of these hormones by a feedback mechanism that allows increased production with the onset of puberty.

Radioimmunoassay

(L *radius,* ray; *immunis,* free, exempt; *assay,* examine, analyze) Technique using radioactive labeling of the material being studied; used for measuring minute constituent quantities of antigen or antibody, hormones, certain drugs, and other substances.

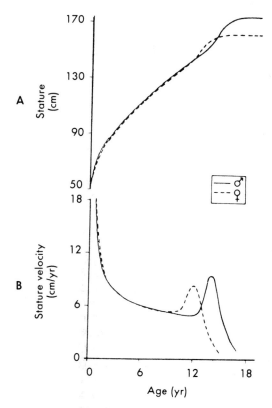

FIG. 8-1 **A,** Growth in stature of typical boy *(solid line)* and girl *(dashed line)*. **B,** Growth velocities at different ages of typical boy *(solid line)* and girl *(dashed line)*.

From Marshall WA: *Clin Endocrinol Metab* 4:4, 1975.

Other theories relate pubertal onset to a change in body composition. An association between menarche and the attainment of a critical body weight has been observed in North American and most European females. It has been theorized that the achievement of the critical body weight of 47.8 kg (105 lb) causes a change in metabolic rate that in turn triggers menarche and initiates the adolescent growth spurt in girls. Another way of stating this relationship is that the attainment of a minimal level of body fatness (17% of body weight) is necessary for the onset of menstruation. Other researchers acknowledge an association between change in body composition and the onset of menarche, but do not view it as a triggering factor of puberty.

Sequence and stages of growth and development. Adolescent growth is characterized by a predictable sequence of stages in sexual maturity, increased height and weight, and changes in body composition. The timing and milestones of pubertal development are summarized in Fig. 8-2. The range of initiation and completion of milestones is listed in years.

Sexual maturity. Beginning with the enlargement of genitalia in males and breast development in females and accompanied by pubic hair distribution, the sexual maturation

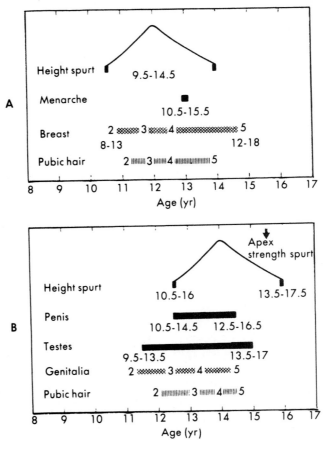

FIG. 8-2   Diagram of sequence of selected events at puberty in girls (**A**) and boys (**B**). *Cross-hatched and small vertical line bars with numbers* refer to developmental stages described in Table 8-1.

From Marshall WA, and Tanner JM: *Arch Dis Child* 45:13, 1970.

of humans can be observed and compared with norms. Table 8-1 describes the detailed stages of that development. In Fig. 8-2 these stages are depicted by the crosshatched and multilined bars with sequence of milestones that make up puberty. The onset of menses (menarche) in females and the completion of genitalia growth in males corresponds with stage 5, or adult status of sexual maturity.

Data have been accumulated to show that during the last century young women have gradually come to experience the menarche at younger ages, the so-called "secular trend." Total maturation probably occurs earlier for males as well. The theory is generally accepted, though records of menstrual age are scarce enough that the basis for its formulation has been questioned.

Height and weight. Throughout the approximately 5 to 7 years of pubertal development, rapid growth continues although a great percentage of height will be gained during the "growth spurt." Like the initiation of puberty, the 18 to 24 month period of the peak **growth velocity** will occur at different ages for different individuals fitting into the sequence of overall sexual development. It occurs earlier for girls than for boys.[1] Following the achievement of sexual maturity, linear growth and weight acquisition continue at a much lower rate and then cease, as shown by the downward slope of the height-spurt curve in Fig. 8-2. For rare females it will continue into the late teens and for males into the 20s. Most females will gain no more than 2 to 3 inches (5.1 to 7.6 cm) after the onset of menses. The rate of weight gain following the menarche is discussed in the later section on adolescent pregnancy (p. 370).

Body composition. The composition of the body changes in the process of maturation. In the prepubertal period the proportion of fat and muscle in males and females tends to be similar (body fat about 15% and 19%, respectively) and lean body mass is about equal

growth velocity
(L *velocitas*, speed) Rate of childhood growth over normal periods of development, as compared with a population standard.

TABLE 8-1   **Stages of Sexual Maturation (Sexual Maturity Ratings)**

Boys	Pubic Hair	Genitalia
Stage 1	None	No change from childhood
Stage 2	Small amount at outer edges of pubis; slight darkening	Beginning penile enlargement; testes enlarged to 5 ml volume; scrotum reddened and changes in texture
Stage 3	Covers pubis	Longer penis; testes 8-10 ml; scrotum further enlarged
Stage 4	Adult type; does not extend to thighs	Larger, wider, and longer penis; testes 12 ml; scrotal skin darker
Stage 5	Adult type; now spread to thighs	Adult penis; testes 15 ml

Girls	Pubic Hair	Breasts
Stage 1	None	No change from childhood
Stage 2	Small amount; downy on labia majora	Breast bud
Stage 3	Increased; darker and curly	Larger; no separation of nipple and areola
Stage 4	More abundant; coarse texture	Increased size; areola and nipple form secondary mound
Stage 5	Adult type; now spread to thighs	Adult distribution of breast tissue; continuous outline

Modified from Tanner JM: *Growth at adolescence,* ed 2, Oxford, 1962, Blackwell Scientific Publications.

for both sexes. During puberty females gain proportionately more fat so that as adults the normal percentage of body fat is about 23% for females and for males it is about 12%. Males during this time gain twice as much muscle as females do. This striking difference in adolescent growth between males and females influences nutritional needs. Because the adolescent male experiences greater gain in bone and lean tissue than the female does, he requires more protein, iron, zinc, and calcium than the female for development of these tissues. Another reason for the male's larger requirements for these nutrients is his greater rate of growth.

Measurement of growth. Knowing the relationship between the milestones of sexual development and physical growth will enable the clinician to assess the progress of growth in an adolescent at a particular time, and give some indication of the extent of future growth. Thus **pubertal development** can be monitored clinically by using weight and height tables and **sexual maturity ratings.** For example, a 16-year-old female who has experienced her menarche and progressed beyond stage 4 of breast development, but who is not as tall as her peers would be considered to be close to her adult height. Excessive or less than normal growth can be detected by plotting height changes on the standard growth grids (see Appendix A). If her height corresponded to the 25th percentile for her age, the physical maturation of the young woman in the example above would be considered to be normal. The major cause of short stature during adolescence is genetically late initiation of puberty, though such conditions as chronic disease and skeletal and chromosomal abnormalities also account for certain children being shorter than normal. Hormonal

Pubertal development
Rapid physical growth and sexual development of puberty

Sexual maturity ratings
Scale defining stages of sexual maturation during puberty.

TABLE 8-2 *Comparison of Erikson's and Piaget's Models for Emotional and Cognitive Development*

Age (years)	Erikson (emotional)	Piaget (cognitive)
0-2	**Phase I** Basic trust versus mistrust	**Sensorimotor period** Learning through senses and manipulation
2-4	**Phase I** Autonomy versus shame and doubt	**Preconceptual period** Classification by a single feature (e.g., size); no concern for contradictions
4-8	**Phase III** Initiative versus guilt	**Initiative thought period** Intuitive classification (e.g., awareness of conservation of mass concept)
8-12	**Phase IV** Industry versus inferiority	**Concrete operations period** Logical thought development; learning to organize
12-20	**Phase V** Ego identity versus role confusion	**Formal operations period** Comprehension of abstract concepts; formation of "ideals"
20 onward	**Phase VI** Intimacy versus isolation	—
Middle adulthood	**Phase VII** Generativity versus stagnation	—
Late adulthood	**Phase VIII** Integrity versus despair	—

imbalances leading to abnormal growth are rare.[1] In the United States malnutrition as a primary cause of short stature is also rare.

Weight can be plotted on a similar grid as height to determine whether an individual is keeping pace with peers or exceeding them in total weight at a particular year of age. Because of the wide variation in weights seen in sample individuals in the adolescent period, some of whom were obese, the frequency distribution represented by the grids cannot be used for evaluation of weight-for-height proportion as it is used for younger children. Evaluation of weight-for-height proportion in adolescents is described in the assessment section (p. 331).

Acne. Initiated by the influence of hormones on the sebaceous glands, acne is a normal characteristic of adolescent development. It occurs in varying degrees of severity in individual teenagers, mediated by factors such as stress and phase of the menstrual cycle. Almost all adolescents have acne, and as many as half of all adolescent contacts with health professionals are associated with dermatologic complaints. Traditionally, dietary factors have been blamed for the appearance of acne. But studies have shown no correlation between ingestion of foods and the appearance or degree of this condition.

Education about the physiologic basis for the development of acne supports teenagers

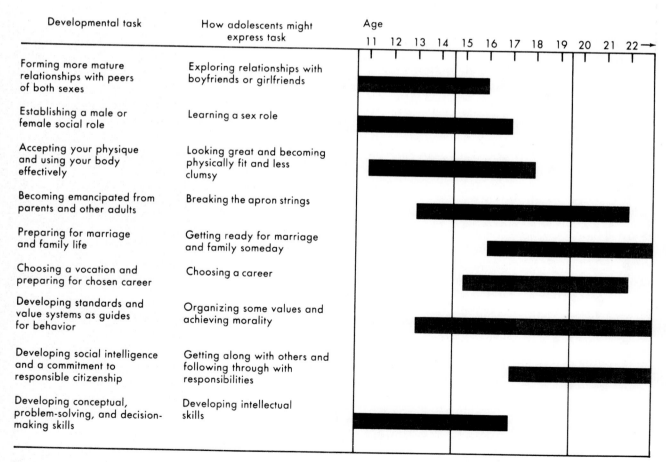

FIG. 8-3 Developmental tasks in adolescence.

Adapted from Thornburg H: *Contemporary adolescence: readings,* ed 2, Monterey, Calif, 1975, Brooks/Cole.

Tretinoin
A form of retinoic acid, a vitamin A derivative, used as a drug in the medical treatment of chronic acne as a topical keratolytic agent (Gr *keras;* horn; *lysis,* dissolution). Keratin is a hard protein; it is the principle constituent of skin, hair, nails, and scar tissue.

in their efforts to control it. Systematic antibiotics given orally and topical applications of benzoyl peroxide and **tretinoin,** as well as special cleansing agents, have been shown to be effective.

It has been suggested that pharmacologic levels of zinc and vitamin A derivatives are useful in treating acne. Low levels of serum zinc have been found in one study among persons suffering most, suggesting that zinc deficiency makes the condition worse. In general, while no research is available to confirm the effect, it would seem that the optimally nourished body will be best able to cope with the development of acne as with many conditions.

Psychosocial Development

Span and scope of adolescence. Adolescence is the term applied to the period of maturation of both mind and body and therefore may be applied to humans before and after as well as during puberty. Along with physical growth, emotional, social, and intellectual development are rapid during adolescence.[2] Milestones in psychologic development of humans are shown in Table 8-2. The ability to use abstract thinking as opposed to the concrete thought patterns of childhood, which the adolescent develops, enables the individual to accomplish these tasks. Planning ahead and connecting facts into

ONE STEP FURTHER

Phases of Adolescent Development

Early adolescence

Challenges parental authority and value system
Holds a fascination with sexuality, although he/she has generally not yet entered into sexual relationships
Compares him/herself with others
Relies greatly on peers for self-esteem
Most comfortable with same-sex peer group
Holds vague and unrealistic plan for career
Deals with the "here and now," and has trouble with the future

Middle adolescence

Continues to challenge parents' authority and shifts to peer group
Attempts to become comfortable with his/her body and is concerned with looking more attractive
Conforms with peers
Begins heterosexual relationships
Begins to develop career plans
Challenges previously taught values and struggles with issues of morality
Capacity and capability for abstracting increases

Late adolescence

Separates him/herself from family and identities; is not dependent upon rebellion from parents
Relies greater on own values while peers have become less important
Prefers intimate, caring relationships
Focuses on future planning for career
Has a sense of perspective and is able to think through problems with alternatives
Begins to develop a degree of financial independence

integrated ideas becomes possible. With the accomplishment of the developmental "tasks of adolescence" as seen in Fig. 8-3, the person is prepared for a role in adult society.

Implications for nutritional issues. Many of the tasks of adolescence relate to the nutritional health of the individual. For example, emotional maturity allows teenagers to develop their own value system. As a result they can choose foods that will enhance their health rather than making their choices by responding to less healthful characteristics of foods as they may have done in childhood. They may go through a time of experimentation while they are learning to make wise choices.

Body image. Developing an image of the physical self that includes an adult body is an intellectual and emotional task intertwined with nutritional issues. Adolescents often feel uncomfortable with rapidly changing bodies. At the same time, being very much affected by influences outside themselves, they want to be like their most perfect peers and the idols of their culture. Stereotypes in the mass media reinforce such images. Teenagers may wish certain body parts were larger and other parts were smaller. They may want to grow faster or slower. These feelings can lead them to try to change their bodies by manipulating their diets, an impulse that certain commercial interests are quick to exploit. Young women who have not developed a mature body image may unnecessarily restrict the amount of food they eat in response to weight gained with the development of secondary sex characteristics. Hoping to achieve the muscular appearance of adult males, young men are tempted to use nutritional supplements. Phases of adolescent development are discussed in the box on p. 322.

NUTRITIONAL REQUIREMENTS
Growth as a Basis for Nutritional Requirements

Limitations of the RDA standard. Studies of the nutritional requirements of adolescents must take into account not only age but also stage of physical maturity.[3] Since such studies are not generally available, the research base on which recommendations are made is limited. The Recommended Dietary Allowances (RDAs) are stated for three adolescent age groups, not related to stages of maturity. The highest levels of nutrients are recommended for the group assumed to be growing at the most rapid rate. Adolescents at the peak of their growth velocity will require large quantities of nutrients. They have been shown to incorporate twice the amount of calcium, iron, zinc, magnesium, and nitrogen into their bodies during the years of the growth spurt compared with that of other years (Table 8-3).

Calculation of needs by height. Dividing the RDA total of nutrient by the centimeters of the reference individual's height provides a quantity of nutrient in units per centimeter that can be applied to any teenager. For example, the RDA for protein for 11- to 14-year-old males is 45 g/day. The reference height is 157 cm. Thus 0.29 g/cm would be recommended. Then the total protein need would be 39 g for the 135 cm male and 54 g for the 185 cm male. This example of variation in size during the teenage years is quite realistic, since persons experience the growth spurt at different ages. Nutrient recommendations will come closest to meeting needs when the largest quantity of nutrient per centimeter is suggested for those experiencing the most rapid growth, even if the age does not coincide with the age at which the highest RDA standard is made.

Specific Nutrient Needs

Energy. The recommended energy intake in the RDA standard for adolescents as shown in Table 8-4 reflects the average needs of teenagers. As well as growth rate, level of exercise will need to be considered in determining the needs of the individual.[4]

Protein. The protein requirement of adolescents has been studied the least of all the age

TABLE 8-3   Daily Increments in Body Content Due to Growth

		Average for Period 10-20 Years (mg)	At Peak of Growth Spurt (mg)
Calcium	M	210	400
	F	110	240
Iron	M	0.57	1.1
	F	0.23	0.9
Nitrogen*	M	320	610 (3.8 g protein)
	F	160	360 (2.2 g protein)
Zinc	M	0.27	0.50
	F	0.18	0.31
Magnesium	M	4.4	8.4
	F	2.3	5.0

*The maintenance needs (2 mg/basal calorie) at 18 years of age are 3500 mg and 2700 mg for males and females, respectively.
From Forbes GB: *Nutritional requirements in adolescence*. In Suskind RM, editor: *Textbook of pediatric nutrition*, New York, 1981, Raven Press.

TABLE 8-4   Recommended Dietary Allowances for Energy for Children and Adolescents (kilocalories per day)

Age (years)	Allowance	Reference Height (cm)	Energy (kcal/cm height)
Children			
7-10	2000	132	15.2
Males			
11-14	2500	157	15.9
15-18	3000	176	17.0
Females			
11-14	2200	157	14.0
15-18	2200	163	13.5

Modified from National Academy of Sciences: *Recommended dietary allowances,* ed 10, Washington, DC, 1989, National Academy Press.

groups. The recommendation is that the energy value of the protein intake should make up 7% to 8% of the total energy consumed. Sex, age, nutritional status, and quality of the dietary protein must be considered in estimating the amount an individual will need. The range of total protein need will be about 39 to 56 g. These amounts are usually obtained in the normal diet, so protein consumption should not be overly emphasized. Protein stores of adolescents should be carefully monitored and supported in situations where nutritional depletion may occur so that physical development will not be impaired.[4]

Calcium. Calcium is an important nutrient in adolescence since the requirement is based on the amount of the mineral needed for skeletal growth. Forty-five percent of total bone growth occurs during this period. The total recommendations are the same for both sexes

TABLE 8-5 *Calculated Iron Requirements for Males and Females at the 3rd, 25th, 75th, and 97th Percentile for Body Weight (from 10-16 years of age)*

	Calculated Iron Requirements (mg)					
Percentile Rating	Daily Dietary Need*		Peak Daily Dietary Need*		Cumulative Need†	
	Male	Female	Male	Female	Male	Female
3rd	6.6	5.1	13.2	10.3	966	751
25th	9.3	5.2	18.6	10.4	1360	772
75th	11.0	5.5	21.9	11.0	1610	794
97th	12.9	5.7	25.8	11.9	1885	836

*Period of adolescent growth spurt.
†Total body iron increment represented by muscle tissue increase during 10-16 year interval.
From McKigney JI, Munro HN, editors: *Nutrient requirements in adolescence*, Cambridge, Mass, 1978, The MIT Press. Copyright © 1978 The MIT Press.

though accumulations are higher for males than for females because of the larger frame males will develop.[4]

Iron. Both males and females have high requirements for iron, as seen in Table 8-5. Males require more iron during adolescence because the buildup of muscle mass is accompanied by greater blood volume. Adolescent females require more than children because they will begin to lose iron monthly with the onset of menses.

Zinc. Zinc is known to be essential for growth as well as sexual maturation and therefore of great importance in adolescence. The retention of zinc increases, especially during the growth spurt, leading to more efficient use of the nutrient in the diet.[4]

Other minerals. The roles of other minerals in the nutrition of adolescents are not well studied. However, magnesium, iodine, phosphorus as well as copper, chromium, cobalt, and fluoride are important. The possibility of interactions between these nutrients cannot be overlooked. The recommendations for safe levels should be followed with moderation so that imbalances will not develop.

Vitamins. Adolescents require high amounts of thiamin, riboflavin, and niacin because of their high energy requirements. Vitamin D is especially needed for rapid skeletal growth. Recommended amounts of vitamins A, E, C, folate, and B_6 are the same as those for adults. Often the quantity of vitamins recommended for adolescents is of necessity **interpolated** from studies in adults and children.[4]

Interpolation
(L *interpolare*, to make new) Process of injecting new interpretation or application of data to expand meaning or use, as in deriving data from one age group and applying it to another.

EATING BEHAVIOR
Typical Nutritional Patterns

Surveys of nutrient intake have shown that adolescents are likely to be obtaining less vitamin A, thiamin, iron, and calcium than recommended. They also ingest more fat, sugar, protein, and sodium than is currently thought to be optimum.[5,6]

While concern is often expressed over the habit of eating between meals, it has been shown that teenagers obtain substantial nourishment from foods eaten outside traditional meals. The choice of foods they make is of greater importance than the time or place of eating. Emphasis should be placed on fresh vegetables and fruits as well as whole grain products to complement the foods high in energy value and protein that they commonly choose.[7]

Irregular Meals

The number of meals teenagers miss and eat away from home increases from early adolescence to late adolescence, reflecting the growing need for independence and time away from home. The evening meal appears to be the most regularly eaten meal of the day. Females are found to skip the evening meal, as well as breakfast and lunch, more often than males.

Breakfast is frequently neglected and is omitted more by teenagers and young adults under 25 years of age than by any other age group in the population. A likely explanation as to why females are more apt to miss breakfast than are males is the pursuit of thinness and frequent attempts at dieting. Many teenage girls believe that they can control their weight by omitting breakfast or lunch. Young women who are dieting should be counseled that this approach is likely to accomplish just the opposite. By midmorning or lunchtime they may be so hungry that they eat more than if they had had at least simple foods in the early morning.

Vegetarian Diets

Adolescents do, on occasion, take on special diets such as vegetarian routines. This can mean anything from eliminating red meat to omitting all animal products (i.e., eggs, fish, poultry, dairy products, and even gelatin). Such diets can be healthful, if planned with care. A sample "vegan" (strict vegetarian) diet is provided in the box on p. 327.

Factors Influencing Eating Behavior

By the time a person reaches adolescence, the influences on eating habits are numerous and the formation of those habits is extremely complex as shown in Fig. 8-4. The growing independence of adolescents, increased participation in social life, and a generally busy schedule of activities have a decided impact on what they eat. They are beginning to buy and prepare more food for themselves and they often eat rapidly and away from home.

Advertising. While the basic foundation for eating habits is found in the family, the influences on eating behavior originating outside the home in modern America are great. Teenagers are very vulnerable to the kind of advertising messages seen in Fig. 8-5. By the time Americans become adolescents they have been influenced by 10 years of television food commercials and the eating habits portrayed in television programs. The average teenager will have watched over a million food commercials, the majority of which are for products with a high concentration of sweetness and fat.

Ease of obtaining ready-to-eat foods. The ease of obtaining food that is ready to eat also influences the eating habits of teenagers. Through vending machines, at movies and sporting events, and at fast-food outlets and convenience groceries food is available at numerous times throughout the day. During the time of their peak growth velocity, adolescents may need to eat often and in large amounts and are able to use foods with a high concentration of energy. However, they will usually need to be more careful of amounts and frequency once growth has slowed.

Nutritional limitations of fast foods. The following factors appear to be the major nutritional limitations of fast-food meals:

- **Calcium, riboflavin, vitamin A.** These essential nutrients are low unless milk or a milkshake is ordered. Extensive use of soft drinks contributes to low intakes of these nutrients in addition to magnesium and vitamin C.[8]
- **Folate, fiber.** There are few sources of these key factors.
- **Fat.** The percent of energy from fat is high in many meal combinations.
- **Sodium.** The sodium content of fast-food meals is high.
- **Energy.** Common meal combinations are excessive in kilocalories when compared with the amounts of nutrients provided.

❖

SAMPLE MENU OF AN ADEQUATE VEGAN DIET FOR A 13-YEAR-OLD

Breakfast
Orange, 1 medium
Oatmeal, ¾ cup
Soymilk, 6 oz
Bread, whole wheat, 1 slice
Jam, 2 tsp

Lunch
Tofu-miso soup with 1 tsp miso, 4 oz tofu
Sandwich of hummus (1 medium pita bread, 2 tsp hummus, ½ cup spinach, 2 slices tomato)
Carrot juice, 6 oz
Figs, dried, 3

Dinner
Casserole of beans (¾ cup brown rice, ½ cup navy beans, 1 tsp safflower oil, 1 cup broccoli, ½ cup yellow squash, ¼ cup onion)
Kale, cooked ¾ cup

Snack
Watermelon, 1 slice
Strawberries, 1 cup
Gorp (¼ cup almonds, ½ oz pumpkin seeds, ¼ cup sunflower seeds, ¼ cup raisins)

From Jacobs C, Dwyer J: Vegetarian children: appropriate and inappropriate diets, *Am J Clin Nutr* 48:811, 1988.

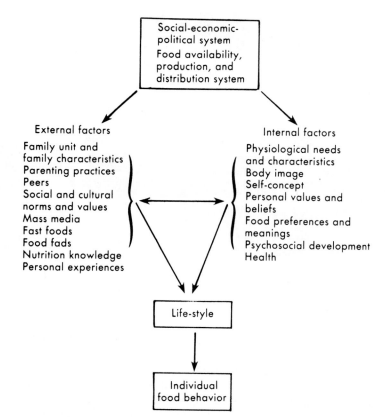

FIG. 8-4   Schematic diagram of factors influencing adolescent food behavior.

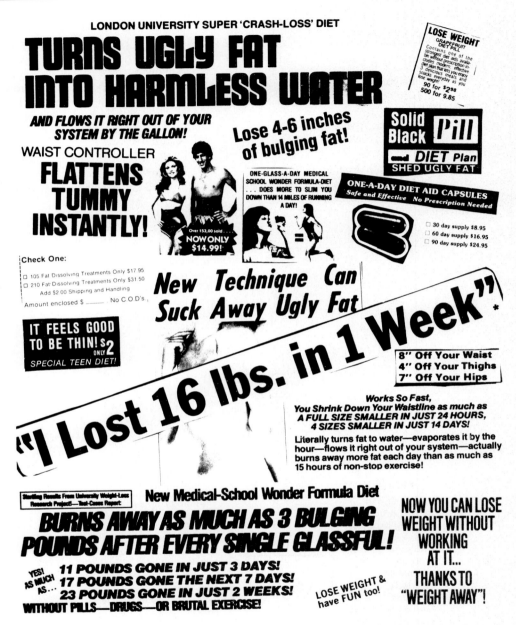

FIG. 8-5 Examples of enticements and advertisements for weight-loss products featured in popular magazines.

Although fast foods can contribute nutrients to the diet, they cannot completely meet the nutritional needs of teenagers. Both adolescents and health professionals should be aware that fast foods are acceptable nutritionally when they are consumed judiciously and as a part of a well-balanced diet.[7] When they become the mainstay of the diet there is cause for concern.[9] A nutrient imbalance may not appear to be a problem until a number of years have gone by, unless some specific problem such as a chronic disease exists. However, evidence is accumulating to show that food intake patterns of teenagers affect their health in later life.[4]

Hypertension and hyperlipidemia. If an adolescent is hypertensive or there is a strong family history of the disease, a diet controlled in sodium and total energy is a part of long-term nutritional care. In the case of hyperlipidemia, fat and energy intake should be controlled. All adolescents should be cautioned against a high intake of sodium, fat, and energy because of the suspected link with cardiovascular disease and should be screened for hyperlipidemia once during adolescence. The following is a guide to the risks of particular levels of blood lipids for ages 2 to 19 years by sex:

	Total cholesterol (mg/dl)	Risk	LDL-cholesterol (mg/dl)	Risk
Males	175-190	Moderate	110-130	Moderate
	>190	High	>130	High
Females	178-200	Moderate	115-140	Moderate
	>200	High	>140	High

Recommended guidelines for monitoring total cholesterol and LDL cholesterol of children and adolescents from high-risk families have recently been issued by the National Cholesterol Education Program (NCEP) and a National Institutes of Health expert panel (see Chapter 7).

Dental Caries and Periodontal Disease

It is becoming apparent that the cause of **dental caries** is a complex process involving the interaction of several factors. The minerals of the tooth enamel are in constant equilibrium with the oral environment. It is necessary therefore to consider not only the presence of fermentable carbohydrate but also such factors as food solubility, mineral composition, and the buffering capacity of the oral environment. Adolescents' propensity to snack on refined carbohydrates is conducive to tooth decay. Since 80% of the average person's total incidence of dental lesions occur in the teenage years, this is the time to encourage habits built on choosing alternatives to sugar-containing foods.

Gingivitis increases in prevalence during the teenage years, and **periodontal disease** often follows. Little is known about the role of nutrition in periodontal disease, although nutritional deficiency, widespread in underdeveloped countries with a high incidence of periodontal disease, has also been implicated. Inadequate intake of these nutrients in the teenage years can have an adverse effect on the health of the gums in later life.

Role of Parents

In order to encourage adolescents to form reasonable eating habits parents should give their children increased responsibility and choice within the range of nourishing foods as they are growing up. By the time they are teenagers they will need some freedom to use the kitchen. This is true for young men as well as for young women.

Substance Use and Abuse

Substance abuse in adolescence is a public health problem of major significance and concern. The substances most widely abused by adolescents are tobacco, smokeless tobacco, alcohol, marijuana, and cocaine. The strongest predictor of drug use by an adolescent is association with a peer group that uses drugs, although poor parenting and drug use by parents are also strong influences. Adolescents who are left alone for long periods of time are more likely to use drugs and to start using them earlier than those who are with families or other positive supervised group activity more of the time. Over 90% of high school seniors have consumed alcohol; in one study one out of seven seniors admitted they had been inebriated once a week. The use of marijuana has been declining in recent years while there has been a steady increase in cocaine use throughout the 1980s. While rates of tobacco use have remained stable since the early 1980s, the rate among females has increased and the age of beginning use has declined for all teenagers. Smokeless tobacco, in the

Dental caries
(L *caries*, "rottenness" Molecular decay or death of hard tissue; disease of the calcified tissue of the teeth resulting from action of microorganisms on carbohydrates, characterized by disintegration of hard outer enamel, followed by breakdown of softer inner dentin material, leaving cavities and exposed soft tissue.

Gingivitis
(L *gingiva*, "gum of the mouth") Inflammation of the gum tissue in the mouth surrounding the base of the teeth.

Periodontal disease
(Gr *Peri*, around; L *dens*, tooth) General term for disease of tissues surrounding the tooth, affecting its integrity and stability and contributing to tooth loss

form of chewing tobacco and snuff, is typically used by male adolescents in rural areas and by young white male athletes, from 7% to 25% in populations studied. It has caused significant oral damage including cancer and thus is cyclical in its relationship to nutritional status.

Overall about 10% to 15% of teenagers have had no experience with drugs and alcohol, 70% to 80% have experimented, 10% to 15% have definable problems, and somewhat less than 1% are chemically dependent, addicted. Cognitive, emotional, and social development is likely to be retarded in the last group.[10]

Impact on nutritional status. Two small studies have been published of nutritional status in drug- or alcohol-abusing teenagers: one study was of a racially mixed group and the other was of a Native American population.[11,12] Deficient *nutrient levels* were not found in blood samples from either group, and neither reported consuming less of the nutrients studied than they needed or than nonusing peers. However, in the study that reported food choices, those of abusers were different from those of controls in that most of the nutrients they consumed came from snack foods and meat products. Fruits, vegetables, and milk were left out of their usual dietary patterns. Thus though the adolescents studied did not have deficiencies that were measured either biochemically or in reported consumption, the long-term effects of their characteristic dietary habits, coupled with exposure to alcohol, would account for the development of the nutritional disorders seen in adult abusers. Studying the nutritional status of 18- to 25-year-old drug abusers would be most useful in the exploration of the natural history of deficiency diseases among alcohol and drug abusers. In summary, it can be said that the effect of substance abuse on nutritional status of any individual depends on the substance, the amount, duration and frequency of use, prior health and nutritional status, stage of physical growth, and nutritional adequacy of the diet consumed.

Identification and referral. Since the incidence of greatest abuse is among 18- to 25-year-old individuals, all health professionals need to be aware of the indicators of drug use so that they can refer adolescents with a definable problem for treatment before they reach a more advanced stage of chemical dependency. These indicators include:

Rash	Dyspnea on exertion
Muscle weakness	Faintness
Vomiting	Hangover
Diarrhea	Blackouts
Stomach pain	Nervousness
Nausea	Depression
Indigestion	Tiredness
Bleeding gums	Insomnia
Sore tongue	Somnolence
Taste loss	Headache
Appetite loss	Seizures
Memory loss	

Nutritional status
(L *status,* condition, situation) Condition of an individual's body tissues and health, especially as related to the nutrients that are essential to the structure, function, and maintenance of body tissues.

Nutritional assessment, intervention, and support are components of the comprehensive physical and psychologic rehabilitative process of adolescent substance abusers.

ASSESSMENT OF NUTRITIONAL STATUS

Teenagers are in a fluctuating state of balance between supplying their bodies with needed nutrients and using up the nutrients. At any one time, this flow is the teenager's nutritional status. Assessment of **nutritional status** is described in Chapter 2. Modification for the adolescent requires use of the sexual maturity ratings and a specific data base with which to compare height, weight, and weight-height proportion.

Anthropometric Data

To evaluate the relationship between the weight and height of an individual adolescent, the detailed tables of the National Health and Nutrition Examination Survey (NHANES), National Center for Health Statistics can be used. An example is shown in Table 8-6; full tables are given in Appendix B. For each 2 cm increment in height at a particular year of age, a range of weights is given. Weight-height values for age and sex between the 25th and the 75th percentiles can be considered to be in the normal range. This range allows for the normal differences in body build of individuals.

In addition, anthropometric data from a skinfold evaluation will yield a more precise assessment of the proportion of fat to muscle and therefore weight to height. For example, a low value for triceps skinfold measurement in an individual above the 75th percentile for weight-height indicates that the adolescent is overweight but not overfat. An assessment of midarm circumference and arm muscle area will confirm the muscular body composition. This type of evaluation is plotted in Fig. 8-6. Anthropometric reference tables are given in Appendixes D, E, and F.

Sexual Maturity Rating

The evaluation of sexual maturity is an essential factor in making a valid nutrition assessment of an adolescent in a normal clinical setting. By knowing the stage of sexual maturity of the adolescent (see Fig. 8-2), it is possible to determine whether the full height has been reached or growth can still occur. Also, it is possible to determine whether the proportion of fat to muscle seen is that which the individual has developed as an adult or has obtained at one stage as a still-developing adolescent. Thus if a young woman at stage 1 of sexual maturity is at the 90th percentile weight-for-height, she will continue to grow in height and has a greater potential to stay within the bounds of normal body composition than has a female of the same age, the same weight-for-height, but who has experienced menarche and is at stage 4 of sexual maturity.

Nutrition Environment

The nutrition environment, the combination of factors that influence the nutritional status, is also an important consideration. Such factors as general medical history,

TABLE 8-6 *Weight in Kilograms of Girls Aged 17 Years at Last Birthday, United States, 1966-1970*

Height (cm)	Percentile						
	5th	10th	25th	50th	75th	90th	95th
145-149.9	38.6	38.8	40.1	45.1	45.7	51.1	51.2
150-154.9	41.6	42.3	44.6	48.9	53.5	59.2	64.1
155-159.9	44.4	45.5	48.7	53.2	57.7	61.6	76.2
160-164.9	46.8	48.0	50.2	55.4	61.5	72.3	82.3
165-169.9	47.9	50.3	55.1	59.3	65.1	69.4	71.6
170-174.9	50.6	52.9	55.5	60.2	65.7	76.1	82.7
175-179.9	54.9	56.7	60.1	61.7	75.2	75.9	83.0

Modified from National Center for Health Statistics: *Height and weight of youths 12-17 years, United States.* In *Vital and health statistics,* series 11, no 124, Health Services and Mental Health Administration, Washington, DC, 1973, US Government Printing Office. Data from the national health survey, US Department of Health, Education, and Welfare, 1973.

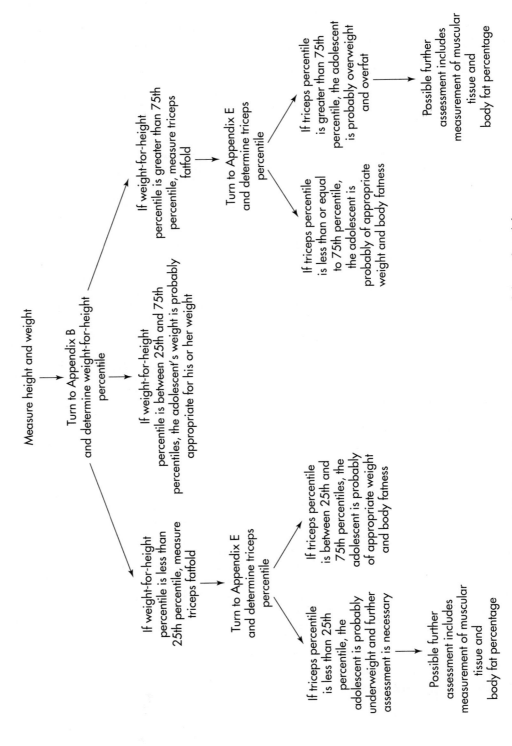

FIG. 8-6 Algorithm for evaluating an adolescent's weight.

TABLE 8-7 *Nutrition Environment Evaluation Guide*

Influences	Key Issues	Significance
Likes and dislikes	Does patient dislike any particular food that is a major source of a specific nutrient (for example, milk is a major source of calcium; citrus fruits of vitamin C; meat of high-quality protein)?	Points out need to explore alternative ways to supply nutrients (for example, substitute cheese and yogurt for milk; broccoli and green peppers for citrus fruit; proper combinations of plant foods for meat)
Environment and attitudes		
Individuals	Does patient express interest in his or her diet?	Gives clues to attitude toward role of nutrition in health care
	Are there any behavioral problems that influence patient's foods choices?	May indicate need to work with other health team members to resolve problem that temporarily precludes nutrition intervention
	Has patient ever followed a special diet? If so, who prescribed it, what type of diet was it, and when was it prescribed? What instructions did patient receive?	Self-prescribed diet may signal inappropriate or unreliable approach toward control of health by diet; points out medical and educational considerations needed in design of care plan
	Does patient think he or she has been following the diet? Is there evidence to substantiate this?	If discrepancy exists, indicates lack of understanding of diet by patient or unwillingness or inability of patient to make dietary changes
	What difficulties if any does patient see in making dietary changes?	Focuses on issues that need consideration in design of individualized care plan
Family	Who purchases and prepares food in home (that is, partially controls patient's food supply)?	Sets scene for type of action plan suitable to patient and family
	Does patient have adequate cooking facilities and equipment or access to other resources?	May indicate need to provide basic nutrition guidelines, including personalized menu plan
	Are there any cultural, regional, or religious factors that affect patient's food choices?	Requires consideration to tailor care plan to individual needs
Peers	How often does patient eat away from home? Where and with whom does patient eat? Are there specific food intake patterns related to peer influences?	Indicates potential influences of peers on food choices; points out potential efficacy of patient- versus family-oriented care plan
Schools	Does patient eat at school? Does patient participate in school feeding programs?	School feeding programs with their standardized composition assure minimal nutrient availability and provide reference for accuracy of reported information

Continued.

TABLE 8-7 *Nutrition Environment Evaluation Guide—cont'd*

Influences	Key Issues	Significance
	Is there anything about school schedule or cafeteria environment that may discourage appropriate nutrient intake?	"Too little time for lunch" or "no one to eat with" may necessitate consultation with other team members or school to resolve lifestyle problems
	Is patient in appropriate grade in school? Has patient received food and nutrition information in school courses?	Gives clues to current knowledge of nutrition and level of intellectual functioning; allows practical planning for educational aspects of care plan
Limited food funds	Is patient or family eligibile for food stamps; Women, Infants, and Children program (WIC); or reduced-price or free school lunch? Do they participate in programs? Does patient or family receive other social assistance?	Indicates family has limited income and may need assistance with food buying and preparation to assure nutritionally adequate diet; points out need to consider referral to appropriate food program or nutrition education resource
Health-related concerns	Does patient have any food allergies or intolerances (as distinguished from dislikes)?	Excludes foods from diet; indicates need to plan and assure adequacy with alternative food choices
	Are there any physical condition affecting ability to consume adequate nutrients (for example, mouth sores, swallowing problems, taste abnormalities)?	Indicates need to consider flavor, consistency, and temperature of food in care plan
	Are there any problems in digestion, absorption, or metabolism that will interfere with nutrient utilization? Will any other therapy (drugs, exercise, radiation) affect nutrient needs?	Indicates need to address these problems in diet preparation

socioeconomic status, medications, alcohol or tobacco use, family attitudes, and peer group food practices all contribute to the adolescent's food choices. Table 8-7 summarizes the significance of each of these influences. **Nutrition assessment** includes the study of both the nutritional status and the nutrition environment of the individual adolescent. The methods described in Chapter 2 will be used to help the health professional understand the effect they have on the adolescent's eating habits. A probing interview by a sensitive nutritionist who has had experience communicating with adolescents will also be required to find out how an individual teenager feels about and manages food.

Nutritional Care Plan

> **Nutritional care plan**
> The person-centered care plan, based on nutritional assessment data and evaluation, for individual nutritional care and education to promote health and prevent or treat disease.

Assessment of all factors in the environment that may influence nutriture is essential if appropriate action to meet needs is going to be initiated as a personal **nutritional care plan.** The extent to which the total nutrition environment is studied depends on the projected use of the nutrition assessment. For example, a great deal of detailed information reflecting

Teenagers and TV: How Do We Increase Physical Activity?

Teenagers from 12 to 17 years of age watch television about 21 hours per week. This estimate does not include any additional hours spent watching videos or playing video or computer games. The sedentary habits of many teens are likely to be contributing to the rising prevalence of obesity in this age group. As many as 30% of teens are obese. The relationship between hours spent watching television and inappropriate body weight gain among adolescents is controversial. Television viewing may be substituting for other activities with a higher energy expenditure and contribute to a positive energy balance. Watching television has been associated with a lowered resting metabolic rate that indirectly may add to weight gain. Increased television viewing could lead to increased consumption of energy dense snacks, raising the total energy intake while limiting energy expenditure in physical activity. All of these factors are likely to be involved. An important goal for nutrition and health educators working with teens should be making available to them physical activities that focus on fun and fitness. School health programs can help students develop patterns of exercise that will provide a foundation for lifelong fitness. After-school or leisure time programs can encourage participation in physical activities that teens will enjoy and that are compatible with their lifestyle and social pattern.

Some suggestions for developing exercise programs for teens are:

- Focus on physical activities that you can do when you are alone or bored: bicycle riding, walking, skating, jogging, aerobic dancing, shooting baskets
- Organize contests in which everyone can participate regardless of their athletic ability: offer prizes for walking, skating, or riding your bicycle a certain distance (maybe 50 miles) or walking or dancing for a certain number of hours (maybe 20 hours) over a certain number of weeks or months
- Emphasize team activities in which everyone on the team is active: basketball, volleyball, soccer, racquetball
- Promote participation rather than winning in team sports; give small prizes or recognition to everyone who plays, not only to the team who wins
- Encourage the formation of small groups to encourage and support each other in exercise activities: "get fit with a friend"
- Favor exercise activities that do not require expensive uniforms or equipment and carry a low risk of injury: walking, jogging, basketball, soccer, volleyball, aerobic dancing

Gortmaker SL, Dietz WH, Cheung LWY: Inactivity, diet, and the fattening of America, *J Am Diet Assoc* 90:1247, 1990.

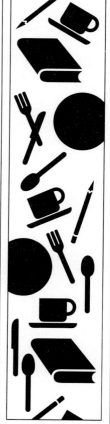
nutritional status is needed for a 13-year-old male with Crohn's disease who is scheduled for a course of **parenteral nutrition.** Information about the nutrition environment would be less vital at this time. However, nutritional care planning for a newly diagnosed 15-year-old female with insulin-dependent diabetes mellitus (IDDM) would require both nutritional status evaluation and assessment of the nutrition environment. Without both components, the care plan cannot adequately address physiologic nutritional needs and the adolescent's ability to meet them.

NUTRITIONAL COUNSELING FOR ADOLESCENTS
Facilitating Change

Attempts to help adolescents improve their nutritional status must be approached with skill, especially because of their growing independence.[13] Nutrition counselors must know

Parenteral nutrition (Gr *para*, beyond, beside; *enteron*, intestine) Nourishment received not through the gastrointestinal tract but rather by an alternate route such as injection into a vein; intravenous feeding of elemental nutrients.

adolescents' physical and psychologic development, lifestyles, and habits as well as appropriate methods of communicating with them.

Strategies for change. Sophisticated strategies to add knowledge, alter attitudes, and change behavior must be used in any setting if the objective is to influence an adolescent's eating habits. Providing knowledge or teaching can be done in a variety of settings from the classroom to the hospital bedside. Altering attitudes is much more difficult and usually demands an individualized experience. Facilitating the adoption of new behavior is even more difficult and requires a lengthy period of time. The adolescent will have to feel positive about any plan before it can succeed. In fact, much effort must be directed toward encouraging the person to want to change before introducing steps to bring the change about.

Personalized counseling. Besides changes in attitude the counselor must impart knowledge in an especially meaningful and individualized manner. Finally, behavior change can be approached in increments that are sufficiently realistic to ensure personal success.

TABLE 8-8   Suggested Members of Health-Care Team to Guide Adolescents in Issues Arising in Pregnancy

Issues	Discipline					
	Obstetrician	Adolescent Medical Specialist	Nurse	Nutritionist	Social Worker	Psychologist
General health and planning of continuous care		X	X	X	X	
Complications of pregnancy	X	X	X	X		
Labor and delivery preparation	X	X	X			
School program					X	X
Economic resources			X		X	
Substance abuse (cessation and education)		X	X	X	X	X
Psychologic adjustment and stress	X	X	X	X	X	X
Development delay			X		X	X
Infant-care education		X	X	X		
Relinquishment counseling			X		X	X
Nutritional care		X	X	X		
Education		X	X	X		
Resource coordination			X	X	X	
Family or marital conflict					X	X

Role of parents. Parents must be appropriately involved in the counseling process. They need help in being supportive, as opposed to being intrusive, as the adolescent makes changes. Both adolescents and their parents must be helped to see the importance of focusing on the process of making change rather than solely on the desired goal of self-care. A sure understanding of both the physical and social sciences, along with a liberal injection of art, are needed in nutrition counseling for adolescents and their parents. It is indeed a challenging field.

The Health Care Team

Adolescent health care is one of the most demanding of clinical problems. As such, it is best handled as a team effort. Any one professional will generally not possess the skills to meet all the client's needs. For example, Table 8-8 lists some of the types of issues that will arise throughout the course of teenage pregnancies with a suggested list of professionals to guide clients in managing these issues. This does not mean that certain problems are the responsibility of any one profession to the exclusion of others. Each professional team member can support and reinforce the messages and guidance provided by other team members. Team conferences aid in coordination of care and team efficiency in meeting identified needs and noting the client's progress in solving various problems. Nutritionists and other professionals who are in positions to influence program planning can help develop clinical teams for the care of adolescents.

EATING DISORDERS

Although recent precise figures are not available, as many as 30% of American teenagers are said to be obese. The number with diagnosed anorexia nervosa or bulimia is growing, and many adolescents with eating disorders remain undiagnosed and untreated. Because

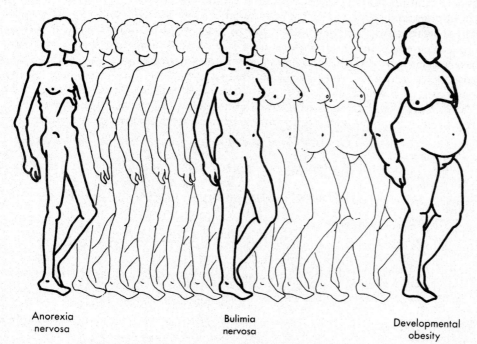

Anorexia
nervosa

Bulimia
nervosa

Developmental
obesity

FIG. 8-7 The spectrum of eating disorders. Although physical conditions vary, underlying psychologic characteristics are held in common across the spectrum.

these disorders are so common among adolescents, health professionals interested in adolescent nutrition must understand them. Eating disorders provide good models for study of other adolescent nutrition problems and their treatment. Therefore, it is valuable to study these disorders in depth.

Spectrum of Eating Disorders in Adolescence

Common characteristics. Eating disorders can best be studied when the physical symptoms are viewed as a spectrum, with developmental obesity at one end and anorexia nervosa at the other (Fig. 8-7). In between are persons at normal and abnormal weights. Along the spectrum these persons hold in common basic underlying psychologic problems that interfere to varying degrees with normal functioning. In developing responses to life, these persons often use food inappropriately. Food-related behaviors and the resulting deviation in weight, the two most obvious aspects of these disorders, are usually the main focus of attention of the person affected, the public, and often the health professional. It is the underlying neurophysical and psychodevelopmental mechanisms, however, that are the essential features of more fundamental study needed by clinicians who are treating the disorders.

Rapid adolescent growth and body image. Because of rapid physical growth and body-image development in adolescence, eating disorders are of special concern at this stage of life. These changes intensify associated self-esteem problems. Anorexia nervosa, for example, is a disorder so tied to body image distortion that it is most commonly seen in adolescence, the period when a person is struggling with self-identity and is most vulnerable to body image problems. Progress in adopting a normal adult body image will be interrupted for the teenager with an eating disorder. Bruch and others have provided classic descriptions of distorted body images in both anorexic and obese adolescents.[14]

Developmental tasks. Teenagers with severe eating disorders fail in varying degrees to accomplish the development tasks of adolescence. The development problems of these persons are summarized in the box on p. 338. The most striking of their problems is failure to develop **autonomy.**

Autonomy
(Gr *autos,* self; *nomos* law) State of functioning independently; self-determination.

Family interaction. In recent years studies of factors contributing to the origin of eating disorders have turned to the structure and interaction of the adolescent's family. Although obese teenagers are a much less homogeneous group than anorexic persons, the family patterns have much in common. Minuchin has described such families as being

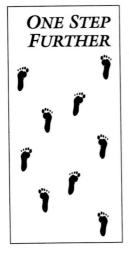

ONE STEP FURTHER

Developmental Problems Associated With Eating Disorders in Adolescents

Inability to develop and use formal operational thought processes, especially in reference to themselves

Inability to experience bodily sensations originating within themselves as "normal" and "valid"

Unrealistic perceptions of body size

Preoccupation with weight and food, reflecting dependence on social opinion and judgment

Failure to normalize eating and exercise patterns

Unrealistic expectations for themselves

Failure to develop autonomy

Difficulty in accomplishing the normal tasks of adolescence

Based on Bruch H: *Eating disorders,* New York, 1973, Basic Books.

psychosomatic.[15] These families are **enmeshed,** rigid, and overprotective with a low tolerance for conflict.

Multifaceted origin. Eating disorders are very complex and may have developed throughout life or appear in the chaotic time of change that is adolescence. Individual and familial, biologic, and psychologic characteristics influenced by the modern social milieu contribute to their origin.

ANOREXIA NERVOSA
Symptoms

The term anorexia nervosa is actually a misnomer.[14] The implication that affected persons have a lack of appetite has been shown to be invalid. Superficially the motivation to be thin keeps the person with anorexia nervosa from eating.[15] In over 100 years of description in the literature, however, a combination of symptoms has come to be recognized as characteristic of the disorder. Although certain of these symptoms may be seen in other disorders, the combination is unique in **anorexia nervosa.** This unique combination of symptoms has been defined by the American Psychiatric Association[16] as follows:

- Refusal to maintain body weight over minimal normal for age and height; loss or failure to gain with maintenance 15% below expected
- Fear of gaining weight or becoming fat, though underweight
- Disturbance in body weight, size, or shape perception: Feels fat or that body parts are fat, though underweight
- Absence of three consecutive menstrual cycles

The above criteria focus more on physical symptoms at the crisis stage than on the underlying psychologic symptoms. Recognition of the psychologic symptoms, however, is of equal importance. The principal psychologic features of anorexia nervosa are "a relentless pursuit of thinness" and "a misuse of the eating function in efforts to solve or camouflage problems that otherwise would appear insolvable," that is, problems resulting from arrested normal development.[14]

Incidence

The majority of persons with anorexia nervosa are adolescents, although it has been seen in other age groups. About 10% of young women are thought to be affected. The disorder has not been commonly seen in males; only 5% to 10% of anorexic teenagers are male. Males who develop the disorder appear to experience anorexia nervosa in essentially the same form as females. Because of the predominance of females in the population seen with anorexia nervosa, the feminine pronoun will be used in this discussion.

Anorexia nervosa occurs predominantly in affluent classes and nations and is supported by a cultural paradox in which food is abundant. Food is used lavishly for purposes other than survival, yet slimness is highly valued. These cultural values are strong internal messages that have great impact on a young adolescent who has not developed autonomy. The lack of a similar value on slimness in males probably accounts for the small number of males seen with the disorder, though the influence of rock stars and other celebrities with excessively thin bodies is beginning to impact the ideals of young males.

Etiology

Theories about the etiology of anorexia nervosa have evolved from the initial psychoanalytic idea that the disease stemmed from an inability to deal with innate sexual drives; through periods when it was ascribed to endocrine deficits and then disturbed patterns of family interaction; to the present when a combination of these biologic,

Enmeshed
To catch, as in a net, and entangle; intertwined family relationships that capture and diminish individual autonomy or self-regard.

Anorexia nervosa
(Gr *anorektos,* without appetite; L *nervosa,* nervous or emotional disorder) A severe psychophysiologic eating disorder, usually seen in girls and young women, in which the person does not lack appetite, as the label would indicate, but is psychologically unable to eat and refuses food, becoming extremely emaciated; a form of self-starvation.

psychologic, and social factors is thought to contribute to the development of the disorders.

Mother-daughter relationship. Bruch's work was the first to incorporate a broader focus than simply the patient and her symptoms.[14] An interaction pattern prevails in which the mother misperceives the needs of her child from infancy on or the child fails to express her needs clearly. In any case the child acquiesces to the mother's misguided ministrations. During the period of infancy and childhood, the daughter is so controlled by her mother that she does not develop a true sense of self as distinguished from her mother.

Effect of adolescence. As adolescence approaches, the body develops and demands for decisions and performance in many areas increase. The teenager panics at her lack of ability to cope independently. She develops rituals related to eating in an effort to be thin and "good." To gain her "independence," the teenager regresses to the period when independence ordinarily begins. In this early stage the principal way of demonstrating growing independence is eating behavior.

Family system. Minuchin's more recent approach describes how not only relationships with the mother but also interrelationships within the family system foster anorexia nervosa.[15] If family members are enmeshed in a system that does not allow development of appropriate roles, the system can produce a variety of psychosomatic problems. The particular direction toward anorexia nervosa may be determined when the main themes of family interaction are related to food, fitness, and appearance.

Biochemical process. The possibility that a biochemical process may be responsible for development of anorexia nervosa continues to be investigated. Although various mechanisms have been proposed, so far none has been shown to be primary or causative. These mechanisms appear to result from psychologic stress, malnutrition, and starvation. The fact that patients and their families fit such characteristic and complex patterns would raise doubt that a single primary physiologic cause exists in most cases. However, it may be found that biochemical factors contribute to development of the disorder.

Psychologic State

The physical manifestations of anorexia nervosa may be sudden, although unrecognized underlying characteristics may have been present previously. Intervention strategies must address both the psychologic and physiologic states of the patient.

Progressive development. From the family's point of view, the anorexic teenager is usually a "model child" until she begins to develop a compulsive attitude about her weight. She has fit into the family unit and met their high expectations. She has worked extremely hard at school, being satisfied with nothing less than excellent grades.

Suddenly the whole family erupts in conflict over her eating behavior. The teenager herself has become troubled about her role in life. She is unable to sustain peer friendships and she is very anxious about relationships with males. She is confused by the need to establish more adult behavior patterns and clings to the rigid standards of childhood. She isolates herself. Life appears to be out of her control. She has conflicting feelings about living as her parents direct, is hurt by their critical comments, and begins to realize that she must assert herself. She takes a stand and will not compromise on her eating and exercise habits. She feels that she is too fat and must be slim to prove that she is a worthy person. She is increasingly preoccupied with her rituals and is angry when her family interferes. She denies her illness.

Distorted perceptions. A wide range of distorted perceptions have been noted, related specifically to body size, sex, hunger, rest, satiety, body temperature, pleasure, control, and to "feeling states" in general. The anorexic teenager has often been described as wishing to stave off adulthood. But the question remains as to whether she wishes to avoid maturation or whether maturation eludes her.

Family problems. Although most families with anorexic teenagers would describe themselves as normal and without problems until the manifestations of anorexia nervosa, these families often have a multitude of problems. The parents may have been dominating and intrusive. They may have overlooked the actual (including nutritional) needs and emotions of their children, even in times when the children have been ill. By adopting a "helpless" stance, the affected children may be thoroughly manipulative and involved in their parents' conflicts. Both parents and children become locked into a system where problems go unresolved and responses are stereotyped.[15]

Physiologic State

In the initial stage of anorexia nervosa, physical symptoms are related to weight, diet, exercise, menses, and nutritional status.

Weight. In some cases the anorexic teenager is overweight when the disorder begins. The anorexic young woman is typically hypersensitive to developing breasts and hips. These young patients often recall a chance statement about their needing to lose weight by a relative or close friend, or a weight reduction plan suggested by a health professional, as the trigger for their initial weight loss behavior.

Diet. The anorexic adolescent usually develops a personal philosophy about her diet, limiting herself by eating food only from certain categories and in certain ways. She may manipulate the fluid or sodium content of her intake. In addition, she may force herself to vomit and misuse laxatives or diuretics to rid herself of food energy and weight. Vomiting may follow episodes of gorging.

Exercise. Exercise rituals are equally varied. Anorexic teenagers include excessive calisthenics and other strenuous activities in their schedules. They may limit rest and use stimulants. They are so frequently involved in junior and senior high school athletics and dancing that coaches and teachers should be educated about the disorder. Good coaches should recognize which of their students may be exercising to their detriment by compulsively training beyond reasonable endurance while losing weight at a rapid rate.

Menses. Although a young woman in a state of starvation would be expected to become amenorrheic, indications are that cessation of the menses occurs in most patients with anorexia nervosa before they have lost sufficient weight and body fat to cause an interruption of the cycle, and lasts beyond the time they have regained weight and body fat.[17,18] Psychologic factors probably contribute to the problem, as well as hormonal disturbances, since stressful states are known to interfere with the endocrine system regulating the menstrual cycle.

Nutritional status. During the initial phase of an anorexic teenager's energy restriction, the body does not exhibit the effects of malnutrition to a measurable degree other than to decrease in weight. Infections are not generally seen. Deficiencies in specific nutrients have not been reported, but they may exist subclinically depending on the food habits of the individual. If weight loss continues unchecked, however, the symptoms of severe starvation may become apparent and additional nutritional problems listed on p. 343 begin to undermine basic health. This state indicates an onset of a crisis.

Intervention Strategies

Initial intervention strategies include early recognition of symptoms, psychotherapy, and nutritional support.

Early recognition of symptoms. A recognition of the developing symptoms is the most important early intervention strategy. A **protocol** for assessing anorexia nervosa and bulimia is provided in Table 8-9. Friends, school personnel, family, and health professionals are among those who observe the growing problems and can take steps to initiate treatment.

Psychotherapy. Individual and family psychotherapy by experienced therapists will

Protocol
(Gr *protokollon,* leaf or tag attached to a rolled papyrus manuscript containing notes as to its contents) A set of governing rules; the plan and procedures for carrying out a scientific study or a person's treatment regimen.

TABLE 8-9   *Issues to Address in a Clinical Assessment of Eating Disorder*

Motivation
Appropriateness of weight goals
Desire to change unhealthful habits
Insight into problem

Emotional/psychological status
Depression
Locus of control
Body image
Self-esteem
Oral expression
Coping skills
Compulsivity
Perfectionism
Independence

Mental function
Intellectual ability
School performance
Attitude toward school
Ability to articulate

Family characteristics
Eating disorders
Other diseases
Natural or other parent
Intrusiveness
Enmeshment
Rigidity
Conflict resolution
Role of food
Exercise patterns
Perceptions of problem
Attempts to intervene
Willingness to participate in therapy

Social relationships
Friends
Social habits
Social skills
Attitude of peers

Eating behavior
Knowledge/acknowledgment of nutritional needs
Meal pattern
Bizarre eating habits
Personal philosophy toward eating
Nutritional adequacy
Control over food supply

Physical status
Signs of bulimia
Signs of starvation
Terminal signs of starvation
Thyroid status (obesity)
Resting heart rate (HR)
Exercise to reach 60% maximum HR

Growth and adiposity
Weight/height/age percentile
Triceps skinfold/age percentile
Arm muscle area/age percentile
Weight/height history
Growth velocity
Maturational stage
Age

Physical activity
Exercise patterns
Hobbies/interests
Personal feeling about exercise

Cachexia
(Gr *kakos,* bad, ill; *hexia,* habit) A profound and grave state of body disorder and deterioration, as seen in cases of advanced malignant disease or starvation, causing gross body weight loss to cadaverous proportions as a result of disordered metabolism.

enable both the affected adolescent and her family to adopt more appropriate roles. It will also help the anorexic teenager to complete the psychologic developmental processes that have been arrested.[14]

Nutritional support. Other than general monitoring of the height and weight, it may not be necessary to treat the patient physically at this stage. Refocusing her attention on the primary emotional and interactional problems rather than the power struggle over food and exercise patterns will often enable the patient to abandon her compulsive striving for thinness. The patient should have access to a professional who can answer her questions about nutrition and make sure that she has the information she needs to begin to regulate her eating patterns to meet her physical needs. Information should be given in the context of the adolescent's desire to change rather than imposed as a rigid system of dietary planning by a professional. The overall disorder should not be defined as solely a nutritional problem, although nutrition counseling is an important component of therapy.

Crisis Stage: Psychologic State

Overall, a lack of progress toward positive family interaction patterns during the initial therapy or continuing avoidance of intervention will often lead to physical and mental deterioration. When the crisis stage of anorexia nervosa develops, severe psychologic and physiologic symptoms appear and intervention must be directed toward the deteriorating condition.

Psychologic effects of starvation. The anorexic teenager in crisis can cause panic in family, friends, and professionals. The family generally sees the adolescent's bizarre eating behavior as the problem and fails to understand the extent of developmental and interactional patterns. As a result, they often seek treatment that does not demand their involvement with the patient in therapy. As she becomes truly **cachectic**, the psychologic changes inherent in starvation, described by Keys in his classic studies, become evident[17]:

- Cognitive processes center around food. Thoughts of food intrude constantly; the major part of the waking hours are spent contemplating it.
- Behavior around food includes toying with it and hoarding, especially during renourishment.
- Coherent creative thinking is impaired.
- Mental function is characterized by apathy, dullness, exhaustion, and depression.
- Interest in sexual function is lacking.

These effects of starvation are superimposed on the anorexic teenager's already disturbed psychologic state. The behavior pattern, distorted perceptions, and weight phobia become more pronounced.

Behavior pattern. Many patients resist what they see as intrusions by professionals. They are secretive and protect the fact that they are carrying out their rituals. Their behavior may otherwise reflect the apathy typically seen in starving people. In obsessional preoccupation they plan menus, read recipes, cook and serve food to others, cut or manipulate food before eating it, and record all that they eat. They usually have a detailed knowledge of the energy value of foods. They may pretend to eat and then hide and dispose of the food. The disturbed adolescent's fear of gaining weight becomes increasingly evident as her weight phobia intensifies.

Crisis Stage: Physiologic State

In the crisis stage of anorexia nervosa, the physiologic state deteriorates with physical signs of starvation, endocrine abnormalities, and undeniable signs of approaching terminal starvation.[19]

Physical signs of starvation. As the crisis stage develops, the individual is unable to take care of herself. The physical state of starvation is now superimposed on the other problems inherent in the disorder. These physical signs of starvation include the following:

Fat-store depletion	**Hirsutism**
Muscle wasting	Thin, dry, brittle hair
Amenorrhea	**Alopecia**
Cheilosis	Degradation of fingernails
Desquamation	**Acrocyanosis**
Dry skin	Postural hypotension

Additional nutritional problems. In addition to the clinical signs, recent research has focused on zinc nutriture, bone mineralization, growth failure, and structural changes in the brain, which result from severe long-term malnutrition in anorectic patients.[20,21] The

Cheilosis
(Gr *cheilos*, lip) A general symptoms of tissue inflammation and breakdown producing swelling and reddening of the lips, a chapped appearance, and fissures at the corners of the mouth; associated with general malnutrition, especially a deficiency of riboflavin.

Hirsutism
(L *hirsutus*, shaggy hair) a condition marked by abundant and excessive hair; abnormal hairiness, especially an adult male pattern of body hair distribution in women.

Alopecia
(Gr *alopekia*, disease in which hair falls out) Baldness; absence of hair from skin areas where it normally is present.

Acrocyanosis
(Gr *akron*, extremity; *kyanos*, blue) Condition due to excessive concentration of reduced hemoglobin in the blood, resulting in arterial unsaturation with oxygen; characterized by cyanosis of extremities with persistent mottled blue or red discoloration of skin on fingers, wrists, toes, and ankles, accompanied by coldness of fingers and toes.

possibility that bone demineralization, growth retardation, and brain structure may prove irreversible to some degree is especially troublesome and warrants further examination.[22-24] The relationship of depressive symptoms and sex role and body image distortion to lowered body weight and the suggestion that less than the expected number of children are born to patients formerly diagnosed with anorexia nervosa are equally disturbing long-term effects of chronic malnutrition. These relationships have serious implications for dancers, gymnasts, and other athletes who keep themselves in a state of starvation, as well as for anoretics.[25-27]

Endocrine abnormalities. The endocrine abnormalities in anorexia nervosa are such that the body essentially reverts to a prepubertal hormonal state. As a result of hypothalamic change, the anorexic adolescent is amenorrheic, is unable to adapt to heat and cold, suffers sleep disturbances, and is unable to conserve body water. There is no interest in sex.

Terminal starvation signs. During the crisis, professionals must monitor the physical state of the patient and take remedial action when there are signs that starvation is approaching a terminal state. The most outstanding of these signs include the following:

- Fluid and electrolyte imbalance indicating inability of the body to maintain homeostasis (dehydration and edema)
- Severe cardiac abnormalities in the absence of electrolyte imbalances, indicating a wasted **myocardium**
- Absence of **ketone bodies** in the urine, indicating a lack of fat stores for metabolic fuel
- Concurrent infection, indicating increasing nutritional needs

Crisis Intervention Strategies

When the anorexic adolescent's condition reaches the crisis stage, hospitalization is necessary to provide comprehensive care involving nutritional therapy.

Hospitalization. For some clinicians, the decision to hospitalize an anorexic patient depends on her reaching a life-threatening physical state. However, if the goal is to renourish the individual so that she will be able to benefit from psychotherapy without semistarvation neurosis, as many authoritative therapists recommend, the anorexic patient must be hospitalized before a critical stage has been reached. The patient can be released from the hospital when she has been nutritionally rehabilitated, usually confirmed by reaching a particular weight-for-height goal (Fig. 8-8).

Comprehensive treatment. Nutritional components of therapeutic regimens for anorexia nervosa in crisis are intertwined with the psychologic aspects of the treatment, and team care is essential. Certain principles can be observed that will apply regardless of the treatment modality. Renourishment obviously will begin with a gradual increase in energy intake.

Diet therapy. In some programs the patient will be allowed to choose anything available on the hospital menu. Other programs impose rules, make additions to what is ordered, or serve a set menu. If a diet is prescribed following the principles established for renourishing malnourished individuals, it should have adequate protein to meet basic needs with additional energy made up of complex carbohydrates and a small amount of fat.

Nutritional supplements. If a patient refuses food, a nutritional supplement, which is prescribed and dispensed as a medicine, has been used. If a life-threatening state is reached at any time, with the patient refusing oral feeding, nourishment by nasogastric tube or parenteral methods may be necessary. These methods will be presented as lifesaving procedures and not as punishment for refusing to eat. Nourishment by mouth is the preferred route and is possible in most cases.

Renourishment edema and body image. Edema generally appears with the renourishment and can be a problem because of the anorexic patient's phobia of weight gain.

Myocardium
heart muscle

Ketone bodies
byproducts of fat metabolism

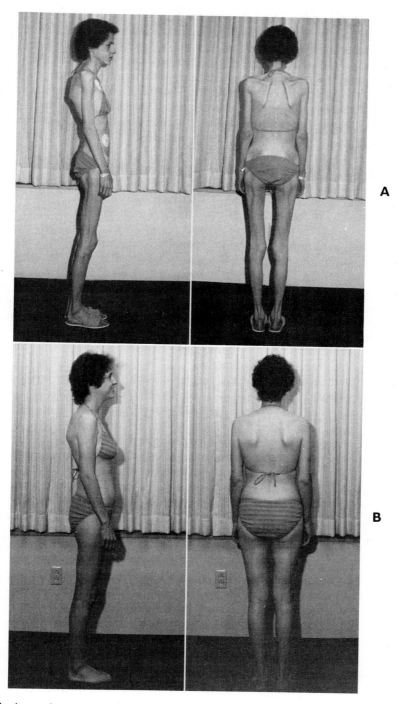

FIG. 8-8 **A,** Anorexic woman before treatment. **B,** Same patient after *gradual* refeeding, nutritional management, and psychologic therapy.

Courtesy Sycamore Hospital, a division of Kettering Medical Center, Dayton, Ohio.

The edema is seen as proof to her that she will "expand" as she feared. Some anticipatory guidance can help her accept such development. Assurance that professionals will aid her in gaining appropriate weight, which is strengthening for her but not forming excess fat, can help desensitize the issue.

Role of the clinical nutritionist. The inclusion of a clinical nutritionist/dietitian on the therapeutic team gives attention to nutritional support care in a manner that does not subvert the psychotherapeutic goal of redirecting the focus of the patient's concern. The nutritionist's knowledge of energy balance as it applies to the individual is needed in determining appropriate weight goals throughout therapy and especially for termination of the hospitalization.

Long-Term Therapy

Psychologic state. The anorexic teenager who has recovered from a starvation crisis by gaining a certain amount of weight to improve her physical state will still have to deal with the developmental arrest that brought her to the crisis, a process that usually requires several years. There will continue to be problems concerning vocational choices and preparation, economic stability, relationships with peers and especially with the opposite sex, weight management, and body image.

Physiologic state. In the long term the anorexic young woman will often experience wide swings in weight from extreme thinness to obesity before she will be able to bring her life into control. She may see herself as somewhat detached from her body and experiment with various food habits before putting food into a more normal perspective. She may keep herself sufficiently thin so that she will not resume her menses. She may feel bloated and have bouts of edema, physical responses to starvation and refeeding, and **carotenemia,** a symptom found in anorexia.

Intervention strategies. In the recovery period the psychotherapeutic goal will be to facilitate normal development in the anorexic teenager, to prepare her for a full adult role in society, and to enable her to function without depending on bizarre eating and exercise habits. She will need information and retraining about food and the physical aspects of life. Many of the techniques described in the section on obesity (p. 361) will be useful. Issues such as the state of nourishment necessary to maintain the menstrual cycle will resurface from time to time as development proceeds. Returning to such issues will enable her to deal more capably with them as time goes on. Guided food experiences in cafeterias, grocery stores, cooking, and entertaining help ready the person for managing food in her environment. The objective is to help the individual put food in a reasonable perspective and give up overfocusing on food out of ignorance. A team consisting of medical, psychologic, and nutrition specialists may provide care, or the care may be left to a single therapist who will be responsible for all aspects of therapy in consultation with other team members.

Outcome. Common features of anorexia nervosa are the strong resistance to treatment and the high incidence of relapse and partial recovery. Some of these patients will manifest varying degrees of the anorexic symptoms in adulthood. Though follow-up criteria have been inconsistently used by researchers, results reported to date indicate that in spite of the fact that weight-for-height proportion improved in about 75% of the patients, menstrual cycles were often unsatisfactorily maintained, ideas about food and weight were disturbed, and psychosocial maladjustment was common.

BULIMIA

First called bulimarexia, **bulimia nervosa** is the most recently recognized eating disorder and is characterized by gorging followed by self-induced vomiting or diarrhea. Although these symptoms may be a part of anorexia nervosa, they also comprise a separate syndrome.

Carotenemia
Condition associated with excess intake or impaired metabolism of carotenoid pigments, especially beta-carotene, resulting in excess carotene in the blood, sometimes to the extent of producing yellowing of the skin resembling jaundice.

Bulimia nervosa
(L *bous,* ox; *limos,* hunger; *nervosa,* nervous or emotional condition) A psychophysiologic eating disorder, seen mainly in girls and young women, marked by alternate gorging on large amounts of food followed by self-induced vomiting and purging with laxatives; weight usually remains fairly stable at a normal amount.

Symptoms

The person suffering from bulimia generally maintains close to normal weight (Fig. 8-7), while gorging (bingeing, eating abnormally large amounts of food) and vomiting or purging (forcing bowels to empty) on a regular basis. The bulimic teenager may have somewhat less severe distortions in body image and less restrictive weight goals than the adolescent with anorexia nervosa. She is often older at age of onset.

APA Criteria

The official diagnostic criteria established by the American Psychiatry Association (APA) includes the following behaviors[16]:

- Recurrent episodes of binge eating, rapid consumption of a large amount of food in a discrete period
- Lack of control over binges
- Regular self-induced vomiting, use of laxatives or diuretics, strict dieting or fasting, or vigorous exercise
- Average of two binge-eating episodes a week for at least 3 months
- Overconcern with body shape and weight

Incidence

The syndrome of bulimia should be differentiated from the recent behavior of many normal adolescent females who occasionally use self-induced vomiting as a means of controlling weight.[28] As many as 20% of college-age females may engage in bulimic behaviors with an estimated 2% to 4% meeting the criteria for diagnosis of bulimia nervosa. A serious condition will be uncontrollable, and the psychologic features of the disorder will impair normal functioning. Bulimia sometimes develops after a serious bout with anorexia nervosa or obesity. The bulimic person is more likely to be fertile than the individual with anorexia nervosa. Therefore, certain young women will be bulimic during pregnancy.

Psychologic State

Separation anxiety is one of the important issues for the bulimic teenager. Her self-esteem is extremely low and is tied to her feelings about her body. She demonstrates excessive need for control and approval. She thinks of herself as physically unattractive, although she is well groomed and has a normally attractive physique. She develops guilt over her habits and her secret feelings of inadequacy. Superficially, she may be very responsible and keep a heavy social schedule. In reality she has few close friends and feels that no one really knows her. In contrast to the more rigid anorexic adolescent, the young woman with bulimia often demonstrates poor impulse control, abuses substances, and becomes easily enraged. By all accounts, the gorging, vomiting, and purging serve to release tension for the sufferers. However, the residual guilt brings renewed tension that perpetuates an uncontrolled cycle. Social isolation is also perpetuated because of the fear that the secret will be found out. If she is pregnant, the bulimic teenager may be committed to protecting the fetus but retain ideas that inhibit normal nourishment of herself, her fetus, and the child after birth.

Physiologic State

Food behavior. The bulimic teenager periodically eats large amounts of food and then voluntarily vomits or purges. Each person with bulimia defines what a binge is for herself. Because of distortions in thinking about food, as little as one doughnut may be thought of as a binge by one person while as much as an entire package of doughnuts may constitute a binge for another. As the duration of the habit extends, it becomes easier for her to vomit. Eventually, the vomiting is a nearly automatic response. In addition, she may take laxatives to purge herself of the energy she has ingested or use diuretics to remove body fluid.

Physical symptoms. As a result of these behaviors, physical symptoms of the bulimic adolescent will include:

- Damage to the teeth
- Irritation of the throat
- Esophageal inflammation (all of the above symptoms from exposure of unprotected tissues to acidic vomitus)
- Swollen salivary glands (from acidic reflux or constant stimulation)
- Broken blood vessels in face (from force of vomiting)
- Cracked, damaged lips
- Rectal bleeding (from overuse of laxatives)

Life-threatening situations are more rare than in anorexia nervosa. They are:

- Dehydration, electrolyte imbalance
- Fistulas or ruptures in upper gastrointestinal tract
- Kidney damage

Concerns during pregnancy are the adverse biochemical environment for the mother and fetus, the mother's abnormal weight gain pattern (weight loss, lack of weight gain, inordinate gain), and the mother's unrealistic ideas about infant feeding.

Intervention Strategies

The techniques most frequently reported in treating bulimia are similar to those used in the long-term recovery period of the person with anorexia nervosa (p. 344). Psychotherapy, nutritional therapy, and care of any pregnancy that may occur must be included.

Psychotherapy. The emphasis of therapy is on freeing the person from guilt, facilitating gains in self-esteem, and helping her deal with anxiety as well as challenging distorted goal-setting based on perfection. Ideally, the young woman's family or partner will be included in the therapy.

Nutritional therapy. While she deals with the psychologic problem, the bulimic individual will still have an eating disorder and will need reeducation to nourish herself properly. Physical and nutritional education can fill gaps in knowledge these teenagers have about their body functions. Over time, myths about weight management can be dispelled and more normal eating habits developed. Because of distorted feelings about food, the bulimic person may feel guilty every time she eats, despite the fact that food is necessary for life. The family often reinforces the guilt by a misguided overfocus on food, thinness, and the physical aspects of life. The bulimic teenager usually restricts her food intake to match the ideal plan she conceives for herself. Binges may thus arise from the natural need for adequate food and the desire for additional gratification.[28]

Role of clinical nutritionist. The clinical nutritionist on the professional team will help the young person with bulimia to see food in a more appropriate context and accept more realistic weight goals using the techniques described in the obesity section (p. 361). Helping her understand the physiologic processes of energy balance and nutrient functions as well as the effects of bingeing, vomiting, and purging as they affect her personally is especially useful. This education, however, must be done gradually in a counseling mode allowing time for alteration of her own rigid system of beliefs. Family and individual psychotherapy will continue concurrently, and it is necessary to deal with the underlying causes of the obsessional food behavior. Group therapy is also used. Strategies for working with a hard-to-reach adolescent are found in the box on p. 349.

Pregnancy care. The bulimic teenager who is pregnant can be helped to accept the idea that the baby she wants must be nourished. She can then be supported in learning to retain

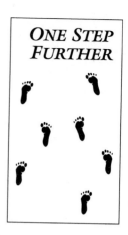

ONE STEP FURTHER

Strategies for Working With a Hard-to-Reach Adolescent

Goal: To reduce the level of stress experienced by the hard-to-reach client:
- Read her behavior as her language
- Complete your introductions as stated earlier
- Respect her coping and provide, gently, words for her behavior so she can link her feelings to the more effective coping mode of verbalizing feelings in a safe environment
- Proceed at a pace that is comfortable for her
- Offer her understanding where she does not understand herself
- Normalize and verbalize feelings by providing balance statements for her to think about
- Recognize her continued resistance and proceed very simply and gently with the information that you believe is essential that she have

those foods that the fetus needs even if she cannot totally give up bingeing and vomiting. She should also be helped in learning to recognize natural hunger signals from her baby after he is born.

OBESITY

At the other end of the physical spectrum of eating disorders is the very obese teenager. Unlike anorexic adolescents, persons who are abnormally heavy do not fit into a homogeneous group and may be carrying excessive weight for a variety of reasons. Factors leading to obesity can be broadly divided into those that are psychologic and those that are physiologic. In any individual a combination of these factors may operate in the development and maintenance of obesity. Because of the cultural response to obesity, the adolescent whose obesity may be physiologically based will generally be subject to many of the same problems as those whose obesity is more psychologically based.

Psychologic Factors

Various psychologic factors are associated with adolescent obesity, whether it develops during earlier childhood or is related to more severe psychiatric disorders.

Developmental obesity. Bruch has described a form of obesity that primarily results from psychologic factors within the family.[14] Thus it is termed developmental obesity. It is an eating disorder comparable to anorexia nervosa in that it originates in the early life of the child. The families of developmentally obese teenagers fit descriptions of the psychosomatic family. The family's attitudes and behavior thus stunt the child's psychologic development and serve as primary causes of the obesity. The obesity itself further inhibits normal development, and this in turn leads to maintenance or increase of body weight. The affected children are made to feel pressure, inappropriate responsibility, and specialness to an abnormal degree in family interactions. They become rigid, isolated, and enmeshed. They develop misperceptions about their basic physical needs and rely on coping skills based on **food abuse.** As obese teenagers, these persons may not develop their full potential as self-competent, well-functioning adults, but they are less likely to experience the complete developmental arrest that the anorexic teenager does.

Body image. The teenager who is overweight is vulnerable to body image disturbances. The type and extent of the disturbance depend on the length of time the person has been heavy, the amount of excessive weight carried, the person's sex, and the life situation surrounding the individual's unique development. For example, teenagers who have been

Food abuse
Misuse and excess eating of food as a reflection of underlying personal needs or problems, rather than in normal quantity and nature as an essential part of good health and enjoyment.

heavy from childhood may react differently than those who have gained weight only during later adolescence. Like anorexic teenagers, many tie thoughts of success or failure to their weight status.

Associated psychologic disorders. In some teenagers, obesity may be associated with severe psychiatric disorders. In others, the overeating behavior may act as an emotionally stabilizing influence helping to maintain the person at a functioning level. Interference in such a situation without substantial support provided can cause the disintegration of the person into an anxious or depressed state.

Cultural and Family Influences

The abundance of food and lack of necessity to expend energy in our society make it very easy for children to gain unwanted weight. In families where food intake and exercise patterns are not appropriate for dealing with this situation, an overweight state can result without other specific psychologic or physiologic origins.

Behavior Patterns in Obese Teenagers

The usual overweight or obese teenager is passive in interactions with others and with the environment. This response further reinforces the weight problem and leads to social isolation, lack of exercise, and disturbed patterns of eating and family interaction.

Social isolation. The passive response pattern of the obese adolescent in contact with others creates social isolation and an increased dependence on the family for relationships, even though the family interaction patterns may be unpleasant and the parents constantly exhibit intrusive and negative attitudes. Adolescents often react to the stigma of obesity by adopting a stereotyped lifestyle with a narrow range of activities.

Sedentary lifestyle. The eating and exercise functions in the lives of obese teenagers generally become distorted. They may never feel comfortable eating in social situations. Their isolation leads them to opt out of many activities that would expend energy. They fear being seen wearing gym clothes or swimsuits or doing physical activities because they feel they are the object of attention and even ridicule. Instead they usually spend an inordinate amount of time in passive pursuits such as watching television or reading. Both of these activities may be paired with eating. Commercial television, especially, fosters this behavior with frequent food-related cues.

Eating patterns. Although many studies of teenagers after they have become obese have shown that on the average they eat no more, and sometimes less, than their normal weight peers, they often have disturbed unstructured patterns of eating. They may eat only in the latter part of the day, feeling nausea when eating earlier, and eat rapidly and indiscriminately.

Family patterns. Parents in some families may be locked into power struggles with their children, attempting in vain to control what they eat. Overanxiety regarding even slight overweight may actually contribute to growing obesity. In other families overeating may be the main theme with most interactions revolving around food.

Physiologic Factors

In certain individuals physiologic factors are principally responsible for their obesity. These factors are summarized in Table 8-10. Two of these underlying factors deserve note here.

Set-point theory. One theory that cannot be overlooked is that certain individuals may be subject to a body weight "set-point." A certain body weight may be physiologically normal for each person, and body characteristics may be tuned to keep the body at that weight.

TABLE 8-10 *Processes Leading to and Sustaining Obesity: Therapeutic Implications*

Process	Therapeutic Implications
Genetic predisposition Certain inherited biochemical, morphologic, and histologic features foster excess storage of energy as fat.	Teach individual to control energy intake and output and to exert any possible control; emphasize the need to be vigilant even if unable to avoid being greater than normal size.
Sodium pump activity Less activity in cells of obese individuals decreases energy usage, making more energy available for storage.	No direct intervention; not known if process is reversible.
Body temperature differences Defect in regulation with failure to maintain normal core temperature by obese individuals increases energy available for storage.	As above.
Adipose tissue lipoprotein lipase activity Rate-limiting enzyme in triglyceride storage is more active in the obese individual, enhancing adipose tissue synthesis.	As above.
Brown adipose tissue activity Responsible for increased facultative thermoclines in animals; also being investigated in humans to no avail so far.	
Insulin resistance Obese bodies are less sensitive to insulin. Resulting hyperinsulinemia tends to maintain obese state.	Exercise improves sensitivity to insulin even without weight loss; insulin resistance is also reversible with weight loss.
Thermogenesis Less energy is spent in obligatory (food processing) or facultative (response to sympathetic nervous system) thermoclines in obese individuals.	Complex carbohydrate increases obligatory thermoclines in some individuals; timing exercise before or after meals increases facultative thermoclines in some.
Adipocyte hypertrophy When energy is available for storage, fat cells enlarge.	Decrease energy available by changing intake/output. Cell size is reduced with energy deficit.

Continued.

TABLE 8-10 *Processes Leading to and Sustaining Obesity: Therapeutic Implications—cont'd*

Process	Therapeutic Implications
Adipocyte hyperplasia When fat cells are filled, new cells will be formed if energy continues to be available for storage.	Already obese individuals can decrease energy available to prevent formation of even more cells. Cell number does not decrease even with energy deficit.
Regional distribution of adipose tissue Typically, males have more central (abdominal) adipose tissue with higher waist/hip ratios than females who have more peripheral (femoral and gluteal) fat with lower waist/hip ratios. Male distribution is associated with diabetes, hypertension, and cardiovascular disease; female distribution is more difficult to change. Difference in cell size and lipoprotein lipase activity in various sites may be important.	Assessing waist/hip ratio helps determine difficulty of achieving weight loss and the harm in remaining obese.
Set point weight Bodies of certain individuals defend high body weights. Others defend low weights or no particular weight.	Decrease excess energy through exercise and substituting complex carbohydrates for fat, so as to reverse any processes that are reversible. If obese adolescents have control of energy intake and output, psychologic support for physiologically sustainable weight is reasonable.

Lower basal energy need. A decreased requirement for the amount of energy used in biochemical reactions may increase the amount of energy available in the systems of some people for storage as fat. Based on present theory, the longer the teenager has been obese and the greater the extent of the obesity, the greater the effect of these factors. The adolescent whose obesity was originally caused by other factors such as social, psychologic, or family influences will, as time passes, have added problems of physiologic obesity. This pattern increases the complexity of the obese state.

Intervention Strategies

An effective program for working with obese teenagers and their families will provide personalized care, giving attention to identifying individual needs and attitudes, setting realistic goals, developing related strategies within a comprehensive approach (see box on p. 362), and evaluating outcome.

Assessment. The individual combination of psychologic and physiologic circumstances by which an individual teenager has become obese must be identified so that intervention can be directed toward specific aspects of the problem. The degree of overweight must be considered. The material in the assessment section, especially Fig. 8-6, may be used to evaluate the size of heavy adolescents. Generally they will be (1) *overweight,* only moderately above weight-height midranges for health; (2) *obese,* about 20% or more above normal weight-height ranges with a higher degree of fatness; and (3) *morbidly obese,* much higher weight for height and a greater amount of fat tissue, associated with multiple health problems. Some of these persons will suffer from hidden eating disorders such as bulimia or anorexia nervosa (recovery stage). The information needed to assess adolescent obesity (Table 8-11) may best be gathered by a team of professionals. Many of these aspects cannot be assessed immediately but will need to be explored over time. Basic initial steps assess physical status and personal attitude.

Physical status. A physical examination will disclose the stage of puberty and rule out any endocrine abnormalities or complications of the obese state. Endocrine disorders are rarely found. Most physiologic abnormalities indicated by clinical laboratory measures that are associated with obesity will respond to weight reduction.

Personal attitude. The most important aspect of initial evaluation is whether the individual is committed to making changes. The teenager's feelings must be assessed initially and at each visit. It is of no value for other persons to have goals related to weight management if the teenager is not ready to change the status quo. The question needs to be, "Are you ready to make changes?" rather than, "Do you want to lose weight?" Many teenagers will answer "yes" to the second question but remain totally passive, the implication being that the process of weight management for them is a passive one in which the professional administers treatment.

Reasons for not starting a weight loss program. A weight loss program should not be instituted if (1) the adolescent has not reached full height, (2) there is a lack of commitment, (3) it is likely to be another in a series of failures harmful to the individual's self-esteem, or (4) the individual is obviously predisposed to obesity by overwhelming physiologic factors. If obese teenagers keep fit, maintain energy equilibrium, and are emotionally healthy, they will be candidates for weight loss only if they understand the physiologic aspects of obesity and are determined to test these aspects in a healthful manner. Those adolescents who are still growing in height should not be encouraged to lose weight because the level of energy restriction required to do so is inadequate to support growth.

Goals. Realistic planning of goals includes a series of short-term steps to the long-term goal.

Short-term goals. Short-term goals need to be based not on changes in weight but on positive changes in food- and exercise-related attitudes and behaviors with appropriate rewards built in. It is especially necessary to build a program around short-term manageable goals related to behavioral change since physiologic factors may make actual weight loss a difficult, long-term achievement. The teenager should be made aware that over the long term an energy deficit will eventually lead to weight loss, however slowly. Working toward improved knowledge, attitudes, or behaviors listed in Table 8-11 is a worthy short-term goal.

Weight goal. The initial weight goal in a weight management program is usually maintenance, that is, cessation of weight gain. In certain situations an even more basic change from rapid gain to slow gain is the more appropriate goal. Immature adolescents who have not completed linear growth can bring weight and, more specifically, percentage of body fat into better proportion with height by holding their weight stable or by reducing gains to a lower rate as height increases. This pattern eliminates nutritional risk to the individual from severe diet restrictions at a time of rapid growth and development. For teenagers who have stabilized their weight and are no longer gaining in height, the next step will be a slow steady loss based on reeducation in the use of energy. A loss of 0.9 kg/week (2 lb/week) should not be exceeded. If this rate appears insignificant to the teenager, point out that it would add up to more than a 45 kg (100 lb) loss over 1 year.

Text continued on p. 359.

ONE STEP FURTHER

Fitness: Testing and Planning Improvement Programs

1. a. Have client sit quietly and relax for 3 to 5 minutes.
    b. Take pulse for 10 seconds.*
    c. Record *resting heart rate (RHR)*: _____
2. a. Find intensity of exercise required to reach *training heart rate (THR)*† and immediately after exercise. THR for teens is 20 to 22 beat/10 sec.‡
    Stop with the exercise that achieves 20 to 22 beats/10 sec. This is the exercise to use initially in the improvement program.

    Intensity increases →

    Run for 5 minutes
    Jog for 5 minutes
    Jog for 2 minutes — walk for 2 minutes — jog for 2 minutes
    Walk uphill or upstairs for 2 to 3 minutes
    Walk for 5 minutes at a more rapid pace
    START   Walk for 5 minutes at a moderate pace

    b. Monitor pulse return toward RHR after each exercise level — it should be below 16 beats/10 sec by 5 minutes.

    _____   _____   _____   _____
    Immediate → 1 minute → 2 minutes → 5 minutes → . . .

3. *Improvement program:* To maintain THR for 15 minutes 4 to 5 days/week:
    a. Work with client to design an individualized program that is comfortable for him or her.
    b. Plan 5-minute warm-up — move at level below the level that maintains THR.
    c. Exercise at intensity that maintains THR.
    d. Five-minute cool down — back to warm-up speed — client should not sit or lie down immediately.
    e. Use a combination of exercise levels and types, if necessary.
    f. If the client is ill, he or she should begin after illness at lower intensity and return slowly to intensify achieved before illness.
4. a. Retest every 3 to 4 weeks.
    b. Increase intensity of exercise to maintain THR.
    c. Client can increase time spent doing the exercise by 5-minute increments, up to 30 minutes.
    d. When client has reached jogging level and maintains it for 6 to 8 weeks, increase THR to 22 to 25 beats/10 sec.
    e. Client can use any aerobic activities (for example, jogging, bicycling, skating, dancing) or combinations that the client prefers.

NOTE: Contraindications for testing and initiating fitness program will be revealed by routine medical history and physical examination.
*10-second time segment is easiest to measure and use.
†*Maximum heart rate (MHR)* is approximately 200 beats/min for persons under 20 years of age (Cumming GR, Everatt D, Hastman L: *Am J Cardiol* 41:69, 1978). THR is 60% of MHR for persons with poor initial fitness, 75% of MHR for persons who are fit (that is, 60% of 200 = 120 beats/min = 20 beats/10 sec [20 to 2 beats/10 sec for normal variation]).
‡An adolescent of normal weight and in reasonable shape may want to start at 22 to 25 beats/10 sec.
From Pipes PL: *Nutrition in infancy and childhood*. St Louis, 1981, Mosby; developed by Scott B and Rees J, Adolescent Program, University of Washington, Seattle, Wash.

TABLE 8-11   Weight Management Assessment

Rate on Scale of 0 to 5 the Contribution to Weight Management
(0 = minimum, 5 = maximum)

	0	1	2	3	4	5

NOURISHMENT
1. Knowledge of
    Meaning of term "calories"
    Role of food in life
    Relationship of energy intake/output
    Major nutrients
        Physiologic role
        Energy value
        Amount needed
        Food sources
        Amount of food needed
    Choosing food in a variety of situations
    Behavior modification techniques
    Appropriate weight/height/age/genetic heritage
2. Attitude
    Acceptance of responsibility for nourishing self
    Commitment to health-promoting habits
        Obtaining appropriate foods
        Nutrition education
3. Eating behavior
    Control of food supply
        Fat content
        Types of food
        Amounts
        Meal pattern
        Between meal eating
        Binges/night eating/other aberrations
    Uses behavior modification techniques
    Eats in social situations
        With family
        Peers
4. Family
    Eating meals together
        Place
        Distractions (TV)
    Serving methods
    Support for weight control via
        Use of food
        Knowledge
        Autonomy allowed to patient to choose food

Continued.

TABLE 8-11 *Weight Management Assessment — cont'd*

	0	1	2	3	4	5

ENERGY TIME MANAGEMENT
1. Knowledge of
   Exercise in energy balance
   Fitness
      Cardiorespiratory
      Muscular
   Exercise
      Aerobic
      Anaerobic
   Monitoring pulse
2. Attitude
   Commitment to exercising regularly
      Without others, equipment, or money if necessary
   Interest in fitness education
   Pleasure in moving
3. Behavior
   Fitness tested
      Program planned
      Program maintained
   Level of fitness
   Relaxation
   Rest/sleep
   Activities shared
      With friends
      With family
   Consciously plans exercise/relaxation/rest
4. Family
   Support of activities
   Family activities
   Understanding of exercise in weight management

PYCHOSOCIAL HEALTH
1. Knowledge of
   Emotional factors in weight management
   Cues to eat
      Internal
      External
   Impact on emotional health of
      Physical activity
      Nourishment
   Responsibility for weight management
   Need to seek guidance for unsolvable problems

TABLE 8-11   Weight Management Assessment—cont'd

	0	1	2	3	4	5
2. Attitude						
Commitment to mental health						
Learning about weight control						
Solving problems						
3. Behavior						
Pleasurable experiences						
Relationships						
Peers						
Family						
Teachers						
Counselors						
School activities						
Social skills						
Intellect						
Insight						
Communication						
Problem solving						
School performance						
Goal setting						
Short term						
Long term						
Self rewards						
4. Emotional Status						
Body image						
Self efficacy						
Locus of control						
Depression versus nondepression						
Sense of humor						
Oral gratification						
Coping skills						
Compulsivity						
Perfectionism						
Independence						
5. Parental						
Perception of weight problem						
Support versus intrusion						
Emotional						
Financial						
Rigidity						
Conflict resolution						
Commitment to treatment						

Continued.

TABLE 8-11 **Weight Management Assessment — cont'd**

OBJECTIVE

Age _____ yr

Length of obesity

	Infancy	Toddler	Early Child-hood	Elementary School	Junior High	Senior High
Reduction at-tempts	Yo-yo	Severe	Diets	Exercise	0	Reasonable
	Anorexia	Bulimia				
Parents	Natural	Adoptive				
	Anorexia	Bulimia	Obesity	Overweight		
Grandparents	Natural	Adoptive				
	Anorexia	Bulimia	Obesity	Overweight		
Maturation (stage)	0	1	2	3	4	5
Menarche	0	+1yr	+2yr	+3yr	+4yr	+5yr
Thyroid screen						
Cholesterol (mg/dl) _____		HDL mg/dl _____			LDL mg/dl _____	
Weight percentile*	>95	95	95-75	75	75-50	50
Height percentile*	95	90	75	50	25	10
Weight/Height percentile*	100-50 lb >95	50-25 lb >95	>95	95	95-75	75
BMI						
TSF percentile†	>95	95	95-75	75	75-50	50
SSF percentile† (male)	>95	95	95-75	75	75-50	50
MAC percentile†	>95	95	95-75	75	75-50	50
AMC percentile†	>95	95	95-75	75	75-50	50
Waist circumference _____inches						
Hips circumference _____inches						
Waist/hip ratio _____						

BMI, body mass index (kg/m^2) (>30 considered obese, 24-27 [females] and 25-27 [males] considered overweight); TSF, triceps skinfold; SSF, subscapular skinfold; MAC, midarm circumference; RHR, resting heart rate; AMA, arm muscle area.

*National Center for Health Statistics: *Height and weight of youths 12-17 years, United States.* In *Vital and health statistics,* series 11, no 124, Health Services and Mental Health Administration, Washington, DC, 1973, US Government Printing Office. Above 75th percentile weight/height/age/sex considered obese if TSF also greater than 75th percentile; 25th-75th percentile weight/height/age/sex considered in normal range (Mahan LK, Rees JM: *Nutrition in adolescents,* St Louis, 1984, Mosby, p 51).

†Standards in Frisancho AR: *Am J Clin Nutr* 34:2540, 1981.

From Rees JM: Management of obesity in adolescence. In Farrow JA, editor: Adolescent medicine, *Med Clin North Am* 74:1285.

TABLE 8-11 *Weight Management Assessment — cont'd*

Exercise to reach 120 beats/min	Slow walk	Moderate walk	Fast walk	Walk up hill	Walk/ jog	Jog
Entry Date _____		+3 mo	+6 mo	+12 mo	+18 mo	+24 mo
Weight _____ lb	+ 10					
	+ 5					
	- 2.5					
	- 5					
	- 10					
	- 15					
Percent body fat _____	+ 3					
	+ 2					
	- 2					
	- 5					
RHR _____	+ 5					
	+ 3					
	- 3					
	- 5					
Height _____ inches	+ 3					
	+ 2					
	+ 1					
AMA _____ mm²	+ 500					
	+ 200					
	+ 100					
	-100					
	-200					

Improvement in any of the physical measures of Table 8-11 constitutes achievement of a long-term goal.

Intervention Strategies: Physiologic Factors

Strategies planned to deal with the physiologic factors of obesity must be based on the laws of **energy exchange** and **balance,** address positive changes in personal food behaviors, avoid the dangers of "crash-diets" and life-threatening situations, and increase physical activity and fitness.[29]

Basic individual energy balance. Whatever the reasons for a teenager being overweight, the method for altering the situation remains the same: decreasing the body's energy intake and increasing the energy output until the appropriate deficit state is established. There is no way of knowing the exact use of energy by a particular body except by testing it over time. To lose weight an energy deficit must be achieved at the cellular

Energy balance
Physiologic aspect of weight management, based on balance between energy intake in food and energy output in physical activity and internal metabolic work.

level. Because this state is not measurable under normal clinical circumstances, there is no set formula that assures weight loss. It is an error to count kilocalories of food energy being eaten and assume that this amount of energy will be available within the biochemical system. Thus a deficit of 3500 kilocalories calculated at the point of intake does not necessarily lead to a loss of 1 lb of body weight. This does not imply that the second law of **thermodynamics** is inoperative, but simply that energy from food may be used in a variety of ways once it is in the body, as indicated previously (Table 8-10). Thus both the physiologic and the psychologic aspects of weight management are unique to the individual.

Eating habits. Each individual teenager must be guided in learning the level of energy intake and output that produces weight gain, loss, and maintenance for them if the treatment is to be effective. An understanding of physiologic factors must be incorporated. The teenager must be made aware that however bleak the physiologic situation appears, the possibility of weight management has not been tested until the individual has control over energy intake and output. There is usually some potential for improvement in the diet that will help even those persons who are physiologically prone to obesity to become more fit and healthy, and to stabilize and perhaps to reduce their weight—in small amounts.

Dietary change. Strategies for dietary change must address the issues of (1) energy and nutrient content of the food intake; (2) circumstances of eating related to timing, place, accompanying social factors, and emotions; and (3) principles of nutrition regarding weight management.

Food use retraining. Specific diets have rarely achieved long-term changes in eating behavior. This result is especially true for teenagers, who tend to rebel against authoritarian techniques and hold a number of negative views about diets. Food use retraining, a series of habit changes planned jointly by the teenager and the therapist and instituted in succession over time, will be more acceptable to most adolescents and is a more realistic way to approach a complex problem.

Time factor. Because eating habits have been developed over a number of years, it is logical that the teenager will need considerable time to make changes. A person cannot suddenly pick up a musical instrument and play it well but will need education, practice, and support to become proficient. Similarly, most teenagers will not be able to learn a new food pattern or "diet" and perfect it immediately. Usually intensive treatment will need to be continued for a year or more to accomplish major dietary changes. Breaking down the problem of food misuse into small components makes change more probable. What habit will be the initial focus, how change will be accomplished, what foods will be eaten, and what motivations and rewards will be effective are developed and clarified in counseling sessions between the therapist and the teenager.

Therapy objective. The nutritional therapist's objective is eventually to focus on each time of day and point of environment where teenagers meet with food and to help them to retrain themselves in the use of food. Most teenagers will have some reasonable habits that can be supported and used as a foundation for the emerging positive patterns.

Self-responsibility. Teenagers will need help at every step to take responsibility for their actions. Coupled with psychologic support, the process can lead to effective change. Even those who are unsuccessful in retraining themselves during the adolescent period will have a model for the future, when they may be able to take greater control. Education regarding the physiologic factors of obesity will help teenagers avoid the harmful quick loss plans to which they are so vulnerable.

Dangers of "crash" diets. A very important component of programs in weight management education involves helping the teenager understand that rapid weight loss by either starvation or too low an energy intake is ineffective. Since the loss is in lean body

Laws of thermodynamics (Gr *Therme,* heat; *dynamis,* power) Basic three laws of physics relating to heat-energy balance: (1) energy like matter is neither created nor destroyed, only constantly transformed and recycled, thus conserving energy in any process; (2) there is always an increase in *entropy* (Gr *entrope,* a turning inward), a measure of the part of heat or other energy form in a system that is not available to perform work, thus entropy increases in all natural (spontaneous and irreversible) processes; and (3) absolute zero in energy balance is unattainable.

mass and fluids, inevitably weight will be regained when usual eating is resumed, and muscle (and the ability to use energy) not fat will have been lost. The deprivation in such a regimen often leads to even greater overeating. Thus the final result of a "crash" diet is often a net gain. It is not difficult to convince those who have had the experience a few times that such practices are ineffective, but it is important to support their impressions by teaching them the physiologic reasons. Teenagers who will not be convinced that such methods and "diet aids" are unhealthy will be deterred from using them by the knowledge that they will not lose *fat*.

Morbid obesity. There are certain life-threatening situations for very obese persons when drastic intervention will be necessary. The physical condition should be monitored to detect any rapid deterioration. The following conditions warrant hospitalization.

- Sudden changes in cardiac or respiratory function
- Inability to move, maintain balance, or travel
- Rapid weight increase because of the above factors
- Inability to fit into furniture and having to rest on floor
- Ulcerations at pressure points and friction areas

As with the anorexic teenager, a period of separation from the family may break up a pernicious cycle leading to physical deterioration. Comprehensive treatment using a modified fast as the dietary component is at present the most practical therapy. Although it is still controversial whether lean body mass can be spared, such dietary methods appear less objectionable than other radical procedures.

Physical activity and fitness. One of the most important concepts of weight management is that energy output must be increased. Individualized exercise programs need to be developed with the obese teenager in order to achieve a gradual increase in physical activity.

The fitness test shown in the box on p. 354 is designed to be a conservative tool that can safely be used with even an extremely obese person. It can be used with or without professional help. Physically, it appears that increasing activity can be rewarding in itself, whereas denying oneself an accustomed food may be more like punishment. In addition to fitness testing and improvement, various strategies can be directed toward increasing energy output by increasing physical activity. These guidelines should be followed. Activities should (1) be built into everyday life, (2) be something the person enjoys or finds useful, (3) not depend on help from others or complex equipment, and (4) not be stressful by causing embarrassing exposure of the body or awkwardness.

Intervention Strategies: Psychologic Factors

Weight management for teenagers should be a total rehabilitation program. It demands a significant length of time and must be individualized. Like the physiologic component, the psychologic component of any weight management problem cannot be overlooked. Activities planned to meet these needs include motivational support, psychotherapy, and counseling.

Motivation. In a short-term situation where the teenager has only a few pounds to lose, the problem is one of motivation. This support can be provided in settings such as schools and many other community settings.

Psychotherapy. With extreme developmental obesity, changes usually require extensive psychotherapeutic intervention. This includes the family when the teenager is living at home.

Counseling. For teenagers falling between these two extremes, a variable degree of supportive counseling will be needed to increase self-acceptance, to decrease stress, to facilitate development, and to enable adolescents to carry out weight management strategies. Teenagers need help in learning to experience the body's signals related to hunger and satiety and to adopt nondestructive coping mechanisms to replace the misuse of food.

Comprehensive Approach

To provide a comprehensive approach to a weight management program for teenagers, attention must be given to additional resources available. These resources include group activities applied with professional guidance, parent education and counseling, and school and community support.

Group activities. Strategies such as camp settings, support groups, peer counseling, social skills and assertiveness training, body awareness experience, physical fitness training, and behavior modification can be used successfully with some individuals. Groups and preplanned programs will help those adolescents with mild, relatively simple problems. *Camps and other groups that provide only for short-term weight loss are detrimental and should be avoided.*

Professional guidance. None of the group settings, however, provide a solution for all aspects of obesity. To be effective, weight management techniques must be applied within the context of ongoing supportive counseling by professionals who assess the specific problems of the individual over time and choose appropriate treatment methods. A team of professionals will be best able to carry out a comprehensive program as described here.

Parent education and counseling. Counseling will enable parents to support their teenagers in learning to manage weight. Education about the physiologic factors involved and rational approaches to management will help dispel myths parents hold. Helping them develop a nonintrusive attitude toward their teenagers is of extreme importance. The counselor can demonstrate this by stressing the need for teenagers, not counselors or parents, to establish their own goals.

School and community support. Although they are rarely in the position to carry out

BE SIZEWISE

*Don't Lose
Your Balance*

Nourishment	**Activities**	**Feelings**
Be good to your body— give it what it needs	Do interesting things— quiet as well as energetic	Learn to know and like yourself
Don't starve or stuff yourself	Take time to relax every day	Have realistic goals for yourself
Know what's in the food you eat	Don't let eating be your only recreation	Don't substitute food for love and companionship
	Do some strenuous activity every day	Build satisfying relationships with your family and friends
	Share active and quiet time with friends	Get help for problems you can't cope with alone

FIG. 8-9 Be sizewise—materials for clinicians, educators, and teenagers.
© American Heart Association of Washington.

therapy because of the complexity of the problem, teachers, school counselors, nurses, coaches, and other community leaders of adolescents have many opportunities to educate and support overweight teenagers. Curriculum materials such as those in Fig. 8-9 have been designed to help adolescents understand the complexity of weight management.

Outcome

Reviews of the outcome of weight management therapies for teenagers are uniformly gloomy. In general such programs are designed as studies of weight loss, when informed workers in the field of adolescent health have stressed the importance of focusing on the other benefits of weight management programs such as increased self-esteem. Added knowledge, increased readiness to work for change, and improved practices are important outcomes of weight management programs for adolescents.

Summary — Eating Disorders

The spectrum of eating disorders affects adolescents physically, psychologically, personally, and socially. Intervention strategies must be directed toward both the nutritional and developmental aspects of these disorders to be effective. Goals must be established in relation to all aspects. Helping teenagers put food into reasonable perspective in their lives will be a principal goal of nutritional therapy. A recognition of the amount of time required for effective intervention is essential for a basic understanding of eating disorders.

PHYSICAL FITNESS AND ATHLETICS
Benefits of Physical Fitness

All teenagers should be encouraged to exercise in ways best suited to their lives. The exercised body is more likely to remain healthy than one that remains sedentary, because historically the human required great energy exchange to obtain food, protect itself, and to survive the elements. The benefits of physical activity include the following[30]:
- Helps maintain optimal body composition
- Improves the possibility of weight loss when that is necessary
- Increases the efficiency of muscle fibers to produce energy
- Increases the efficiency of hormones (insulin, lipoprotein lipase, epinephrine) to regulate energy metabolism
- Decreases the production of lactic acid, which interferes with energy production
- Strengthens the heart, lungs, and circulatory system
- Increases levels of HDL over LDL and decreases levels of some triglycerides
- Raises rates of basal metabolism
- Helps control appetite

Lack of Fitness

Health care workers are increasingly called upon to help teenagers incorporate fitness into their lives as the energy requirements of modern life decrease.[31] Only about 50% of young people today are regularly involved in vigorous exercise. When tested, 30% of males and more than 50% of females 6 to 17 years of age cannot do even a single pull-up.[31]

Elements of Fitness

Each teenager should participate in activities that maintain the elements of fitness: body composition; cardiorespiratory function; and muscular strength, endurance, and flexibility. Raising the heart rate to at least 50% but no more than 75% of maximum for 15 minutes, with 5 minutes warm-up and cool-down, at least 3 days a week will maintain cardiorespiratory fitness. This process is incorporated in the testing and improvement protocol given (see the box on p. 354). The maximum heart rate of adolescents has been shown to be about 200. This number can be used until age 20, when the usual calculation for adults, subtracting the age from 220 to derive the maximum heart rate, can begin. Stressful exercise is unnecessary and undesirable. Continuous gradual improvement and maintenance are effective. A few well-chosen calisthenics will maintain muscular strength, flexibility, and endurance. Adolescents who participate in sports as well as those who do not should develop personal programs to assure fitness is maintained between seasonal participation in organized programs.

Nutritional Requirements for Athletics

Adolescent athletes require specific nutritional support, primarily to maintain normal growth and physiologic maturation in spite of the physical stress. Energy is the basic factor in this process. The amount of additional energy needed will depend on the intensity, duration, and type of exercise being done (Table 8-12).

Sources of energy. Energy is best utilized if it is supplied as **carbohydrate.** An additional 6 to 7 g of protein per day is sufficient in a muscle-building phase. Thereafter 2 to 3 g of protein per day above the daily recommmended allowance will support body maintenance in most athletes. Abnormally high levels of protein are counterproductive, leading to dehydration as the body rids itself of nitrogenous waste products. The need for carbohydrate rather than protein as fuel to build muscle is one of the most misunderstood principles among adolescent athletes.

Weight management. Weight should be gained or lost following safe, effective methods described here. To successfully support normal growth, weight should be maintained at an optimal level long term rather than be subjected to seasonal, or especially, weekly manipulation as is often urged by coaches of wrestling and crew during competition. The development pattern of skeletal growth and weight gain must be considered. Two problems in this area are common among teenage athletes who become too thin while trying to reduce the percentage of body fat: (1) females interrupt their menses, and (2) males stunt their **linear growth.** Anabolic steroids taken by males to increase weight cause stunting of growth and disturbed development of secondary sex characteristics.

Supplements. An increased dietary intake should provide sufficient amounts of nutrients, making supplements unnecessary. Supplementation of nutrients in amounts above those recommended has not resulted in benefits during competition. Of the vitamins and minerals, iron is particularly important to young athletes because "sports anemia" is associated with reduced oxygenation; the B vitamins are essential in energy production.[32]

Anabolic steroids. Many young adolescents (estimated at 5% to 10% by those studying the incidence) use **anabolic steroids.** Use is apparently greater among male athletes who say they use them to increase muscle, size, strength, speed, and to improve personal appearance and athletic performance. The research shows that young people who use these substances lack appropriate knowledge of the profound effects they have on the whole body.[33] Studies of the effects on adolescents are not available.

Short-term events. A light workout one day before competition, combined with increased dietary carbohydrate, mainly starches, will assure a supply of liver and muscle glycogen to support the athlete during a short-term event. On the day of competition eliminate roughage, fats, and gas-forming foods from the diet to decrease discomfort and untimely need for elimination. If several short-term events are held in one day, additional carbohydrate will provide energy. Otherwise stores should be sufficient. Fluid replacement follows the same principles given below for long-term events.

Long-term events. For longer events that last at least 1 hour, supplies of body fuel and fluids will need attention.

Carbohydrate fuel
Basic organic carbon compound in food (starches and sugars) that is the primary and most efficient form of body fuel for energy, especially for building body muscles.

Linear growth
(L *linearis,* a line) Linear measure of growing body length; height.

Anabolic steroids
(Gr *Anabole,* a building of construction) Any of a group of synthetic derivatives of testosterone, the male sex hormone, having pronounced anabolic (tissue building) properties; a drug used in clinical medicine to promote growth and repair body tissues in debilitating illness. Widespread illegal abuse of the drug by some athletes and body builders harms health.

TABLE 8-12 **Calorie Requirements in Adolescence***

Age	Recommended Daily Allowances (calories per pound per day)			Health Fitness†	Competitive‡			Long Endurance§		
	Low Calorie	Median Calorie	High Calorie		Weight Loss	Weight Stable	Weight Gain	Weight Loss	Weight Stable	Weight Gain
Males										
11-14	20	27	37	+2	+2	+7	+12	+19	+24	+29
15-18	14	19	27	+2	+1	+5	+8	+13	+16	+20
Females										
11-14	15	22	30	+2	+0	+5	+10	+14	+19	+24
15-18	10	17	25	+1½	+0	+4	+8	+12	+16	+20

*Note: The amounts listed are given in ranges to account for variability of body build and maturational level within an age group. For additional calorie needs for sports to achieve weight maintenance, add figures listed to the daily calorie needs per pound per day. Weight loss or gain is based on 1-lb change per week, with the object of losing body fat or gaining lean muscle mass. These figures are estimates and may need to be adjusted for the individual. Competitive and long endurance sports are not recommended for 4- to 10-year-olds.

†Based on an average amount of calories expended for four 30-minute periods of exercise per wk.
‡Based on an average amount of calories expended for six 2-hour practices per week.
§Based on an average amount of calories expended for seven 3.5-hour practices per week plus three 4-hour competitive events per month.
From Nevin-Folino NL: *Sports nutrition in children and adolescents.* In Queen PM, Lang CE, editors: *Handbook of Pediatric Nutrition,* 1993, Aspen.

Glycogen loading
Practice among athletes in endurance events of increasing intake of complex carbohydrates in days before the event to increase glycogen storage for energy reserve fuel during the event.

Body fuel stores. Modified **glycogen loading** before a long-term event will improve not only liver storage but also muscle reserves. Glucose can be taken after the event begins to spare liver glycogen stores, but it should not be ingested just before an event because it impairs lipid mobilization.

Fluids and electrolytes. Body fluid–electrolyte balance is very important during long-term events, indeed throughout athletic training and competition.[30] Exaggerated shifts in fluids and electrolytes due to strenuous exercise are intensified by environmental temperatures and the sweat of exertion. Water must be replaced at the level of 1 pint for each pound of body weight lost in any exercise or training session. Thus fluid must be available to keep up with thirst during events and may have to be replaced at levels beyond thirst in the post-event period. Electrolytes and additional glucose can be obtained by using natural juices and fluids made with specified concentrations. The maximal sugar content for an efficient replacement drink is 2.0 to 2.5 g of sugar per decaliter. The need for replacing fluids will vary according to loss due to the event and climate. It is unnecessary for athletes trying to keep warm on the sidelines of a soccer game in a cold northern climate to drink electrolyte-rich fluids designed for sweat-inducing events in tropical conditions.

Overall nutritional goals. Maintaining appropriate weight for height is a good general guide to dietary adequacy as long as the foods eaten to attain that weight are nutrient rich. Obtaining sufficient food may prove difficult for teenage athletes whose days may be filled from early morning to late evening with practices as well as normal activities including classes and study assignments. Parents, coaches, and school officials need to support teenagers by helping them plan specifically to obtain adequate acceptable foods at times when rigorous schedules allow them to eat.

ADOLESCENT PREGNANCY
Developmental Issues

Teenage pregnancy must be studied in the light of the highly dynamic nature of adolescence. Both the psychologic and the physical status of the adolescent have implications for the course of any pregnancy. The many interactions of factors in adolescent development and in reproduction have great clinical significance for all aspects of the pregnancy, including the nutritional aspect.[34] Indeed, adolescents are changing so profoundly that pregnancy for the younger, less mature teenager will be different from that of the older, more mature adolescent.

Less mature teenagers will be more dependent on others and less able to act and make decisions on their own. They will be more **narcissistic** and less able to comprehend the needs of others. These young women will be less realistic, engage in more fantasy and wishful thinking, and have less insight into their own behaviors and motives (see the box on p. 368). In general, younger teenagers will have fewer intellectual and physical skills to cope with any situation, especially a complex reproductive experience. Many of the difficulties related to pregnancy in adolescence stem from this immaturity. As development advances, a person is able to carry out reproduction and child rearing in a more normal, less problem-fraught way. As seen in Fig. 8-10, the timeline of events in teenage pregnancy has great potential for affecting the nutritional well-being of the adolescent.

Narcissism
Self-love; drawn from Narcissus, a character in Greek mythology who saw his image mirrored in a pool of water and fell in love with his own reflection.

Gynecologic age
(Gr *gynaikos*, women) Length of time from onset of menses to present time of conception.

Reproduction During Adolescence

The pregnant adolescent's nutritional needs are influenced by many factors. Primary influences are her growth and nutrient stores, her **gynecologic age,** and her preconception nutritional status.

Adolescent growth and nutrient stores The assumption that pregnant adolescents need a supply of nutrients to support their own growth along with that of the growing fetus

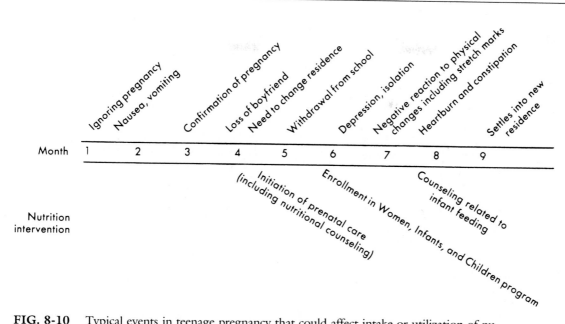

FIG. 8-10 Typical events in teenage pregnancy that could affect intake or utilization of nutrients.

has been questioned. Because hormone levels are high in pregnancy, even the slower adolescent growth that usually follows menarche may not occur. According to recent studies growth does continue to some degree during adolescent pregnancy.[35] Whether actual growth continues for an adolescent who becomes pregnant, she will have experienced rapid growth more recently than her adult counterparts. There will have been less opportunity for storage of nutrients. Thus there may be greater physiologic risk to young women who conceive in menarche.

Gynecologic age. The number of years between the onset of menses and conception is calculated to derive the gynecologic age. Those adolescents who are more sexually mature, that is, of greater gynecologic age, share a vulnerability to physiologic stresses but appear to have no more physically-based complications than do adult women. It is the young women of lower gynecologic age who carry more risk and need more nutritional support. The number of adolescents who become pregnant in the first 2 years following menarche will be relatively small because most of them will not be ovulating during that time even though they are menstruating. Those who do become pregnant, however, are of great concern to clinicians and researchers in this area.

Nutritional status at conception. Pregnant adolescents who are of young gynecologic age and malnourished at the time of conception are at double risk. They appear to have the greatest need for nutrients to support a pregnancy and maintain optimal health themselves.[36]

Hazards to the Mother

Given the complexity of pregnancy in the adolescent period, it is logical to question how these young women fare during pregnancy. They have more complications, a higher risk of maternal mortality, and more problems in personal psychologic development and education that carry implications for economic well-being (see the box on p. 369).

Complications. The variety of complications often described for the teenage mother during gestation include:

ONE STEP FURTHER

Expectations vs. Reality

Pregnant adolescents often find their expectations are quite different from the reality of motherhood.

EXPECTATION	REALITY
Life with baby	
Life with baby will be wonderful.	Life with baby isn't wonderful.
Baby will meet their emotional needs.	Baby doesn't meet emotional needs. Baby may even interfere with their own need-meeting.
They won't be lonely anymore.	They may be even more lonely with the demands and limitations of a baby.
Parenting	
Parenting is easy (based on baby-sitting experience). They will manage.	Parenting is not easy. The 24-hr responsibility is overwhelming.
Others (e.g., partner, family) will help them.	Many are parenting alone. There are limited resources for teen parents. Many are not ready to accept help, education, role modeling, etc.
Self-esteem	
Self-esteem will increase with pregnancy and parenthood. They now have a role.	Self-conscious about body changes. Society disapproves. Self-esteem decreases. Baby takes attention away from them.
Relationships	
Her parents will be upset, but supportive. They will care for the teen mom and her baby.	Many have family support, but some parents reject or do not support on their terms.
Relationship with partner will improve or he'll come back.	Some live common-law or are married. Relationship with partner is often strained and he frequently leaves.
Friendships will continue as they are.	Life is different from peers. They become isolated from friends.
Finances	
Somebody will provide welfare.	Welfare is not sufficient, and mothers are unable to manage. Many do not know how to budget.
Some plan to be self-sufficient (finish school, get a job).	Self-sufficiency takes a long time. Often they don't have energy and/or the organizational skills to continue or reenter school/work.
Housing	
Want to find affordable, safe, clean housing to live on their own.	Landlords can be biased against single moms, children, and tenants on welfare. Rent may be too expensive to afford.
Goals	
Motherhood will make life meaningful.	Life may prove to be no more meaningful.
Tend not to have long-term goals.	Difficult to follow through, even on short-term goals.

Modified from Browne C, Urback M: Pregnant adolescents: expectations vs. reality, *Can J Public Health,* June 1989.

❖

> ### RISKS ASSOCIATED WITH ADOLESCENT PREGNANCY
>
> - *Maternal risks*
>   Pregnancy-induced hypertension
>   Premature labor
>   Intrauterine growth retardation
>   Anemia
>   Maternal mortality
>   Increased incidence of cephalopelvic dispro-
>   portion
> - *Neonatal risks*
>   Increased perinatal mortality
>   Increased neonatal mortality
>   Prematurity
>
>   Lack of access to pediatric health care
>   services
>   Poor parenting skills
> - *Psychosocial risks for mother and baby*
>   Failure to complete education
>   Unemployment
>   Poverty
>   Dependence upon public assistance
>   Poor job satisfaction
>   Marital instability
>   Greater number of children per mother

- First and third trimester bleeding
- Anemia
- Difficult labor and delivery
- **Cephalopelvic disproportion**
- Pregnancy-induced hypertensive disorders including **preeclampsia** and eclampsia
- Infections

Of these complications, the most common physical problem is infection, while the most common serious complication is preeclampsia. Preeclampsia usually occurs in the third trimester and is manifested in increased weight gain, fluid retention, high blood pressure, and proteinuria; it does not appear to run a different course in pregnant teenagers than in older women. Some researchers point out that it is a disease of first pregnancies. By and large, data support this observation. In addition, the harmful effects of preeclampsia, or the more serious state of eclampsia, may be greater in teenagers. Damage to the cardiovascular and renal systems initiated with a first pregnancy early in life and intensified by insults such as other pregnancies can increase the risk of developing renal and cardiovascular problems with increasing age.

Maternal mortality. The serious burden of maternal mortality is also a problem. The rate is 2½ times greater for mothers under 15 years of age than for those 20 to 24 years of age.

Effect on normal developmental steps. Apart from the physical sequelae, pregnancy often affects teenagers' psychologic development, education, and ability to gain economic independence. Clearly these developmental steps are difficult to achieve in any case, and for many adolescents pregnancy is not a cause of failure but a coinciding event. The situations responsible for early pregnancy often remain unresolved, and many teenage mothers have additional pregnancies before the adolescent years are over.

Hazards to the Infant

Infants born to teenage mothers suffer a higher incidence of morbidity and mortality in the perinatal period than infants of older mothers. Problems seen more frequently include[36]:

- Prematurity
- Stillbirth
- Low birth weight (the major hazard in adolescent pregnancy)

**Cephalopelvic dispro-
portion**
(Gr *kephale,* head; *pyelos,* an oblong trough,
pelvis) Relationship
of fetal head to size of
the maternal pelvis.

Preeclampsia
(Gr *pre-,* before; *ek-
lampein,* to shine forth)
Abnormal condition
of late pregnancy
marked by rather sud-
den hypertension and
increased edema, usu-
ally accompanied by
proteinuria; may
progress to more se-
vere stage of
preeclampsia with con-
vulsions and coma.

- Perinatal and infant deaths
- Physical deformities

It is difficult to compare the likelihood of these problems occurring in infants born to teenage versus older mothers, or to younger versus older teenage mothers. But it is generally agreed that the problems do occur in a considerable number of teenage pregnancies. For example, the incidence of low birth weight is far greater when the mothers are adolescent.

Weight Gain

Specific requirements. There is evidence that adolescents need to gain substantial weight during gestation to deliver optimal weight infants. Their infants will be somewhat smaller than the infants born to adult women with the same gestational weight gain.[37,38] For example, when adolescents gain from 26 to 35 lb, the incidence of low birth weight (under 2500 g, or 5.5 lb) is 6.3%, equivalent to the incidence for adult women who have gained 21 to 25 lb.[39] The incidence of fetal mortality and morbidity are thus linked to weight gain, because they are linked to low birth weight.

The continuing growth and development of the adolescent may account for the extra weight that is needed. Table 8-13 shows the amount of weight a young woman could be expected to gain in the 9-month period corresponding to her gynecologic age if she were not pregnant. That amount plus the amount she would have to gain to be normal weight for her height and age if she is underweight probably constitute the extra amount she will gain in pregnancy.[40] Some authors refute this idea, theorizing (1) that teenagers may retain extra weight following delivery if they gain more than adult women, and (2) that their infants may be small in a natural adaptation to the less mature maternal biologic state of the adolescent and therefore not at risk simply because their birth weights are lower.[41,42] Many questions about the gestational weight gain of adolescents remain to be answered by future research including:

- Is delivery of an infant weighing 3000 to 4000 g between 39 and 41 weeks gestation an optimal outcome for adolescent as well as adult young women?
- Is weight gain controlled by the biologic makeup in adolescence so it would not be possible for a young woman to gain more weight even if it was well known that achieving a certain range of weight gain would allow her to deliver an optimal weight infant?
- If adolescent mothers retain larger amounts of body fat as a result of gaining at a higher rate than adult women, is the adverse effect to the mother of potentially retaining 5 lb extra, for example, more serious than the actual risk to an infant born at a lower than optimal birth weight after a pregnancy during which the adolescent mother gained less than optimal weight?

TABLE 8-13 **Approximate 9-Month Increments in Weight of Postmenarcheal Women**

Postmenarcheal Year	lb	kg
1	8	3.45
2	5	2.0
3	2	.90
4 and 5	1.32	.60

Data from Frisch RE: *Hum Biol* 48:353, 1976.

Rate of gain. The latest recommendations from the National Academy of Sciences suggests that, depending on their prepregnant weight status, women gain at the following rates in the last two trimesters of pregnancy:

Normal weight	.361-.529 (.440 average) kg/week
Underweight	.386-.588 (.490 average) kg/week
Overweight	.218-.386 (.300 average) kg/week

The committee recommended that adolescents gain at the upper end of these ranges, but felt there was not sufficient evidence to make separate recommendations for teenage mothers. Other recommendations of this report are discussed in Chapter 4.[43]

Evidence is accumulating to show that the average rate of gain by adolescents in the final trimesters of pregnancy is on the average above .500 kg/week. In one study a group of multiethnic adolescent mothers who delivered term infants with a mean birth weight of 3258 g (calculated from data given) gained at the rate of .505 to .531 kg/week (50th percentile) during the last 18 weeks of pregnancy. The 75th percentile was .692 to .893 kg/week.[44] To decrease the number of infants weighing less than optimal, the average rate would have to be greater. As it was, 5% of the term infants following relatively uncomplicated pregnancies weighed under 2500 g, in the category of high risk.

In summary, the evidence does not suggest that the natural gain of adolescents should be restricted to levels recommended for adult women. The upper limit of optimal needs to be established because some young women will need to exercise control in order not to gain in excess of that needed to improve infant size at birth.

Assessment and Management of Nutrition

Risk factors. For nutrition services to be provided efficiently and effectively, pregnant teenage clients should be screened for those risk factors most closely linked to poor outcomes. At this point, significant factors include the following:

- Low gynecologic age
- Low prepregnancy weight for height, or other significant evidence of malnutrition
- Low pregnancy weight gain
- Infections during pregnancy
- Excessive pregnancy weight gain
- Excessive weight-for-height at conception
- Anemia

Other risk factors gathered from history include the following:

- Unhealthy lifestyle (including use of tobacco, drugs, and alcohol)
- Unfavorable reproductive history
- Chronic diseases or eating disorders

Overall assessment of the pregnant teenager follows more or less the general pattern for assessment of all pregnant women, as discussed in Chapter 4.

Nutrient needs. A summary of recommended amounts of nutrients is provided in Table 8-14. It combines the allowance for pregnancy in adult women with the amounts recommended for nonpregnant adolescents. A clinically practical way of assuring nutrient adequacy is to encourage the pregnant adolescent to gain the recommended amount of weight by consuming nutrient-rich foods. Sources of protein, calcium, iron, micronutrients, and dietary fiber are important. Contact with health professionals during prenatal care provides many important opportunities to teach adolescents about feeding themselves and their families. A clinical protocol for nutritional management of adolescent pregnancy is provided in the box on p. 373.

Economic and psychosocial needs. The economic instability of pregnant adolescents makes it impossible to assume that they will have an adequate food supply. The impact of

TABLE 8-14 *Recommended Dietary Allowances for Pregnant Adolescent Females*

| Nutrient | Age (reference height) | | | |
| | 11-14 years (157 cm) | | 15-18 years (163 cm) | |
	RDA	RDA/cm	RDA	RDA/cm
Energy (kcal)*	2500	15.9	2500	15.3
Protein (g)	56	0.38	54	0.36
Calcium (mg)	1200	7.6	1200	7.4
Phosphorus (mg)	1200	7.6	1200	7.4
Iron (mg)	30	0.19	30	0.18
Magnesium (mg)	300	2.0	320	2.1
Iodine (μg)	175	1.1	175	1.1
Zinc (mg)	15	0.09	15	0.09
Vitamin A (μg RE)	800	5.1	800	4.9
Vitamin D (μg)	10	0.06	10	0.06
Vitamin E (mg α-TE)	10	0.06	10	0.06
Ascorbic acid (mg)	60	0.38	70	0.43
Niacin (mg NE)	17	0.11	17	0.10
Riboflavin (mg)	1.6	0.01	1.6	0.01
Thiamin (mg)	1.5	0.01	1.5	0.01
Folate (μg)	400	2.3	400	2.5
Vitamin B_6 (mg)	2.0	0.01	2.1	0.01
Vitamin B_{12} (μg)	2.2	0.01	2.2	0.01

*Second and third trimester.
Modified from Food and Nutrition Board, National Research Council: *Recommended dietary allowances,* ed 10, Washington, DC, 1989, National Academy of Sciences.

lifestyle, economics, and other stressful issues on the nutritional well-being of young pregnant women is great and must be acknowledged in any program to improve their nutritional status. A summary of these issues is provided in the box on p. 374. Above all, the stage of social and emotional development will determine the mother's ability to cope with all aspects of reproduction.

Involving the father of the infant. When the partner of the younger pregnant woman is available, he should be included in counseling sessions to build mutual nutritional support for the pregnancy. Specific outreach to the father can be beneficial. If he is employed or in school, an effort should be made to see him at least occasionally. This effort will be especially important if for some reason he is interfering with the young woman's ability to nourish herself. Sharing what is known about the father's contribution to the outcome of pregnancy helps some adolescent males become more interested in maintaining healthy living habits.

Individualized counseling. To be effective, the clinician must work within the context of an individualized counseling relationship with the young pregnant adolescent and her partner.[36] The counselor will not "prescribe" but make practical suggestions and give support for changing of the teenagers' habits, usually in small increments, throughout the pregnancy.

Benefits of nutrition counseling. The benefits of nutrition counseling will generally be seen more in the long term than in a particular pregnancy. Prenatal care is one of the best opportunities to present sound nutritional information to a vulnerable group of

Protocol for Assessment and Management of Normal Teenage Pregnancy

Initial evaluation (if possible)

Review intake material, social and lifestyle history

Review clinical data
  Height and weight
  Gynecologic age
  Physical signs of health
  Expected delivery date

Review laboratory data
  Hematocrit or hemoglobin
  Urinalysis

Begin to build relationship with the client (and partner if available)

Assess client's perspective of nutrition issues

Assess attitude about, and acceptance of, prepregnancy weight and feelings about weight gain during pregnancy

Assess intake patterns using dietary methodology best suited to client and professional

Make preliminary assessment of food resources and refer to supportive agencies if necessary

Check for nausea and vomiting and suggest possible remedy

Discuss supplemental vitamins and minerals

Make initial plan that sets priorities for issues

Come to agreement with patient about any initial changes and steps to take; have client state plan as she perceives it

Determine client understanding of relation between nutrition and health

Do initial anthropometrics, calculate reasonable weight gain

Second visit

Check on referrals to other agencies

Discuss results of initial evaluation and suggest any changes necessary in dietary patterns (use printed materials as appropriate)

Do any further investigations when necessary

Laboratory studies
  For specific diagnosis of anemia:
    Protoporphyrin heme or serum ferritin
    Serum or red cell folate
    Serum vitamin B_{12}

Further probing of dietary habits if necessary

Monitor weight gain; discuss projected weight gain for following visit and total for gestation

Assess and address issues affecting nutritional status in order of priority for the individual
  Activity level
  Appetite changes
  Pica, food cravings, and aversions
  Allergies/food intolerances
  Supplementation practices (prescribed and self-selected)

Subsequent visits

Monitor and support appropriate weight gain; include discussion of fitness and encourage habitual safe exercise

Support upgrade in nutritional pattern in support of the woman and the developing infant; augment knowledge of principles of nutrition; continue to address issues affecting nutritional status

Check for heartburn, small food-intake capacity, and elimination problems; suggest dietary interventions

Begin preliminary discussion and comparison of advantages/disadvantages of breastfeeding and formula feeding

Final prenatal visit(s)

Discuss infant feeding if client will keep infant

If breastfeeding is chosen, provide preliminary guidance about breastfeeding practices

If formula feeding is chosen, discuss product selection and preparation; define important details about feeding techniques

Postpartum visits

Help client to understand safe methods of managing weight following delivery

Review infant feeding practices and infant growth; provide assistance when problems are identified

ONE STEP FURTHER

ONE STEP FURTHER

Issues in Adolescent Pregnancy That Influence Nutritional Well-Being

Acceptance of the pregnancy

Desire to carry out successful pregnancy
Acceptance of responsibility (even if child is to be relinquished)
Clarification of identity as mother separate from her own mother
Realistic acceptance versus fantasy and idealization

Food resources

Family meals (timing, quantity, quality, responsibility)
Self-reliance
School lunch
Fast-food outlets
Socially related eating
Food assistance (WIC program and others)
Mobilization of all resources

Body image

Degree of acceptance of an adult body
Maturity in facing bodily changes throughout pregnancy

Living situation

Acceptance by living partners and extended family
Role expectations of living partners
Financial support
Facilities and resources
Ethnic group (religious, cultural, and social patterns)
Emancipation versus dependency
Support system versus isolation

Relationship with the father of child

Presence or absence of father
Quality of relationship
Influence on decision making
Contribution to resources
Influence on mother's nutritional habits and general lifestyle
Understanding of physiologic processes
Tolerance of physical changes in pregnancy and physical needs of mother and child

Influence on child feeding

Peer relationships

Support from friends
Influence on nutritional knowledge and attitudes
Influence on general lifestyle

Nutritional state

Weight-for-height proportion
Maturational state
Tissue stores of nutrients
Reproductive and contraceptive history
Physical health
History of dietary patterns and nutritional status, including weight-losing schemes
Present eating habits
Complications of pregnancy (nausea and vomiting)
Substance use
Activity patterns
Need for intensive remediation

Prenatal care

Initiation of and compliance with prenatal care
Dependability of supporting resources
Identification of risk factors

Nutritional attitude and knowledge

Prior attitude toward nutrition
Understanding of role of nutrition in pregnancy
Knowledge of foods as sources of nutrients and of nutrients needed by the body
Desire to obtain adequate nutrition
Ability to obtain adequate nutrition and to control food supply

Preparation for child feeding

Knowledge of child-feeding practices
Attitude and decisions about child feeding
Responsibility for feeding
Understanding the importance of the bonding process
Support from family and friends

teenagers. Even if they seek care late in pregnancy and miss appointments, for most of them these contacts constitute the greatest input of health care during their adolescence.

Energy and nutrient intake. Helping pregnant adolescents follow the suggested rate of gain can ensure sufficient energy intake to support the pregnancy and the mother's own developmental needs. Following the guidelines dramatically demonstrates in just a few months the possibility of exerting personal control over eating, as well as the effect on both weight and nutritional status, in a way the teenager can understand. There is great appeal in discussing with adolescents the effects of various events on their bodies and on the growing fetus. Learning about the physiologic needs of both her own body and her developing infant can be the teenager's impetus for upgrading the quality of her diet to keep pace with the increase in energy intake needed to support adequate weight gain. Repeated counseling sessions to review those needs may motivate the young mother to try new foods to obtain additional sources of nutrients. Attention to nutritional health in the prenatal period can become a model for taking responsibility for feeding a family. The young woman can gain experience in the use of community resources to obtain food for herself and her family.

In summary, nutrition counseling in prenatal care for teenagers can accomplish the following goals:

1. Serve as a model for exerting control over what a person eats with visible results in terms of the optimal weight gain pattern and the quality of foods contributing to it.
2. Be an impetus for trying new foods.
3. Serve as a model for taking responsibility and using community resources to feed a family.

The nutrition counselor will be most effective when working within a clinical program designed specifically for adolescents. Such programs have been shown to improve overall outcome in adolescent pregnancy.[36] A case study of two teenage pregnancies is provided in the box below.

CASE STUDY

Two Teenage Pregnancies

Two adolescent females in the same grade become pregnant. One is 16.5 years of age: her menses began at age 14, and her weight for height is below the 5th percentile. The other pregnant adolescent is 15 years of age: her menses began at age 9, and her weight for height is at the 50th percentile.

Questions for analysis
1. Describe the theoretical difference in nutritional needs of the two adolescents.
2. Which one should be given clinical priority? Why?
3. If neither young woman sought prenatal care, what might you expect as the outcome for the respective infants? Why?

Summary

The physical and psychosocial gains in development are rapid and all encompassing in the adolescent period of human life. The parameters of physical growth are the basis for determining nutritional needs. Eating behavior is influenced to a great extent at this time by the developing body image and, as a result of breaking ties with the family, by the total culture. Thus if health professionals hope to help adolescents improve their nutritional patterns they must use appropriate tactics. They will need to sort out fact and reality in terms of the realistic role of nutrition in health and behavior. Emphasis must be placed on physical fitness as an important way to help all adolescents balance energy intake and output.

In eating disorders the overall objective is to help the individual put the eating function into proper perspective. The athlete must obtain sufficient nourishment to support a growing body that is subjected to stress. In chronic diseases the diet must eliminate nutrients that cause symptoms and be supplemented if necessary to allow growth to continue. If a pregnancy should occur, the adolescent will need support in nourishing herself and her developing infant during a chaotic time. While a great deal is still unknown about nutritional needs of adolescents, the growing interest in this age group should stimulate the research necessary to close gaps in our knowledge.

Review Questions

1. Define the terms *adolescence* and *puberty*. Explain how they are related.
2. Draw the growth velocity curve for males and females from birth to adulthood and describe the implications of different stages on the nutritional needs of humans.
3. Discuss the reasons for not using commonly available growth grids to assess weight/height proportion in adolescents and the alternate database that is appropriate.
4. Describe ways in which psychologic development influences nutritional status of adolescents.
5. Discuss the commonalities and differences of specifically recognized syndromes across the spectrum of eating disorders.
6. Describe how you would set up a comprehensive weight management program for teenagers in a community where none had ever existed before.
7. It has been proposed that adolescents need to gain more weight during pregnancy than adult women do. What aspects of adolescent growth and development lead to the idea that these larger gains are beneficial?

References

1. Tanner JM: *Foetus into man,* Cambridge, Mass, 1978, Harvard University Press.
2. Newman B, Newman P: *Adolescent development,* Columbus, Ohio, 1986, Merrill Press.
3. McKigney JL, Munro HN, editors: *Nutrient requirements in adolescence,* Cambridge, Mass, 1976, Massachusetts Institute of Technology Press.
4. Gong E, Heald FT: *Diet, nutrition, and adolescence.* In Shils M, Young VR, editors: *Modern nutrition in health and disease,* ed 7, Philadelphia, 1988, Lea & Febiger.
5. Witschi JC et al: Sources of fat, fatty acids, and cholesterol in the diets of adolescents, *J Am Diet Assoc* 90:1429, 1990.
6. Read MH et al: Adolescent compliance with dietary guidelines: health and education implications, *Adolescence* 23:567, 1988.
7. Bigler-Doughten S, Jenkins MR: Adolescent snacks: nutrient density and nutritional contribution to total intake, *J Am Diet Assoc* 87:1678, 1987.
8. Guenther PM: Beverages in the diets of American teenagers, *J Am Diet Assoc* 86:493, 1986.

9. Portnoy B, Christenson GM: Cancer knowledge and related practices: results from the National Adolescent Student Health Survey, *J School Health* 59:218, 1989.

10. Farrow JA, Adolescent chemical dependency. In Farrow JA, editor: Adolescent medicine, *Med Clin North Am* 74:1265, 1990.

11. Farrow JA et al: Health, developmental, and nutritional status of adolescent alcohol and marijuana abusers, *Pediatrics* 79:218, 1987.

12. Story M, Van Zyl York P: Nutritional status of Native American adolescent substance users, *J Am Diet Assoc* 87:1680, 1987.

13. Story M, Resnick MD: Adolescents' views on food and nutrition, *J Nutr Educ* 18:188, 1986.

14. Bruch H: Developmental considerations of anorexia nervosa and obesity, *Can J Psychiatry* 26:212, 1981.

15. Minuchin S et al: *Psychosomatic families: anorexia nervosa in context,* Cambridge, Mass, 1978, Harvard University Press.

16. *Diagnostic and statistical manual of mental disorders,* ed 3, Washington, DC, 1980, American Psychiatric Association.

17. Keys A et al: *The biology of human starvation,* vol I and II, Minneapolis, 1950, University of Minnesota Press.

18. Meyer AE et al: Psychoendocrinology of remenorrhea in the late outcome of anorexia nervosa, *Psychother Psychosom* 45:174, 1986.

19. Commerci G: Eating disorders. In Farrow JA, editor: Adolescent medicine, *Med Clin North Am* 74:1293, 1990.

20. Bachrach LK et al: Decreased bone density in adolescent girls with anorexia nervosa, *Pediatrics* 86:440, 1990.

21. Nussbaum M et al: Cerebral atrophy in anorexia nervosa, *J Pediatr* 96:867, 1980.

22. Rigotti NA et al: The clinical course of osteoporosis in anorexia nervosa: a longitudinal study of cortical bone mass, *J Am Med Assoc* 265:1133, 1991.

23. Nussbaum MP et al: Blunted growth hormone responses to clonidine in adolescent girls with early anorexia nervosa: evidence for an early hypothalmic defect, *J Adol Med* 18:145, 1990.

24. Dolan RJ et al: Structural brain changes in patients with anorexia nervosa, *Psychol Med* 18:349, 1988.

25. Laessle RG et al: Depression as a correlate of starvation in patients with eating disorders, *Biol Psychiatry* 23:719, 1988.

26. Steiger H et al: Relationship of body-image distortion to sex-role identification, irrational cognitions, and body weight in eating-disoriented females, *J Clin Psychol* 45:61, 1989.

27. Brinch M et al: Anorexia nervosa and motherhood: reproduction pattern and mothering behavior of 50 women, *Acta Psychiatr Scand* 77:611, 1988.

28. Polivy J, Herman CP: Diagnosis and treatment of normal eating, *J Consult Clin Psychol* 55:635, 1987.

29. Rees JM: Management of obesity in adolescents. In Farrow JA, editor: Adolescent medicine, *Med Clin North Am* 74:1275, 1990.

30. McArdle WD et al: *Exercise physiology: energy, nutrition, and human performance,* ed 2, Philadelphia, 1986, Lea & Febiger.

31. Gortmaker SL et al: Inactivity, diet, and the fattening of America, *J Am Diet Assoc* 90:1247, 1990.

32. American Medical Association and American Dietetic Association: *Targets for adolescent health: adolescent nutrition and physical fitness,* Chicago, 1991, Am Med Assoc.

33. Johnson MD et al: Anabolic steroid use by male adolescents, *Pediatrics* 83:921, 1989.

34. Story M, editor: *Nutrition management of the pregnant adolescent: a practical reference guide,* Washington, DC, 1990, MCH National Clearinghouse.

35. Scholl TO et al: Maternal growth during pregnancy and decreased infant birth weight, *Am J Clin Nutr* 51:790, 1990.

36. Rees JM et al: Position of the American Dietetic Association: nutrition management of adolescent pregnancy, and technical support paper, *J Am Diet Assoc* 89:900, 1989.

37. Haiek L, Lederman SA: The relationship between maternal weight for height and term birth weight in teens and adult women, *J Adol Health Care* 10:16, 1988.

38. Frisancho AR et al: Developmental and nutritional determinants of pregnancy outcome among teenagers, *Am J Phys Anthropol* 66:247, 1985.

39. Taffel S, National Center for Health Statistics: *Maternal weight gain and the outcome of pregnancy,* United States, 1980, Vital and Health Statistics, Series 21, No 44, DHHS Pub No (PHS) 86-1922, Washington, DC, June 1986, US Government Printing Office.

40. Rosso P, Lederman SA: *Nutrition in the pregnant adolescent.* In Winick M, editor: *Adolescent nutrition,* New York, 1982, John Wiley & Sons.

41. Garn SM, Petzold AS: Characteristics of the mother and child in teenage pregnancy, *Am J Dis Child* 137:365, 1983.

42. Stevens-Simon C, McAnarney ER: Adolescent maternal weight gain and low birth weight: a multifactorial model, *Am J Clin Nutr* 47:948, 1988.

43. Institute of Medicine, National Academy of Sciences: *Nutrition during pregnancy,* Washington, DC, 1990, National Academy Press.

44. Hediger ML et al: Rate and amount of weight gain during adolescent pregnancy: associations with maternal weight-for-height and birth weight, *Am J Clin Nutr* 52:793, 1990.

Further Reading

Arquitt AB et al: Dehydroepiandrosterone sulfate, cholesterol, hemoglobin, and anthropometric measures related to growth in male adolescents, *J Am Diet Assoc* 91:575, 1991.
This study investigates the relationship of nutritional status and biochemical and physical

markers of maturation in adolescent males.

Expert Panel on Population Strategies for Blood Cholesterol Reduction, *National Cholesterol Education Program: executive summary,* NIH Pub No 90-3047, Washington, DC, 1990, US Department of Health and Human Services.

This expert panel report provides recommendations for promoting healthy eating patterns in all Americans including adolescents, with the goal of lowering blood cholesterol of individuals and reducing the average cholesterol level throughout the population, in turn reducing risks of atherosclerosis and coronary heart disease.

Heald FP: Atherosclerosis during adolescence. In Farrow JA, editor: Adolescent medicine, *Med Clin North Am* 74:1321, 1990.

This author reviews the evidence for development of atherosclerotic lesions in early life and discusses the need to assess and treat adolescents in order to prevent further damage.

Moore DC: Body image and eating behavior in adolescent girls, *Am J Dis Child* 142:1114, 1988.

Moore DC: Body image and eating behavior in adolescent boys, *Am J Dis Child* 144:475, 1990.

In these twin articles, the author reports results of surveys regarding dissatisfaction with weight and shape, and the attempts by both males and females to change their bodies.

Thibault L, Roberge AG: The nutritional status of subjects with anorexia nervosa, *Int J Vitam Nutri Res* 57:447, 1987.

These authors report the relationship of nutritional deficiencies in the diets of 25 anorexic patients and discuss these findings in relation to symptoms of the disorder.

Queen PM, Lang CE: *Handbook of pediatric nutrition,* Gaithersburg, Md, 1993, Aspen Publishers.

Carruth BR, Skinner JD: *Adolescent nutrition education,* Theme issue, *J Nutr Educ* 20:6, December, 1988.

Story MS: *Nutrition management of the pregnant adolescent: a practical reference guide,* March of Dimes Birth Defects Foundation, USDHHS, USDA, Washington, DC, 1990.

9 Nutrition and the Aging Adult

Eleanor D. Schlenker

Basic Concepts

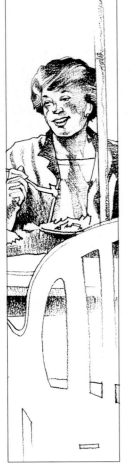

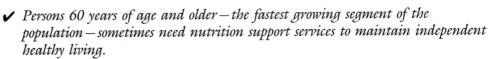

✔ *Persons 60 years of age and older — the fastest growing segment of the population — sometimes need nutrition support services to maintain independent healthy living.*

✔ *Aging brings a gradual decline in normal physiological functions.*

✔ *Energy needs decrease with age but protein, vitamin, and mineral needs do not decrease, making nutrient density important in meal planning.*

✔ *Vitamins and minerals are the nutrients most likely to be lacking in an older person's diet; they are also most adversely affected by multiple medications, both over-the-counter and prescription drugs.*

✔ *Numerous social, physiological, and economic factors influence food and nutrient intake in older people.*

*T*he number of older people in our society is increasing rapidly. One in eight Americans is age 65 or older. By the year 2030 it will be one in four.[1] One of the fastest growing segments within the older population is the 85 and older group. These population shifts have far-reaching implications across our society, from public discussions of health care costs and the need for health care reform to increasing efforts by food manufacturers to develop preprepared products that will be attractive to older consumers. This increase in number of older people presents both a challenge and a responsibility to the health professional. Nutrition and food programs that promote continuing physical and mental well-being in healthy older people will become increasingly important. Specialized nutrition services designed to maintain the highest level of independence and functional capacity possible must be developed for those older people in declining health.

In this chapter we look at the changing nutrient needs of the aging population. We explore the environmental, personal, and health factors that influence them. We seek effective intervention strategies based on sensitive evaluation of each older person as an individual.

DEMOGRAPHIC ASPECTS OF AGING
Population Trends

In the United States age 65 is often used as a benchmark to characterize the older population—those who have "retired." But **chronological age** does not measure physical health or zest for life. Also, individuals continue to change as they age so that 65-year-olds differ markedly from 90-year-olds. To recognize these changes United States census reports group older Americans into the following three age categories:

- Age 65 to 74—the young-old
- Age 75 to 84—the old-old
- Age 85 and over—the oldest-old

As the over-65 group increases in number, it will increase also in diversity. Those men and women age 85 and over are more likely to have serious health problems and depend on others for care whereas the young-old may still be employed. An increasing proportion of the older population will be African-American and Hispanic as these elderly groups are increasing at a faster rate than white elderly.[1]

Changes in Life Expectancy

Nature of the changes. **Life expectancy** is the average remaining years of life for a person of a given age. The dramatic increase in life expectancy in this century occurred primarily in infancy and childhood. For men life expectancy at birth increased from 48 years to 72 years since 1900; for women life expectancy increased from 51 to 79 years.[2] However, despite improvements in medical care, life expectancy at age 65 has increased only 4 years in men and 7 years in women over this time period. Thus the growth of the older population does not reflect an increase in maximal lifespan but instead reflects the extended lifespan of those individuals who in the past would have died in infancy or childhood.

Influencing factors. Gains in life expectancy have not been equal among all groups. Women can expect to live longer than men, and white persons can expect to live 6 to 8 years longer than black persons.[2] Increased smoking among women may reduce their life expectancy, as death rates from lung cancer continue to climb and now exceed death rates from breast cancer. Level of education and income influence accessibility to health care and are related to life expectancy. These latter factors may contribute to the lower life expectancy of African-Americans.

Causes of death. The three most common causes of death are heart disease, cancer, and **cerebral hemorrhage** (stroke).[1] All three causes are related to degenerative changes associated with aging and the environment. In contrast, the leading cause of death in 1900 was infectious diseases such as pneumonia and influenza, now controlled with antibiotic drugs. A lifestyle based on a diet moderate in sucrose, fat, and sodium, with no smoking, limited or no use of alcohol, and regular exercise can delay the onset of chronic disease and improve the health status of the expanding older population.

Socioeconomic Characteristics of the Aging Population

At one time the general public associated old age with poor health, illness, and disability. This view led to the assumption that the majority of older people lived in institutions. In fact 95% of the aged live within the community with a spouse, other family member or friend, or alone; only 5% are in long-term care facilities.[1] Living arrangements differ between older men and older women. Most older men are married and live with their spouse. In contrast over half of older women are widows and 41% live alone. Living situation can contribute to the food problems of older people. An aged widow who lives in a rural area and cannot drive may depend on relatives or friends for transportation to a food store.

Chronological age
Age of an individual based on the number of years lived compared, for example, with biological age, the relative age of a person based on physiological capacity and measurements.

Life expectancy
The average remaining years a person of a given age, sex, and race may expect to live, based on statistical population averages.

Cerebral hemorrhage
Rupture of an artery in the brain, cerebrovascular accident (CVA), stroke.

Older women, older persons living alone, and those age 85 and over are more likely to be poorly nourished because of lower income. Usually couples have a more adequate income than single individuals. Black and Hispanic elderly persons are more likely than white elderly persons to be poor. Government programs such as food stamps or **congregate meals** (p. 413) can help those with limited money for groceries.

NUTRITION AND THE LIFESPAN

Since antiquity, people have been searching for potions to preserve health and prolong life. Ponce de Leon came to the New World seeking the "fountain of youth." Francis Bacon, who lived from 1591 to 1626, was the first to recommend scientific evaluation of the relationship between diet and longevity. He advocated a frugal diet and encouraged the study of people in various climates and living situations to determine those characteristics that influence lifespan. Unfortunately, Bacon's recommendations for research are only beginning to receive attention.

Animal Studies

Researchers have evaluated the influence of various diet patterns on aging changes and length of life in experimental animals. Several general concepts have emerged from these studies.

Energy intake. Energy intake controls not only the general increase in body size of an animal but also the rate of maturation and aging. Animals fed diets restricted in kilocalories yet adequate in protein, vitamins, and minerals beginning at weaning and continuing through adulthood live 40% longer than those given unlimited access to food; **chronic diseases** such as kidney disease and heart disease also appear at a later age in the energy-restricted animals.[3] Energy restriction also delays biochemical alterations such as the age-related decline in the immune system. Reducing energy intake after the completion of physiological growth and attainment of sexual maturity still increases the lifespan and delays chronic disease in experimental animals.

Rate of growth. Protein intake in addition to total energy intake influences both rate of growth and survival.[3] In experimental animals, diets high in energy and protein result in rapid growth, large body size and weight, and early onset of degenerative disease. The suggestion that rapid growth and increased body weight accelerate the aging process has serious implications for humans in light of current growth patterns. Today's children are taller, heavier, and reach puberty at earlier ages than did previous generations. In experimental animals, regular physical exercise slows the rate of growth, lowers body weight, and increases the lifespan. Regular physical exercise may slow the aging process in humans.

Human Studies

Limited information is available to evaluate the influence of lifelong dietary habits on health and longevity. Studies that collected detailed information at one point in time did not follow subjects at regularly scheduled intervals nor did they continue to collect information over an extended period of years. Following the same individual over time—a **longitudinal study**—is necessary to evaluate the influence of diet and lifestyle on physiological and biochemical aging.

Longitudinal studies. Longitudinal studies evaluating diet and exercise patterns and subsequent morbidity and mortality indicate that good eating habits and continued physical activity contribute to health and survival in middle age and beyond. Several studies conducted in different parts of the country serve as examples.

Michigan study. Nutrient intake influenced physical well-being and length of life in a longitudinal study of 100 Michigan women who ranged in age from 40 to 85 years when

---

Congregate meals
Group meals for older adults, served in a social setting in the community and funded by Title III-C of the Older Americans Act.

Chronic disease
(Gr *chronos*, time) Diseases of aging or of long duration for which there is no cure.

Longitudinal study
Study of persons or populations over a long period of time to measure effects of specific factors on the aging process and incidence and course of disease.

first evaluated.[4] Over the next 7 years, mortality was higher in those who consumed diets containing less than 40% of the RDA for one or more nutrients. Nutrients most frequently deficient were calcium, vitamin A, and ascorbic acid. Twenty-four years after the first interview dietary records were collected from the surviving women.[5] Mean intake of total energy, fat, and carbohydrate had decreased by 25%, although protein, vitamin, and mineral levels (with the exception of calcium) met or exceeded 67% of the RDA. Protein, fat, and carbohydrate provided 18%, 35%, and 47% of total energy, respectively. Foods high in simple carbohydrate and fat but low in other nutrients were consumed in lesser amounts. Fruits, vegetables, milk products, and breads and cereals were emphasized. A decrease in energy intake to accommodate a reduced level of physical activity with continued emphasis on the protective foods appears to be a successful dietary model for the transition from middle to advanced age.

California study. An ongoing study that began with 7000 adults living in Alameda, California, examines the influence on mortality of the following health practices — adequate sleep, regular meals (including breakfast), desirable body weight, not smoking, limited or no use of alcohol, and regular physical activity.[6] After 5 years it was evident that poor health practices resulted in earlier death, whereas good health habits led to longer life. Men who followed at least five of the health practices had a life expectancy 11 years longer than men who followed three or less. For women the comparable difference in life expectancy was 7 years. These practices continued to influence health at age 70 and beyond. Those adults following three or less of these practices were twice as likely to be physically disabled compared with those following six or more, regardless of their health status when the study began. These findings support the idea that **nutrition education** and intervention activities benefit even those already old.

Georgia centenarian study. A new study evaluates the food patterns of elderly people in Georgia, including 22 centenarians.[7] It was found that only 5% of the centenarians have to avoid any particular foods because of abdominal distress; however, 37% have trouble biting or chewing certain foods. Mean energy intake of the centenarians was 1581 kcal and 42% of kilocalories came from fat. It is interesting to note that all of these people had stable body weights throughout adulthood despite their rather high fat intakes. Continued observation of this group can provide insight as to the dietary needs and preferences of individuals in extreme old age.

Body weight studies. Life insurance standards used to evaluate the body weight of individuals as compared with their peers of similar height and sex have been used to predict mortality risk. The general conclusion drawn from these statistics is the greater the deviation between actual body weight and standard weight (the body weight of policy holders who lived the longest), the greater the risk of death.

Patterns of overweight differ according to age, sex, and ethnic group. National Health and Nutrition Examination Survey (NHANES II) data suggest that prevalence of overweight is similar in black and white men between the ages of 30 and 69, although increasing slightly with age (24% of those ages 30 to 39 and 28% of those ages 60 to 69 are overweight).[8] In women the situation is quite different. The percentage of white women who are overweight increased from 21% in the 30- to 39-year-old group to 36% in the 60- to 69-year-old group. Among black women, the percentage overweight in these age groups is 36% and 61%, respectively. Thirty-four percent of the Mexican-American men in both age categories were overweight and 40% and 60% of the younger and older women, respectively.

The association between overweight, chronic disease, and mortality risk at older ages remains controversial. Obese men between the ages of 20 and 45 are at high risk for hypertension, diabetes mellitus, and high blood lipids; however, these problems also increase among the nonobese as they age. Nevertheless, a 30-year follow-up of 5500 men and women in Framingham, Massachusetts, indicated that relative weights 10%

Nutrition education
The process of helping individuals obtain the knowledge, skills, and motivation needed to make appropriate food choices for positive health throughout life.

to 30% above standard weight had an adverse effect on longevity among those over age 65.[9] Although women tend to be more resistant to the hazards of overweight, the Framingham women more than 30% overweight had an increased risk of cardiovascular disease.

A complicating factor when reviewing the mortality risk of overweight versus underweight older people is smoking habits.[10] Underweight in persons age 60 and over is often associated with smoking, and death is more likely to occur within a few years. Among older nonsmokers **mortality rates** are lower in underweight men as compared to overweight men. Optimal body weights for older people are within 10% of the average weight for their age, height, and sex. However, the average weights for older people are still 10 to 15 pounds higher than for younger people of the same sex and height.[9] A major consideration in the dietary management of elderly persons is prevention of inappropriate weight gain.

Mortality rate
Total number of deaths in a specific category divided by the total number of deaths in the total population.

BIOLOGIC ASPECTS OF AGING
The Aging Process

In general terms the study of aging includes all changes in body structure and function that occur over the lifespan as a result of growth, maturation, and **senescence**. In our context, aging refers to the time-dependent biological and physiological changes that begin about age 30 and are degenerative in their effect. The pattern and sequence of changes associated with normal aging are always the same, although the rate at which changes occur differs from one person to another. For example, muscle mass, which comprises a very small proportion of body weight in the infant, increases steadily throughout childhood and early adulthood and then declines in middle and old age. Both genetic and environmental factors influence the rate of aging. Individuals with long-lived parents are more likely to survive beyond age 70. Environmental factors such as irradiation or level of nutrition influence lifespan in experimental animals. In humans, environmental stress that increases one's risk of chronic disease also increases the rate of aging.

Senescence
(L *senescere,* to grow old) Normal process or condition of growing old.

Cellular Level Changes

No one knows exactly how the aging process takes place, but changes are observed first in the cell. Among cell types that continue to divide throughout their normal lifespan (e.g., skin cells or the mucosal cells lining the gastrointestinal tract) the rate of division slows as the cell nears the end of its normal lifespan and, eventually, stops. Cells from species with shorter lifespans undergo fewer divisions than those from species with longer lifespans. Cells from an older human donor will undergo fewer divisions than those from a younger human donor. Although the older person will always have some cells that are rapidly dividing, they will be fewer in number and the total cell count will be reduced. A reduced number of **parietal cells** within the **gastric** mucosa causes the decrease in hydrochloric acid secretion observed in some older people.

Parietal cells
(L *parietes,* wall) Cells lining the stomach that secrete hydrochloric acid; chief cells.

Gastric
(Gr *gaster,* stomach) Pertaining to the stomach.

Organ Level Changes

Highly differentiated cells including brain, kidney, and muscle do not continue to divide throughout life but do undergo functional changes with time, and some cells die. As a result the organ systems become less efficient as fewer cells remain to carry on normal body functions. The aging cell is less able to synthesize important molecules required for hormonal or neural control or the induction of enzymes. Consequently, specialized organs and tissues are less able to respond to environmental stimuli and there is a breakdown in the coordination of body systems that work together to carry out physiological functions.

PHYSIOLOGIC ASPECTS OF AGING
Brain and Neural Control

Functional changes. Both structural and biochemical changes contribute to functional alterations in the aging brain. There is general agreement that neurons are lost in advanced age (estimates of losses range as high as 20% to 40%), although questions regarding changes in brain weight are still unresolved. Neither cell number nor brain weight appears to be related to the diagnosis of **senile dementia of the Alzheimer type (SDAT)**. Blood flow through the aging brain decreases as a result of vascular changes, contributing to a decline in cerebral function.

Neurotransmitters. Decreased synthesis of **neurotransmitters** (e.g., dopamine, serotonin, or acetylcholine) required for the conduction of nerve impulses has been observed in older people. The most striking reductions in neurotransmitter levels occur in the hypothalamus and cerebral cortex; these areas of the brain control psychomotor skills and cognitive function, activities that exhibit age-related alterations. **Parkinson's disease,** a disorder of the central nervous system occurring among older persons, is thought to relate to the altered metabolism of dopamine. The muscle rigidity, tremors, and shuffling gait associated with this disease can be improved with treatment with levodopa.

Organic brain syndrome. Brain disorders that lead to behavior changes and mental deterioration increase with age. Loss of cells, changes in the physical arrangement of cells, or atherosclerosis of the brain blood vessels can lead to progressive and irreversible **dementia**. Brain disorders increase in prevalence after age 80. SDAT is distinguished by the younger age of onset—before age 65. High aluminum levels in brain cells are the result not the cause of SDAT; use of aluminum cooking utensils is not associated with the development of this disorder. As the disease progresses patients become less able to care for themselves and no longer recognize family members or friends. Changes occur in eating behavior as patients forget how to use eating utensils, and, for example, may try to eat soup with a fork. Eventually, they lose all ability to feed themselves.

Coordination of Physiologic Functions

Response to stimuli. One characteristic of physiologic aging is decreased ability to respond to changes in the environment. Organ systems respond more slowly to changes in the external environment such as changes in room temperature. The return to homeostasis following a challenge to the internal environment such as the rise in blood glucose after a high carbohydrate meal also requires a longer period of time.

The age-related decline in physiologic function has been evaluated in the men participating in the Baltimore Longitudinal Study of Aging (BLSA).[11] This study has been ongoing for almost 30 years, and each subject returns every 2 years for reevaluation. This makes it possible for the researchers to observe when changes occur in each individual and to compare men of different ages. The loss in functional capacity of important organ systems between ages 30 and 80 is presented in Fig. 9-1. The degree of loss is influenced by the level of coordination required among one or more organ systems. Nerve conduction velocity exhibits less change than resting cardiac output requiring both neural and muscular control. Renal function declines by 50%.

Response to added demand. As a system becomes more complex, impairment becomes more obvious. An older person may walk with comparative ease on a level surface but find it difficult to climb stairs. In spite of decrements in physiologic functions most older people get along quite well on a day-to-day basis. However, when extreme demands are placed on the system such as occurs in strenuous exercise or severe illness or when organ tissue losses are excessive, problems of **functional disability** become evident.

Senile dementia of the Alzheimer type (SDAT)
A type of senile dementia first described by German physician Alois Alzheimer (1864-1915); causes progressive, irreversible degenerative changes in the brain, resulting in loss of neuromuscular function and mental capacity.

Neurotransmitter
(Gr *neuron*, nerve: L *trans*, through, across; *missio*, a sending) A large group of over 40 different chemical substances including compounds as diverse as acetylcholine, various hormones, and several amino acids, which function as essential chemical messengers for sending (or inhibiting) nerve impulses across synapses of connecting nerve endings.

Parkinson's disease
A neurological disorder described by English physician James Parkinson (1755-1824) and characterized by tremor, muscular rigidity, and abnormally decreased motor function and mobility.

Dementia

(L *de* + *mens,* mind) Progressive organic mental disorder causing changes in personality, disorientation, deterioration in intellectual function, and loss of memory and judgment; dementia caused by drug overdose, electrolyte or fluid imbalance, or insulin shock will be reversed on treatment; dementia caused by injury or degenerative changes in brain tissue is not reversible.

Functional disability

Disability that interferes with activities of daily living, such as bathing, dressing, shopping, preparing meals, or eating.

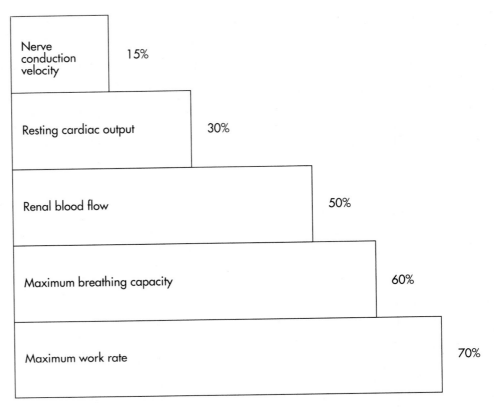

Nerve conduction velocity	15%
Resting cardiac output	30%
Renal blood flow	50%
Maximum breathing capacity	60%
Maximum work rate	70%

FIG. 9-1   Loss in physiological function between ages 30 and 80. These changes in physiological function were observed in men participating in the BLSA.

Data from Shock NW et al: *Normal human aging: The Baltimore Longitudinal Study of Aging,* NIH Pub No 84-2450, Washington, DC, 1984, US Government Printing Office.

Endocrine System

Information describing age-related changes in hormone levels or the mechanisms involved is limited. Blood levels of some hormones such as aldosterone decrease, whereas others such as thyroxin (T_4) remain the same. Decreased hormone secretion can result from either diminished synthesis or release. Reduced utilization of a hormone or slowed excretion will limit hormone release through feedback mechanisms. Current research is looking at hypothalamus-pituitary regulation of hormone secretion, storage, and release. The aged hypothalamus is less sensitive to messages received and may play a role in altered endocrine function.

Cardiovascular System

Functional changes. Age-related changes in the heart and circulatory system involve both structure and function. The work load of the heart increases as a result of increased peripheral resistance caused by atherosclerotic deposition and loss of arterial elasticity. At the same time the effectiveness of the heart muscle as a pump is reduced as the strength of contraction is diminished. Resting **cardiac output** falls as the volume of blood pumped with each stroke decreases. Subsequently, blood flow through the coronary arteries supplying nutrients to the heart muscle itself is compromised. Thus the work load on the heart increases as nutrients become less available. As a consequence, the aged heart is much

Cardiac output

Total amount of blood pumped by the heart per minute (average value is approximately 5 liters).

less tolerant of either physiological or emotional stress. This intolerance points to the importance of medical evaluation of older persons before they begin an intensive exercise program.

Hypertension. Changes in cardiovascular function contribute to the age-related rise in blood pressure observed in both sexes. Hypertension is a significant medical and nutritional problem among older persons. Effective management requires body weight management, some level of sodium limitation, exercise, and reduced alcohol intake. In a national survey 54% of those between the ages of 65 and 74 had systolic pressures above 140 mm Hg or diastolic pressures above 90 mm Hg.[12] Black elderly had the highest prevalence (72%). High blood pressure increases substantially the risk of stroke, coronary heart disease, and renal failure.

Renal System

Functional changes. Kidney function deteriorates with age because of a loss of nephrons and a 30% decrease in blood flow, a consequence of reduced cardiac output.[11] Because the **glomerular filtration rate** is slowed, it takes longer to clear drugs or metabolic wastes from the blood. On that basis excessive protein intakes resulting in high blood urea nitrogen levels or megadoses of water-soluble vitamins should be avoided. The aged kidney is less able to form concentrated urine so adequate fluid intake is essential. In the **nephron** tubule, glucose, plasma proteins, ascorbic acid, and other nutrients are less efficiently reabsorbed while drug metabolites and H^+ ions are less efficiently excreted.

Water balance. Fluid regulation and water balance are serious issues in the nutritional management of older people. Dehydration leads to seriously elevated electrolyte levels and is an ever-present danger in bed-bound elderly patients who are unable to drink without help. Water balance is also a problem in relatively healthy elderly. A recent study evaluating fluid intake in younger and older people reported that the older subjects had a decreased sense of thirst.[13] After 6 hours of fluid deprivation not only did they experience less feeling of thirst, they also drank considerably less water than was needed for fluid replacement once water became available. At the same time the older kidney is less able to respond to **antidiuretic hormone** (ADH) to reduce the amount of fluid lost in the urine. On the other extreme some prescription drugs induce release of ADH and contribute to **water intoxication**. Therefore records of fluid intake become very important in the care of debilitated older persons with limited access to water.

Pulmonary System

Structural changes in the lung bring about a loss of alveolar surface area and a decrease in elasticity. Although total lung capacity does not change, the proportion of alveolar space ventilated with each breath and thus the total surface area for gas exchange decreases. Gas exchange is less efficient because of the decreased permeability of the alveolar membranes and a reduced blood flow. **Oxyhemoglobin** saturation of arterial blood is lower in advanced age, making oxygen transfer to the tissues more difficult. The reduced ability to effectively increase oxygen intake becomes a significant factor in exercise or physiological stress.

Gastrointestinal Function

Functional changes. There is little evidence to support the generally held concept that advancing age results in dysfunction of the stomach, small intestine, and colon. However, gastrointestinal discomforts including nausea, heartburn, and constipation increase in frequency. Such symptoms often relate to poor eating and bowel habits, mental anxiety, or side effects of commonly used drugs. Gastrointestinal distress does not necessarily indicate malabsorption. Persons with no discomfort may absorb nutrients poorly, whereas others with persistent distress may absorb nutrients normally.[14]

Glomerular filtration rate
A measure of the amount of blood filtered by the cup-like glomerulus at the head of each kidney nephron per unit of time (ml/min)

Nephron
(Gr *nephros*, kidney) The structural and functional unit of the kidney where waste products are removed from the blood plasma and urine is formed.

Antidiuretic hormone (ADH)
Hormone secreted by the posterior pituitary gland in response to body stress or a decrease in blood volume. It acts on the distal tubules of the kidney's nephrons to cause water reabsorption and thus protect vital body water; also called vasopressin.

Water intoxication
An abnormal increase in the amount of water in the body; sodium concentration of body fluids is lowered causing confusion, stupor, seizures, and harmful effects on the central nervous system.

Oxyhemoglobin
Hemoglobin with bound oxygen for transport of oxygen from the lungs to the cells for vital metabolic work.

Swallowing problems. Changes in muscle innervation and reduced secretion of saliva (xerostomia) can cause difficulty in swallowing, particularly in frail aged persons. Fear of choking may result in food refused and progressive weight loss. General dehydration or certain drugs causing dry mouth can add to this problem. Older people should eat only when seated in an upright position. Being fed in a **supine** position increases the risk of food aspiration and pneumonia.

Bowel problems. Constipation, a problem for many older people, is related to low fluid intake, a diet low in fiber and bulk, medications, and a general lack of exercise. Interviews with 211 frail, homebound elderly people revealed that 45% had problems with constipation and 11% viewed this as a major health problem.[15] Many older people believe that a daily bowel movement is essential. True constipation is characterized by (1) fewer than two bowel movements per week, (2) persistent difficulty in passing stools, (3) bleeding with bowel movements, or (4) pain with bowel movements. Any bleeding from the rectum should be reported to a physician immediately.

Laxative abuse. Individuals with normal bowel function who do not have a daily bowel movement sometimes turn to laxatives in an effort to relieve the perceived problem. After the purging effect of the laxative, normal bowel movements may not resume the following day. This reinforces the idea that the individual is constipated and results in a vicious cycle. Use of laxatives over a prolonged period results in loss of normal bowel function. Diets generous in whole grain breads and cereals and fruits and vegetables, along with an adequate fluid intake (1500 to 2000 ml daily), contribute to the formation of large, soft stools and more frequent bowel movements.

Enzyme Secretion for Digestion and Absorption

Digestive secretions. For the most part, a lack of digestive enzymes does not impair the absorption of nutrients in healthy older people. Because digestive enzymes are normally secreted at levels substantially above what is required, reduced enzyme levels are still sufficient to break down all food consumed into the forms required for absorption.

One alteration in digestive function that is prevalent in the older population is **atrophic gastritis,** a chronic inflammation of the stomach lining. Both the total volume and hydrochloric acid concentration of gastric juice and the volume of pepsin secreted are reduced. In a group of community-living Boston elderly 40% of those above age 80 were found to have atrophic gastritis.[14] This alteration in the normal acid environment of the stomach interferes with the absorption of iron, calcium, vitamin B_{12}, vitamin B_6, and folacin. A rise in pH also permits increased growth of bacteria, leading to further mucosal damage and malabsorption. Another change that may occur in the gastric mucosa is reduced secretion of intrinsic factor, resulting in vitamin B_{12} deficiency. In the small intestine pancreatic enzymes and bile are usually present in sufficient amounts to allow normal breakdown of carbohydrate, fat, and protein.

Lactose intolerance. Reduced lactase levels have been evaluated in relation to the low milk consumption of some older persons. It appears that psychological attitudes toward milk are as important, if not more so, than physiological factors in lactose intolerance. Malabsorption was not related to the incidence of digestive symptoms reported by older people following ingestion of a lactose-containing or a lactose-free beverage.[16] Over half of the malabsorbers reported drinking more than one glass of milk each day, suggesting that factors in addition to lactose malabsorption influence low milk consumption in this age group.

Nutrient Digestion and Absorption

Protein, carbohydrate, and fat. Although the process of digestion and absorption is slowed with age, carbohydrate and protein are not handled differently by older as compared with younger individuals. Common monosaccharides are efficiently absorbed. Similarly, healthy older people do not lose greater amounts of protein through the gastrointestinal tract than younger people when given levels of 1.0 g/kg body weight. On normal intakes the absolute amount of fat absorbed does not change with age. Generally, neutral fat (triglyceride) comprises only a minor portion of fecal fat with fatty acids being the predominant fat. Some older individuals, when fed high levels of fat (100 g per day), do excrete more undigested fat than younger individuals, with the likely cause being lower pancreatic lipase levels.[17]

Vitamins and minerals. Age-related alterations in vitamin and mineral absorption are poorly understood. These nutrients are studied usually in relation to nutritional status or deficiency; their absorption is discussed in later sections.

NUTRIENT REQUIREMENTS OF OLDER PEOPLE
Recommended Dietary Allowances

The Recommended Dietary Allowances (RDA) as applied to older people are quite controversial.[18] Several issues pertaining to the current RDA are described below.

Heterogeneity of older adults. Because there have been very few studies of older people, the RDA for persons over age 50 have been extrapolated from those for young adults. For most nutrients the RDA are the same for younger adults, ages 25 to 50, and older adults age 51 and over. There are no adjustments in recommended intakes beyond age 51, although persons 50 to 60 years old have different needs than those 80 to 90 years old.

Physiological changes. Young adults differ from older adults in body composition, physiological function, and metabolic adaptation. Physiological changes in gastric secretions influence digestion and absorption and may increase the need for particular nutrients. Estrogen withdrawal following menopause alters calcium absorption levels and bone metabolism. Reduced ability of the renal system to excrete waste contraindicates excessive intakes of nutrients.

Disease interaction. Chronic diseases influence nutrient requirements both as a result of the disease process and the drugs prescribed in therapeutic management. **Diuretics** used to treat hypertension can deplete body potassium, **pyridoxine**, folacin, or zinc levels, depending on the particular drug. One researcher has advocated the development of formulas based on prescription drug use and disease complications to establish nutritional risk and recommended nutrient intakes in older persons.[19] When evaluating nutrient needs it is important to consider each older client as an individual and look at general health, amount of physical activity, and presence or absence of chronic disease.

The current RDAs for people ages 25 to 50 and 51 and over differ for iron, thiamin, riboflavin, and niacin.[18] The iron allowance is reduced from 15 mg to 10 mg for women above age 50 because of the cessation of menstruation and associated iron loss. The recommended intakes of thiamin, riboflavin, and niacin are lower for men and women in response to the perceived decrease in energy requirements after age 50.

Energy Needs

Energy needs decrease with age based on changes in the **resting energy expenditure** (REE) and physical activity levels. In an older sedentary adult the REE represents 60% to 75% of the total energy expenditure.[20] Physical activity plays a major role in maintaining energy balance in the older person, and the kilocalories expended vary according to individual activity patterns.

Resting energy expenditure (REE). The REE is affected by sex, age, body size, thyroid status, and body composition, but the major influence is the amount of lean body mass. Women at all ages have lower resting energy needs per unit of body height and

Diuretic
(Gr *diouretikos*, promoting urine) A drug that decreases the reabsorption of water in the renal tubule and increases loss of water through the urine; some types of diuretics induce loss of body sodium and potassium along with fluid.

Pyridoxine
Chemical name for vitamin B_6, named for its ringlike structure.

Resting energy expenditure (REE)
An estimate of the minimum amount of energy required by the body to maintain itself when the individual is resting and awake; in general practice the REE is usually calculated from a formula using individual factors of weight, height, age, and sex.

weight because of their higher proportion of body fat and lower proportion of lean body mass. REE decreases about 24% in men and 15% in women between the ages of 20 and 60 as lean body mass is lost.[20] Decreases in the REE in later life generally do not relate to impaired thyroid function.

Data from the BLSA (see p. 385) indicate that basal energy needs continue to decline beyond age 60.[20] Basal energy expenditure is 1541 kcal/day for healthy 60-year-olds and 1369 kcal/day for healthy 80-year-olds of normal weight. However, when basal energy expenditure was calculated on the basis of kilocalories per kilogram body weight, there was very little difference between the two age groups (19.8 versus 18.7 kcal/kg body wt/day). These data support the idea expressed earlier that the differences in basal energy expenditure in men and women of differing ages are related to the differences in their lean body mass.

Developing the Energy Requirement

Components of the energy requirement. The two major components of the total energy **requirement** are the REE and the energy expenditure in physical activity. The thermic effect of food contributes rather little to the total energy requirement. Information from the BLSA indicates that energy expended in physical activity declines most sharply in young adulthood, rather than in later life. Daily energy expenditure decreased by 40 kcal between ages 35 and 44, 17 kcal between ages 55 and 64, and 24 kcal between ages 75 and 84.[21] This decrease in energy expenditure in middle age no doubt contributes to the weight gain that occurs in that period and points to the need for a regular exercise program that continues throughout adulthood.

Recommended energy intakes. Before 1989 the RDA for energy specified two age categories beyond age 50: one included ages 51 to 75 and the other included ages 76 and over.[18] The recommended energy intake was adjusted downward in the older group to accommodate an anticipated decrease in energy expenditure. The most recent RDA grouped all persons over age 50 with the explanation that a continuing decrease in energy expenditure with advancing age is neither inevitable nor desirable (Table 9-1). A recent study of 15 healthy older men whose average age was 69 found that the current RDA significantly underestimated the energy requirements of these older people.[22] These men expended more energy carrying out the routine physical tasks related to daily living than was assumed in the usual calculations. Moving about seems to require more effort in older people with reduced muscle coordination.[23] These standards need to be reevaluated in light of the growing numbers of healthy, active elderly people.

Problems with low energy intake. Many older individuals, especially those for whom physical activity is difficult, have energy intakes below those recommended. In NHANES

Requirement
The amount of a nutrient that when fed to a human or animal prevents the appearance of deficiency symptoms and maintain health.

TABLE 9-1 Recommended Energy Intakes for Persons Over Age 50

	Women	Men
Body weight (kg)*	65	77
Body height (cm)*	160	173
Kcal/kg body wt	30	30
Kcal/day	1900	2300
Range of intake (variation of 20%)	1520-2280	1840-2760

Modified from Food and Nutrition Board, National Research Council: *Recommended dietary allowances*, ed 10, Washington, DC, 1989, National Academy Press.
*Body weight and height are the reference values for this age group.

III mean energy intakes were 2110 kcal/day and 1578 kcal/day, respectively, for men and women 60 to 69 years of age.[24] For men and women age 80 and older, energy intakes dropped to 1776 kcal/day and 1329 kcal/day, respectively. Energy intake strongly influences intakes of vitamins and minerals. Among 691 older people in Boston, those with low energy intakes (less than 22 kcal/kg body wt) were more likely to consume inadequate amounts of vitamin B_6, folacin, calcium, and zinc.[25]

Physical Activity and Fitness

Physical fitness is the state in which a person's muscular, cardiovascular, and respiratory systems have the ability to respond to physical work with rapid recovery and minimal fatigue. Decreases in fitness occur as a result of smoking, lack of exercise, and age-related deterioration. Regular exercise leads to improved functional capacity that enhances the individual's ability to carry on household duties and personal care and maintain the highest level of independence possible. Regular exercise also increases energy expenditure and contributes to body weight management.

Activity, aging, and skeletal muscle. At the present time researchers are evaluating the influence of both physical activity and age on the loss of skeletal muscle that occurs over adulthood. Although we have assumed that this decrease in muscle mass resulted from metabolic changes associated with aging, it now appears that the decrease in physical activity over adulthood may be a major cause. Muscle disuse leads to not only a decrease in the absolute amount of skeletal muscle but also a decrease in strength of the remaining muscle. Muscle strength and muscle mass are factors in both the distance an older person can walk and the speed.[26] Loss of muscle strength is a cause of falls in older people that further impede mobility if fractures occur.

Types of physical training. Physical fitness is enhanced by endurance and strength training, and both have advantages for elderly people. Endurance training using the large muscles, for example, walking, improves cardiovascular and respiratory response and has a positive effect on body composition and serum lipids. Walking several hours each week leads to a measurable decrease in body fat and improved abdominal-hip ratio. The accompanying increase in energy expenditure can help to prevent an unwanted increase in body weight or allow an increased food intake supplying needed protein, vitamins, and minerals.

The value of strength training for elderly people has been gaining increasing attention. Strength training involves increasing the force or weight against which a muscle must push or pull. Not only does this training reverse the loss of strength in existing muscle, it also restores muscle that has been lost by increasing the size of existing muscle fibers. A strength training program with elderly people up to 96 years of age demonstrated an increase of 9% in the leg muscle area and an improvement in the ability to walk without help.[26] Strength training also causes an increase in energy expenditure by as much as 15%. It is suggested that older people in a strength training program have a protein intake of at least 1.0 g per kg body weight.

Physical activity counseling is important for older adults. Even modest increases in activity are likely to be beneficial. At the same time safety is an overriding issue when working with an elderly person who is considering an exercise program. Abrupt, overly strenuous activity for those who have been sedentary is dangerous for the heart and the large muscles. Most injuries among those exercising for health reasons are caused by excessive activity after a long period of muscle disuse. Walking short distances and gradually increasing the distance covered is a safe way to begin exercise. Strength training must be supervised by a health professional with experience in working with older people. All older people entering a fitness program should discuss it with their physician beforehand.

Essential Fatty Acids

Currently, there is no RDA for the essential fatty acids. Linoleic acid and arachidonic acid are important components of cell membranes. Linoleic acid, an omega-3 fatty acid, is a substrate for the synthesis of eicosapentaenoic acid and docosahexaenoic acid, both of which can also be obtained from fatty fish (see p. 52 in Ch. 3 for discussion of omega-3 fatty acids). Linoleic acid also can be converted to arachidonic acid, which does not need to be obtained from food when sufficient linoleic acid is available. Efforts to control fat and energy levels can result in low intakes of linoleic acid. Moreover, intakes of linoleic acid may still remain low when fat intake is high. In a French nursing home linoleic acid intake equalled only 4 g per day, although fat provided 40% of total kilocalories.[27] Younger people living in that community obtained 12 g of linoleic acid per day on a similar intake of fat. The nursing home residents also had lower serum concentrations of arachidonic acid, leading those researchers to suggest that the metabolic conversion of linoleic acid to arachidonic acid may be less efficient in older people. Including at least one tablespoon of vegetable oil in the daily diet helps provide needed amounts of linoleic acid.

Protein Requirements

Protein needs of adults. Even well-nourished adults appear to lose body nitrogen as a function of age. It is estimated that total body nitrogen decreases from 1320 g in the young adult to 1070 g in the aged adult. **Skeletal muscle** contributes a major portion of the protein that is lost with lesser amounts coming from vital organs such as the heart or liver. Muscle mass comprises 45% of body weight in the young adult but only 27% of body weight beyond age 70. As a result of this loss of muscle **protein turnover** shifts in location from the muscle to the **visceral organs**.

The change in body nitrogen content has led to different interpretations as to the protein requirements of older people. A decrease in skeletal muscle and organ mass could reduce the need for protein and amino acids. On the other hand, an inadequate intake of nitrogen throughout adulthood could be responsible for the observed loss in body nitrogen. Evaluations of protein requirements in the elderly have not completely resolved this question.

Evaluating protein requirements. The method used to evaluate protein requirements in older adults is the nitrogen balance method. Nitrogen balance studies evaluate the level of dietary protein that must be consumed to replace **obligatory nitrogen losses** and achieve nitrogen balance. The balance method also measures the ability of the older individual to effectively use the protein being fed. Obligatory nitrogen losses are higher in men than women because of their higher proportion of muscle and lower proportion of body fat. Obligatory nitrogen losses calculated on the basis of lean body mass are higher in older than in younger individuals as a result of the shift in protein turnover from the muscle to the visceral organs.

A recent study evaluated nitrogen balance in 12 older people ranging in age from 56 to 80 years.[28] One group was given 0.8 g/kg body wt/day of protein (the current RDA) and the other group was given 1.6 g/kg body wt/day (two times the current RDA). The group receiving the current RDA for protein was in **negative nitrogen balance** (depleting body protein stores) over the study period, whereas the group receiving two times the RDA for protein was in positive balance (storing protein) (Fig. 9-2). Those researchers estimated the protein intake required by older people to maintain nitrogen equilibrium to be 1.0 g/kg body wt/day. According to this study a safe protein intake for elderly adults would be 1.0 to 1.25 g/kg body wt/day.[28] It appears that the current RDA for protein, even good quality protein, is not adequate to assure positive protein status in many older adults.

Skeletal muscle
Muscles attached to skeletal bones for control of body movements; major component of lean body mass.

Protein turnover
The metabolic process in the body by which proteins are being constantly synthesized, broken down, and the resulting amino acids resynthesized into new proteins.

Visceral organs
(L *viscus*, large body organ) Large internal organs of the body located in the chest and abdomen.

Obligatory nitrogen loss
The lowest level of nitrogen excretion that can be reached by an individual despite all body conservation mechanisms.

Negative nitrogen balance
Situation in which the amount of nitrogen consumed is less than the amount of nitrogen lost through all excretory routes resulting in a net loss of body nitrogen.

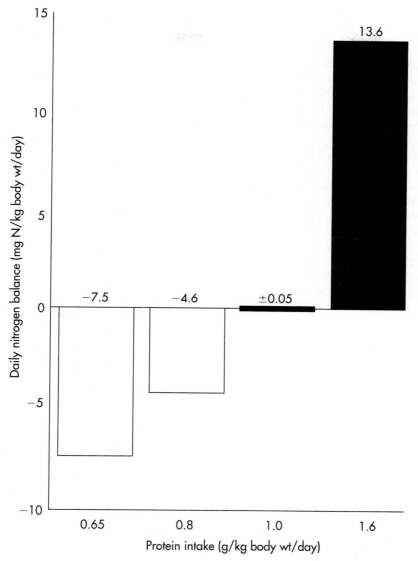

FIG. 9-2   Retention and loss of nitrogen in older people given increasing amounts of egg protein. The level of protein required for nitrogen balance has been calculated to be 1.0 g per kg of body weight.

From Campbell WW et al: Increased protein requirements in elderly people: new data and retrospective assessments, *Am J Clin Nutr* 60:501, 1994 and Uauy R, Scrimshaw NS, Young VR: Human protein requirements: nitrogen balance response to graded levels of egg protein in elderly men and women, *Am J Clin Nutr* 31:779, 1978.

Factors influencing protein requirements. The inability of older persons to achieve nitrogen balance on test diets may relate to the type and level of protein they consumed in the months prior. When given self-selected diets, older people can maintain nitrogen balance on lower levels of protein than when given test diets. Emotional and physical stress increase protein requirements. Inflammation and infection lead to loss of body protein stores mediated in part by the stress response of the adrenal **corticosteroid** hormones.

Corticosteroid
(L *corticix*, bark, shell) Any of the steroids affecting carbohydrate, fat, and protein metabolism that are produced in the outer region (cortex) of the adrenal glands in response to stimulus by the adrenocorticotropic hormone (ACTH) from the pituitary gland, or any of their synthetic derivatives. These compounds include glucocorticoids affecting glucose metabolism and mineralcorticoids affecting electrolyte (Na^+) concentration and fluid-electrolyte balance.

Factors influencing protein utilization. Classic studies describe the protein-sparing action of carbohydrate and point to the need for sufficient kilocalories to support the use of dietary protein for tissue growth or repair. When kilocalories are limited, protein metabolism is compromised regardless of protein intake. The inability of some older individuals to maintain nitrogen balance on what would seem to be adequate levels of protein may relate to the energy value of the diet. The recommended energy intake for people over age 50 is 30 kcal/kg body wt/day (see Table 9-1)[18]; however, dietary surveys of healthy elderly persons indicate that intakes are as low as 22 to 25 kcal/kg body wt/day.[25] Using physical activity to allow greater flexibility in energy intake should be a priority in nutritional counseling of older persons.

Amino acid requirements. The amino acid requirements of older persons are poorly defined. Tryptophan requirements appear to decrease with age, but threonine and valine requirements seem to increase. When requirements are calculated on the basis of lean body mass, however, older people have a greater need for the essential amino acids than do younger people.

Protein-energy malnutrition (PEM). The older person with a debilitating disease and a poor diet has low nutrient reserves and is particularly vulnerable to overt malnutrition. These circumstances no doubt contribute to the poor nutritional status observed in some institutionalized elderly persons who had a disability and consequently inadequate meals before entering the health care facility. PEM is sometimes difficult to identify in an aged population because assessment standards specific to older people have not been developed. Also, chronic diseases can bring about physiological or biochemical changes that interfere with nutritional evaluation (e.g., fluid retention in cardiac failure can mask a loss in body weight). Serum albumin levels appear to be the most reliable indicator of PEM in the older adult.

Protein intake. Protein intake is adequate in many older Americans, but protein status is income-related. Low income people are more likely to have low intakes. NHANES II reported that 10% of higher-income women 65 to 74 years of age consumed less than two thirds of the RDA, whereas 25% of lower-income women consumed less than that amount.[29] At greatest risk are those consuming inadequate levels of both protein and energy. Over 50% of the lower-income women had less than two thirds of the recommended level of kilocalories. Inadequate energy intake results in less efficient use of the protein that is available.

VITAMIN REQUIREMENTS OF OLDER PEOPLE
Fat-Soluble Vitamins

Micelle
(L *micella,* small body)
A microscopic colloid particle of fat and bile formed in the small intestine as the initial stage of fat absorption.

Absorption of the fat-soluble vitamins requires pancreatic lipase and bile for breaking down dietary fat and "packaging" it in fat **micelles** for transport. Thus older persons with gallbladder disease or reduced secretion of pancreatic enzymes who have impaired fat absorption may also absorb the fat-soluble vitamins poorly.

Vitamin A and vitamin E. Advancing age does not increase the requirement for vitamin A or hinder its absorption. In fact, vitamin A may be more easily absorbed by older people. When deficient serum levels are detected, they usually relate to low intake and respond to dietary improvement. But questions have been raised about the advisability of long-term use of concentrated vitamin A supplements by the elderly. Healthy older people in Boston who took vitamin A supplements containing over 10,000 IU (about two times the RDA) for at least 5 years had elevated levels of serum retinyl esters and of particular enzymes that suggested possible liver damage; however, no evidence of toxicity was observed in New Mexico elderly consuming supplements of these levels.[30] Many older persons also routinely consume vitamin E supplements at levels of 50 to 100 times the RDA. Although there is currently no evidence of toxicity resulting from high intakes of vitamin E, it appears that vitamin E supplements enhance vitamin A storage in the liver. This emphasizes the need for caution among those consuming high levels of both vitamins.

Mean intakes of vitamin A for persons above age 60 exceed the RDA, but individual intakes are influenced by ethnic background. NHANES III reported that about half of older white men and women met the RDA for vitamin A.[31] In contrast nearly half of black and Mexican-American elderly consumed *less than 60%* of the RDA. Dietary intake can be influenced by income since dark green and deep yellow vegetables and fruits high in beta carotene (provitamin A) tend to be expensive, especially in the winter months. Hispanic people are thought to be particularly vulnerable to low vitamin A intakes because of their limited use of fruits and vegetables rich in carotenes; however, Hispanic elderly generally have normal serum retinol levels.[32] Vitamin E is also a problem among older people. For white men and women ages 60 to 69, the **median** vitamin E intake in alpha tocopherol equivalents was about 75% of the RDA. Black and Hispanic men and women of this age had a median intake about 50% of the RDA. Megadoses of vitamin E (80 times the RDA) have been shown to stimulate the immune system and production of T-cells in generally healthy older people, although the long-term response to vitamin E supplementation is not known.[33] Such levels of vitamin E should not be consumed without constant medical supervision.

Vitamin D. The vitamin D status of older people based on dietary intake or serum vitamin D metabolite levels is less than optimal. Dietary sources make only a limited contribution to the vitamin D requirement. In older people in North America and Europe the average vitamin D intake is about 2.5 μg (50% of the RDA).[34] Serum vitamin D metabolite levels are lower in winter, emphasizing the importance of sunlight in meeting body needs. Although age-related changes in the skin reduce the older person's ability to synthesize vitamin D, this source remains important in maintaining adequate vitamin D status. Appropriate levels of either dietary vitamin D or sun exposure offer some degree of protection against hip fracture in elderly women. A lack of vitamin D that decreases calcium absorption and subsequently increases serum parathyroid hormone (PTH) levels indirectly causes a mobilization of calcium from the bone. Older women who raised their total vitamin D intake to 500 IU per day suppressed this rise in PTH levels that occurs in cold winter months when exposure to sunlight is minimal.[34] Preventing seasonal vitamin D deficiency is one way to preserve bone mass.

Webb and coworkers evaluated vitamin D requirements in nursing home residents who had very little exposure to sunlight.[35] They found that a daily supplement of 10 μg (400 IU) was sufficient to maintain adequate levels of **calcitriol**. The current RDA of 5 μg (200 IU)[18] did not preserve optimal vitamin D status in this population. At the same time older people should not consume supplements containing greater than 10 μg in light of the potential toxicity of vitamin D.

The trend toward using calcium supplements rather than consuming dairy products as calcium sources contributes to poor dietary intakes of vitamin D. One cup of milk supplying about 300 mg of calcium will also provide 100 IU of vitamin D.

Water-Soluble Vitamins

Thiamin, riboflavin, and niacin. Thiamin, riboflavin, and niacin, members of the vitamin B complex, act as coenzymes in energy metabolism. Thus their RDAs are based on energy intake and decrease in response to lower energy needs. Nevertheless, higher intakes sufficient to maintain optimum biochemical enzyme indices are beneficial. In a study of older Irish women those given a thiamin supplement of 10 mg daily to raise serum enzymes to appropriate levels had an improved appetite and sense of physical well-being as compared with those given a **placebo**.[36] Riboflavin requirements appear to increase

Median
The middle value in a series of numbers, so that half of the numbers are below the median and half of the numbers are above.

Calcitriol
Activated hormone form of vitamin D. [1,25 $(OH)_2 D_3$], 1,25,dihydroxycholecalciferol.

Placebo
An inactive substance such as water or sugar used in nutritional studies to compare the effects of an inactive substance with the effects of the test nutrient or compound.

when older people participate in physical training, leading to the suggestion that the RDA for riboflavin remain the same throughout adulthood.[19] Poor status for thiamin or riboflavin usually relates to low dietary intake or excessive alcohol consumption. Black and Hispanic older people have lower intakes of riboflavin based on their lower consumption of dairy products.

Vitamin C. Ascorbic acid metabolism differs in older men compared with older women; older men have lower plasma levels despite intakes equal to or higher than those of older women. An important measurement in ascorbic acid metabolism is the total body pool that is estimated to reach a maximum at a plasma concentration of about 1.0 mg/dl. Older men require intakes of 150 mg/day to reach that plasma level, with no further increase at higher levels of intake. Older women reach a plasma concentration of 1.0 mg/dl on intakes of 75 to 80 mg/day and attain a maximum plasma concentration of 1.3 mg/dl at an intake of 280 mg/day.[37] This difference could relate to the higher proportion of lean body mass in men.[38] On intakes that equal the current RDA (60 mg) older men have plasma concentrations below 0.4 mg/dl, which is the critical level used to identify individuals at risk of deficiency. This finding indicates that the ascorbic acid RDA for older men should be reevaluated.

In older people, socioeconomic status influences ascorbic acid status. Those people with lower incomes are more likely to have deficient serum ascorbic acid levels and lower intakes of vitamin C-rich fruits and vegetables. Ascorbic acid is lost if cooked vegetables are held at serving temperature for long periods of time, which can occur in quantity meal programs. Citrus fruits are a better choice of vitamin C under those circumstances.

Vitamin B$_6$. Vitamin B$_6$ (pyridoxine) is a problem nutrient for many older persons. Both serum levels and the activity levels of red blood cell enzymes requiring vitamin B$_6$ as a cofactor are lower in older versus younger adults. In a study of 198 elderly people living in the community, 36% of the women and 18% of the men had intakes below 67% of the RDA.[39] Moreover, prescription drugs sometimes interfere with vitamin B$_6$ absorption.

Recent work at the Human Nutrition Research Center on Aging in Boston indicated that the vitamin B$_6$ *requirement* of healthy elderly men is 1.96 mg and of healthy elderly women is 1.90 mg.[40] This report points to a serious discrepancy between the current RDA for vitamin B$_6$ for persons above age 50 and the apparent requirement. This is especially critical for women, as their apparent requirement of 1.90 mg actually exceeds their RDA of 1.6 mg. The RDA for men of 2.0 mg does not provide any measure of safety based on the apparent requirement of 1.96 mg. While further work continues, a dietary goal for older adults should be a daily intake of at least 2.0 mg.

Decreased use of meat, poultry, or fish because of chewing problems or financial constraints lowers vitamin B$_6$ intake. Frail elderly persons with low energy intakes may not be able to meet requirements through food only and may need a supplement. Because vitamin B$_6$ is easily destroyed by heat processing, preprepared foods can be relatively poor sources. Potatoes and other vegetables are good sources of this vitamin.

Folacin. Folacin deficiency in older persons is associated with poor dietary intake, atrophic gastritis resulting in **achlorhydria**, use of antacids or prescription drugs that interfere with folate absorption or utilization, and alcoholism. Although folacin absorption is decreased in those with low gastric acid levels, it has been speculated that folacin-synthesizing bacteria that grow in the upper small intestine when gastric acid is reduced may provide a compensatory source of the vitamin.[14] Overt deficiency is seldom seen in healthy, financially advantaged older people even on daily intakes of 200 μg. Elderly black and Hispanic persons are at particular risk of folacin deficiency if their use of citrus fruits and fresh dark green vegetables is infrequent. Cooking practices contribute to folacin deficiency

Achlorhydria

(L *a-*, negative; *chlorhydria*, hydrochloric acid) Absence or reduced amounts of hydrochloric acid in the gastric secretions.

if vegetables are boiled for long periods of time and the vitamin destroyed.

Vitamin B₁₂. Intrinsic factor secreted by the gastric mucosa is required for the absorption of vitamin B₁₂. Lack of intrinsic factor causes vitamin B₁₂ deficiency and over time degenerative changes in the brain and spinal cord bringing mental deterioration and altering cognitive function, personality, and physical coordination. In atrophic gastritis, intrinsic factor and gastric acid levels are lowered as is subsequent vitamin B₁₂ absorption. Vitamin B₁₂ absorption is impaired in older adults with low gastric acid levels because gastric acid is required to release food-bound vitamin B₁₂ and make it available for absorption.

A recent survey of 548 surviving members of the Framingham Heart Study found that serum **cobalamin** levels decrease with age among even healthy elderly people (Fig. 9-3).[41] Low serum cobalamin levels were found in 40% of the elderly group (ages 67 to 90) as compared with 18% of the young group. Moreover, 12% of the older group had elevated serum methylmalonic acid concentrations. Methylmalonic acid accumulates when vitamin B₁₂ is no longer available as a coenzyme to support the conversion of methylmalonyl coenzyme A to succinyl coenzyme A within the citric acid cycle. Those researchers concluded that many older people, regardless of serum vitamin B₁₂ levels, are metabolically deficient in vitamin B₁₂.

Cobalamin
(Ger *kobold,* mine) A term for the cobalt-containing portion of the vitamin B₁₂ molecule.

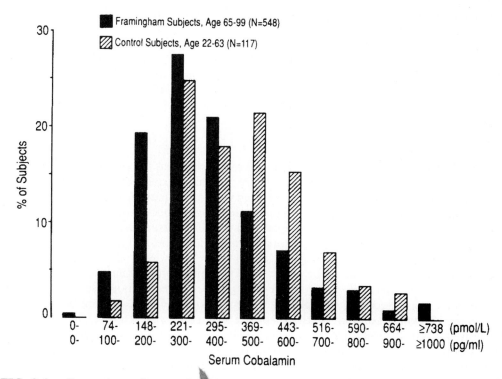

FIG. 9-3   Comparison of serum vitamin B₁₂ levels in community-living elderly people and younger people. The majority of the elderly people had serum levels at the lower end of the distribution; more of the younger people had serum levels at the middle and upper end of the distribution.

From Lindenbaum J et al: Prevalence of cobalamin deficiency in the Framingham elderly population, *Am J Clin Nutr* 60:2, 1994.

MINERAL REQUIREMENTS OF OLDER PEOPLE
Iron

Iron absorption. Absorption of iron, a complicated and inefficient process in people of all ages, is even more difficult in older people with altered gastrointestinal secretions. Hydrochloric acid is necessary to reduce iron from the ferric form found in food to the ferrous form necessary for absorption. Antacids that raise gastric pH levels and certain drugs (e.g., cholestyramine) that bind inorganic iron decrease iron uptake. A liberal intake of fiber promoting normal bowel function can lower iron absorption. Nevertheless, most healthy older people can maintain adequate iron status on intakes approximating the RDA. Moreover, older blood donors are able to increase the percentage of iron absorbed in response to reduced body iron stores.

Iron requirements. After menopause in women and after age 50 in men, body iron stores begin to increase. By age 70, iron stores average 800 mg in women (increased from 300 mg before menopause) and 1200 mg in men. Daily iron losses in the form of desquamated cells are estimated to be less than 1.0 mg per day in older men and nonmenstruating women. This loss can be replaced easily on an intake of 10 mg per day. Pathological conditions such as peptic ulcers and undiagnosed cancer or excessive aspirin use leading to continual blood loss through the gastrointestinal tract can significantly deplete iron reserves. Low level blood loss may not be detected in a **guaiac** test of the stools for occult (hidden) blood. Nevertheless this test should immediately follow any diagnosis of iron deficiency.

> **Guaiac**
> A compound used in laboratory tests to determine the presence of occult blood as in the feces.

Older women are vulnerable to poor iron intake based on their relatively low energy intakes. As iron can be obtained from fortified cereal products, nutrition education should include combining foods to best advantage to support iron absorption. At the same time we need to caution older persons to avoid multiple daily servings of cereal products fortified at a level of 15 mg of iron per serving and intended to meet the iron requirement of the menstruating female.

Calcium and Phosphorus

Control of calcium metabolism. Calcium metabolism has important implications for both nutritional and physical health. To ensure normal function of the heart and nervous system, serum calcium levels must be maintained within very narrow limits (9 to 11 mg/dl). A decrease in serum calcium levels or an increase in serum phosphorus levels triggers the release of PTH, which restores serum calcium by (1) releasing calcium from the bone (resorption), (2) increasing calcium absorption in the intestine, and (3) increasing calcium reabsorption in the kidney.

Estrogen appears to balance the action of PTH in promoting bone calcium release and exerts a positive effect on bone before menopause. After menopause and estrogen withdrawal, bone becomes increasingly sensitive to PTH and calcium mobilization accelerates. As bone resorption continues to raise serum calcium levels, less PTH is released, lowering calcium absorption in the intestine. Thus loss of body calcium increases while net absorption decreases. If this process continues unabated, bone density and strength will be lost and susceptibility to fracture will increase. Estrogen also supports bone health by stimulating the conversion of vitamin D to calcitriol, thereby increasing calcium absorption. The subsequent decrease in calcium absorption after estrogen withdrawal further exacerbates calcium release from the bone.

Calcium requirement. The daily calcium intake required to prevent calcium loss in postmenopausal women remains controversial. The Food and Nutrition Board has taken the position that calcium intakes above the current RDA of 800 mg do not consistently prevent bone loss.[18] On the other hand, some researchers have demonstrated that calcium intakes of 1000 mg to 1500 mg per day can actually increase bone density in postmenopausal women.[42-44] A total calcium intake of at least 1000 mg daily would seem to be a prudent goal for older women. Current intakes of older people from all ethnic groups fall well below this goal. White men and women age 60 to 69 who participated in NHANES III had median intakes of 734 mg and 660 mg, respectively.[31] Hispanic men of this age had a median intake of 810 mg, but median intakes in older Hispanic women and older black men fell to 490 mg. Older black women had the lowest calcium intakes with a median intake of 399 mg. This median value indicates that half of these black women had intakes *less* than 399 mg. Dairy products low in fat can provide both calcium and the necessary vitamin D and support a prudent diet.

Chromium

Chromium is an important nutrient for maintaining normal glucose metabolism, since it facilitates the interaction of insulin with its receptor site on the cell membrane. Chromium intake and absorption are relatively low in all age groups. Healthy older Canadians on self-selected diets had chromium intakes ranging from 21 μg to 274 μg per day with a mean intake of 96 μg.[45] Those with the highest intakes were drinking large quantities of tea, reported to be a good source. The current recommendation for an Estimated Safe and Adequate Daily Dietary Intake is 50 to 200 μg per day. An American diet containing 1600 kcal was found to supply only 25 μg of chromium; an energy intake of 2300 kcal provided 33 μg.[18] In light of the low energy intakes of many older persons, it is likely that chromium intake falls well below the recommended minimum in a significant segment of this population.

Zinc

Dietary zinc levels are influenced by total energy intake, total money spent for food, and food selection. Older men with energy intakes of 1800 kcal consumed about 10.6 mg of zinc (RDA = 15 mg). Older women consuming 1300 kcal took in only 7.2 mg of zinc or 60% of the RDA.[46] In the average American diet about 40% of the zinc is provided by meat, fish, and poultry, which are relatively expensive items in the food budget. The most common food source is beef. A diet based on dairy products and highly processed breads and cereals will be low in zinc. A recent evaluation of menus served in adult boarding homes for elderly people found that 60% provided less than two thirds of the RDA for zinc.[47] Another population at particular risk for zinc deficiency is older vegetarians whose primary sources of zinc are low in bioavailability. Foods high in phytate reduce total zinc absorption regardless of the zinc level present in the overall diet.

Zinc plays important roles in taste, wound healing, and the immune response. Each of these functions is altered in certain older people; however, zinc supplementation does not reverse these changes in persons with adequate zinc status.[46] Moreover, self-medication with zinc supplements can actually depress immune function and lower HDL-cholesterol levels. Optimum zinc intake is particularly important for healing **decubitus ulcers** or recovering from surgery.

Decubitus ulcer
A bedsore caused by prolonged pressure on the skin and tissues covering a bony area; occurs in elderly people who are confined to bed or immobilized.

Fluid Intake

Water is supplied to the body through food, liquids, and water of oxidation. In younger people the thirst mechanism ensures an adequate fluid intake, whereas a diminished sensitivity to dehydration and reduced sensation of thirst substantially lowers spontaneous fluid intake in older people. The disabled individual who cannot drink without help is particularly vulnerable to low fluid intake and acute dehydration. Those elderly people subject to incontinence may make a conscious effort to restrict fluids to avoid embarrassment. Patients given high protein supplements will become dehydrated if fluids are limited. Unless diagnosed with cardiac or renal complications, older people should drink a minimum of six to eight glasses of fluid each day.[13]

NUTRITIONAL AND CHRONIC DISORDERS IN THE AGED
Carbohydrate Metabolism and Glucose Tolerance

Glucose tolerance, the ability to metabolize a standard dose of glucose, deteriorates with age. In younger individuals abnormal glucose tolerance is associated with the development of diabetes mellitus. In older individuals the separation between disease-related pathology and normal aging is less clear.

Blood glucose levels. Fasting blood glucose levels are not higher in older people than in younger people. However, 2 hours after consuming 50 g of glucose under standard conditions, blood glucose levels remain higher in older persons. Many factors contribute to this alteration in glucose tolerance. The age-related decrease in lean body mass and increase in body fat play a role as excessive fatness contributes to impaired glucose tolerance in all age groups. Physical activity promotes energy metabolism in the skeletal muscle and glucose uptake for fuel. Conversely, bed rest or a sedentary lifestyle reduces glucose movement into the skeletal muscle cell and thereby increases **postprandial** blood glucose levels. Potassium depletion resulting from poor intake or prolonged use of certain diuretics will impair glucose tolerance as potassium ions are required to move glucose into the cell.

Physiological aspects. In diabetes mellitus there is a lack of the active form of insulin required to facilitate both the entry and metabolism of glucose in the cell. This is not the case in older persons with age-related changes in glucose tolerance. In fact, insulin levels are often higher in older people; but the fat cells in older people are generally larger than the fat cells in normal weight younger people, and enlarged fat cells are less sensitive to the action of insulin. In 652 healthy men ranging in age from 43 to 85 years, those with high BMI and abdominal-hip ratio had higher fasting and postprandial insulin levels.[48] It is advantageous to maintain normal serum insulin levels as **hyperinsulinemia** is a risk factor for both NIDDM and cardiovascular disease. Weight reduction with a loss of abdominal fat and physical exercise can improve glucose tolerance and ameliorate excessively high serum insulin levels.

Diet effects. Diets high in complex carbohydrate and fiber improve glucose tolerance in older persons. Fiber slows the rate at which glucose moves into the blood from the small intestine, thereby lowering blood glucose levels after eating. Diets low in carbohydrate appear to contribute to the deterioration in glucose tolerance associated with aging.

Bone Disorders in the Aging Adult

Loss of bone. Loss of bone mass in middle and old age has been observed in prehistoric skeletons from the year 2000 B.C. Osteoporosis (porous bone) is the clinical syndrome associated with the absolute decrease in bone mineral and bone matrix. It results in bone pain, spinal deformity, and bone fractures that occur spontaneously (with no fall or trauma). At about age 30, women begin to lose bone and over their adult life lose as much as 35% of their **cortical bone** and 50% of their **trabecular bone**; men lose only about two thirds as much.[49] All people lose bone as they age, but not all develop osteoporosis. Bone is lost from the spine, hip, and femur. Loss of bone and bone strength increases susceptibility to fracture and possible disability. The incidence of spontaneous hip fractures is such that by age 90, one in three women and one in six men will have a fracture.[49] The resulting immobility can change one's lifestyle. For example, an older woman may be forced to give up her home and go live with a family member or enter a long-term care

Postprandial
Following a meal.

Hyperinsulinemia
(Gr *hyper* + L *insula*, island) An excessively high level of insulin in the blood.

Cortical bone
(Gr *corticis*, bark, shell) Long bones of the body extremities with heavy outer cortex layer.

Trabecular bone
(L *trabs*, a little beam) General term for small meshwork of bones at end of the long bones forming attached joints; also part of the connecting network between vertebrae.

facility after breaking her hip. Spinal deformities such as **kyphosis** increase in advanced age as bone loss continues.

Osteoporosis and osteomalacia. Osteoporosis is the most common bone disorder in older persons. Bone mass is decreased, but there is no change in the chemical ratio of mineral to protein matrix. Remaining bone is normal, there is just less of it. Once thought to be relatively inactive, bone is now recognized to be an active tissue that undergoes constant remodeling throughout life. While old bone is being broken down at one location by osteoclasts, the cells that dissolve bone mineral and matrix, new bone is being formed at another location by osteoblasts, the cells that synthesize the protein matrix and accumulate the bone mineral. With aging this process becomes uncoupled, and bone is resorbed at a faster rate than it can be replaced. Impaired calcium absorption contributes to this disorder.

Osteomalacia (adult rickets) is caused by a vitamin D deficiency and low absorption of calcium. Bone density is decreased because of poor mineralization of the available protein matrix. Among older people vitamin D problems can relate to (1) low vitamin D intake and no exposure to sunlight, (2) malabsorption of ingested vitamin D, or (3) liver or renal disease that interferes with the conversion of vitamin D to calcitriol. These two bone disorders are illustrated in Fig. 9-4.

Factors influencing bone health. Many factors affect bone loss (see the box on p. 402). The most obvious predisposing factor to bone loss is being female. The relative bone mass remaining at older ages is influenced by the total amount of bone laid down during periods of growth, pointing to the importance of appropriate calcium intakes in childhood and adolescence. Men at all ages have greater bone mass than women and lose bone less rapidly. Black people have more bone than white people and are less likely to develop osteoporosis. Lifestyle choices including exercise level and use of cigarettes or alcohol influence bone mass. Hormonal imbalances accelerate bone loss.

Prevention of osteoporosis. No effective treatment now exists for replacing bone that has been lost. Thus prevention of bone loss is the key, beginning with adolescent girls and women of all ages (see Chapter 3). Avoiding cigarette smoking and excessive use of alcohol will retard bone loss. Regular physical exercise promotes bone health. The pull of gravity and body weight exerted on the bone preserves bone tissue; in fact, weightlessness, as occurs in space flight, leads to rapid loss of bone mineral and matrix. Prolonged bed rest has the same effect. Even general inactivity contributes to calcium loss. Older persons who exercise infrequently experience a higher rate of bone loss when compared with those who exercise several times a week. Walking is an effective way to preserve bone mass.

Raising calcium intake to at least 800 mg daily helps preserve bone mass in women who are 5 years or more beyond menopause but is less effective immediately after cessation of

Kyphosis
(Gr *kyphos,* hunchbacked) An abnormal outward curvature of the upper back resulting from age-related bone loss from the vertebrae.

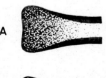
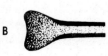

A

B

C

FIG. 9-4 Normal bone, osteoporosis, and osteomalacia **A,** Normal bone. **B,** Osteoporosis in which there is a reduced amount of bone of normal composition. **C,** Osteomalacia in which the amount of bone is normal but the composition is abnormal with reduced mineral density.

❖

CHARACTERISTICS ASSOCIATED WITH LOWER BONE MASS

Genetic
Female
White or Asian race
Family history of bone disease
Extremely short or tall stature

Physiological or Hormonal
Hyperparathyroidism
Hyperthyroidism
Diabetes mellitus
Premature menopause
Leanness

Environmental
Low calcium intake
High phosphorus intake
Limited exposure to sunlight
Limited physical activity
High caffeine intake
Use of alcohol
Smoking

Resorption
(L *resorbere,* to swallow again) The process by which bone is lost; the mineral crystals are dissolved, and the protein matrix is broken down and removed.

menstruation.[43] Estrogen replacement therapy reduces the activity of the osteoclasts and thereby slows bone loss but may increase one's risk of cancer.[44] Boron, an ultratrace element found in fruits and vegetables, appears to support bone health and is a current area of research. Calcitriol, the active vitamin D hormone, is being evaluated as a therapeutic measure to reduce the risk of osteoporosis. Fluoride at low levels supports the formation of bone crystals that are resistant to **resorption**; unfortunately, the use of fluoride supplements to stimulate the formation of new bone has been unsuccessful.[50]

Use of calcium supplements. Media attention to the risks of bone loss and bone fractures has led to mass marketing of calcium supplements. Although selection of high-calcium foods with high bioavailability should be a first priority in nutrition counseling, some older people do not consume dairy products because of lactose intolerance or cultural food preferences. Recommendations when choosing calcium supplements should address the following:

- Bioavailability of the calcium—calcium carbonate, lactate, gluconate, or citrate malate (used to fortify orange juice) are all reasonably well absorbed if consumed with a meal.
- Cost—which form or brand will provide the most calcium per tablet at the lowest cost?
- Safety—supplements containing bone meal or derived from other natural sources are often high in lead or aluminum; if using products with vitamin D added, avoid total vitamin D intakes exceeding 400 IU (10 μg) per day.
- Level of calcium per tablet—those containing above 500 mg per tablet should be avoided, as they can result in gastrointestinal discomfort or constipation.

Nutritional Anemia

Anemia
(Gr *a-,* negative; *haima,* blood) Blood condition marked by a decrease in number of circulating red blood cells or amount of hemoglobin, or both.

Anemia refers to changes in either the number or characteristics of the erythrocyte that results in a decrease in the oxygen-carrying capacity of the blood. The subsequent oxygen deficit in the tissues causes an increased heart rate, shortness of breath, and weakness. Unfortunately, these symptoms are often thought typical of older people and go unnoticed as anemia develops.

Iron-deficiency anemia. The most common anemia in older people is iron-deficiency anemia. Blood loss through the gastrointestinal tract is a frequent and critical cause of iron deficiency in elderly people (see p. 398). Healthy older people have hemoglobin levels similar to those of healthy younger people, but several trends are apparent. In men hemoglobin levels decrease with age and prevalence of anemia is higher after age 65. Women have lower hemoglobin levels throughout the child-bearing years, but iron status levels improve when menstruation ceases. Aged black persons, particularly women, are more likely to have hemoglobin levels below 12 g/dl.[51] In general older people have reduced numbers of red blood cells compared with established standards, however, the red blood cells produced have a normal hemoglobin concentration.

Erythropoiesis is less efficient in advanced age because of changes in the bone marrow. Protein-energy malnutrition further depresses red blood cell production. Chronic low-grade infection associated with fever, inflammation, or renal disease interferes with the release of iron for hemoglobin synthesis. This produces an anemia characterized by a reduced number of red blood cells normal in size and hemoglobin content and low serum iron levels. This anemia, sometimes referred to as the anemia of chronic disorders, is highly resistant to treatment.

Treatment of iron-deficiency anemia requires careful evaluation. Administering supplemental iron to persons who in fact have an anemia caused by folacin or vitamin B_{12} deficiency has serious consequences, as the lack of vitamin B_{12} and progressive neural damage continue. Self-medication with iron supplements above the RDA of 10 mg is dangerous and can lead to **hemochromatosis** and liver damage.

Megaloblastic anemia. A **megaloblastic anemia** arising from a vitamin B_{12} deficiency occurs in less than 1% of the population, but the average age at onset is 60 years. It was given the name "pernicious" anemia because its persistent downward course led to death. The age-related decline in serum vitamin B_{12} levels is not a consistent predictor of vitamin B_{12} deficiency or onset of pernicious anemia. If vitamin B_{12} is poorly absorbed and body stores are being depleted, serum levels can be expected to decline; however, many people with serum levels below normal, observed over time, do not develop overt anemia. Conversely, older patients with normal erythrocytes can have neurological and behavioral changes resulting from vitamin B_{12} deficiency that in some instances improve with vitamin B_{12} supplementation.[52]

Increasing numbers of older people are being given intramuscular injections of vitamin B_{12} as a preventive measure. Those diagnosed with and treated for pernicious anemia must be made aware of the need to return for continued treatment to prevent subsequent deterioration.

DRUG-NUTRIENT RELATIONSHIPS
Drug Use in Aging Adults

Older people comprise about 12% of the general population, but they use about 35% of all prescription drugs.[53] This is not surprising because many chronic diseases associated with aging are managed with prescription drugs. Hypertension, heart disease, and diabetes mellitus are the most commonly diagnosed medical conditions among older people. Osteoarthritis is also a prevalent ailment. Over two thirds of older people take at least one prescription drug daily, and many who have multiple health problems take six or more.[53]

Older persons are particularly vulnerable to adverse nutritional effects from both prescription and nonprescription drugs. Nutritional status may already be jeopardized by less than optimal nutrient intake. Chronic diseases necessitate long-term drug therapy with the potential for gradual depletion of existing nutrient reserves. The growing trend toward polypharmacy or multiple drug use compounds nutritional effects. Moreover, most drugs have been tested on younger individuals who have different rates of drug absorption, metabolism, and excretion, based on differences in body composition and renal function.

Hemochromatosis
(Gr *haima*, blood; *chroma*, color) Disorder of iron metabolism characterized by excess iron deposits in the tissues, especially in the liver and pancreas; results from iron overload caused by prolonged use of iron supplements or multiple blood transfusions.

Megaloblastic anemia
(Gr *mega*, great size; *blastos*, embryo, germ) Anemia caused by faulty production of abnormally large immature red blood cells, due to a deficiency of vitamin B_{12} or folacin.

Mechanisms of Drug-Nutrient Actions

Interference with normal processes. Drugs can interfere with nutrients at the point of ingestion, absorption, utilization, or excretion. Food intake may decrease because of drugs that depress appetite or cause nausea or vomiting. Interference with the secretion of digestive enzymes or gastric acid or alterations in pH or transit time by particular drugs prevents the digestion of foods into the nutrient forms required for absorption. Competition for binding sites on the intestinal mucosa will reduce nutrient uptake. Some drugs prevent the conversion of a vitamin into its active form, thereby negating its metabolic function. Other drugs form insoluble complexes with nutrients. In general vitamins and minerals are most affected.

Depletion of nutrient reserves. Nutrient depletion is most likely to occur with a drug that inhibits absorption or with a drug taken for an extended period of time. A drug that acts as a vitamin **antagonist** or affects a nutrient such as folacin that participates in a variety of metabolic processes impairs biochemical function. Finally, nutritional effects of drugs are more serious in individuals with preexisting malnutrition. Those with marginal nutritional status who consume multiple drugs over periods of years are at greatest risk of nutrient depletion.

Nutritional Aspects of Drugs

Effects of prescription drugs. The drugs most frequently prescribed for older persons are diuretics and cardiac drugs, drugs for disorders of the central nervous system, agents to manage diabetes mellitus, and analgesics to manage osteoarthritis.[53] Digoxin, which stimulates the heart and is used to treat cardiac failure, causes **anorexia** and nausea and a syndrome identified as cardiac cachexia. Particular diuretics that promote the excretion of water and sodium also promote the loss of potassium. Medicines used to control convulsions and seizures increase the need for vitamin D.

Effects of nonprescription drugs. Because over-the-counter (OTC) drugs are easily obtained and commonly used, they are often perceived to be without risk. Use of these drugs may not be reported to a physician, creating the possibility of a dangerous interaction with a prescription drug. Also, dosage may be increased above that recommended if the desired effect is not achieved.

The most commonly used OTC drug is aspirin (acetylsalicylic acid) used for arthritis, headache, and muscle pain. Prolonged use can induce iron-deficiency anemia through irritation of the gastrointestinal mucosa and subsequent blood loss. Gastrointestinal drugs also are used regularly by many elderly people. Continuous use of laxatives depletes sodium and potassium and can lead to chronic diarrhea. Mineral oil, sometimes used as a **cathartic**, interferes with the absorption of fat soluble vitamins. Sodium bicarbonate and other antacids increase gastric pH, inactivating thiamin and hindering the absorption of iron, calcium, and folacin. Aluminum hydroxide-containing antacids bind phosphate and are known to cause phosphate depletion and accelerate bone loss.

Use of vitamin and mineral supplements. Many elderly people regularly use vitamin and mineral supplements. In a Wisconsin study of 2152 individuals ranging in age from 43 to 86 years, 44% of those age 65 and over used a supplement but only 34% of those below age 65 did.[54] However, the supplements chosen do not always provide the nutrients that are in shortest supply. Although calcium intake is frequently low relative to the RDA, calcium supplements were chosen by less than half of the supplement users in the Wisconsin study. Of concern should be the excessive use of vitamin-mineral supplements. Among healthy older people in New Mexico some individuals were routinely consuming five times or more the recommended levels of vitamins A and D, intakes that over prolonged periods are potentially toxic.[55]

Antagonist
(Gr *antagonisma*, struggle) Agent that has an opposite, conflicting, or inhibiting action to another substance.

Anorexia
(Gr *a*, orexis not appetite) Loss of appetite.

Cathartic
(Gr *katharsis*, cleansing) A substance used to empty the bowel; a laxative.

Addictive Behaviors in the Older Adult

Alcohol or drug dependencies are believed to be fairly common among the elderly but frequently undetected. Dementia and depression, consequences of alcohol or drug dependence, are associated also with medical conditions and age-related changes in neurological status, thus the health professional may overlook the true cause. When substance abuse is identified, appropriate interventions include counseling, support groups, and substance-free structured environments.

Abuse of alcohol. Estimates of the elderly believed to have drinking problems vary greatly from less than 5% to over 60%. It is believed that 15% to 20% of institutionalized elderly have or had an alcohol problem.[56] Physical and emotional distress, loneliness, and bereavement all contribute to increased use of alcohol. Among 691 older persons in Boston, 43% of the men and 28% of the women consumed alcohol at least once over the 3-day record period, but general use decreased with age.[25] As people grow older, their tolerance to alcohol decreases and adverse side effects increase, even in chronic alcoholics. The risk of nutritional deficiency arising from long-term use of prescription or OTC drugs is markedly increased by excessive drinking or when prior alcoholism has depleted nutrient stores. Also, alcohol interacts with some drugs and conditions to worsen the negative effects. High alcohol intake decreases serum potassium levels, putting the cardiac patient on digitalis at risk of toxicity. The alcohol abuser with IDDM can become hypoglycemic as alcohol interferes with **gluconeogenesis**.

Abuse of drugs. The use of illicit drugs is relatively uncommon in the elderly population, although this problem will grow as younger users move into older age categories. However, the abuse of prescribed medications is becoming more prevalent as sedatives, **psychotropic** drugs, and analgesics are used to treat a greater variety of conditions. One report indicated that 21% of nursing home residents were being given potentially addictive drugs such as **barbiturates** or narcotics for relief of pain.[56] Caregivers may overmedicate individuals with dementia to make them docile and easier to control. Older people at home using mood-altering drugs on a regular basis to relieve temporary depression or anxiety may consume increasing amounts as tolerance to the drug develops. Social withdrawal and the inability to perform household tasks may be the consequences of inappropriate use. Combining alcohol and psychotropic medications is particularly dangerous, resulting in delirium, muscle weakness, and serious medical complications.

FOOD SELECTION PATTERNS OF OLDER PEOPLE
Environmental Factors

Lifestyle changes. In the older adult food patterns reflect lifelong attitudes and habits as influenced by the changing environment. To better understand the influence of lifestyle, health, and economic status on the food choices of older people, review the examples in Table 9-2. These factors can act both individually and in combination with others. The older woman who has taken pride in "cooking from scratch" may have to rely on preprepared items or home-delivered meals if her worsening arthritis makes food preparation difficult. For older people on a fixed pension, increasing health care expenses will reduce the amount of money available for food. Solving the food problems of older people often involves seeking alternatives as living situations and resources change and things have to be done differently.

Dietary adequacy. Changes in living situation or income level contribute to poor nutrient intake in some older people, but this is not true for all older people. The stereotype of the old person who subsists on tea and toast is not substantiated by survey data from the United States or Europe. Although there are isolated cases that do follow this pattern,

Gluconeogenesis
(Gr *gleukos*, sweetness; *neos*, new; *gennan*, to produce) Production of glucose from noncarbohydrate molecules such as amino acids from protein and the glycerol portion from the breakdown of fats.

Psychotropic
(Gr *psyche* + *trepein*, to turn) To exert an effect on the mind, altering behavior, mental activity, or emotional experience.

Barbiturate
(Saint Barbara, drug discovered on day of the saint, 1864) Drug used to reduce anxiety or induce sleep; sometimes used to treat disorders causing convulsions.

TABLE 9-2   *Influences on Food Choices of Older People*

Psychological Factors	Physiological Factors	Socioeconomic Factors
Social activity	Appetite	Age
Self-esteem	Taste acuity	Sex
Nutrition knowledge	Olfactory acuity	Income
Perceived health benefit	Dental status	Cooking facilities
Loneliness	Prescribed diets	Daily schedule
Bereavement	Chronic disease	Retirement/leisure time
Symbolism of food	Food intolerance	Education
Mental awareness	Health status	Distance to food store
Food likes/dislikes	Physical disability	Availability of transportation
Food beliefs	Physical exercise	Availability of familiar foods
	Use of drugs	
	Vision level	

they are not typical of this age group. The mere fact that an older person has survived to an advanced age indicates an ability to select a reasonably adequate diet over a lifetime.

Changes in Lifelong Food Patterns

Decreased energy intakes and nutrient density. Normal aging is accompanied by a decrease in the quantity of food consumed. According to NHANES III, mean daily intake in men decreased 1249 kcal over adulthood, from 3025 kcal at ages 20 to 29 to 1776 kcal at ages 80 and over.[24] Among women energy intake decreased by 628 kcal, from 1957 kcal to 1329 kcal over this age range. Older persons may compensate for their lower energy intakes by choosing foods more carefully, as indicated by the fact that intakes of vitamin A actually increased between ages 20 and 80, from 1026 RE to 1207 RE among men, and from 786 RE to 1083 RE among women. Unfortunately, this pattern does not hold true for all nutrients. Zinc intakes decreased by 20% to 30% over this age range. If older persons decrease their energy intakes by consuming less of all foods, rather than selectively reducing their intakes of items lower in **nutrient density**, the overall quality of the diet suffers.

Nutrient density
The protein, vitamin, or mineral content of a food expressed in relation to its energy (caloric) content.

Changes in food availability. Changes in agriculture, food preservation, and food processing over the past 50 years have multiplied the food items now available to the consumer. Frozen orange juice and frozen entrees designed for reheating in a microwave oven were unheard of during the early adult years of people now age 60 and over. The adoption of new food items by older adults suggests that nutritious foods not formerly a part of the diet may be accepted if introduced in a positive way.

Psychologic Aspects of Food Selection

Eating alone. Throughout life eating is a social activity. Loss of spouse or friends brings a loss of eating companions for the older individual who may now be regularly eating alone for the first time. It is important to recognize, however, that some older people are content living and eating alone and may have done so most of their lives, whereas others are very lonely and dependent. Mental depression or a need for attention may be expressed as a food problem and lead to significant weight loss.

Retirement. Retirement brings a change in lifestyle for both single adults and couples. For couples, both are at home and can participate in meal planning and preparation. Among one group of retired couples not only did husbands participate in food-related decisions but their participation also had nutritional implications.[57] The greater the

Nutrition Programs for the Elderly: Increasing Nutrient Density

Good nutrition plays a major role in keeping older people healthy and functioning. Many elderly Americans, however, are not eating as well as they should. For some it may be a matter of not eating appropriate foods and for others of not eating at all. A recent government report estimated that as many as one million older people living in their own homes may be malnourished. (See text for a discussion of the factors that can lead to poor food intake in the elderly.) Both congregate and home-delivered meals funded by Title III-C of the Older Americans Act contribute significantly to the food intake of many older people in the community. Careful attention to both the quantity and the nutrient density of the food provided may prevent the development of malnutrition in older people dependent on these meals.

Current regulations require that all Title III-C meals conform to the Dietary Guidelines for Americans and that each meal provide one third of the RDA. Based on the RDAs for men and women over age 50, a meal providing about one third of the day's energy needs should contain about 600 to 800 kcal. Although a diet containing no more than 30% fat is recommended for healthy adults, it is sometimes appropriate to allow a higher level of fat in Title III-C meals. Weight loss is a serious threat for older persons with chronic disease. Also, sauces and gravies help to maintain temperature and moisture in foods that must be transported. Finally, for many elderly people the Title III-C meal at noon is their major meal of the day, justifying a higher level of all nutrients. All meals should be planned to maximize nutrient density. Some suggestions are given below.

Main dish

Recipes including meat, fish, poultry, eggs, legumes, and peanut butter are good sources of protein, vitamin B_6, iron, and zinc; dishes made with cheese and milk supply protein, riboflavin, and calcium (if a dairy food is the major source of protein, iron and zinc will need to be supplied elsewhere in the meal).

Fruits and vegetables

Emphasize dark green and deep yellow vegetables and fruits, citrus, bananas, and potatoes to provide the carotenoids, vitamin B_6, ascorbic acid, folacin, potassium, magnesium, and fiber.

Enriched or whole grains

Popular whole grains include whole wheat bread, corn bread, and bran or oatmeal muffins; use whole grain toppings on casseroles or fruit desserts to contribute important vitamins and minerals.

Dessert

Choose plain fruit or baked fruit, pudding, custard, ice cream or baked products made with whole grains, raisins, sweet potatoes, pumpkin, and bananas; these add protein, iron, calcium, carotenoids, and other vitamins and minerals.

Milk

Offer lowfat or buttermilk to increase consumption; nonfat dry milk or cheese can be used to fortify soups, sauces, or mashed potatoes.

All nutrition programs are expected to ensure that their meals meet nutritional guidelines. Unfortunately, many programs do not have a nutritionist or dietitian to develop their menus or monitor food safety, meal costs, and overall food quality. If meals are to include the highest appropriate level of nutrients possible, the input of nutrition professionals is essential.

From Rhodes SS, editor: *Effective meal planning for the elderly nutrition program,* Chicago, 1991, American Dietetic Association; US Department of Health and Human Services: *Food and nutrition for life: malnutrition and older Americans,* Report by the Assistant Secretary for Aging, Administration on Aging, Washington, DC, December 1994.

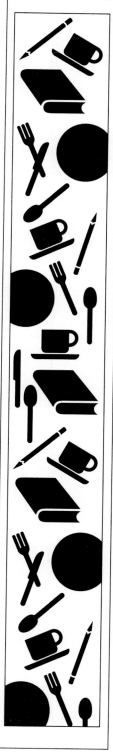

STRATEGIES FOR NUTRITION EDUCATION

husband's involvement in meal planning and food purchasing the better the diet. Nutrition education programs are often directed toward women, but leaders should make an effort to involve men. Men may be less bored with food activities and therefore more receptive and strongly influence food decisions within a retired family.

Mental disorders. Mental disorders and organic brain syndrome can cause confusion, irritability, and dementia. These individuals may forget to eat or attempt to eat nonedible substances. Patients with senile dementia often need to be fed. With these groups it is advantageous to have the main meal at noon, the time when they are most alert and attentive to food intake.

Physiologic Aspects of Food Selection

Sensory changes. The majority of older people in the community describe their appetite as good to excellent, but anorexia is a common side effect of many prescription drugs.[58] Taste and smell influence our selection and enjoyment of food. Sensitivity to the four basic tastes — sweet, sour, salty, and bitter — declines with age, although the effect of these changes on actual food tastes is not well understood. Even healthy older adults have a diminished sense of smell, which also influences taste. Dentures, poor oral hygiene, and certain prescription drugs contribute to **dysgeusia**, unpleasant or disordered taste. The addition of flavor enhancers (intense flavor mixtures added to foods) can compensate for sensory and olfactory losses and improve food palatability and acceptance. Retirement home residents (average age, 85 years) were found to consume more protein foods over a 3-week period when flavor enhancers were added and their intakes of protein, thiamin, and zinc were improved.[59] The tendency of older people to oversalt may be an attempt to strengthen flavor when taste is altered.

Dental problems. Periodontal disease, gingivitis, and tooth loss are thought to alter dietary patterns in older people, particularly in those who are **edentulous** (without any teeth). Economic difficulties can prevent the elderly from seeking professional services for preparation or repair of dentures. In general, lack of dentures influences the enjoyment of eating more than it does actual nutrient intake. Dairy products, eggs, ground beef, and well-cooked chicken and fish provide high quality protein for those with chewing problems. Fruit juices, peeled fresh fruit, and steamed vegetables are good sources of vitamins A and C and folacin.

Physical health. Older adults with limited vision or impaired mobility find it difficult to shop for groceries or prepare meals. Moving about the kitchen requires intense effort for a person who must grasp a cane or walker. Poor eyesight will preclude reading nutrition labels or package directions. Peeling vegetables or fruit is painful or even impossible for a person whose hands are crippled with arthritis. These problems increase an elderly person's dependence on preprepared items that often are high in sodium and fat and low in vitamins and trace minerals. Nutrition education programs should assist older people in making healthful choices from the preprepared foods available.

Special diets. Health problems or multiple risk factors for chronic disease sometimes necessitate a prescribed diet limited in energy, fat, sodium, or cholesterol. Diets also may be self-prescribed such as diets to alleviate arthritis obtained from a friend or salesperson. Elderly people need to be apprised of the dangers of following a "diabetic," low fat, or weight loss regimen that is not appropriate for them.

Living Arrangements and Food Intake

Cooking facilities. Older people living in their own homes usually have a working stove, oven, and refrigerator for food storage and preparation. Those who live in rented rooms with no kitchen privileges are forced to eat in restaurants or elsewhere. They may heat

---

Dysgeusia

(Gr *dys*, bad; *geusis*, taste) Abnormally perverted sense of taste or bad taste in the mouth.

Periodontal disease

(Gr *peri*, around + *odove*, tooth) Inflammation and breakdown of tissues and ligaments that surround the tooth and hold it in place; periodontal disease is often the cause of tooth loss in older people.

Gingivitis

(L *gingiva*, gum + Gr *itis*, inflammation) Condition of red, swollen and bleeding gums; can result from accumulation of plaque on the teeth or vitamin deficiency; sometimes occurs with diabetes mellitus.

Edentulous

(L *e*, without; *dens*, tooth) Absence of natural teeth.

foods on a hotplate or use a heating coil to heat water for soup or beverages. A small toaster oven or a microwave oven is a good investment for a person cooking for only one or two.

Food shopping. Lack of access to a grocery store is a problem for some older adults. In suburban or rural areas stores can be at some distance, requiring either a car or a ride. In urban settings an older person may have to ride a bus or walk to the store (Fig. 9-5). During winter months ice and snow create added difficulties for the elderly person who must carry bundles home. For inner city elderly the nearest store is often a convenience store with high prices and limited selection, since supermarkets in downtown areas are closing because of poor profit margins. Grocery delivery or shopping services are valuable programs for senior centers or volunteer community agencies.

Household size. It is true that older people who live and eat alone are not always motivated to prepare adequate meals; however, other lifestyle and personal factors including sex, age, economic status, and health status also have an influence. Davis and coworkers evaluated household size and dietary quality in over 4400 older adults who participated in the National Food Consumption Survey of the U.S. Dept. of Agriculture.[60] In women over age 64 living alone did not increase the likelihood of a poor diet; in fact 21% of the married women had poor diets but only 17% of the single women. The situation was completely reversed among the oldest men. One fourth of the single men over age 74 had poor diets, but only 9% of the married men. Older men may find it difficult to prepare their own meals as this was not expected of them as young adults.

Another important finding was that total energy intake was the most important factor in determining overall dietary quality. Those with poor diets also spent less money for food and were more likely to be in poor health (Table 9-3). The older people with diets low in nutrients did not make poorer food choices, they consumed less food in general. Older people living alone may skip meals if they are sick and have no one to help with food preparation. Congregate or home-delivered meals (see p. 413) may increase total food consumption among older people in poor health or with less money for food.

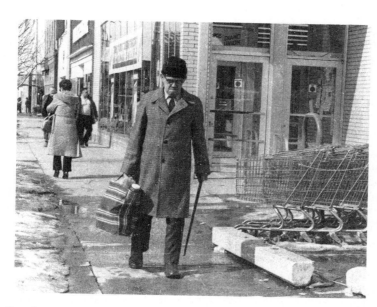

FIG. 9-5   Carrying groceries home from the store is a difficult task for older people.

TABLE 9-3 *Factors Affecting Dietary Quality in Older People*

	Men		Women	
	High Quality Diet	Poor Quality Diet	High Quality Diet	Poor Quality Diet
Energy intake (kcal)	2136	1222	1593	934
Money spent for food per week	$19.42	$16.09	$19.02	$15.70
Participants in poor health	29%	51%	32%	45%

Modified from Davis MA et al: Living arrangements and dietary quality of older US adults, *J Am Diet Assoc* 90:1667, 1990.

Economic Aspects of Food Selection

In general the average income of people over age 64 is increasing faster than that of people age 64 and under.[61] This statistic, however, obscures the fact that many older individuals live in poverty. Elderly women and minority elderly are more likely to be poor. Being poor influences food patterns in the following ways:

- Low income elderly have less money to spend for food
- Low income elderly are less likely to own a car and depend on nearby food stores that may have higher prices
- Low income elderly are more likely to live in the inner city or in a rural area where food is more expensive

Food stamps are available to older people meeting specific income guidelines. Food stamps increase food buying power and can improve dietary quality. Unfortunately, eligible older people are less likely to obtain food stamps than eligible younger people. Older persons may be less well informed about the program, may lack transportation to the appropriate office to enroll, or may not apply because of pride. Older households spend a larger proportion of their total income on food when compared with younger households, but people age 75 and over spend only half as much money per person for food as the general population.[61] Overall the elderly spend less money on food away from home. It is interesting to note, however, that McDonald's estimates that 30% of their customers are above age 60.[61]

Ethnic Diversity and Food Selection

Black elderly. Both income and ethnic group influence food selection and nutrient intake in older adults. Food records from NHANES III revealed that older black adults have lower **mean** intakes of energy, protein, and several important vitamins and minerals than older white adults (Table 9-4).[24,31] In an earlier survey black men and women above age 60 had higher intakes of vitamin A than white men and women of this age.[29] Older black families may have been eating more servings of cooked greens high in carotenes. Black women above age 70 consume the least amount of food, which may relate to their economic situation since 47% of elderly black women have incomes below the **poverty line.**[61]

Mexican-American elderly. For elderly Mexican-American women in Texas preferences for traditional ethnic foods rather than income influenced their food choices.[62] Foods eaten frequently were flour tortillas, legumes, poultry, eggs, and organ meats. They added saturated fats in cooking and had high intakes of sugar. Dairy foods, deep yellow fruits, and dark green vegetables were seldom used. Nutrient intakes obtained from a national

Mean
Mathematical term for the average numerical value of a group of numbers.

Poverty line
The minimum income required to provide the basic necessities of food, clothing, and shelter for an individual or family as determined by a US government agency.

TABLE 9-4   *Mean Nutrient Intakes in Older People From Several Ethnic Groups*

	White		Black		Mexican-American	
	Men	Women	Men	Women	Men	Women
Energy (kcal)	2118	1602	1882	1402	1963	1297
Protein (g)	85	64	78	56	78	56
Fat (g)	81	60	73	53	73	46
Vitamin A (RE)	1301	1116	914	959	1171	714
Vitamin C (mg)	106	112	87	105	111	84
Folacin (µg)	335	285	259	240	327	207
Calcium (mg)	895	743	609	477	837	606
Iron (mg)	16.8	13.2	13.2	10.6	14.6	10.6
Zinc (mg)	13.4	9.9	10.4	7.9	10.6	8.4

Data from US Department of Health and Human Services: *Energy and macronutrient intakes of persons ages 2 months and over in the United States: Third National Health and Nutrition Examination Survey*, Phase I, 1988-91, Advance Data from Vital and Health Statistics, Number 255, October 24, 1994, Hyattsville, Md, National Center for Health Statistics and US Department of Health and Human Services: *Dietary intake of vitamins, minerals, and fiber of persons age 2 months and over in the United States: Third National Health and Nutrition Examination Survey*, Phase I, 1988-91, Advance Data from Vital and Health Statistics, Number 258, November 14, 1994, Hyattsville, Md, National Center for Health Statistics.

sample of elderly Mexican-Americans reflect the selection of good protein sources such as poultry but also the need to increase servings of foods rich in zinc and for women vitamin A (see Table 9-4).[31]

Asian-American elderly. The Asian-American population has a low incidence of heart disease and diabetes mellitus. However, a recent dietary study of 169 Chinese elderly, 90 Korean elderly, and 50 Japanese elderly residing in a senior apartment complex found some serious nutrient deficiencies.[63] Over half of the Chinese and Korean women were consuming less than two thirds of the RDA for calcium. Energy intakes were low and vitamins A and C and riboflavin were problem nutrients in these women. All of the men and the Japanese women tended to have better diets. These elderly Asian-Americans had not adopted American food patterns; they continued to prefer their ethnic foods.

It is important to understand and respect the traditional food habits of older people who belong to particular ethnic groups. Recognizing the need to preserve these cultural patterns can help support the development of appropriate programs that meet the social and health needs of individual groups.

Food Selection Patterns and Nutrition Intervention

Food frequency patterns of older people reported from NHANES II indicate that bread and ready-to-eat cereals (both enriched and whole grain) are consumed regularly.[64-65] Eggs and luncheon meats were the most common foods from the meat or protein group. Orange juice, bananas, lettuce, and potatoes were the fruits and vegetables included most regularly in meal planning. Milk was used frequently but in relatively low amounts, possibly as a whitener in coffee and tea. Immediately apparent is the absence of a dark green leafy vegetable or other source of folacin and sources of precursors of vitamin A. Orange juice adds ascorbic acid, some folacin, and potassium to the diet, and bananas supply both potassium and vitamin B_6. Increased use of milk and other dairy products is needed, and whole grain products should be encouraged. Alternatives to luncheon meats, often high in fat and sodium and low in other nutrients, should be explored.

Nutrition education and dietary intervention for older adults can take place in senior centers, senior housing complexes, physician's offices, or health care facilities. An important source of nutrition information is the nutrition label. In fact the food label is used more frequently than any other source of nutrition information including newspaper or magazine articles, television programs, or materials from government agencies.[66] The consumer who is most likely to read food labels is a woman age 55 or older. Use of food labels tends to decrease in later years, most likely as a result of changes in vision. Individuals

---

The Warning Signs of poor nutritional health are often overlooked. Use this checklist to find out if you or someone you know is at nutritional risk.

DETERMINE YOUR NUTRITIONAL HEALTH

Read the statements below. Circle the number in the yes column for those that apply to you or someone you know. For each yes answer, score the number in the box. Total your nutritional score.

	YES
I have an illness or condition that made me change the kind and/or amount of food I eat.	2
I eat fewer than 2 meals per day.	3
I eat few fruits or vegetables, or milk products.	2
I have 3 or more drinks of beer, liquor or wine almost every day.	2
I have tooth or mouth problems that make it hard for me to eat.	2
I don't always have enough money to buy the food I need.	4
I eat alone most of the time.	1
I take 3 or more different prescribed or over-the-counter drugs a day.	1
Without wanting to, I have lost or gained 10 pounds in the last 6 months.	2
I am not always physically able to shop, cook and/or feed myself.	2
	TOTAL

Total Your Nutritional Score. If it's —

0-2   **Good!** Recheck your nutritional score in 6 months.

3-5   **You are at moderate nutritional risk.** See what can be done to improve your eating habits and lifestyle. Your office on aging, senior nutrition program, senior citizens center or health department can help. Recheck your nutritional score in 3 months.

6 or more   **You are at high nutritional risk.** Bring this checklist the next time you see your doctor, dietitian or other qualified health or social service professional. Talk with them about any problems you may have. Ask for help to improve your nutritional health.

These materials developed and distributed by the Nutrition Screening Initiative, a project of:

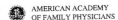 AMERICAN ACADEMY OF FAMILY PHYSICIANS

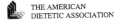 THE AMERICAN DIETETIC ASSOCIATION

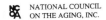 NATIONAL COUNCIL ON THE AGING, INC.

Remember that warning signs suggest risk, but do not represent diagnosis of any condition. Turn the page to learn more about the Warning Signs of poor nutritional health.

FIG. 9-6   Determine Your Nutritional Health Checklist.

From *Nutrition Screening Initiative*, American Academy of Family Physicians, American Dietetic Association, National Council on Aging, Ross Products Division, Abbott Laboratories.

on special diets, whether self-initiated or prescribed by a health professional, are more likely to pay attention to the food label when choosing products. Guidance in using the food label should always be a part of nutrition education for older adults.

Nutrition Screening Initiative

An important task for the nutrition professional is the identification of those elderly people who have a less than optimum nutrient intake. When these individuals are identified, nutrition intervention can prevent any further nutrient-related deterioration in health. The Nutrition Screening Initiative is a national effort to promote the identification of older people at risk and was developed through a joint effort of the American Dietetic Association, the American Academy of Family Physicians, and the National Council on the Aging. A panel of experts developed and field tested a checklist of factors that are related to nutritional status in older people (Fig. 9-6).[67] Older adults with scores of 6 or higher are more likely to have low nutrient intakes and increased risk of chronic disease. They should be referred to a nutrition or other health professional for functional and nutritional assessment, diet planning, and information regarding appropriate social and food support services (see below). The Determine Your Nutritional Health checklist can be administered wherever older people are found and is a good starting point for discussing nutrition and health. It should be completed at least once yearly to identify any nutrition-related problems that may be developing.

NUTRITION PROGRAMS FOR OLDER PEOPLE
Nutrition and the Continuum of Care

The continuum of care refers to the range of nutrition, health, social, and personal services required to support independent living and personal well-being at the highest possible level. These support services provide **long-term care** in institutional or community settings. In a community setting nutrition support services provided by family members, neighbors, or community agencies allow the older person with some limitation of activity to continue to live independently. Such services may take the form of a ride to the grocery store or delivery of meals by a community agency. Congregate meals that provide both a nutritious meal and a social experience help to maintain health and well-being in the relatively fit adult.

Long-term care
Medical, health, personal, or homemaking services provided within an institution or in the community for older adults with some limitation of activity who are no longer able to completely care for their own needs.

National Nutrition Program for the Elderly (Title III-C)

Basic authorization. The Older Americans Act of 1965, as amended, is the major legislation providing programs for persons age 60 and over. When establishing the nutrition program in 1972, Congress directed attention to elderly persons who might not eat adequately because of the following:
- Cannot afford to do so
- Lack the skills to select and prepare nourishing meals
- Have limited mobility that hinders shopping and cooking
- Feel rejected and lonely and lack incentive to cook and eat alone

The congregate meal program, funded under **Title III-C** of the Older Americans Act was intended to make meals available at little or no cost in a social setting. It operates through meal sites in community or recreation centers, municipal buildings, public housing, senior citizens centers, or churches. Meals are served 5 days a week in urban settings but fewer days in rural locations. Important criteria in selecting a location are accessibility and familiarity to the older people in the community. Close to 150 million congregate meals are served each year.[68] See the box on p. 414 that describes a potential client for a congregate meal program in an urban community.

Title III-C
The statute of the Older Americans Act authorizing congregate and home-delivered meals for people 60 years of age and over.

CASE STUDY

The Needs of an Elderly Woman Living Alone

Miss Evans has just celebrated her 80th birthday. She is 65 inches tall, weighs 158 pounds, and has no major health problems other than arthritis. She uses aspirin regularly for pain. Miss Evans lives in a subsidized high-rise apartment complex for senior citizens with a small efficiency kitchen. She has a two-unit range top, small oven, and small refrigerator but very limited storage space for frozen or shelf-stable items. She prepares all her own meals and eats alone. She usually has toast and coffee for breakfast and either a bowl of cereal or a peanut butter sandwich for lunch. She does not drink any milk except with her cereal but is fond of cheese. She makes a lot of stews, often buying chicken when it is on sale. She likes all fruits and vegetables but uses mostly canned items because they are cheaper than fresh. The amount of money she can spend for food is very limited. She likes whole wheat bread although her favorite brand is higher in cost than other breads. Miss Evans had been shopping about twice a week at a supermarket located about one mile from her apartment, traveling by bus. Since a recent fall, she is afraid to ride the bus alone, and now her nephew shops for her once every 2 weeks. In between she buys necessary items at a convenience store about one city block from her apartment, but the prices there are much higher. She has been feeling very tired lately and has lost her appetite, although she has well-fitting dentures and is able to eat anything she wishes. She weighs herself every week and noticed that she lost 5 pounds over the past month.

Questions for analysis
1. What are the socioeconomic or lifestyle factors that influence Miss Evan's food intake?
2. What are the physiological factors that may influence her food intake?
3. Which nutrients appear to be lacking in her dietary pattern?
4. What would you recommend to improve her food intake?
5. What are some food programs that would assist Miss Evans in remaining independent?

Since the congregate meal program was begun, the older population has changed both in age and general characteristics. There are more people age 75 and over, and these individuals are more likely to be frail, chronically ill, and homebound. To meet this emerging need, amendments to the Older Americans Act have authorized increased funds for home-delivered meals. About 40% of the meals now funded under Title III-C are home-delivered. This represents about 100 million meals per year.[68]

Home-Delivered Meals

General organization. Meal delivery programs have been developed by community nonprofit organizations and health and social service agencies such as hospitals, churches, nursing homes, and visiting nurses associations. Most receive some funding through the Older Americans Act. Meals are delivered by volunteers who often pay their own transportation costs. Meal delivery programs operate on weekdays and deliver a hot meal at noon and sometimes a cold meal also to be eaten later. Some programs include additional food on Friday to provide for weekend days. But a recent survey of 430 meal delivery programs revealed that less than half provide weekend meals.[69] Those programs that do usually deliver additional frozen meals to be used on nondelivery days. Programs in areas with a high proportion of minority elderly are the least likely to offer weekend meals. No program provides meals on all days or for all meals of the day.

Eligibility requirements. Older people can request meal delivery directly or be referred by a family member, physician, visiting nurse, nutrition professional, outreach worker, or social worker. Programs receiving Title III-C funding require that (1) recipients be age 60 or over and (2) recipients be unable to leave their homes because of disability or other extenuating circumstance. A two-person household may be in need of home-delivered meals if one person is so burdened caring for an invalid spouse that he or she has little time, incentive, or energy to prepare adequate meals. Implementation of the **diagnosis-related group** (DRG) guidelines has resulted in the earlier release of older patients from medical facilities and a dramatic increase in requests for home-delivered meals.

Innovative approaches to food delivery. As the number of homebound elderly continues to escalate, the cost of daily meal delivery is rapidly becoming prohibitive. Meal delivery in rural areas is especially burdensome in cost and has the added problem of maintaining foods at appropriate temperatures over an extended delivery time. One alternative to daily delivery of hot meals is weekly delivery of several frozen meals. This also allows recipients to choose what they want to eat on a particular day and at what time. For homebound persons who are able to move about within their homes, groceries can supplement either frozen or hot meals. Canned, dehydrated, and freeze-dried foods, fruit, and milk are appropriate supplementary foods for weekends or other nondelivery days. Analysis of the relative cost-effectiveness and cost-benefit of alternative food delivery systems should be a priority as we seek to improve community-based, long-term care.

> **Diagnosis related group (DRG)**
> A US government cost-containment management classification scheme for predesignation of Medicare payments based on specific diagnosis categories of disease.

Nutrition Standards for Meals Programs

Meals provided under Title III-C funding are expected to contain one third of the RDA for persons over age 50. If two or three meals are provided, the total for the day should equal 67% or 100% of the RDA, respectively, thereby allowing some flexibility within individual meals. Limited funding and a lack of professionally trained personnel make modified diets impractical in most locations. The meal provided for all participants is likely to be acceptable for those following a diabetic plan or those who must limit their fat intake if portion size is controlled, skim milk is available, and fruit is offered as an alternative to a high caloric dessert. General modifications limiting sodium and sugar are a potential benefit to all participants. Because weight loss is a serious threat to many elderly people, menus containing up to 35% of total kilocalories as fat are generally appropriate in meal programs for the elderly.[70]

Nutrition Program Evaluation

Congregate meals. Kohrs and coworkers evaluated the impact of congregate meals on the nutritional status of 466 rural elderly persons.[71] They reported that menus provided considerably more than one third of the RDA for many nutrients calculated. For women the meals contained at least 80% of the RDA for protein, vitamins A and C, and riboflavin, and at least 40% of the RDA for energy, calcium, iron, and the B vitamins. For men the protein, vitamins A and C, and energy content of the menus was between 40% and 67% of the RDA. Women who lived alone and older people with limited educations and lower incomes consumed a greater share of their daily nutrients at the meal site. For elderly people living in poverty, the negative effect of low income on dietary nutrient quality was ameliorated by the congregate meal. Calcium and vitamin A, nutrients often in short supply in the diets of older people, were most influenced by participation.

Home-delivered meals. Homebound elderly with physical disabilities are at high risk for poor diets. A California study evaluated the daily nutrient intake of 48 urban and 47 rural elderly people between the ages of 60 and 94 who were receiving home-delivered meals.[72] About 50% of the participants needed help with cooking, and 77% needed help with grocery shopping. Although mean intakes of many nutrients met or exceeded the RDA, mean intakes of energy, vitamin B_6, calcium, copper, magnesium, and zinc fell below. Also, the diets of many individuals were low in several nutrients; 25% of the recipients had intakes below two thirds of the RDA for up to 12 nutrients. Home-delivered meals allow homebound elderly to enjoy a greater variety of food; however, one delivered meal each day will not raise intakes of important nutrients to desired levels if other meals are sparse.

Summary

People above age 60 are increasing in number faster than any other segment of the population. Chronic diseases including heart disease, cancer, and stroke have become the major causes of death as the development of antibiotics has reduced dramatically the deaths resulting from infectious diseases. Normal aging and the effects of chronic disease bring about changes in major organ systems and declining heart, renal, and pulmonary function. Loss of skeletal muscle contributes to the observed decline in resting energy metabolism. These physiological changes influence the energy and nutrient requirements of the aging adult. Unfortunately, the nutrient needs of both healthy and physically impaired older people are poorly understood; the current RDAs for those above age 50 have been extrapolated from the recommendations for young adults and overlook the differences between the various age groups. Current research studies suggest that the present RDAs for protein, pyridoxine, and vitamin D are too low to maintain optimum status in relatively healthy elderly people. Intakes of calcium at levels above the RDA of 800 mg may reduce bone loss and the risk of osteoporosis and bone fractures. The major factor influencing dietary adequacy in older people is total energy intake. Loneliness, poverty, physical disability, and gastrointestinal side effects of prescription and over-the-counter drugs can reduce food intake. Inappropriate use of alcohol or psychotropic drugs can negatively affect food intake and nutrient utilization. Community nutrition programs funded under the Older American Act, including congregate and home-delivered meals, make positive contributions to the nutritional status of elderly participants.

Review Questions

1. What factors have led to the significant increase in life expectancy that has occurred since 1900? Why has life expectancy at age 65 not changed to the same extent over this period?
2. Describe several physiological changes that occur with normal aging. What is a nutritional implication of each?
3. What are some limitations of the current RDAs for older persons? How do the RDAs for persons over age 50 differ from those for younger adults?
4. What are the components of the energy requirement? How and why do they change with aging? What are the problems associated with low energy intake?
5. The requirements for protein, vitamin D, vitamin B_6, and vitamin B_{12} may increase in older adulthood. What evidence do we have to support this idea? What foods would you recommend to ensure appropriate intake and utilization of these nutrients?
6. Explain the difference between osteoporosis and osteomalacia. What are the physiological and dietary factors that are associated with the development of

osteoporosis? What recommendations would you give to a postmenopausal woman who is concerned about her bone health?

7. Describe the mechanisms by which drugs can adversely affect nutritional status. Describe two addictive behaviors that occur in older people. What circumstances might lead to these behaviors?

8. How do age, energy intake, sex, physical disability, poverty, household size, and ethnic group influence nutrient intake in older people? Who is most vulnerable?

9. Describe several types of community nutrition programs that serve older people. What levels of nutrient intake are provided by each?

10. You receive a telephone call from a woman who is concerned about her elderly mother who appears to have an inadequate diet. What screening tool could you use to assess the mother's nutritional risk? What questions would you ask? What recommendations would you offer to improve nutrient intake if needed?

References

1. US Senate Special Committee on Aging: *Aging America: trends and projections (annotated)*, Serial No 101-J, Washington, DC, 1990, US Government Printing Office.

2. US Department of Health and Human Services: *Vital statistics of the United States, 1989, Life tables*, Vol II, Sec 6, DHHS Pub No (PHS) 93-1104, Hyattsville, Md, 1992, US Public Health Service.

3. Masoro EJ, Shimokawa I, Yu BP: Retardation of the aging processes in rats by food restriction, *Ann N Y Acad Sci* 621:337, 1991.

4. Kelley L, Ohlson MA, Harper LJ: Food selection and well-being of aging women, *J Am Diet Assoc* 33:466, 1957.

5. Schlenker ED: *Nutritional status of older women*, PhD dissertation, Michigan State University, East Lansing, Mich, 1976.

6. Breslow L, Breslow N: Health practice and disability: some evidence from Alameda County, *Prev Med* 22:86, 1993.

7. Johnson MA et al: Nutritional patterns of centenarians, *Int J Aging Hum Dev* 34(1):57, 1992.

8. US Department of Health and Human Services: *Nutrition monitoring in the United States. Chartbook I. Selected findings from the National Nutrition Monitoring and Related Research Program*, DHHS Pub No (PHS) 93-1255-2, 1993, Hyattsville, Md, US Public Health Service.

9. Van Itallie TB, Lew EA: *Health implications of overweight in the elderly*. In Prinsley DM, Sandstead HH, editors: *Nutrition and aging: progress in clinical and biological research*, vol 326, New York, 1990, Alan R Liss.

10. Harris T et al: Body mass index and mortality among nonsmoking older persons, *JAMA* 259 (10):1520, 1988.

11. Shock NW et al: *Normal human aging: The Baltimore Longitudinal Study of Aging*, NIH Pub No 84-2450, Washington, DC, 1984, US Government Printing Office.

12. National High Blood Pressure Education Program Working Group: National high blood pressure education program working group report on hypertension in the elderly, *Hypertension* 23:275, 1994.

13. Rolls BJ, Phillips PA: Aging and disturbances of thirst and fluid balance, *Nutr Rev* 48:137, 1990.

14. Russell RM: Changes in gastrointestinal function attributed to aging, *Am J Clin Nutr* 55:1203S, 1992.

15. Wolfsen CR et al: Constipation in the daily lives of frail elderly people, *Arch Fam Med* 2:853, 1993.

16. Rorick MH, Scrimshaw NS: Comparative tolerance of elderly from differing ethnic backgrounds to lactose-containing and lactose-free dairy drinks: A double-blind study, *J Gerontol* 34:191, 1979.

17. Werner I, Hambraeus L: *The digestive capacity of elderly people*. In Carlson, LA, editor: *Nutrition in old age*, Symposia Swedish Nutrition Foundation X, Stockholm, 1972, Almqvist and Wiksell.

18. Food and Nutrition Board: *Recommended Dietary Allowances,* ed 10, Washington, DC, 1989, National Academy of Sciences.

19. Blumberg J: Nutrient requirements of the healthy elderly—should there be specific RDAs, *Nutr Rev* 52:515, 1994.

20. James WPT, Ralph A, Ferro-Luzzi A: *Energy needs of the elderly: a new approach.* In Munro HN, Danford DE, editors: *Nutrition, aging, and the elderly, human nutrition, a comprehensive treatise,* vol 6, New York, 1989, Plenum Press.

21. Elahi VK et al: A longitudinal study of nutritional intake in men, *J Gerontol* 38:162, 1983.

22. Roberts SB et al: What are the dietary energy needs of elderly adults, *Int J Obesity* 16:969, 1992.

23. Voorrips LE et al: Energy expenditure at rest and during standardized activities: a comparison between elderly and middle-aged women, *Am J Clin Nutr* 58:15, 1993.

24. US Department of Health and Human Services: *Energy and macronutrient intakes of persons ages 2 months and over in the United States: Third National Health and Nutrition Examination Survey, Phase I, 1988-91, Advance Data from Vital and Health Statistics,* Number 255, Oct. 24, 1994, Hyattsville, Md, National Center for Health Statistics.

25. McGandy RB et al: Nutritional status survey of healthy noninstitutionalized elderly: Nutrient intakes from three-day diet records and nutrient supplements, *Nutr Res* 6:785, 1986.

26. Evans WJ: Exercise, nutrition, and aging, *J Nutr* 122:796, 1992.

27. Asciutti-Moura LS et al: Fatty acid composition of serum lipids and its relation to diet in an elderly institutionalized population, *Am J Clin Nutr* 48:980, 1988.

28. Campbell WW et al: Increased protein requirements in elderly people: new data and retrospective assessments, *Am J Clin Nutr* 60:501, 1994.

29. US Department of Health and Human Services: *Dietary intake source data: United States 1976-80,* DHHS Pub No (PHS) 83:1681, Washington, DC, 1983, US Government Printing Office.

30. Stauber PM et al: A longitudinal study of the relationship between vitamin A supplementation and plasma retinol, retinol esters, and liver enzyme activities in a healthy elderly population, *Am J Clin Nutr* 54:878, 1991.

31. US Department of Health and Human Services: *Dietary intake of vitamins, minerals, and fiber of persons ages 2 months and over in the United States: Third National Health and Nutrition Examination Survey, Phase I, 1988-91, Advance Data from Vital and Health Statistics,* Number 258, Nov. 14, 1994, Hyattsville, Md, National Center for Health Statistics.

32. Looker AC, Johnson CL, Underwood BA: Serum retinol levels of persons aged 4 to 74 years from three Hispanic groups, *Am J Clin Nutr* 48:1490, 1988.

33. Meydani SN et al: Vitamin E supplementation enhances cell-mediated immunity in healthy elderly subjects, *Am J Clin Nutr* 52:557, 1990.

34. Dawson-Hughes B et al: Effect of vitamin D supplementation on wintertime and overall bone loss in healthy postmenopausal women, *Ann Intern Med* 115:505, 1991.

35. Webb AR et al: An evaluation of the relative contributions of exposure to sunlight and of diet to the circulating concentrations of 25-hydroxyvitamin D in an elderly nursing home population in Boston, *Am J Clin Nutr* 51:1075, 1990.

36. Smidt LJ et al: Influence of thiamin supplementation on the health and general well-being of an elderly Irish population with marginal thiamin deficiency, *J Gerontol* 46:M16, 1991.

37. VanderJaqt DJ, Garry PJ, Bhagavan HN: Ascorbic acid intake and plasma levels in healthy elderly people, *Am J Clin Nutr* 46:290, 1987.

38. Blanchard J: Effects of gender on vitamin C pharmacokinetics in man, *J Am Coll Nutr* 10:453, 1991.

39. Manore MM et al: Plasma pyridoxal 5-phosphate concentration and dietary vitamin B_6 intake in free-living, low-income elderly people, *Am J Clin Nutr* 50:339, 1989.

40. Ribaya-Mercado JD et al: Vitamin B_6 requirements of elderly men and women, *J Nutr* 121:1062, 1991.

41. Lindenbaum J et al: Prevalence of cobalamin deficiency in the Framingham elderly population, *Am J Clin Nutr* 60:2, 1994.

42. Reid IR et al: Effect of calcium supplementation on bone loss in postmenopausal women, *N Engl J Med* 328:460, 1993.

43. Dawson-Hughes B: Calcium supplementation and bone loss: a review of controlled clinical trials, *Am J Clin Nutr* 54:2745, 1991.

44. Aloia JF et al: Calcium supplementation with and without hormone replacement therapy to prevent postmenopausal bone loss, *Ann Intern Med* 120:97, 1994.

45. Gibson RS et al: Dietary chromium and manganese intakes of a selected sample of Canadian elderly women, *Hum Nutr Appl Nutr* 39A:43, 1985.

46. Sandstead H et al: Zinc nutriture in the elderly in relation to taste acuity, immune response, and wound healing, *Am J Clin Nutr* 36:1046, 1982.

47. Goren S, Siverstein LJ, Gonzales N: A survey of food service managers of Washington State boarding homes for the elderly, *J Nutr Elderly* 12(3):27, 1993.

48. Parker DR et al: Relationship of dietary saturated fatty acids and body habitus to serum insulin concentrations: The Normative Aging Study, *Am J Clin Nutr* 58:129, 1993.

49. Riggs BL, Melton LJ: Involutional osteoporosis, *N Engl J Med* 314:1676, 1986.

50. Riggs BL et al: Clinical trial of fluoride therapy in postmenopausal osteoporosis women: extended observations and additional analysis, *J Bone Miner Res* 9:265, 1994.

51. US Department of Health and Human Services: *Nutrition monitoring in the United States: an update report on nutrition monitoring,* DHHS Pub No (PHS) 89-1255, Hyattsville, Md, 1989, US Government Printing Office.

52. Lindenbaum J et al: Neuropsychiatric disorders caused by cobalamin deficiency in the absence of anemia or macrocytosis, *N Engl J Med* 318:1720, 1988.

53. Chrischilles EA et al: Use of medications by persons 65 and over: data from the established populations for epidemiologic studies of the elderly, *J Gerontol* 47(5):M137, 1992.

54. Mares-Perlman JA et al: Nutrient supplements contribute to the dietary intake of middle- and older-aged adult residents of Beaver Dam, Wisconsin, *J Nutr* 123:176, 1993.

55. Garry PJ et al: Nutritional status in a healthy elderly population: dietary and supplemental intakes, *Am J Clin Nutr* 36(2):319, 1982.

56. Solomon K et al: Alcoholism and prescription drug abuse in the elderly: St Louis University Grand Rounds, *J Am Geriatr Soc* 41:57, 1993.

57. Schafer RB, Keith PM: Social-psychological factors in the dietary quality of married and single elderly, *J Am Diet Assoc* 81:30, 1982.

58. US Department of Health and Human Services: *Health: United States, 1990,* DHHS Pub No (PHS) 91-1232, Hyattsville, Md, 1991, US Government Printing Office.

59. Schiffman S, Warwick ZS: Effect of flavor enhancement of foods for the elderly on nutritional status: food intake, biochemical indices, and anthropometric measures, *Physiol Behav* 53:395, 1993.

60. Davis MA et al: Living arrangements and dietary quality of older US adults, *J Am Diet Assoc* 90:1667, 1990.

61. Senauer B, Asp E, Kinsey J: *Food trends and the changing consumer,* St. Paul, Minn, 1991, Eagen Press.

62. Bartholomew AM et al: Food frequency intakes and sociodemographic factors of elderly Mexican-Americans and nonHispanic whites, *J Am Diet Assoc* 90:1693, 1990.

63. Kim KA et al: Nutritional status of Chinese, Korean, and Japanese-American elderly, *J Am Diet Assoc* 93:1416, 1993.

64. Murphy SP, Everett DF, Dresser CM: Food group consumption reported by the elderly during the NHANES I Epidemiologic Followup Study, *J Nutr Educ* 21:214, 1989.

65. Fanelli MT, Stevenhagen KS: Characterizing consumption patterns by food frequency methods: core foods and variety of foods in diets of older Americans, *J Am Diet Assoc* 85:1570, 1985.

66. Bender MM, Derby BM: Prevalence of reading nutrition and ingredient information on food labels among adult Americans: 1982-1988, *J Nutr Ed* 24(6):292, 1992.

67. White JV et al: Nutrition screening initiative: development and implementation of the public awareness checklist and screening tools, *J Am Diet Assoc* 92:163, 1992.

68. O'Shaughnessy C: *Older Americans Act nutrition program: CRS report for Congress,* Congressional Research Service, Washington, DC, Jan. 19, 1990.

69. Balsam AL et al: Weekend home-delivered meals in elderly nutrition programs, *J Am Diet Assoc* 92:1125, 1992.

70. Rhodes SS, editor: *Effective menu planning for the elderly nutrition program,* Chicago, 1991, The American Dietetic Association.

71. Kohrs MB, O'Hanlon P, Eklund D: Title VII nutrition program for the elderly: contribution to one day's dietary intake, *J Am Diet Assoc* 72:487, 1978.

72. Stevens DA, Grivetti LE, McDonald RB: Nutrient intake of urban and rural elderly receiving home-delivered meals, *J Am Diet Assoc* 92:714, 1992.

Further Readings

Butterworth DE et al: Exercise training and nutrient intake in elderly women, *J Am Diet Assoc* 93:653, 1993.

This article describes a study of nutrient intake patterns in sedentary elderly women as compared with those who began a program of moderate exercise involving walking or calisthenics. Implications for nutrition counseling of sedentary and physically active older people are discussed.

Nevitt MC, Cummings SR, and the Study of Osteoporotic Fractures Research Group: Type of fall and risk of hip and wrist fractures: the study of osteoporotic fractures, *J Am Geriatr Soc* 41:1226, 1993.

Exercise and strength training appear to reduce falls and the likelihood of a bone fracture in elderly people. This study provides an interesting analysis of these relationships with recommendations for patient education.

Barrett-Connor E, Chun Chang J, Edelstein SL: Coffee-associated osteoporosis offset by daily milk consumption: The Rancho Bernardo Study, *JAMA* 271:280, 1994.

Caffeine intake in coffee has been associated with low bone mass. This study describes how increased milk consumption can offset that loss.

Blumberg JB: Changing nutrient requirements in older adults, *Nutr Today* 27(5):15, 1992.

This review discusses recent evidence that supports a reconsideration of the Recommended Dietary Allowances for older people.

Davis SA et al: Living arrangements and dietary quality of older US adults, *J Am Diet Assoc* 90:1667, 1990.

This article provides a comprehensive discussion of the many sociologic and economic factors that influence nutrient intake in people age 55 and over in the United States.

Goldberg JP, Gershoff SN, McGandy RB: Appropriate topics for nutrition education for the elderly, *J Nutr Educ* 22:303, 1990.

This article is a source of many good ideas for nutrition education topics and methods of presentation when working with older people.

Popkin BM, Haines PS, Patterson RE: Dietary changes in older Americans, 1977-1987, *J Am Diet Assoc* 55:823, 1992.

This article provides an overview of the changes in dietary choices by older people that have occurred over this 10-year period and the implications for nutrition education.

Kim I et al: Vitamin and mineral supplement use and mortality in a US cohort, *Am J Public Health* 83:546, 1993.

Those who promote inappropriate use of vitamin and mineral supplements often suggest that this practice will prevent illness or death. This study examined supplement use and subsequent mortality in a US adult population.

Levenson DI, Bockman RS: A review of calcium preparations, *Nutr Rev* 52(7):221, 1994.
This article provides a review of all aspects of calcium supplements including both positive and adverse physiological effects, bioavailability, and medical conditions that affect their use.

Astrand PO: Physical activity and fitness, *Am J Clin Nutr* 55(Suppl):1231S, 1992.
This article came from a symposium on Aging: Nutrition and the Quality of Life. It provides an overview of strength and endurance training, their physiological effects in reducing chronic disease risk, and prescriptions for exercise in the elderly.

Jackson TM: Nutrition research and the elderly, US Administration on Aging Symposium, *Nutr Rev* 52 (No 8, Part II):S1-S53, 1994.
This issue of Nutrition Reviews is devoted to nutritional issues and concerns of the elderly including nutrient requirements, food preferences, nutrition screening, and disease prevention.

Physical Growth
NCHS Percentiles

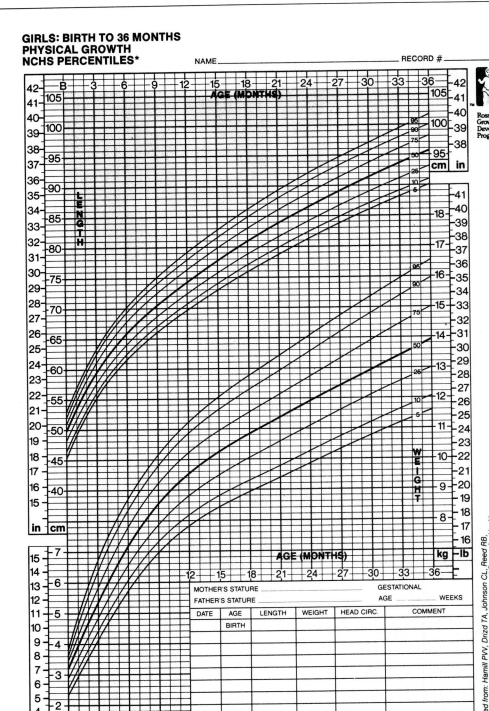

GIRLS: BIRTH TO 36 MONTHS
PHYSICAL GROWTH
NCHS PERCENTILES*

NAME _____ RECORD # _____

*Adapted from: Hamill PVV, Drizd TA, Johnson CL, Reed RB, Roche AF, Moore WM: Physical growth: National Center for Health Statistics percentiles. AM J CLIN NUTR 32:607-629, 1979. Data from the Fels Research Institute, Wright State University School of Medicine. Yellow Springs, Ohio.

© 1982 ROSS LABORATORIES

Ross
Growth &
Development
Program

MOTHER'S STATURE _____ GESTATIONAL
FATHER'S STATURE _____ AGE _____ WEEKS

DATE	AGE	LENGTH	WEIGHT	HEAD CIRC.	COMMENT
	BIRTH				

BOYS: BIRTH TO 36 MONTHS
PHYSICAL GROWTH
NCHS PERCENTILES*

NAME_____ RECORD #_____

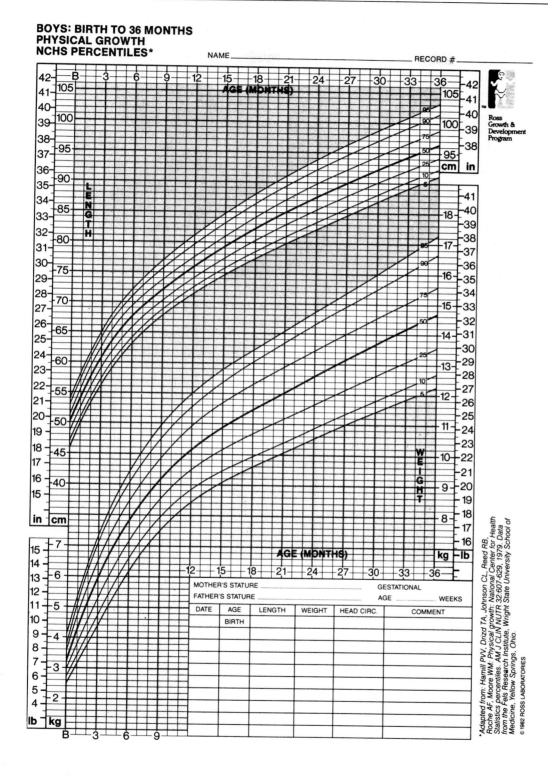

MOTHER'S STATURE _____ GESTATIONAL
FATHER'S STATURE _____ AGE _____ WEEKS

DATE	AGE	LENGTH	WEIGHT	HEAD CIRC.	COMMENT
	BIRTH				

Ross
Growth &
Development
Program

Adapted from: Hamill PVV, Drizd TA, Johnson CL, Reed RB, Roche AF, Moore WM: Physical growth: National Center for Health Statistics percentiles. AM J CLIN NUTR 32:607-629, 1979. Data from the Fels Research Institute, Wright State University School of Medicine, Yellow Springs, Ohio.

GIRLS: BIRTH TO 36 MONTHS
PHYSICAL GROWTH
NCHS PERCENTILES*

NAME _____   RECORD # _____

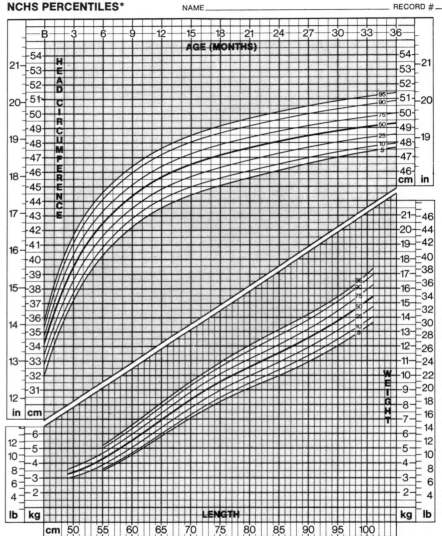

*Adapted from: Hamill PVV, Drizd TA, Johnson CL, Reed RB, Roche AF, Moore WM: Physical growth: National Center for Health Statistics percentiles. AM J CLIN NUTR 32:607-629, 1979. Data from the Fels Research Institute, Wright State University School of Medicine, Yellow Springs, Ohio.

© 1982 ROSS LABORATORIES

DATE	AGE	LENGTH	WEIGHT	HEAD CIRC.	COMMENT

Recommend the formulation you prefer
with the name you trust

SIMILAC®
SIMILAC® WITH IRON
SIMILAC® WITH WHEY
Infant Formulas

The ISOMIL® System of
Soy Protein Formulas

ADVANCE®
Nutritional Beverage

ROSS LABORATORIES
COLUMBUS, OHIO 43216
Division of Abbott Laboratories, USA

G106/JUNE 1983   LITHO IN USA

BOYS: BIRTH TO 36 MONTHS
PHYSICAL GROWTH
NCHS PERCENTILES*

NAME _____   RECORD # _____

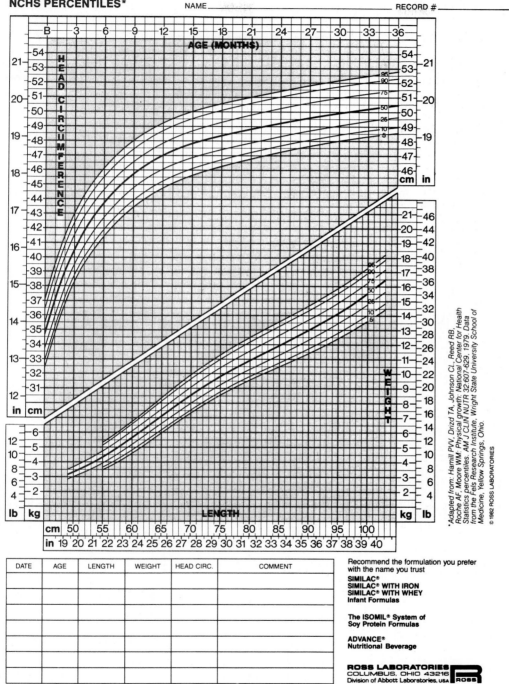

Adapted from: Hamill PVV, Drizd TA, Johnson CL, Reed RB, Roche AF, Moore WM. Physical growth: National Center for Health Statistics percentiles. AM J CLIN NUTR 32:607-629, 1979. Data from the Fels Research Institute, Wright State University School of Medicine, Yellow Springs, Ohio.
© 1982 ROSS LABORATORIES

DATE	AGE	LENGTH	WEIGHT	HEAD CIRC.	COMMENT

GIRLS: 2 TO 18 YEARS
PHYSICAL GROWTH
NCHS PERCENTILES*

NAME_____ RECORD #_____

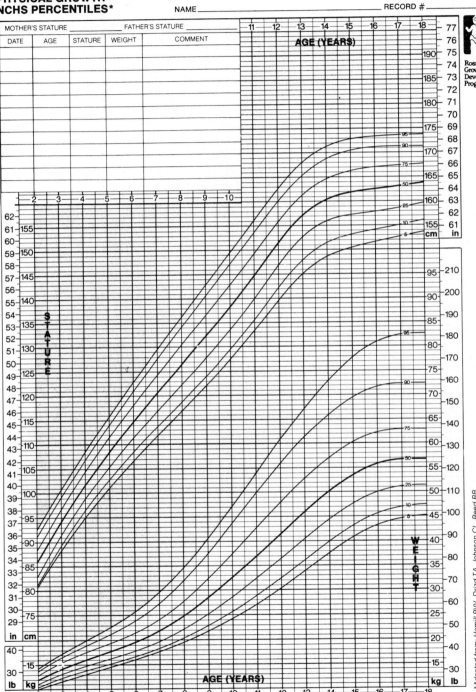

Adapted from: Hamill PVV, Drizd TA, Johnson CL, Reed RB, Roche AF, Moore WM: Physical growth: National Center for Health Statistics percentiles. AM J CLIN NUTR 32:607-629, 1979. Data from the National Center for Health Statistics (NCHS) Hyattsville, Maryland.

© 1982 ROSS LABORATORIES

Ross
Growth &
Development
Program

BOYS: 2 TO 18 YEARS
PHYSICAL GROWTH
NCHS PERCENTILES*

NAME _____ RECORD # _____

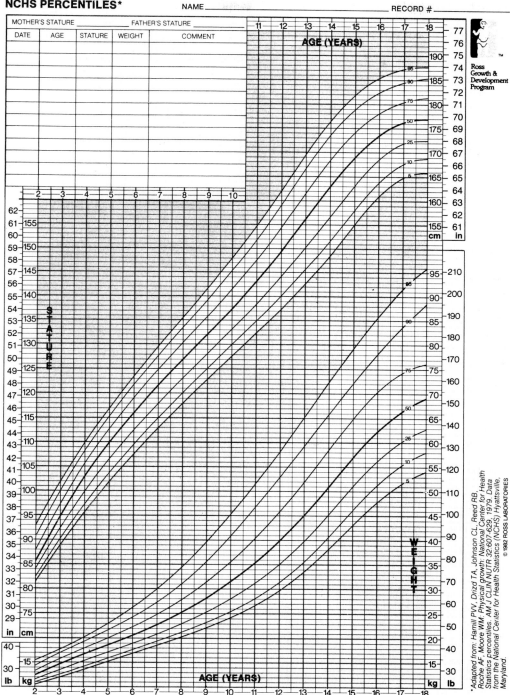

Ross
Growth &
Development
Program

GIRLS: PREPUBESCENT
PHYSICAL GROWTH
NCHS PERCENTILES*

NAME_____ RECORD #_____

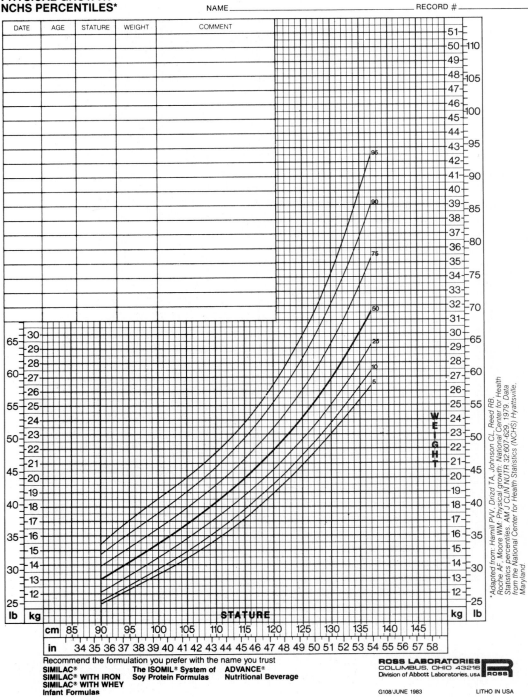

DATE	AGE	STATURE	WEIGHT	COMMENT

STATURE

cm 85 90 95 100 105 110 115 120 125 130 135 140 145

in 34 35 36 37 38 39 40 41 42 43 44 45 46 47 48 49 50 51 52 53 54 55 56 57 58

*Adapted from: Hamill PVV, Drizd TA, Johnson CL, Reed RB, Roche AF, Moore WM: Physical growth: National Center for Health Statistics percentiles. AM J CLIN NUTR 32:607-629, 1979. Data from the National Center for Health Statistics (NCHS) Hyattsville, Maryland.

© 1982 ROSS LABORATORIES

Recommend the formulation you prefer with the name you trust

SIMILAC®
SIMILAC® WITH IRON
SIMILAC® WITH WHEY
Infant Formulas

The **ISOMIL®** System of
Soy Protein Formulas

ADVANCE®
Nutritional Beverage

ROSS LABORATORIES
COLUMBUS, OHIO 43216
Division of Abbott Laboratories, USA

G108/JUNE 1983   LITHO IN USA

**BOYS: PREPUBESCENT
PHYSICAL GROWTH
NCHS PERCENTILES***

NAME_____ RECORD #_____

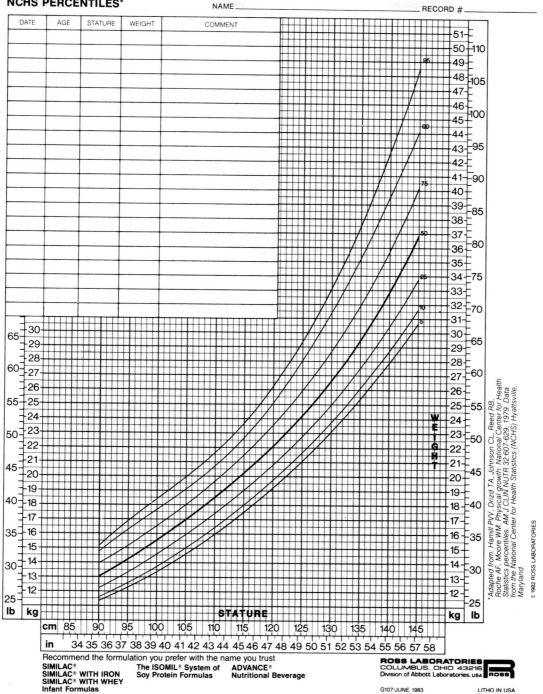

DATE	AGE	STATURE	WEIGHT	COMMENT

Adapted from: Hamill PVV, Drizd TA, Johnson CL, Reed RB, Roche AF, Moore WM: Physical growth: National Center for Health Statistics percentiles. AM J CLIN NUTR 32:607-629, 1979. Data from the National Center for Health Statistics (NCHS) Hyattsville, Maryland.

© 1982 ROSS LABORATORIES

Recommend the formulation you prefer with the name you trust

SIMILAC®
SIMILAC® WITH IRON
SIMILAC® WITH WHEY
Infant Formulas

The ISOMIL® System of
Soy Protein Formulas

ADVANCE®
Nutritional Beverage

ROSS LABORATORIES
COLUMBUS, OHIO 43216
Division of Abbott Laboratories, USA **ROSS**

G107/JUNE 1983   LITHO IN USA

B

Weight-Height of Youths 12 to 17 Years of Age

Weight-Height of Youths at 12 Years (kg/cm)

									Percentile				
Sex and Height	n	N	$\overline{X}$	s	$s_{\overline{x}}$	5th	10th	25th	50th	75th	90th	95th	
MALE						IN KILOGRAMS							
Under 130 cm	5	15	*	*	*	*	*	*	*	*	*	*	
130.0-134.9 cm	4	8	*	*	*	*	*	*	*	*	*	*	
135.0-139.9 cm	34	111	32.50	3.741	0.727	26.6	27.6	30.2	31.6	34.7	37.7	39.4	
140.0-144.9 cm	80	241	34.28	3.635	0.601	28.1	30.0	31.8	34.1	36.5	38.6	40.7	
145.0-149.9 cm	123	386	39.27	6.243	0.615	32.1	33.2	35.7	38.2	40.9	46.1	52.5	
150.0-154.9 cm	156	513	42.90	6.314	0.480	34.9	36.1	38.2	42.1	46.0	51.6	56.3	
155.0-159.9 cm	135	432	47.35	7.551	0.769	38.3	39.4	41.9	46.2	50.5	57.4	61.9	
160.0-164.9 cm	65	201	50.82	8.735	1.388	42.1	42.7	44.9	48.4	56.0	61.1	67.1	
165.0-169.9 cm	29	88	55.75	8.811	2.031	43.3	46.4	49.0	54.4	59.9	68.3	76.6	
170.0-174.9 cm	8	21	62.37	4.503	1.993	54.0	58.1	60.1	61.0	66.0	69.1	69.5	
175.0-179.9 cm	3	10	*	*	*	*	*	*	*	*	*	*	
180.0-184.9 cm	1	2	*	*	*	*	*	*	*	*	*	—	
185.0-189.9 cm	—	—	—	—	—	—	—	—	—	—	—	—	
190.0-194.9 cm	—	—	—	—	—	—	—	—	—	—	—	—	
195.0 cm and over	—	—	—	—	—	—	—	—	—	—	—	—	
FEMALE													
Under 130 cm	—	—	—	—	—	—	—	—	—	—	—	—	
130.0-134.9 cm	3	10	*	*	*	*	*	*	*	*	*	*	
135.0-139.9 cm	12	44	29.41	3.372	0.914	25.0	25.0	26.4	28.9	32.1	34.1	34.2	
140.0-144.9 cm	32	116	38.30	7.314	1.194	28.8	30.6	33.3	36.8	41.4	49.2	55.1	
145.0-149.9 cm	72	258	39.78	6.205	0.975	31.8	32.8	35.5	38.5	42.8	48.3	50.6	
150.0-154.9 cm	147	517	44.00	7.421	0.677	34.4	35.8	38.9	42.8	47.4	52.9	57.4	
155.0-159.9 cm	144	525	48.74	8.369	0.714	37.9	39.2	43.0	46.8	53.8	60.7	63.5	
160.0-164.9 cm	95	336	53.06	8.010	0.658	42.5	43.9	47.2	51.1	57.2	65.6	69.6	
165.0-169.9 cm	31	117	54.89	7.022	1.384	43.9	47.1	50.4	53.1	59.7	64.5	71.3	
170.0-174.9 cm	11	42	63.66	14.501	6.214	48.7	50.1	50.8	56.7	82.2	86.0	86.1	
175.0-179.9 cm	—	—	—	—	—	—	—	—	—	—	—	—	
180.0-184.9 cm	—	—	—	—	—	—	—	—	—	—	—	—	
185.0-189.9 cm	—	—	—	—	—	—	—	—	—	—	—	—	
190.0-194.9 cm	—	—	—	—	—	—	—	—	—	—	—	—	
195.0 cm and over	—	—	—	—	—	—	—	—	—	—	—	—	

n, sample size; *N*, estimated number of youths in population in thousands; $\overline{X}$, mean; *s*, standard deviation; $s_{\overline{x}}$, standard error of the mean. From National Center for Health Statistics: *Height and weight of youths 12-17 years, United States.* In *Vital and health statistics*, series 11, no 124, Health Services and Mental Health Administration, Washington, DC, 1973, US Government Printing Office.

Weight-Height of Youths at 13 Years (kg/cm)

Sex and Height	n	N	$\bar{X}$	s	$s_{\bar{x}}$	5th	10th	25th	50th	75th	90th	95th
								Percentile				
								IN KILOGRAMS				
MALE												
Under 130 cm	—	—	—	—	—	—	—	—	—	—	—	—
130.0–134.9 cm	2	5	*	*	*	*	*	*	*	*	*	*
135.0–139.9 cm	6	25	32.62	5.624	7.716	27.2	27.6	28.9	31.0	34.9	43.1	43.2
140.0–144.9 cm	18	56	36.54	5.852	1.607	30.0	30.5	32.1	36.1	39.2	41.7	53.2
145.0–149.9 cm	65	204	39.03	5.270	0.662	32.4	33.9	36.1	37.9	41.2	44.5	46.4
150.0–154.9 cm	99	312	42.58	6.724	0.865	34.8	36.2	37.9	41.0	45.5	49.4	61.0
155.0–159.9 cm	131	421	47.27	7.482	0.717	37.8	39.2	41.7	45.8	51.1	58.7	61.7
160.0–164.9 cm	125	393	53.01	9.324	0.916	41.5	43.7	46.9	50.4	58.2	64.4	72.5
165.0–169.9 cm	91	285	55.92	8.560	0.833	46.3	47.5	49.3	53.6	59.4	69.0	75.0
170.0–174.9 cm	63	215	62.01	10.362	1.033	51.2	51.6	53.7	60.1	67.0	76.0	85.0
175.0–179.9 cm	19	68	67.92	12.085	3.428	56.3	57.9	60.1	63.3	70.3	88.3	89.0
180.0–184.9 cm	5	15	*	*	*	*	*	*	*	*	*	*
185.0–189.9 cm	—	—	—	—	—	—	—	—	—	—	—	—
190.0–194.9 cm	—	—	—	—	—	—	—	—	—	—	—	—
195.0 cm and over	—	—	—	—	—	—	—	—	—	—	—	—
FEMALE												
Under 130 cm	—	—	—	—	—	—	—	—	—	—	—	—
130.0–134.9 cm	1	3	*	*	*	*	*	*	*	*	*	*
135.0–139.9 cm	—	—	—	—	—	—	—	—	—	—	—	—
140.0–144.9 cm	15	51	37.13	7.317	2.259	26.6	27.5	30.5	36.7	40.1	44.5	56.1
145.0–149.9 cm	47	165	42.23	6.880	0.888	34.7	35.6	38.2	40.5	44.2	53.6	57.6
150.0–154.9 cm	98	329	44.32	7.029	0.787	35.6	36.5	39.2	42.9	47.3	53.7	57.9
155.0–159.9 cm	152	499	49.75	8.757	0.699	39.1	39.9	43.8	48.4	53.8	61.0	65.9
160.0–164.9 cm	156	515	53.16	8.399	0.522	41.2	43.9	47.7	52.2	57.0	63.8	68.5
165.0–169.9 cm	86	284	58.17	9.125	0.921	46.2	47.4	52.2	58.1	61.5	69.3	76.2
170.0–174.9 cm	24	87	58.11	13.209	2.343	46.2	47.1	48.4	52.9	65.3	68.6	96.8
175.0–179.9 cm	3	10	*	*	*	*	*	*	*	*	*	*
180.0–184.9 cm	—	—	—	—	—	—	—	—	—	—	—	—
185.0–189.9 cm	—	—	—	—	—	—	—	—	—	—	—	—
190.0–194.9 cm	—	—	—	—	—	—	—	—	—	—	—	—
195.0 cm and over	—	—	—	—	—	—	—	—	—	—	—	—

Weight-Height of Youths at 14 Years (kg/cm)

IN KILOGRAMS

Sex and Height	n	N	$\bar{X}$	s	$s_{\bar{x}}$	Percentile						
						5th	10th	25th	50th	75th	90th	95th
MALE												
Under 130 cm	—	—	—	—	—	—	—	—	—	—	—	—
130.0-134.9 cm	—	—	—	—	—	—	—	—	—	—	—	—
135.0-139.9 cm	2	7	*	*	*	*	*	*	*	*	*	*
140.0-144.9 cm	3	13	*	*	*	*	*	*	*	*	*	*
145.0-149.9 cm	11	42	40.51	1.829	0.644	36.9	38.6	39.6	40.6	42.0	42.5	42.7
150.0-154.9 cm	45	135	43.63	6.277	1.182	36.2	37.0	39.0	41.4	48.0	51.7	55.3
155.0-159.9 cm	83	261	47.42	7.822	0.872	37.7	38.7	41.8	46.1	51.2	58.0	62.7
160.0-164.9 cm	96	299	52.28	6.785	0.584	42.5	44.0	47.5	52.1	56.3	61.5	65.1
165.0-169.9 cm	134	432	58.07	9.416	1.054	47.7	49.3	51.6	55.4	62.3	70.6	75.7
170.0-174.9 cm	144	435	62.37	11.516	1.095	49.7	51.0	55.0	59.4	65.6	79.2	86.3
175.0-179.9 cm	71	228	65.54	9.704	1.306	50.9	55.1	58.5	64.7	69.9	74.5	84.0
180.0-184.9 cm	25	81	72.44	13.014	2.298	59.6	60.0	65.1	69.4	77.0	83.0	94.3
185.0-189.9 cm	3	9	*	*	*	*	*	*	*	*	*	*
190.0-194.9 cm	1	3	*	*	*	*	*	*	*	*	*	*
195.0 cm and over	—	—	—	—	—	—	—	—	—	—	—	—
FEMALE												
Under 130 cm	—	—	—	—	—	—	—	—	—	—	—	—
130.0-134.9 cm	—	—	—	—	—	—	—	—	—	—	—	—
135.0-139.9 cm	1	2	*	*	*	*	*	*	*	*	*	*
140.0-144.9 cm	2	6	*	*	*	*	*	*	*	*	*	*
145.0-149.9 cm	17	52	42.00	5.879	1.683	32.0	35.3	36.3	42.3	47.5	49.5	51.1
150.0-154.9 cm	64	196	48.26	6.797	0.926	37.7	39.2	42.5	47.9	53.3	55.9	58.8
155.0-159.9 cm	157	508	51.35	7.705	0.520	42.1	43.4	46.3	49.6	55.6	62.2	64.3
160.0-164.9 cm	186	603	54.59	8.810	0.707	43.0	45.0	48.4	53.0	59.7	66.7	70.7
165.0-169.9 cm	114	372	58.46	10.185	0.955	45.9	47.5	52.1	56.8	61.8	70.5	76.4
170.0-174.9 cm	36	121	64.37	15.821	2.814	49.2	52.1	56.2	59.8	70.5	72.9	99.4
175.0-179.9 cm	7	28	61.33	5.496	2.620	51.7	52.0	57.7	59.8	64.6	70.2	70.6
180.0-184.9 cm	2	7	*	*	*	*	*	*	*	*	*	*
185.0-189.9 cm	—	—	—	—	—	—	—	—	—	—	—	—
190.0-194.9 cm	—	—	—	—	—	—	—	—	—	—	—	—
195.0 cm and over	—	—	—	—	—	—	—	—	—	—	—	—

Weight-Height of Youths at 15 Years (kg/cm)

							Percentile (IN KILOGRAMS)					
Sex and Height	n	N	$\bar{X}$	s	$s_{\bar{x}}$	5th	10th	25th	50th	75th	90th	95th
MALE												
Under 130 cm	—	—	—	—	—	—	—	—	—	—	—	—
130.0-134.9 cm	—	—	—	—	—	—	—	—	—	—	—	—
135.0-139.9 cm	—	—	—	—	—	—	—	—	—	—	—	—
140.0-144.9 cm	1	2	*	*	*	*	*	*	*	*	*	*
145.0-149.9 cm	10	30	45.72	8.582	3.550	35.7	39.2	42.6	44.7	46.0	48.7	76.1
150.0-154.9 cm	34	99	52.81	10.552	1.695	40.3	43.1	46.7	49.2	56.7	69.6	76.3
155.0-159.9 cm	71	206	53.01	8.417	0.986	42.7	44.1	46.9	51.5	56.3	65.3	68.8
160.0-164.9 cm	132	404	57.72	8.503	0.819	48.0	48.8	53.1	56.4	61.3	67.1	73.3
165.0-169.9 cm	176	574	62.88	8.464	0.633	51.6	53.4	56.7	61.9	67.2	72.9	78.1
170.0-174.9 cm	118	374	65.80	9.457	1.045	53.1	55.6	59.7	64.3	69.5	80.2	89.2
175.0-179.9 cm	51	144	72.00	11.928	1.724	54.6	60.3	64.4	70.2	68.4	84.4	96.6
180.0-184.9 cm	14	48	74.21	15.035	5.200	58.3	58.5	62.9	70.7	84.6	92.4	110.8
185.0-189.9 cm	6	15	83.39	16.431	10.332	66.4	66.7	69.6	73.8	103.0	105.7	106.2
190.0-194.9 cm	—	—	—	—	—	—	—	—	—	—	—	—
195.0 cm and over	—	—	—	—	—	—	—	—	—	—	—	—
FEMALE												
Under 130 cm	—	—	—	—	—	—	—	—	—	—	—	—
130.0-134.9 cm	—	—	—	—	—	—	—	—	—	—	—	—
135.0-139.9 cm	—	—	—	—	—	—	—	—	—	—	—	—
140.0-144.9 cm	2	5	*	*	*	*	*	*	*	*	*	*
145.0-149.9 cm	15	51	47.91	7.875	3.623	36.0	39.4	42.1	45.4	52.7	55.7	66.3
150.0-154.9 cm	69	242	49.69	8.895	1.190	39.1	40.6	44.3	48.1	52.8	60.5	68.3
155.0-159.9 cm	111	400	51.52	8.473	0.934	41.4	43.5	46.3	50.8	55.1	59.8	65.2
160.0-164.9 cm	137	509	57.03	10.828	0.875	45.1	47.3	50.2	55.0	60.2	71.7	77.7
165.0-169.9 cm	109	398	60.71	10.357	1.053	47.5	49.3	55.1	58.4	65.7	74.1	81.0
170.0-174.9 cm	49	188	65.27	10.730	1.880	49.7	53.6	57.2	61.2	71.6	85.3	86.4
175.0-179.9 cm	7	23	63.30	8.872	4.807	49.7	49.9	53.8	62.4	71.1	71.9	79.2
180.0-184.9 cm	3	26	*	*	*	*	*	*	*	*	*	*
185.0-189.9 cm	1	3	*	*	*	*	*	*	*	*	*	*
190.0-194.9 cm	—	—	—	—	—	—	—	—	—	—	—	—
195.0 cm and over	—	—	—	—	—	—	—	—	—	—	—	—

Weight-Height of Youths at 16 Years (kg/cm)

Sex and Height	n	N	$\bar{X}$	s	$s_{\bar{x}}$	5th	10th	25th	50th	75th	90th	95th
								IN KILOGRAMS — Percentile				
MALE												
Under 130 cm	—	—	—	—	—	—	—	—	—	—	—	—
130.0–134.9 cm	—	—	—	—	—	—	—	—	—	—	—	—
135.0–139.9 cm	—	—	—	—	—	—	—	—	—	—	—	—
140.0–144.9 cm	1	1	*	*	*	*	*	*	*	*	*	*
145.0–149.9 cm	4	12	*	*	*	*	*	*	*	*	*	*
150.0–154.9 cm	11	33	49.89	7.323	3.572	42.0	42.2	44.7	46.8	54.4	59.8	67.2
155.0–159.9 cm	32	108	53.09	6.459	1.273	44.2	44.9	48.2	51.4	58.0	60.9	66.1
160.0–164.9 cm	87	275	59.39	9.178	0.981	48.5	49.8	52.7	58.0	63.9	69.3	75.9
165.0–169.9 cm	166	552	62.66	7.556	0.629	51.6	53.8	57.5	61.6	67.1	73.1	78.0
170.0–174.9 cm	149	511	67.33	9.018	0.856	56.3	58.2	61.0	65.4	72.5	80.1	83.8
175.0–179.9 cm	72	227	72.38	12.485	1.993	58.3	59.3	64.4	68.9	76.5	90.2	96.9
180.0–184.9 cm	29	95	81.06	14.268	3.265	63.7	66.6	69.7	78.4	90.3	97.0	111.4
185.0–189.9 cm	30	10	*	*	*	*	*	*	*	*	*	*
190.0–194.9 cm	2	7	*	*	*	*	*	*	*	*	*	*
195.0 cm and over	—	—	—	—	—	—	—	—	—	—	—	—
FEMALE												
Under 130 cm	—	—	—	—	—	—	—	—	—	—	—	—
130.0–134.9 cm	—	—	—	—	—	—	—	—	—	—	—	—
135.0–139.9 cm	2	5	*	*	*	*	*	*	*	*	*	*
140.0–144.9 cm	10	33	52.58	8.198	3.191	43.9	44.1	44.9	51.0	54.5	72.0	72.1
145.0–149.9 cm	57	178	51.79	10.457	1.053	41.4	42.0	45.8	48.9	54.1	61.5	83.3
150.0–154.9 cm	117	354	53.20	7.766	0.734	44.0	45.6	48.4	51.6	56.4	61.9	69.0
155.0–159.9 cm	160	547	57.71	11.129	1.246	46.1	47.3	51.5	55.5	61.2	69.5	75.1
160.0–164.9 cm	122	450	61.72	11.998	0.802	47.1	48.8	53.3	59.1	67.3	78.7	86.7
165.0–169.9 cm	53	170	63.61	8.734	1.126	52.9	53.8	58.1	62.1	66.8	73.8	84.2
170.0–174.9 cm	14	45	72.55	15.012	5.224	58.6	58.8	61.7	65.9	80.6	99.1	105.5
175.0–179.9 cm	1	2	*	*	*	*	*	*	*	*	*	*
180.0–184.9 cm	—	—	—	—	—	—	—	—	—	—	—	—
185.0–189.9 cm	—	—	—	—	—	—	—	—	—	—	—	—
190.0–194.9 cm	—	—	—	—	—	—	—	—	—	—	—	—
195.0 cm and over	—	—	—	—	—	—	—	—	—	—	—	—

Weight-Height of Youths at 17 Years (kg/cm)

Sex and Height	n	N	$\bar{X}$	s	$s_{\bar{x}}$	5th	10th	25th	50th	75th	90th	95th
									Percentile			
MALE							IN KILOGRAMS					
Under 130 cm	—	—	—	—	—	—	—	—	—	—	—	—
130.0–134.9 cm	—	—	—	—	—	—	—	—	—	—	—	—
135.0–139.9 cm	—	—	—	—	—	—	—	—	—	—	—	—
140.0–144.9 cm	—	—	—	—	—	—	—	—	—	—	—	—
145.0–149.9 cm	—	—	—	—	—	—	—	—	—	—	—	—
150.0–154.9 cm	1	3	*	*	*	*	*	*	*	*	*	*
155.0–159.9 cm	11	39	54.63	9.397	3.414	43.8	46.4	48.2	49.7	57.8	69.9	73.2
160.0–164.9 cm	25	81	57.75	6.503	1.355	49.7	51.1	52.5	56.9	61.6	70.1	70.8
165.0–169.9 cm	63	248	62.57	8.344	1.224	50.2	53.2	56.4	61.5	66.9	72.7	77.3
170.0–174.9 cm	115	396	67.06	11.163	0.704	53.3	55.5	59.5	64.6	71.9	80.9	91.6
175.0–179.9 cm	151	537	68.37	9.907	0.831	56.9	58.9	61.5	66.5	73.6	79.4	88.4
180.0–184.9 cm	80	297	73.31	12.454	1.335	59.6	61.0	65.1	71.2	78.4	91.8	102.7
185.0–189.9 cm	36	133	76.03	9.171	1.301	62.4	66.3	70.5	75.3	80.8	90.3	92.9
190.0–194.9 cm	7	25	81.40	10.985	7.588	62.9	62.9	67.8	87.3	90.3	90.6	90.6
195.0 cm and over	—	—	—	—	—	—	—	—	—	—	—	—
FEMALE												
Under 130 cm	—	—	—	—	—	—	—	—	—	—	—	—
130.0–134.9 cm	—	—	—	—	—	—	—	—	—	—	—	—
135.0–139.9 cm	—	—	—	—	—	—	—	—	—	—	—	—
140.0–144.9 cm	2	5	*	*	*	*	*	*	*	*	*	*
145.0–149.9 cm	8	26	43.49	3.939	1.604	38.6	38.8	40.1	45.1	45.7	51.1	51.2
150.0–154.9 cm	43	151	49.96	6.508	0.827	41.6	42.3	44.6	48.9	53.5	59.2	64.1
155.0–159.9 cm	103	385	54.71	9.903	0.775	44.4	45.5	48.7	53.2	57.7	61.6	76.2
160.0–164.9 cm	133	506	57.79	10.620	1.028	46.8	48.0	50.2	55.4	61.5	72.3	82.3
165.0–169.9 cm	116	433	60.63	10.117	1.182	47.9	50.3	55.1	59.3	65.1	69.4	71.6
170.0–174.9 cm	51	186	62.18	9.132	1.407	50.6	52.9	55.5	60.2	65.7	76.1	82.7
175.0–179.9 cm	12	47	65.76	8.405	2.229	54.9	56.7	60.1	61.7	75.2	75.9	83.0
180.0–184.9 cm	1	2	*	*	*	*	*	*	*	*	*	*
185.0–189.9 cm	—	—	—	—	—	—	—	—	—	—	—	—
190.0–194.9 cm	—	—	—	—	—	—	—	—	—	—	—	—
195.0 cm and over	—	—	—	—	—	—	—	—	—	—	—	—

Weight-Height of Youths at 12 Years (lb/in)

Sex and Height	n	N	$\bar{X}$	s	$s_{\bar{x}}$	Percentile						
						5th	10th	25th	50th	75th	90th	95th
						IN POUNDS						
MALE												
Under 51.18 in	5	15	*	*	*	*	*	*	*	*	*	*
51.18-53.15 in	4	8	*	*	*	*	*	*	*	*	*	*
53.15-55.12 in	34	111	71.65	8.248	1.603	54.6	60.8	66.6	69.7	76.5	83.1	86.9
55.12-57.09 in	80	241	75.57	8.014	1.325	61.9	66.1	70.1	75.2	80.5	85.1	89.7
57.09-59.06 in	123	386	86.58	13.764	1.356	70.8	73.2	78.7	84.2	90.2	101.6	115.7
59.06-61.02 in	156	513	94.58	13.920	1.058	76.9	79.6	84.2	92.8	101.4	113.8	124.1
61.02-62.99 in	135	433	104.39	16.647	1.695	84.4	86.9	92.4	101.9	111.3	126.5	136.5
62.99-64.96 in	65	201	112.04	19.257	3.060	92.8	94.1	99.0	106.7	123.5	134.7	147.9
64.96-66.93 in	29	88	122.91	19.425	4.478	95.5	102.3	108.0	119.9	132.1	150.6	168.9
66.93-68.90 in	8	21	137.50	9.927	4.394	119.0	128.1	132.5	134.5	145.5	152.3	153.2
68.90-70.87 in	3	10	*	*	*	*	*	*	*	*	*	*
70.87-72.83 in	1	2	*	*	*	*	*	*	*	*	*	*
72.83-74.80 in	—	—	—	—	—	—	—	—	—	—	—	—
74.80-76.77 in	—	—	—	—	—	—	—	—	—	—	—	—
76.77 in and over	—	—	—	—	—	—	—	—	—	—	—	—
FEMALE												
Under 51.18 in	—	—	—	—	—	—	—	—	—	—	—	—
51.18-53.15 in	3	10	*	*	*	*	*	*	*	*	*	*
53.15-55.12 in	12	44	64.84	7.434	2.015	55.1	55.1	58.2	63.7	70.8	75.2	75.4
55.12-57.09 in	32	116	84.44	16.125	2.632	63.5	67.5	73.4	81.1	91.3	108.5	121.5
57.09-59.06 in	72	258	87.70	13.680	2.150	70.1	72.3	78.3	78.9	94.4	106.5	111.6
59.06-61.02 in	147	517	97.00	16.361	1.493	75.8	78.9	85.8	94.4	104.5	116.6	126.5
61.02-62.99 in	144	525	107.45	18.451	1.574	83.6	86.4	94.8	103.2	118.6	133.8	140.0
62.99-64.96 in	95	336	117.00	17.659	1.451	93.7	96.8	104.1	112.7	126.1	144.6	153.4
64.96-66.93 in	31	117	121.01	15.481	3.051	96.8	103.8	111.1	117.1	131.6	142.2	157.2
66.93-68.90 in	11	42	140.35	31.969	13.700	107.4	110.5	112.0	125.0	181.2	189.6	189.8
68.90-70.87 in	—	—	—	—	—	—	—	—	—	—	—	—
70.87-72.83 in	—	—	—	—	—	—	—	—	—	—	—	—
72.83-74.80 in	—	—	—	—	—	—	—	—	—	—	—	—
74.80-76.77 in	—	—	—	—	—	—	—	—	—	—	—	—
76.77 in and over	—	—	—	—	—	—	—	—	—	—	—	—

Weight-Height of Youths at 13 Years (lb/in)

Sex and Height	n	N	X̄	s	$s_{\bar{x}}$	Percentile IN POUNDS 5th	10th	25th	50th	75th	90th	95th
MALE												
Under 51.18 in	—	—	—	—	—	—	—	—	—	—	—	—
51.18-53.15 in	2	5	*	*	*	*	*	*	*	*	*	*
53.15-55.12 in	8	25	71.91	12.399	17.011	60.0	60.8	63.7	68.3	76.9	95.0	95.2
55.12-57.09 in	18	56	80.56	12.902	3.543	66.1	67.2	70.8	79.6	86.4	91.9	117.3
57.09-59.06 in	65	204	86.05	11.618	1.460	71.4	74.7	79.6	83.6	90.8	98.1	102.3
59.06-61.02 in	99	312	93.87	14.824	1.907	76.7	79.8	83.6	90.4	100.3	108.9	134.5
61.02-62.99 in	131	421	104.21	16.495	1.581	83.3	86.4	91.9	101.0	112.7	129.4	136.0
62.99-64.96 in	125	393	116.87	20.556	2.019	91.5	96.3	103.4	111.1	128.3	142.0	159.8
64.96-66.93 in	91	285	123.28	18.872	1.837	102.1	104.7	108.7	118.2	131.0	152.1	165.3
66.93-68.90 in	63	215	136.71	22.844	2.277	112.9	113.8	118.4	132.5	147.7	167.6	187.4
68.90-70.87 in	19	68	149.72	26.643	7.557	124.1	127.6	132.5	139.6	155.0	194.7	196.2
70.87-72.83 in	5	15	*	*	*	*	*	*	*	*	*	*
72.83-74.80 in	—	—	—	—	—	—	—	—	—	—	—	—
74.80-76.77 in	—	—	—	—	—	—	—	—	—	—	—	—
76.77 in and over	—	—	—	—	—	—	—	—	—	—	—	—
FEMALE												
Under 51.18 in	—	—	—	—	—	—	—	—	—	—	—	—
51.18-53.15 in	1	3	*	*	*	*	*	*	*	*	*	*
53.15-55.12 in	—	—	—	—	—	—	—	—	—	—	—	—
55.12-57.09 in	15	51	81.86	16.131	4.980	58.6	60.6	67.2	80.9	88.4	98.1	123.7
57.09-59.06 in	47	165	93.10	15.168	1.958	76.5	78.5	84.2	89.3	97.4	118.2	127.0
59.06-61.02 in	98	329	97.71	15.496	1.735	78.7	80.5	86.4	94.6	104.3	118.4	127.6
61.02-62.99 in	152	499	109.68	19.306	1.541	86.2	88.0	96.6	106.7	118.6	134.5	145.3
62.99-64.96 in	156	515	117.20	18.517	1.151	90.8	96.8	105.2	115.1	125.7	140.7	151.0
64.96-66.93 in	86	284	128.24	20.117	2.031	101.9	104.5	115.1	128.1	135.6	152.8	168.0
66.93-68.90 in	24	87	128.11	29.121	5.165	101.9	103.8	106.7	116.6	144.0	151.2	213.4
68.90-70.87 in	3	10	*	*	*	*	*	*	*	*	*	*
70.87-72.83 in	—	—	—	—	—	—	—	—	—	—	—	—
72.83-74.80 in	—	—	—	—	—	—	—	—	—	—	—	—
74.80-76.77 in	—	—	—	—	—	—	—	—	—	—	—	—
76.77 in and over	—	—	—	—	—	—	—	—	—	—	—	—

Weight-Height of Youths at 14 Years (lb/in)

						Percentile						
						IN POUNDS						
Sex and Height	n	N	X̄	s	$s_{\bar{x}}$	5th	10th	25th	50th	75th	90th	95th
MALE												
Under 51.18 in	—	—	—	—	—	—	—	—	—	—	—	—
51.18-53.15 in	—	7	*	*	*	*	*	*	*	*	*	*
53.15-55.12 in	2	13	*	*	*	*	*	*	*	*	*	*
55.12-57.09 in	3	42	89.31	4.032	1.420	81.4	85.1	87.3	89.5	92.6	93.7	94.1
57.09-59.06 in	11	135	96.19	13.838	2.606	79.8	81.6	86.0	91.3	106.8	114.0	121.9
59.06-61.02 in	45	261	104.54	17.245	1.922	83.1	85.3	92.2	101.6	112.9	127.9	138.2
61.02-62.99 in	83	299	115.26	14.958	1.288	93.7	97.0	104.7	114.9	124.1	135.6	143.5
62.99-64.96 in	96	432	128.02	20.759	2.324	105.2	108.7	113.8	122.1	137.4	155.6	166.9
64.96-66.93 in	134	435	137.50	25.388	2.414	109.6	112.4	121.3	131.0	145.0	165.2	185.2
66.93-68.90 in	144	228	144.49	21.394	2.879	112.2	121.5	129.0	142.6	154.1	174.1	190.3
68.90-70.87 in	71	81	159.70	28.691	5.066	131.4	132.3	143.5	153.0	170.9	183.0	207.9
70.87-72.83 in	25	9	*	*	*	*	*	*	*	*	*	*
72.83-74.80 in	3	3	*	*	*	*	*	*	*	*	*	*
74.80-76.77 in	1	—	—	—	—	—	—	—	—	—	—	—
76.77 in and over	—	—	—	—	—	—	—	—	—	—	—	—
FEMALE												
Under 51.18 in	—	—	—	—	—	—	—	—	—	—	—	—
51.18-53.15 in	—	—	—	—	—	—	—	—	—	—	—	—
53.15-55.12 in	1	2	*	*	*	*	*	*	*	*	*	*
55.12-57.09 in	2	6	*	*	*	*	*	*	*	*	*	*
57.09-59.06 in	17	52	92.59	12.961	3.710	70.5	77.8	80.0	93.3	104.7	109.1	112.7
59.06-61.02 in	64	196	106.40	14.985	2.042	83.1	86.4	93.7	105.6	117.5	123.2	129.6
61.02-62.99 in	157	508	113.21	16.987	1.146	90.8	95.7	102.1	109.3	122.6	137.1	141.8
62.99-64.96 in	186	603	120.35	19.423	1.559	94.8	99.2	106.7	116.8	131.6	147.0	155.0
64.96-66.93 in	114	372	128.88	22.454	2.105	101.2	104.7	114.9	125.2	136.2	155.4	168.4
66.93-68.90 in	36	121	141.91	34.879	6.204	108.5	114.9	123.9	131.8	155.4	160.7	219.1
68.90-70.87 in	7	28	135.21	12.117	5.776	114.0	114.6	127.2	131.8	142.4	154.8	155.6
70.87-72.83 in	2	7	*	*	*	*	*	*	*	*	*	*
72.83-74.80 in	—	—	—	—	—	—	—	—	—	—	—	—
74.80-76.77 in	—	—	—	—	—	—	—	—	—	—	—	—
76.77 in and over	—	—	—	—	—	—	—	—	—	—	—	—

Weight-Height of Youths at 15 Years (lb/in)

| | | | | | | Percentile (IN POUNDS) | | | | | | |
Sex and Height	n	N	$\bar{X}$	s	$s_{\bar{x}}$	5th	10th	25th	50th	75th	90th	95th
MALE												
Under 51.18 in	—	—	—	—	—	—	—	—	—	—	—	—
51.18–53.15 in	—	—	—	—	—	—	—	—	—	—	—	—
53.15–55.12 in	—	—	—	—	—	—	—	—	—	—	—	—
55.12–57.09 in	—	—	—	—	—	—	—	—	—	—	—	—
57.09–59.06 in	1	2	*	*	*	*	*	*	*	*	*	*
59.06–61.02 in	10	30	100.80	18.920	7.826	78.7	86.4	93.9	98.5	101.4	107.4	167.8
61.02–62.99 in	34	99	116.43	23.263	3.737	88.8	95.0	103.0	108.5	125.0	153.4	168.2
62.99–64.96 in	71	206	116.87	18.556	2.174	94.1	97.2	103.4	113.5	124.1	144.0	151.7
64.96–66.93 in	132	404	127.25	18.746	1.806	105.8	107.6	117.1	124.3	135.1	147.9	161.6
66.93–68.90 in	176	574	138.63	18.660	1.396	113.8	117.7	125.0	136.5	148.2	160.7	172.2
68.90–70.87 in	118	374	146.06	20.849	2.304	117.1	122.6	131.6	141.8	153.2	176.8	196.7
70.87–72.83 in	51	144	158.73	26.297	3.801	120.4	132.9	142.0	154.8	172.8	186.1	213.0
72.83–74.80 in	14	48	163.61	33.147	11.464	128.5	129.0	138.7	155.9	186.5	203.7	244.3
74.80–76.77 in	6	15	183.84	36.224	22.778	146.4	147.0	153.4	162.7	227.1	233.0	234.1
76.77 in and over	—	—	—	—	—	—	—	—	—	—	—	—
FEMALE												
Under 51.18 in	—	—	—	—	—	—	—	—	—	—	—	—
51.18–53.15 in	—	—	—	—	—	—	—	—	—	—	—	—
53.15–55.12 in	—	—	—	—	—	—	—	—	—	—	—	—
55.12–57.09 in	2	5	*	*	*	*	*	*	*	*	*	*
57.09–59.06 in	15	51	105.62	17.361	7.987	79.4	86.9	92.8	100.1	116.2	122.8	146.2
59.06–61.02 in	69	242	109.55	19.610	2.624	86.2	89.5	97.7	106.0	116.4	133.4	150.6
61.02–62.99 in	111	400	113.58	18.680	2.059	91.3	95.9	102.1	121.0	121.5	131.8	143.7
62.99–64.96 in	137	509	125.73	23.872	1.929	99.4	104.3	110.7	121.3	132.7	158.1	171.3
64.96–66.93 in	109	398	133.84	22.833	2.322	104.7	108.7	121.5	128.8	144.8	163.4	178.6
66.93–68.90 in	49	188	143.90	23.656	4.145	109.6	118.2	126.1	134.9	157.9	188.1	190.5
68.90–70.87 in	7	23	139.55	19.559	10.598	109.6	110.0	118.6	137.6	156.1	158.5	174.6
70.87–72.83 in	3	26	*	*	*	*	*	*	*	*	*	*
72.83–74.80 in	1	3	*	*	*	*	*	*	*	*	*	*
74.80–76.77 in	—	—	—	—	—	—	—	—	—	—	—	—
76.77 in and over	—	—	—	—	—	—	—	—	—	—	—	—

Weight-Height of Youths at 16 Years (lb/in)

Sex and Height	n	N	$\bar{X}$	s	$s_{\bar{x}}$	Percentile (IN POUNDS)						
						5th	10th	25th	50th	75th	90th	95th
MALE												
Under 51.18 in	—	—	—	—	—	—	—	—	—	—	—	—
51.18-53.15 in	—	—	—	—	—	—	—	—	—	—	—	—
53.15-55.12 in	—	—	—	—	—	—	—	—	—	—	—	—
55.12-57.09 in	—	—	—	—	—	—	—	—	—	—	—	—
57.09-59.06 in	1	1	*	*	*	*	*	*	*	*	*	*
59.06-61.02 in	4	12	*	*	*	*	*	*	*	*	*	*
61.02-62.99 in	11	33	109.99	16.145	7.875	92.6	93.0	98.5	103.2	119.9	131.8	148.2
62.99-64.96 in	32	108	117.04	14.240	2.807	97.4	99.0	106.3	113.3	127.9	134.3	145.7
64.96-66.93 in	87	275	130.93	20.234	2.163	106.9	109.8	116.2	127.9	140.9	152.8	167.3
66.93-68.90 in	166	552	138.14	16.658	1.387	113.8	118.6	126.8	135.8	147.9	161.2	172.0
68.90-70.87 in	149	511	148.44	19.881	1.887	124.1	128.3	134.5	144.2	159.8	176.6	184.7
70.87-72.83 in	72	227	159.57	27.525	4.394	128.5	130.7	142.0	151.9	168.7	198.9	213.6
72.83-74.80 in	29	95	178.71	31.456	7.198	140.4	146.8	153.7	172.8	199.1	213.8	245.6
74.80-76.77 in	3	10	*	*	*	*	*	*	*	*	*	*
76.77 in and over	2	7	*	*	*	*	*	*	*	*	*	*
FEMALE												
Under 51.18 in	—	—	—	—	—	—	—	—	—	—	—	—
51.18-53.15 in	—	—	—	—	—	—	—	—	—	—	—	—
53.15-55.12 in	—	—	—	—	—	—	—	—	—	—	—	—
55.12-57.09 in	2	5	*	*	*	*	*	*	*	*	*	*
57.09-59.06 in	10	33	115.92	18.074	7.035	96.8	97.2	99.0	112.4	120.2	158.7	158.9
59.06-61.02 in	57	178	114.18	23.054	2.322	91.3	92.6	101.0	107.8	119.3	135.6	183.6
61.02-62.99 in	117	354	117.29	17.121	1.618	97.0	100.5	106.7	113.8	124.3	136.5	152.1
62.99-64.96 in	160	547	127.23	24.535	2.747	101.6	104.3	113.5	122.4	134.9	153.2	165.6
64.96-66.93 in	122	450	136.07	26.451	1.768	103.8	107.6	117.5	130.3	148.4	173.5	191.1
66.93-68.90 in	53	170	140.24	19.255	2.482	116.6	118.6	128.1	136.9	147.3	173.7	185.6
68.90-70.87 in	14	45	159.95	33.096	11.517	129.2	129.6	136.0	145.3	177.7	218.5	232.6
70.87-72.83 in	1	2	*	*	*	*	*	*	*	*	*	*
72.83-74.80 in	—	—	—	—	—	—	—	—	—	—	—	—
74.80-76.77 in	—	—	—	—	—	—	—	—	—	—	—	—
76.77 in and over	—	—	—	—	—	—	—	—	—	—	—	—

Weight-Height of Youths at 17 Years (lb/in)

Sex and Height	n	N	$\bar{X}$	s	$s_{\bar{x}}$	Percentile IN POUNDS						
						5th	10th	25th	50th	75th	90th	95th
MALE												
Under 51.18 in	—	—	—	—	—	—	—	—	—	—	—	—
51.18-53.15 in	—	—	—	—	—	—	—	—	—	—	—	—
53.15-55.12 in	—	—	—	—	—	—	—	—	—	—	—	—
55.12-57.09 in	—	—	—	—	—	—	—	—	—	—	—	—
57.09-59.06 in	1	3	*	*	*	*	*	*	*	*	*	*
59.06-61.02 in	11	39	120.44	20.717	7.527	96.6	102.3	106.3	109.6	127.4	154.1	161.4
61.02-62.99 in	25	81	127.32	14.337	2.987	109.6	112.7	115.7	125.4	135.8	154.5	156.1
62.99-64.96 in	63	248	137.94	18.395	2.699	110.7	117.3	124.3	135.6	147.5	160.3	170.4
64.96-66.93 in	115	396	147.84	24.610	1.552	117.5	122.4	131.2	142.4	158.5	178.4	202.2
66.93-68.90 in	151	537	150.73	21.841	1.832	125.4	129.9	135.6	146.6	162.3	175.0	194.9
68.90-70.87 in	80	297	161.62	27.456	2.943	131.4	134.5	143.5	157.0	172.8	202.4	226.4
70.87-72.83 in	36	133	167.62	20.219	2.868	137.6	146.2	155.4	166.0	178.1	199.1	204.8
72.83-74.80 in	7	25	179.46	24.218	16.729	138.7	138.7	149.5	192.5	199.1	199.7	199.7
74.80-76.77 in	—	—	—	—	—	—	—	—	—	—	—	—
76.77 in and over	—	—	—	—	—	—	—	—	—	—	—	—
FEMALE												
Under 51.18 in	—	—	—	—	—	—	—	—	—	—	—	—
51.18-53.15 in	—	—	—	—	—	—	—	—	—	—	—	—
53.15-55.12 in	—	—	—	—	—	—	—	—	—	—	—	—
55.12-57.09 in	2	5	*	*	*	*	*	*	*	*	*	*
57.09-59.06 in	8	26	95.88	8.684	3.536	85.1	85.5	88.4	99.4	100.8	112.7	112.9
59.06-61.02 in	43	151	110.14	14.348	1.823	91.7	93.3	98.3	107.8	117.9	130.5	141.3
61.02-62.99 in	103	385	120.61	21.832	1.709	97.9	100.3	107.4	117.3	127.2	135.8	168.0
62.99-64.96 in	133	506	127.41	23.413	2.266	103.2	105.8	110.7	122.1	127.2	159.4	181.4
64.96-66.93 in	116	433	133.67	22.304	2.606	105.6	110.9	121.5	130.7	143.5	153.0	157.9
66.93-68.90 in	51	186	137.08	20.133	3.102	111.6	116.6	122.4	132.7	144.8	167.8	182.3
68.90-70.87 in	12	47	14.98	18.530	4.914	121.0	125.0	132.5	136.0	165.8	167.3	183.0
70.87-72.83 in	1	2	*	*	*	*	*	*	*	*	*	*
72.83-74.80 in	—	—	—	—	—	—	—	—	—	—	—	—
74.80-76.77 in	—	—	—	—	—	—	—	—	—	—	—	—
76.77 in and over	—	—	—	—	—	—	—	—	—	—	—	—

C Andres Age-Specific Weight-Height Table for Adults and the Elderly*

Height	Weight Range for Men and Women by Age (Years) in Pounds†				
	25	35	45	55	65
ft−in					
4−10	84-111	92-119	99-127	107-135	115-142
4−11	87-115	95-123	103-131	111-139	119-147
5−0	90-119	98-127	106-135	114-143	123-152
5−1	93-123	101-131	110-140	118-148	127-157
5−2	96-127	105-136	113-144	122-153	131-163
5−3	99-131	108-140	117-149	126-158	135-168
5−4	102-135	112-145	121-154	130-163	140-173
5−5	106-140	115-149	125-159	134-168	144-179
5−6	109-144	119-154	129-164	138-174	148-184
5−7	112-148	122-159	133-169	143-179	153-190
5−8	116-153	126-163	137-174	147-184	158-196
5−9	119-157	130-168	141-179	151-190	162-201
5−10	122-162	134-173	145-184	156-195	167-207
5−11	126-167	137-178	149-190	160-201	172-213
6−0	129-171	141-183	153-195	165-207	177-219
6−1	133-176	145-188	157-200	169-213	182-225
6−2	137-181	149-194	162-206	174-219	187-232
6−3	141-186	153-199	166-212	179-225	192-238
6−4	144-191	157-205	171-218	184-231	197-244

*Values in this table are in pounds for height without shoes and weight without clothes. To convert inches to centimeters, multiply by 2.54, to convert pounds to kilograms, multiply by 0.455.
†Data from Andres R: Gerontology Research Center, National Institute of Aging, Baltimore, Md.

D Mid-Upper Arm Circumference Percentiles (cm)

	Female					Male				
Age (years)	5th	25th	50th	75th	95th	5th	25th	50th	75th	95th
1	13.8	14.8	15.6	16.4	17.7	14.2	15.0	15.9	17.0	18.3
2	14.2	15.2	16.0	16.7	18.4	14.1	15.3	16.2	17.0	18.5
3	14.3	15.8	16.7	17.5	18.9	15.0	16.0	16.7	17.5	19.0
4	14.9	16.0	16.9	17.7	19.1	14.9	16.2	17.1	18.0	19.2
5	15.3	16.5	17.5	18.5	21.1	15.3	16.7	17.5	18.5	20.4
6	15.6	17.0	17.6	18.7	21.1	15.5	16.7	17.9	18.8	22.8
7	16.4	17.4	18.3	19.9	23.1	16.2	17.7	18.7	20.1	23.0
8	16.8	18.3	19.5	21.4	26.1	16.2	17.7	19.0	20.2	24.5
9	17.8	19.4	21.1	22.4	26.0	17.5	18.7	20.0	21.7	25.7
10	17.4	19.3	21.0	22.8	26.5	18.1	19.6	21.0	23.1	27.4
11	18.5	20.8	22.4	24.8	30.3	18.6	20.2	22.3	24.4	28.0
12	19.4	21.6	23.7	25.6	29.4	19.3	21.4	23.2	25.4	30.3
13	20.2	22.3	24.3	27.1	33.8	19.4	22.8	24.7	26.3	30.1
14	21.4	23.7	25.2	27.2	32.2	22.0	23.7	25.3	28.3	32.3
15	20.8	23.9	25.4	27.9	32.2	22.2	24.4	26.4	28.4	32.0
16	21.8	24.1	25.8	28.3	33.4	24.4	26.2	27.8	30.3	34.3
17	22.0	24.1	26.4	29.5	35.0	24.6	26.7	28.5	30.8	34.7
18	22.2	24.1	25.8	28.1	32.5	24.5	27.6	29.7	32.1	37.9
19-25	21.1	24.7	26.5	29.0	34.5	26.2	28.8	30.8	33.1	37.2
25-35	23.3	25.6	27.7	30.4	36.8	27.1	30.0	31.9	34.2	37.5
35-45	24.1	26.7	29.0	31.7	37.8	27.8	30.5	32.6	34.5	37.4
45-55	24.2	27.4	29.9	32.8	38.4	26.7	30.1	32.2	34.2	37.6
55-65	24.3	28.0	30.3	33.5	38.5	25.8	29.6	31.7	33.6	36.9
65-75	24.0	27.4	29.9	32.6	37.3	24.8	28.5	30.7	32.5	35.5

Data derived from the Health and Nutrition Examination Survey data of 1971-1974, using same population samples as those of the National Center for Health Statistics (NCHS) growth percentiles for children. Adapted from Frisancho AR: New norms of upper limb fat and muscle areas for assessment of nutritional status, *Am J Clin Nutr* 34:2540, 1981.

E Triceps Skinfold Percentiles (mm)

Age (years)	Female					Male				
	5th	25th	50th	75th	95th	5th	25th	50th	75th	95th
1	6	8	10	12	16	6	8	10	12	16
2	6	9	10	12	16	6	8	10	12	15
3	7	9	11	12	15	6	8	10	11	15
4	7	8	10	12	16	6	8	9	11	14
5	6	8	10	12	18	6	8	9	11	15
6	6	8	10	12	16	5	7	8	10	16
7	6	9	11	13	18	5	7	9	12	17
8	6	9	12	15	24	5	7	8	10	16
9	8	10	13	16	22	6	7	10	13	18
10	7	10	12	17	27	6	8	10	14	21
11	7	10	13	18	28	6	8	11	16	24
12	8	11	14	18	27	6	8	11	14	28
13	8	12	15	21	30	5	7	10	14	26
14	9	13	16	21	28	4	7	9	14	24
15	8	12	17	21	32	4	6	8	11	24
16	10	15	18	22	31	4	6	8	12	22
17	10	13	19	24	37	5	6	8	12	19
18	10	15	18	22	30	4	6	9	13	24
19-25	10	14	18	24	34	4	7	10	15	22
25-35	10	16	21	27	37	5	8	12	16	24
35-45	12	18	23	29	38	5	8	12	16	23
45-55	12	20	25	30	40	6	8	12	15	25
55-65	12	20	25	31	38	5	8	11	14	22
65-75	12	18	24	29	36	4	8	11	15	22

Data derived from the Health and Nutrition Examination Survey data of 1971-1974, using same population samples as those of the National Center for Health Statistics (NCHS) growth percentiles for children. Adapted from Frisancho AR: New norms of upper limb fat and muscle areas for assessment of nutritional status, *Am J Clin Nutr* 34:2540, 1981.

Mid-Upper Arm Muscle Circumference Percentiles (cm)

Age (years)	Female					Male				
	5th	25th	50th	75th	95th	5th	25th	50th	75th	95th
1	10.5	11.7	12.4	13.9	14.3	11.0	11.9	12.7	13.5	14.7
2	11.1	11.9	12.6	13.3	14.7	11.1	12.2	13.0	14.0	15.0
3	11.3	12.4	13.2	14.0	15.2	11.7	13.1	13.7	14.3	15.3
4	11.5	12.8	13.8	14.4	15.7	12.3	13.3	14.1	14.8	15.9
5	12.5	13.4	14.2	15.1	16.5	12.8	14.0	14.7	15.4	16.9
6	13.0	13.8	14.5	15.4	17.1	13.1	14.2	15.1	16.1	17.7
7	12.9	14.2	15.1	16.0	17.6	13.7	15.1	16.0	16.8	19.0
8	13.8	15.1	16.0	17.1	19.4	14.0	15.4	16.2	17.0	18.7
9	14.7	15.8	16.7	18.0	19.8	15.1	16.1	17.0	18.3	20.2
10	14.8	15.9	17.0	18.0	19.7	15.6	16.6	18.0	19.1	22.1
11	15.0	17.1	18.1	19.6	22.3	15.9	17.3	18.3	19.5	23.0
12	16.2	18.0	19.1	20.1	22.0	16.7	18.2	19.5	21.0	24.1
13	16.9	18.3	19.8	21.1	24.0	17.2	19.6	21.1	22.6	24.5
14	17.4	19.0	20.1	21.6	24.7	18.9	21.2	22.3	24.0	26.4
15	17.5	18.9	20.2	21.5	24.4	19.9	21.8	23.7	25.4	27.2
16	17.0	19.0	20.2	21.6	24.9	21.3	23.4	24.9	26.9	29.6
17	17.5	19.4	20.5	22.1	25.7	22.4	24.5	25.8	27.3	31.2
18	17.4	19.1	20.2	21.5	24.5	22.6	25.2	26.4	28.3	32.4
19-25	17.9	19.5	20.7	22.1	24.9	23.8	25.7	27.3	28.9	32.1
25-35	18.3	19.9	21.2	22.8	26.4	24.3	26.4	27.9	29.8	32.6
35-45	18.6	20.5	21.8	23.6	27.2	24.7	26.9	28.6	30.2	32.7
45-55	18.7	20.6	22.0	23.8	27.4	23.9	26.5	28.1	30.0	32.6
55-65	18.7	20.9	22.5	24.4	28.0	23.6	26.0	27.8	29.5	32.0
65-75	18.5	20.8	22.5	24.4	27.9	22.3	25.1	26.8	28.4	30.6

Values derived by formula calculation. Data derived from the Health and Nutrition Examination Survey data of 1971-1974, using same population samples as those of the National Center for Health Statistics (NCHS) growth percentiles for children. Adapted from Frisancho AR: New norms of upper limb fat and muscle areas for assessment of nutritional status, *Am J Clin Nutr* 34:2540, 1981.

G

Clinical Signs and Symptoms of Various Nutrient Deficiencies

Area of Examination	Sign/Symptom	Potential Nutrient Deficiency
Hair	Alopecia	Zinc, essential fatty acids
	Easy pluckability	Protein, essential fatty acids
	Lackluster	Protein, zinc
	"Corkscrew" hair	Vitamin C, vitamin A
	Decreased pigmentation	Protein, copper
Eyes	Xerosis of conjunctiva	Vitamin A
	Corneal vascularization	Riboflavin
	Keratomalacia	Vitamin A
	Bitot's spots	Vitamin A
Gastrointestinal tract	Nausea, vomiting	Pyridoxine
	Diarrhea	Zinc, niacin
	Stomatitis	Pyridoxine, riboflavin, iron
	Cheilosis	Pyridoxine, iron
	Glossitis	Pyridoxine, zinc, niacin, folate, vitamin B_{12}
	Magenta tongue	Riboflavin
	Swollen, bleeding gums	Vitamin C
	Fissured tongue	Niacin
	Hepatomegaly	Protein
Skin	Dry and scaling	Vitamin A, essential fatty acids, zinc
	Petechiae, ecchymoses	Vitamin C, vitamin K
Skin – cont'd	Follicular hyperkeratosis	Vitamin A, essential fatty acids
	Nasolabial seborrhea	Niacin, pyridoxine, riboflavin
	Bilateral dermatitis	Niacin, zinc
Extremities	Subcutaneous fat loss	Kilocalories
	Muscle wastage	Kilocalories, protein
	Edema	Protein
	Osteomalacia, bone pain, rickets	Vitamin D
	Arthralgia	Vitamin C
Hematologic	Anemia	Vitamin B_{12}, iron, folate, copper, vitamin E, vitamin K
	Leukopenia, neutropenia	Copper
	Low prothrombin, prolonged clotting time	Vitamin K
Neurologic	Disorientation	Niacin, thiamin
	Confabulation	Thiamin
	Neuropathy	Thiamin, pyridoxine, chromium
	Paresthesia	Thiamin, pyridoxine, vitamin B_{12}
Cardiovascular	Congestive heart failure, cardiomegaly, tachycardia	Thiamin
	Cardiomyopathy	Selenium

From Ross Laboratories.

Normal Biochemical Levels for Nutrients and Test Measurements

Biochemical Indicators of Good Nutrition Status

Nutrient or Measurement	Test	Normal or Acceptable Levels	
		Men	Women
Iron	Hemoglobin (g/100 ml)	≥14.0	≥12.0
	Infants (under 2 years)	≥10.0	≥10.0
	Children (6-12 years)	≥11.5	≥11.5
	Pregnancy (2nd trimester)		≥11.0
	(3rd trimester)		≥10.5
Protein	Serum albumin (g/100 ml)	≥3.5	≥3.5
Normal lipid metabolism	Serum cholesterol (mg/100 ml)	<200	<200
	Serum triglyceride (mg/100 ml)	<250	<250
Normal carbohydrate metabolism	Serum glucose (mg/100 ml)	75-110	75-110
Sodium	Serum sodium (mEq/L)	130-150	130-155
Potassium	Serum potassium (mEq/L)	3.5-5.3	3.5-5.3
Vitamin A	Plasma vitamin A (μg/100 ml)	>20	>20
Vitamin C	Serum vitamin C (mg/100 ml)	≥0.3	≥0.3
Riboflavin	Erythrocyte glutathione peroxidase (% stimulation of activity by added riboflavin cofactor)	<20	<20
Vitamin B_6	Tryptophan load test—increase in excretion of xanthurenic acid (mg/day)	<25	<25
Folate	Serum folate (nanogram/ml)	>6.0	>6.0
Thiamin	Urinary thiamin (μg/g creatinine)	>65	>65
Zinc	Plasma zinc (μg/100 ml)	80-115	80-115

Some information obtained from Roe DA: *Drug-induced nutritional deficiencies,* Westport, Conn, 1976, AVI Press; and Sauberlich HE, Skala HH, and Dowdy RP: *Laboratory tests for the assessment of nutritional status,* Cleveland, 1974, CRC Press, Inc.

I

Recommended Nutrient Intakes for Canadians

Age	Sex	Energy (kcal)	Thiamin (mg)	Riboflavin (mg)	Niacin NE	n-3 PUFA (g)	n-6 PUFA (g)
0-4 months	Both	600	0.3	0.3	4	0.5	3
5-12 months	Both	900	0.4	0.5	7	0.5	3
1 year	Both	1100	0.5	0.6	8	0.6	4
2-3 years	Both	1300	0.6	0.7	9	0.7	4
4-6 years	Both	1800	0.7	0.9	13	1.0	6
7-9 years	M	2200	0.9	1.1	16	1.2	7
	F	1900	0.8	1.0	14	1.0	6
10-12 years	M	2500	1.0	1.3	18	1.4	8
	F	2200	0.9	1.1	16	1.2	7
13-15 years	M	2800	1.1	1.4	20	1.5	9
	F	2200	0.9	1.1	16	1.2	7
16-18 years	M	3200	1.3	1.6	23	1.8	11
	F	2100	0.8	1.1	15	1.2	7
19-24 years	M	3000	1.2	1.5	22	1.6	10
	F	2100	0.8	1.1	15	1.2	7
25-49 years	M	2700	1.1	1.4	19	1.5	9
	F	1900	0.8	1.0	14	1.1	7
50-74 years	M	2300	0.9	1.2	16	1.3	8
	F	1800	0.8*	1.0*	14*	1.1*	7*
75+ years	M	2000	0.8	1.0	14	1.1	7
	F†	1700	0.8*	1.0*	14*	1.1*	7*
Pregnancy (additional)							
1st Trimester		100	0.1	0.1	0.11	0.05	0.3
2nd Trimester		300	0.1	0.3	0.22	0.16	0.9
3rd Trimester		300	0.1	0.3	0.22	0.16	0.9
Lactation (additional)		450	0.2	0.4	0.33	0.25	1.5

NE, niacin equivalents; *PUFA,* polyunsaturated fatty acids.
*Level below which intake should not fall.
†Assumes moderate physical activity.
From Scientific Review Committee: *Nutrition recommendations,* Ottawa, 1990, Health and Welfare.

Summary Examples of Recommended Nutrient Intake Based on Age and Body Weight Expressed as Daily Rates

Age	Sex	Weight (kg)	Protein (g)	Vitamin A RE	Vitamin D (μg)	Vitamin E (mg)	Vitamin C (mg)	Folate (μg)	Vitamin B_{12} (μg)	Calcium (mg)	Phosphorus (mg)	Magnesium (mg)	Iron (mg)	Iodine (μg)	Zinc (mg)
0-4 months	Both	6.0	12*	400	10	3	20	25	0.3	250†	150	20	0.3‡	30	2‡
5-12 months	Both	9.0	12	400	10	3	20	40	0.4	400	200	32	7	40	3
1 year	Both	11	13	400	10	3	20	40	0.5	500	300	40	6	55	4
2-3 years	Both	14	16	400	5	4	20	50	0.6	550	350	50	6	65	4
4-6 years	Both	18	19	500	5	5	25	70	0.8	600	400	65	8	85	5
7-9 years	M	25	26	700	2.5	7	25	90	1.0	700	500	100	8	110	7
7-9 years	F	25	26	700	2.5	6	25	90	1.0	700	500	100	8	95	7
10-12 years	M	34	34	800	2.5	8	25	120	1.0	900	700	130	8	125	9
10-12 years	F	36	36	800	2.5	7	25	130	1.0	1100	800	135	8	110	9
13-15 years	M	50	49	900	2.5	9	30	175	1.0	1100	900	185	10	160	12
13-15 years	F	48	46	800	2.5	7	30	170	1.0	1000	850	180	13	160	9
16-18 years	M	62	58	1000	2.5	10	40§	220	1.0	900	1000	230	10	160	12
16-18 years	F	53	47	800	2.5	7	30§	190	1.0	700	850	200	12	160	9
19-24 years	M	71	61	1000	2.5	10	40§	220	1.0	800	1000	240	9	160	12
19-24 years	F	58	50	800	2.5	7	30§	180	1.0	700	850	200	13	160	9
25-49 years	M	74	64	1000	2.5	9	40§	230	1.0	800	1000	250	9	160	12
25-49 years	F	59	51	800	2.5	6	30§	185	1.0	700	850	200	13	160	9
50-74 years	M	73	63	1000	5	7	40§	230	1.0	800	1000	250	9	160	12
50-74 years	F	63	54	800	5	6	30§	195	1.0	800	850	210	8	160	9
75+ years	M	69	59	1000	5	6	40§	215	1.0	800	1000	230	9	160	12
75+ years	F	64	55	800	5	5	30§	200	1.0	800	850	210	8	160	9
Pregnancy (additional)															
1st Trimester			5	0	2.5	2	0	200	1.2	500	200	15	0	25	6
2nd Trimester			20	0	2.5	2	10	200	1.2	500	200	45	5	25	6
3rd Trimester			24	0	2.5	2	10	200	1.2	500	200	45	10	25	6
Lactation (additional)			20	400	2.5	3	25	100	0.2	500	200	65	0	50	6

RE, retinol equivalents.
*Protein is assumed to be from breast milk and must be adjusted for infant formula.
†Infant formula with high phosphorus should contain 375 mg of calcium.
‡Breast milk is assumed to be the source of the mineral.
§Smokers should increase vitamin C by 50%.
From Scientific Review Committee: *Nutrition recommendations,* Ottawa, 1990, Health and Welfare.

J

Food Guide: Exchange Lists for Meal Planning (1986 Revision)

The *exchange system of dietary control,* developed by two professional organizations—the American Dietetic Association and the American Diabetes Association—is based on a simple grouping of common foods according to generally equivalent nutritional values. This system may be used for any situation requiring caloric and food value control.

The foods are divided into six basic groups (with subgroups), called the "exchange lists." Each food item within a group or subgroup contains about the same food value as other food items in that group, allowing for exchange within groups, thus providing for variety in food choices as well as food value control. Hence the term *food exchanges* is sometimes used to refer to food choices or servings. The total number of "exchanges" per day depends on individual nutritional needs, based on normal nutrition standards. Although there is some variation in the composition of foods within the exchange groups, for simplicity the following values for carbohydrate, protein, fat, and kilocalories are used.

Exchange Lists

Food Groups	Carbohydrate (g)	Protein (g)	Fat (g)	Kcal
Starch/Bread	15	3	Trace	80
Meat				
Lean	—	7	3	55
Medium-fat	—	7	5	75
High-fat	—	7	8	100
Vegetable	5	2	—	25
Fruit	15	—	—	60
Milk				
Skim	12	8	Trace	90
Low-fat	12	8	5	120
Whole	12	8	8	150
Fat	—	—	5	45

List 1: Starch/Bread List

Whole grain foods have about 2 g fiber per serving. Foods containing 3 g fiber per serving or more are marked with the symbol *.

Cereals/grains/pasta

*Bran cereals, concentrated	⅓ cup
*Bran cereals, flaked (such as Bran Buds, All Bran)	½ cup
Bulgur (cooked)	½ cup
Cooked cereals	½ cup
Cornmeal (dry)	2½ tbsp
Grapenuts	3 tbsp
Grits (cooked)	½ cup
Other ready-to-eat unsweetened cereals	¾ cup
Pasta (cooked)	½ cup
Puffed cereal	1½ cup
Rice, white or brown (cooked)	⅓ cup
Shredded Wheat	½ cup
*Wheat germ	3 tbsp

Dried beans/peas/lentils

*Beans and peas (cooked; such as kidney, white, split, black-eyed)	⅓ cup
*Lentils (cooked)	⅓ cup
*Baked beans	¼ cup

Starchy vegetables

*Corn	½ cup
*Corn on cob, 6 inches long	1
*Lima beans	½ cup
*Peas, green (fresh, frozen, or canned)	½ cup
*Plantain	½ cup
Potato, baked	1 small (3 oz)
Potato, mashed	½ cup
Squash, winter (acorn, butternut)	¾ cup
Yam, sweet potato, plain	⅓ cup

Bread

Bagel	½ (1 oz)
Bread sticks, crisp (4 inches long × ½ inch)	2 (⅔ oz)
Croutons, low fat	1 cup
English muffin	½
Frankfurter bun or hamburger bun	½ (1 oz)
Pita (6 inches across)	½
Plain roll, small	1 (1 oz)
Raisin, unfrosted	1 slice (1 oz)
*Rye, pumpernickel	1 slice (1 oz)
Tortilla, 6 inches across	1
White (including French, Italian)	1 slice (1 oz)
Whole wheat	1 slice (1 oz)

Crackers/snacks

Animal crackers	8
Graham crackers (2½ inches square)	3
Matzoth	¾ oz
Melba toast	5 slices
Oyster crackers	24
Popcorn (popped, no fat added)	3 cups
Pretzels	¾ oz
Rye crisp (2 inches × 3½ inches)	4
Saltine-type crackers	6
Whole wheat crackers, no fat added (crisp breads, such as Finn, Kavli, Wasa)	2-4 slices (¾ oz)

Starch foods prepared with fat (count as 1 starch/bread serving + 1 fat)

Biscuit (2½ inches across)	1
Chow mein noodles	½ cup
Corn bread (2 inch cube)	1 (2 oz)
Cracker, round butter type	6
French fried potatoes (2 to 3½ inches long)	10 (1½ oz)
Muffin, plain, small	1
Pancake (4 inches across)	2
Stuffing, bread (prepared)	¼ cup
Taco shell (6 inches across)	2
Waffle (4½ inch square)	1
Whole wheat crackers, fat added (such as Triscuits)	4-6 (1 oz)

List 2: Meat and Meat Substitutes List

To reduce fat intake, choose items mainly from the lean and medium-fat groups, using more fish and poultry (with skin removed) as meat choices, and trimming fat from all meats. Items having 400 mg sodium or more per exchange are marked with the symbol **. None of the items on this list contributes fiber to the diet. One exchange is equal to the amount listed for each item. In the case of meat, for example, a serving may be 2-3 exchanges (2-3 oz).

Lean meat and substitutes

Beef	USDA Good or Choice grades of lean beef, such as round, sir-loin, and flank steak; tenderloin; and chipped beef**	1 oz
Pork	Lean pork, such as fresh ham; canned, cured, or boiled ham**; Canadian bacon**; tenderloin	1 oz
Veal	All cuts except for veal cutlets (ground or cubed)	1 oz
Poultry	Chicken, turkey, Cornish hen (without skin)	1 oz
Fish	All fresh and frozen fish	1 oz
	Crab, lobster, scallops, shrimp, clams (fresh or canned in water**)	2 oz
	Oysters	6 medium
	Tuna** (canned in water)	¼ cup
	Herring (uncreamed or smoked)	1 oz
	Sardines (canned)	2 medium
Wild game	Venison, rabbit, squirrel	1 oz
	Pheasant, duck, goose (without skin)	1 oz
Cheese	Any cottage cheese	¼ cup
	Grated parmesan	2 tbsp
	Diet cheeses** (less than 55 kcal/oz)	1 oz
Other	95% fat-free luncheon meat	1 oz slice
	Egg whites	3 whites
	Egg substitutes (less than 55 kcal/¼ cup)	¼ cup

Medium-fat meat and substitutes

Beef	Ground beef, roast (rib, chuck, rump), steak (cubed, porterhouse, T-bone), and meatloaf (most beef products are in this category)	1 oz
Pork	Chops, loin roast, Boston butt, cutlets (most pork products fall into this category)	1 oz
Lamb	Chops, leg, and roast (most lamb products fall into this category)	1 oz
Veal	Cutlet (ground or cubes, unbreaded)	1 oz
Poultry	Chicken (with skin), domestic duck or goose (well-drained of fat), ground turkey	1 oz
Fish	Tuna** (canned in oil and drained)	¼ cup
	Salmon** (canned)	¼ cup
Cheese	Skim or part-skim cheeses, such as:	
	Ricotta	¼ cup
	Mozzarella	1 oz
	Diet cheeses** (56-80 kcal/oz)	1 oz
Other	86% fat-free luncheon meat**	1 oz
	Egg (high in cholesterol, limit to 3/week)	1
	Egg substitutes (56-80 kcal per ¼ cup)	¼ cup
	Tofu (2½ × 2¾ × 1 inch)	4 oz
	Liver, heart, kidney, sweetbreads (high in cholesterol, limit use)	1 oz

High-fat meat and substitutes (these items are high in saturated fat, cholesterol, and kilocalories; limit to 3 times/week)

Beef	USDA Prime cuts, ribs; corned beef**	1 oz
Pork	Spareribs, ground pork, pork sausage**	1 oz
Lamb	Ground lamb patties	1 oz
Fish	Any fried fish product	1 oz
Cheese	Regular cheeses**, such as American, Blue, Swiss	1 oz
Other	Luncheon meat**, such as bologna, salami, pimento loaf	1 oz slice
	Sausage**, such as Polish, Italian	1 oz
	Knockwurst, smoked	1 oz
	Bratwurst**	1 oz
	Frankfurter** (turkey or chicken)	1 frank (10/lb)
	Frankfurter** (beef, pork, or combination) (count as 1 high-fat meat + 1 fat)	1 frank (10/lb)
	Peanut butter	1 tbsp

List 3: Vegetable List

Unless otherwise noted, one vegetable exchange is 1 cup raw vegetable or ½ cup cooked vegetable or vegetable juice. Vegetables containing 400 mg sodium or more per serving are marked with the symbol **. Fresh and frozen vegetables have less added salt. Canned vegetables contain more salt, but rinsing will help remove much of it. In general, vegetables contain 2-3 g dietary fiber per serving. Starchy vegetables are found in the Starch/Bread List. Other free vegetables are in the Free Food List.

Artichoke (½ medium)	Mushrooms, cooked
Asparagus	Okra
Beans (green, wax, Italian)	Onions
Bean sprouts	Pea pods
Beets	Peppers (green)
Broccoli	Rutabaga
Brussels sprouts	Sauerkraut**
Cabbage	Spinach
Carrots	Summer squash (crookneck)
Cauliflower	Tomato (1 large)
Eggplant	Tomato/vegetable juice
Greens (collard, mustard, turnip)	Turnips
Kohlrabi	Water chestnuts
Leeks	Zucchini

List 4: Fruit List

Fruits containing 3 g dietary fiber or more per serving are marked with the symbol *. Portions are usual serving sizes of commonly eaten fruits.

Fresh, unsweetened frozen, and unsweetened canned fruit

Apple (raw, 2 inches across)	1 apple
Applesauce (unsweetened)	½ cup
Apricots (medium, raw)	4 apricots
Apricots (canned)	½ cup or 4 halves
Banana (9 inches long)	½ banana
*Blackberries (raw)	¾ cup
*Blueberries (raw)	¾ cup
Canteloupe (5 inches across)	⅓ melon
Canteloupe (cubes)	1 cup
Cherries (large, raw)	12 cherries
Cherries (canned)	½ cup
Figs (raw, 2 inches across)	2 figs

Fruit cocktail (canned)	½ cup
Grapefruit (medium)	½ grapefruit
Grapefruit (segments)	¾ cup
Grapes (small)	15 grapes
Honeydew melon (medium)	⅛ melon
Honeydew melon (cubes)	1 cup
Kiwi fruit (large)	1 kiwi fruit
Mandarin oranges (segments)	¾ cup
Mango (small)	½ mango
*Nectarine (1½ inches across)	1 nectarine
Orange (2½ inches across)	1 orange
Papaya (small cubes or balls)	1 cup
Peach (2¾ inches across)	1 peach
Peach (slices)	¾ cup
Peaches (canned)	½ cup or 2 halves
Pear	½ large pear or 1 small
Pears (canned)	½ cup or 2 halves
Persimmon (medium, native)	2 persimmons
Pineapple (raw, cubes)	¾ cup
Plum (raw, 2 inches across)	2 plums
*Pomegranate	½ pomegranate
*Raspberries (raw)	1 cup
*Strawberries (raw, whole)	1¼ cups
Tangerine (2½ inches across)	2 tangerines
Watermelon (cubes or balls)	1¼ cup

Dried fruit

*Apples	4 rings
*Apricots	7 halves
Dates	2½ medium
*Figs	1½
*Prunes	3 medium
Raisins	2 tbsp

*Fruit juice

Apple juice or cider	½ cup
Cranberry juice cocktail	⅓ cup
Grapefruit juice	⅓ cup
Grape juice	⅓ cup
Orange juice	½ cup
Pineapple juice	½ cup
Prune juice	⅓ cup

List 5: Milk List

Milk may be used alone or in combination with other foods. See the Combination Foods List.

Skim and very lowfat milk

Skim or nonfat milk	1 cup
½% milk	1 cup
1% milk	1 cup
Lowfat buttermilk	1 cup
Evaporated skim milk	½ cup
Dry nonfat milk	⅓ cup
Plain nonfat yogurt	8 oz

Lowfat milk

2% milk	1 cup
Plain lowfat yogurt (with added nonfat milk solids)	8 oz

Whole milk (more than 3¼% butterfat; limit use)

Whole milk	1 cup
Evaporated whole milk	½ cup
Whole plain yogurt	8 oz

List 6: Fat List

Measure carefully; use mainly unsaturated fats. Sodium content varies widely, so check labels.

Unsaturated fats

Avocado	⅛ medium
Margarine	1 tsp
Margarine, diet	1 tbsp
Mayonnaise	1 tsp
Mayonnaise, reduced kcal	1 tbsp
Nuts and seeds	
Almonds, dry roasted	6 whole
Cashews, dry roasted	1 tbsp
Pecans	2 whole
Peanuts	20 small or 10 large
Walnuts	2 whole
Other nuts	1 tbsp
Seeds, pine nuts, sunflower (shelled)	1 tbsp
Pumpkin seeds	1 tsp
Oil (corn, cottonseed, safflower, soybean, sunflower, olive, peanut)	1 tsp
Olives	10 small or 5 large
Salad dressing, mayonnaise type	2 tsp
Salad dressing, mayonnaise type, low kcal	1 tbsp
Salad dressing (all varieties)	1 tbsp
Salad dressing, low kcal	2 tbsp
(2 tbsp low-calorie salad dressing is a free food)	

Saturated fats

Butter	1 tsp
Bacon	1 slice
Chitterlings	½ oz
Coconut, shredded	2 tbsp
Coffee whitener, liquid	2 tbsp
Coffee whitener, powder	4 tsp
Cream (light, coffee, table)	2 tbsp
Cream, sour	2 tbsp
Cream (heavy, whipping)	1 tbsp
Cream cheese	1 tbsp
Salt pork	¼ oz

Free Foods

Any food or drink containing less than 20 kcal/serving is "free." If a serving size is given, 2-3 servings per day are sufficient. Higher fiber* or sodium** foods are indicated. Use *nonstick pan spray* for cooking as desired.

Drink

Bouillon** or broth, fat-free
Bouillon, low sodium
Carbonated drinks, sugar-free
Carbonated water
Club soda
Cocoa powder, unsweetened   1 tbsp
Coffee/Tea
Drink mixes, sugar-free
Tonic water, sugar-free

Condiments

Catsup   1 tbsp
Horseradish
Mustard
Pickles**, dill, unsweetened
Salad dressing, low kcal   2 tbsp
Taco sauce   1 tbsp
Vinegar

Seasonings

Basil (fresh)
Celery seeds
Cinnamon
Chili powder
Chives
Curry
Dill
Flavoring extracts
    (vanilla, almond, walnut, butter)
Garlic, fresh and powder
Herbs, spices
Hot pepper sauce and flakes
Lemon, juice and zest (outer skin)
Lemon pepper
Lime, juice and zest
Mint, fresh leaves
Onion powder
Oregano
Paprika
Parsley
Pepper
Pimento
Soy sauce**
Soy sauce, low sodium—"lite"
Wine, used in cooking   ¼ cup
Worcestershire sauce

Fruits

Cranberries, unsweetened   ½ cup
Rhubarb, unsweetened   ½ cup

Vegetables

Cabbage
Celery
Chinese cabbage*
Cucumber
Green onion
Hot peppers
Mushrooms
Radishes
Zucchini*

Salad greens

Endive
Escarole
Lettuce
Romaine
Spinach

Sweet substitutes

Candy, hard, sugar-free
Gelatin dessert, sugar free
Gum, sugar-free
Jam/Jelly, sugar-free   2 tsp
Pancake, syrup, sugar-free   1-2 tbsp
Sugar substitutes
    (saccharin, aspartame)
Whipped topping   2 tbsp

Combination Foods

Check the *American Dietetic Association/American Diabetes Association Family Cookbooks* and the *American Diabetes Association Holiday Cookbook* for many recipes and much information, including combination foods.

Food	Amount	Exchanges
Casserole, homemade	1 cup (8 oz)	2 starch, 2 medium-fat meat, 1 fat
Cheese pizza**, thin crust	¼ of 10 inch	2 starch, 1 medium-fat meat, 1 fat
Chili beans* **	1 cup (8 oz)	2 starch, 2 medium-fat meat, 2 fat
Chow mein* ** (without noodles or rice)	2 cups	1 starch, 2 vegetables, 2 lean meat
Macaroni and cheese**	1 cup	2 starch, 1 medium-fat meat, 2 fat
Spaghetti and meatballs (canned)	1 cup	2 starch, 1 medium-fat meat, 1 fat
Sugar-free pudding (made with skim milk)	½ cup	1 starch

Soup

Food	Amount	Exchanges
Bean* **	1 cup	1 starch, 1 vegetable, 1 lean meat
Chunky, all varieties**	10¾ oz can	1 starch, 1 vegetable, 1 medium-fat meat
Cream** (made with water)	1 cup	1 starch, 1 fat
Vegetable** or broth**	1 cup	1 starch

Beans used as a meat substitute

Food	Amount	Exchanges
Dried beans*, peas*, lentils* (cooked)	1 cup	2 starch, 1 lean meat

Foods for Occasional Use

Food	Amount	Exchanges
Angel food cake	¹⁄₁₂ cake	2 starch
Plain cake, no icing	¹⁄₁₂ cake or 3 in square	2 starch, 2 fat
Cookies	2 small (¾ in across)	1 starch, 1 fat
Frozen fruit yogurt	⅓ cup	1 starch
Gingersnaps	3	1 starch
Granola	¼ cup	1 starch, 1 fat
Granola bars	1 small	1 starch, 1 fat
Ice cream, any flavor	½ cup	1 starch, 2 fat
Ice milk, any flavor	½ cup	1 starch, 1 fat
Sherbet, any flavor	¼ cup	1 starch
Snack chips**, all varieties	1 oz	1 starch, 2 fat
Vanilla wafers	6 small	1 starch, 1 fat

K Dietary Fiber and Kilocalorie Values for Selected Foods

Foods	Serving	Dietary fiber (g)	Kcal
Breads and cereals			
All Bran	⅓ cup	8.5	70
Bran (100%)	½ cup	8.4	75
Bran Buds	⅓ cup	7.9	75
Corn Bran	⅔ cup	5.4	100
Bran Chex	⅔ cup	4.6	90
Cracklin' Oat Bran	⅓ cup	4.3	110
Bran Flakes	¾ cup	4.0	90
Air-popped popcorn	1 cup	2.5	25
Oatmeal	1 cup	2.2	144
Grapenuts	¼ cup	1.4	100
Whole-wheat bread	1 slice	1.4	60
Legumes, cooked			
Kidney beans	½ cup	7.3	110
Lima beans	½ cup	4.5	130
Vegetables, cooked			
Green peas	½ cup	3.6	55
Corn	½ cup	2.9	70
Parsnip	½ cup	2.7	50
Potato, with skin	1 medium	2.5	95
Brussels sprouts	½ cup	2.3	30
Carrots	½ cup	2.3	25
Broccoli	½ cup	2.2	20
Beans, green	½ cup	1.6	15
Tomato, chopped	½ cup	1.5	17
Cabbage, red & white	½ cup	1.4	15
Kale	½ cup	1.4	20
Cauliflower	½ cup	1.1	15
Lettuce (fresh)	1 cup	0.8	7
Fruits			
Apple	1 medium	3.5	80
Raisins	¼ cup	3.1	110
Prunes, dried	3	3.0	60
Strawberries	1 cup	3.0	45
Orange	1 medium	2.6	60
Banana	1 medium	2.4	105
Blueberries	½ cup	2.0	40
Dates, dried	3	1.9	70
Peach	1 medium	1.9	35
Apricot, fresh	3 medium	1.8	50
Grapefruit	½ cup	1.6	40
Apricot, dried	5 halves	1.4	40
Cherries	10	1.2	50
Pineapple	½ cup	1.1	40

Adapted from Lanza E, Butrum RR: A critical review of food fiber analysis and data, *J Am Diet Assoc* 86:732, 1986.

Exercise Levels With Age, Nutrition, Fluid, and Health Assessment Guidelines

Definitions	Examples (Not Inclusive)	Recommended Age
1. **Routine:** The duration of the activity is less than 20 minutes, and it may or may not reach 60% of maximum heart beat rate.	Recess play, casual walking, recreational noncontinual sport (i.e., T-ball, volleyball)	Minimum activity level for any age
2. **Health Fitness:** 60% to 80% of maximum heart beat rate is achieved for greater than 20 minutes at least three times per week for a minimum of 6 months. The activity should involve muscular strength and flexibility.	Brisk walking, jogging, running, cycling, hiking, swimming, dancing	Preferred level for any age
3. **Competitive Sports:** An activity less than or equal to 6 months that consists of team involvement, preseason training, and competing either as a team member or individually at an intramural or interschool level.	Swimming, gymnastics, diving, volleyball, wrestling, sprinting, relay, football, soccer, basketball, tennis, field hockey, cross country	Junior high age and above
3a. **Competitive <6 months:** Short endurance—intense activity that lasts for 20 minutes or less.	As above	Junior high age and above
3b. **Competitive <6 months:** Long endurance—activity, intense or nonintense, that lasts for longer than 20 minutes.	As above	High school age and above
4. **Competitive Sports:** Longer than 6 months. Same as above Competitive, but usually involved at a personal level other than school.	Same as 3 above, but may include state or national competition	High school age and above
4a. **Competitive 6 months:** Short endurance—same as above.	As above	
4b. **Competitive 6 months:** Long endurance—same as above.	As above	
5. **Performing:** An activity that requires dedicated practice (several times a week) to perform with a group or individually a routine lasting anywhere from 5 min to 1 hr (or longer) in competition or performance.	Ballet, dance, or gymnastics	Junior high age and above as determined by a physician
6. **Marching Band:** Involvement with a band that competes or performs in marching or choreographed performance. Includes preseason training as well as competition or performance.	High school marching or competing bands	Junior high age and above
7. **Seasonal:** Intramural involvement with a team or individual activity not based heavily on winning but just participation. Practice required. May or may not last longer than 20 minutes three or more times a week, but activity is not sustained longer than 2 or 3 months.	Soccer, softball, swimming lessons	All ages

Nutrition Comments	Fluid Intake	Recommended Health Assessment
Normal nutrition for age from the basic food groups	Normal for age	Yearly routine exam from a pediatrician or physician for all age children.
Normal nutrition for age from the basic food groups. If desired weight for height, possibly more calories.	Good hydration, especially in adverse weather. Normal requirements for age plus replacement of lost fluid from activity.	Yearly routine exam from a pediatrician or physician for all age children. Education from a physician or health professional on healthy practices (diet, fluid, injury prevention, warm-up and cool-down techniques, etc.). Immediate attention from an appropriate health professional for an injury or insult.
Nutrition assessment, recommendations, and education, preferably from a registered dietitian for an individual's season intake to achieve weight and body composition for the sport. Recommendations will be dependent on type of activity, duration, and intensity.	Pre-event, event, and post-event (or pre-practice and postpractice) hydration. Good hydration at other times. Electrolyte replacement may be needed if heavy sweating occurs or in adverse weather conditions.	Preparticipation assessment by a health team consisting of a physician, dietitian, nurse or nurse practitioner, and possibly a physical therapist. Examination as well as education should be given to students at this time. Immediate attention from an appropriate health professional for any injury or insult during the sports season.
2 g protein/kg for growing athletes 1 g protein/kg for mature athletes May need carbohydrate during the event if long in duration (>4 hr). Modified carbohydrate loading (normal diet, intense exercise 7-4 days before, high carbohydrate diet 3-1 days before event) no more than 2-3 times per year.	Electrolyte replacement needs assessed and replacement given if necessary.	
Same as 3 above	Same as 3 above	As above. It is very important that a physician determine that the maturation age of the participant is appropriate for the sport.
Nutrition assessment, recommendations, and education provided, preferably by a registered dietitian due to the usually restricted intake to achieve desired weight for performance	Normal hydration and replacement of lost fluids from practice or performance	Preparticipation assessment by a physician, dietitian, and possibly an orthopedist or physical therapist. Injury attention as in competitive sports.
Nutrition assessment, recommendations, and education, preferably from a registered dietitian in a group setting, or individually if necessary.	As above in 3a, 3b	Same as above in 2 or 3a, 3b. Nutrition attention by a registered dietitian if the participant is less than 85% or greater than 120% of desired weight for height.
As in 2 above.	As above in 3a, 3b	Preparticipation assessment by a pediatrician or physician, as in 2 above. Nutrition attention by a registered dietitian if the participant is less than 85% or greater than 120% of desired weight for height.

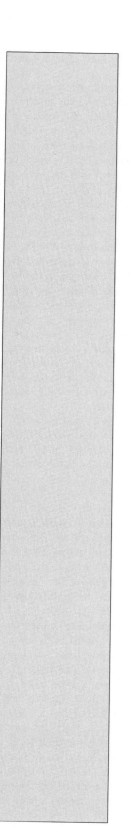

Glossary

Abscissa (L *ab,* from; *scindere,* to cut) Usually the horizontal X line used as a base of reference in graphing relative data. When suitable values are assigned to both of the two lines of the graph, the horizontal X axis or ordinates and the bisecting vertical Y axis or abscissas, corresponding data with reference to the other can be plotted.

Acetaldehyde Chemical compound, intermediate metabolic product in the breakdown of alcohol by liver enzymes.

Achlorhydria (L *a-,* negative; *chlorhydria,* hydrochloric acid) Absence or reduced amounts of hydrochloric acid in the gastric secretions.

Acne (Gr *achne,* chaff) Common inflammation (*acne vulgaris*) of the pilosebaceous (L *pilus,* hair; *sebum,* suet; thick semifluid secretion composed of fat and epithelial cell debris) glands of the skin, mainly on the face, chest, and back. Precise cause unknown, but suggested factors include hormones, stress, heredity, and bacteria; usually self-limiting after the physiologic stress of puberty.

Acrocyanosis (Gr *akron,* extremity; *kyanos,* blue) Condition characterized by cyanotic discoloration, coldness, and sweating of the extremities, especially the hands, caused by arterial spasm that is usually precipitated by cold or emotional stress.

Acronym (Gr *acros,* topmost, foremost; *-onym,* word, name) A word or name formed from the initial letters or groups of letters of words in a set series.

Addiction (L *addictio,* a giving over, surrender, being enslaved to) State of being enslaved to some undesirable practice that is physically or psychologically habit-forming to the extent that its cessation causes severe trauma.

Adenoidal pad (Gr *adenos,* gland; *eidos,* form) Normal lymphoid tissue in the nasopharynx of children.

Adenosine triphosphate (ATP) The high energy compound formed in the cell, called the "energy currency" of the cell due to the binding of energy in its high-energy phosphate bonds for release for cell work as these bonds are split.

Adipocytes (L *adipis,* fat; *kytos,* hollow vessel, cell) Fat cells.

Adipose tissue (L *adipis,* fat, lard) Loose connective tissue in which fat cells (adipocytes) accumulate and are stored.

Affective goal Communication goal related to processes of feelings and desires, attitudes and values.

Alopecia (Gr *alopekia,* disease in which hair falls out) Baldness; absence of hair from skin areas of the body where it normally is present.

Alveoli (L *alveus,* hollow) Small sac-like formations; thin-walled chambers in the lungs surrounded by networks of capillaries through whose walls exchange of carbon dioxide and oxygen takes place.

Alveoli (L *alveus,* hollow) Small sac-like outpouching areas in the mammary gland, secretory units that produce and secrete milk.

Alzheimer-type senile dementia (ATSD) A type of senile dementia first described by German physician Alois Alzheimer (1864-1915); progressive, irreversible degenerative changes in the brain, resulting in loss of neuromuscular function and mental capacity.

Amenorrhea (Gr *a-,* negative; *men,* month; *rhoia,* flow) Absence of menses. Nutritional amenorrhea results from extreme weight loss and malnutrition, as in eating disorders such as anorexia nervosa.

Amino acids (*amino,* the monovalent chemical group -NH2) Carriers of the essential element nitrogen; structural units of protein, specific amino acids being linked in specific sequence by peptide chains to form specific proteins.

Amylase (Gr *amylon,* starch; *-ase,* enzyme suffix) Group name for enzymes that act on starch to render successively smaller and smaller molecules of dextrins and maltose, for example, salivary amylase (ptyalin) and pancreatic amylase (amylopsin). The generic group name amylase is now more widely used for any starch-splitting enzyme.

Anabolic steroids (Gr *anabole,* a building or construction) Any of a group of synthetic derivatives of testosterone, the male sex hormone, having pronounced anabolic (tissue building) properties; a drug used in clinical medicine to promote growth and repair of tissues in debilitating illness. Widespread illegal abuse of the drug by some athletes and body builders harms their health.

Anabolism Metabolic process by which body tissues are built.

Anemia (Gr *a-,* negative; *haima,* blood) Blood condition marked by a decrease in number of circulating red blood cells, hemoglobin, or both.

Anorexia: (Gr *a, orexis* not appetite) Loss of appetite.

Anorexia nervosa (Gr *anorektos,* without appetite; L *nervosa,* nervous or emotional disorder) A severe psychophysiologic eating disorder, usually seen in girls and young women, in which the person does not lack appetite, as the label would indicate, but is psychologically unable to eat and refuses food, becoming extremely emaciated; a form of self-starvation.

Antagonist (Gr *antagonisma,* struggle) Agent that has an opposite, conflicting, or inhibiting action to another substance.

Antepartum (L, *anto,* before; *partum,* parting, a separate part) Period of gestation before onset of maternal labor and birth of the infant.

Anthropometry (Gr *anthropos,* man, human; *metron,* measure) The science and procedures that deal with measurement of the size, weight, and proportional dimensions of the human body.

Antibodies Immune system components, specific immunoglobulins, especially secretory IgA in the bowel and upper respiratory mucosa that destroy invading antigens.

Antidiuretic hormone (ADH) Hormone secreted by the posterior pituitary gland in response to body stress. It acts on the distal tubules of the kidney's nephrons to cause water reabsorption and thus protect vital body water; also called *vasopressin.*

Antigen (antibody + Gr *gennan,* to produce) Any disease agent such as toxins, bacteria, viruses, and other foreign substances, whose presence stimulates the production of antibodies of the immune system to combat and destroy them.

Antioxidant (Gr *anti-,* against; *oxys,* keen) A substance that inhibits oxidation of polyunsaturated fatty acids and formation of free radicals in the cells.

Antirachitic (Gr *anti-,* against; *rachitis,* a spinal disorder) An agent that is therapeutically effective against rickets, a nutritional deficiency disease affecting childhood bone development, in which vitamin D is lacking.

Aorta Main large trunk blood vessel from the heart, leading down the center of the body through the chest and upper abdomen from which the systemic arterial blood system proceeds.

Apgar score A scale developed by American anesthesiologist Virginia Apgar (1909-1974), by which an infant's condition is defined at 1 minute and 5 minutes after birth by scoring the heart rate, respiratory effort, muscle tone, reflex irritability, and color.

Apocrine (Gr *apokrinesthai,* to be secreted) A type of glandular secretion in which the end portion of the secreting cell is removed with the secretory product.

Areola (L *areola,* area, space) Pigmented area surrounding the nipple of the human breast.

Ascorbic acid Chemical name for vitamin C, based on its antiscorbutic function in prevention of the deficiency disease scurvy.

Atherosclerosis (Gr *athere,* gruel; *skleros,* hard) Condition characterized by gradual formation, beginning in childhood in genetically predisposed individuals, of fatty cheese-like streaks that develop into hardened plaques in the intima or inner lining of major blood vessels such as coronary arteries, eventually in adulthood cutting off blood supply to the tissue served by the vessel; the underlying pathology of coronary heart disease.

Atherosclerotic lesions Characteristic lesions, called athromas; the fatty raised streaks and plaques that signal atherosclerosis, the underlying cardiovascular disease associated with elevated levels of serum lipids, especially cholesterol, and related risk factors such as smoking, obesity, and hypertension.

Atrophic gastritis A chronic inflammation of the stomach causing damage to the mucosal lining and reduced secretion of hydrochloric acid and in some cases intrinsic factor; loss of intrinsic factor and the inability to absorb vitamin B_{12} leads to pernicious anemia.

Autonomy (Gr *autos,* self; *nomos,* law) State of functioning independently; self-determination.

Axis (L *axis,* axle, central line) One of two coordinates (the other called abscissa) used as a frame of reference between values in graphing data; usually the vertical Y axis, also called ordinate axis.

Barbiturate: (Saint Barbara, drug discovered on day of the saint, 1864) Drug used to reduce anxiety or induce sleep; sometimes used to treat disorders causing convulsions.

Basal oxygen consumption Amount of oxygen intake to meet basal metabolic needs; a means of measuring basal metabolic rate (BMR). Comparative metabolic measures in current use are derived by formula calculation using individual factors of weight, height, age, and sex: basal energy expenditure (BEE), and resting energy expenditure (REE).

Basic four food groups A simple general food guide issued by the U.S. Department of Agriculture, using a grouping of commonly used foods and agricultural products for planning a day's balanced meals: breads/cereals, vegetables/fruits, milk and dairy products, and meat, with recent suggested food item revisions to reduce fats and sugars.

Behavioral goal Communication goal related to processes of changing behavior.

Bile (L *bilis,* bile) A fluid secreted by the liver and transported to the gallbladder for concentration and storage; released into duodenum upon entry of fat to facilitate enzymatic fat digestion by acting as an emulsifying agent.

Bioavailability Amount of a nutrient ingested in food that is absorbed and thus available to the body for metabolic use.

Blastocyst (Gr *blastos,* germ; *kystis,* sac, bladder) A stage in the development of the embryo in which the cells are arranged in a single layer to form a hollow sphere.

Body compartment The collective quantity of a particular vital substance in the body, for example, the mineral compartment, composed mainly of the skeletal bone mass.

Body composition The relative sizes of the four body compartments that make up the physical body—lean body mass, fat, water, and mineral mass.

Body mass index A calculated assessment of body mass based on weight and height: BMI = weight (kg) divided by height (m)^2.

Botulism A serious, often fatal, form of food poisoning from ingesting food contaminated with the powerful toxins of the bacteria *Clostridium botulinum.* The toxin blocks transmission of neural impulses at the nerve terminals, causing gradual paralysis and death when affecting respiratory muscles. Most cases result from eating carelessly home-canned food, so that all such foods should be boiled at least 10 minutes before eating. Cases reported in infants have been related to eating spore-containing honey, so honey should not be fed to infants.

Bradycardia (Gr *bradys,* slow; *kardia,* heart) A slow heart beat, evidenced by slowing of the pulse rate to less than 60 beats/min.

Brush border Vast array of microvilli covering each villus on the absorptive surface of the small intestine, holding nutrients ready for absorption within an unstirred layer of water and facilitating their absorption with a greatly expanded surface area. So named because they appear as the bristles of a brush when viewed with an electron microscope.

Buffering capacity Function of the body's main buffer system, composed of two balancing partners, an acid partner (carbonic acid) and a base partner (sodium bicarbonate), that act together to buffer or neutralize any incoming acid or base to maintain the necessary degree of acidity and alkalinity in the body fluids that is compatible with life and health.

Bulimia nervosa (L *bous,* ox; *limos,* hunger; *nervosa,* nervous or emotional condition) A psychophysiologic eating disorder, seen mainly in girls and young women, marked by alternate gorging on large amounts of food followed by self-induced vomiting and purging with laxative; weight usually remains fairly stable at a normal amount.

Cachexia (Gr *kakos,* bad, ill; *hexia,* habit) A profound and grave state of body disorder and deterioration, as seen in cases of advanced malignant disease or starvation, causing gross body weight loss to cadaverous proportions as a result of disorder metabolism.

Calcitonin (L *calx,* lime, calcium; *tonus,* balance) A polypeptide hormone secreted by the thyroid gland in response to hypercalcemia, which acts to lower both calcium and phosphate in the blood.

Calcitriol Activated hormone form of vitamin D [1,25(OH)$_2$D$_3$]—1,25,dihydroxycholecalciferol.

Candida albicans (L *candidus,* glowing white) Most frequent agent of *candidiasis,* a yeast-like fungus infecting moist tissue areas of the body, involving skin, vaginal, and oral mucosa.

Carbohydrate fuel Basic organic carbon compound in food (starches and sugars) that is the primary and most efficient form of body fuel for energy, especially for building body muscles.

Carboxypeptidase (L *carbo-,* coal, carbon—fundamental element in all organic compounds) The chemical group *carboxyl*—COOH—at the end of the carbon chain identifies the compound as an organic acid. The end of this term, *-peptidase,* indicates a protein-splitting enzyme, which together with the first part means that this is an enzyme that acts on the peptide bond of the terminal amino acid having a free-end carboxyl group.

Cardiac output Total amount of blood pumped by the heart per minute.

Carnitine A naturally occurring amino acid ($C_7H_{15}NO_3$) formed from methionine and lysine, required for transport of long-chain fatty acids across the mitochondrial membrane where they are oxidized as fuel substrate for metabolic energy.

Carotenemia Condition associated with excess intake or impaired metabolism of carotenoid pigments, especially beta-carotene, resulting in excess carotene in the blood, sometimes to the extent of producing a yellowing of the skin resembling jaundice.

Carotenoids Any of a group of red and yellow pigments chemically similar to and including carotene found in dark green and yellow vegetables and fruits.

Casein hydrolysate formula Infant formula with base of hydrolyzed casein, major milk protein, produced by partially breaking down the casein of cow's milk into smaller peptide fragments, making a product that is more easily digested.

Catabolism Metabolic process by which body tissue is broken down.

Catalyst (Gr *katalysis,* dissolution) A substance, such as enzymes and their component trace elements, that controls specific cell metabolism reactions but is not changed or consumed itself in the reaction as are the specific substrates on which it works.

Cathartic (Gr *katharsis,* cleansing) A substance used to empty the bowel; a laxative.

Celiac disease (Gr *koilia,* belly) A malabsorption diarrheal disease of intestinal mucosa caused by an abnormal reaction to gluten in certain grains such as wheat; infantile form marked by extreme wasting, growth retardation, and celiac crisis.

Cephalopelvic disproportion (Gr *kephale,* head; *pyelos,* an oblong trough, pelvis) Relationship of fetal head to size of the maternal pelvis.

Cerebral hemorrhage Rupture of an artery in the brain; cerebrovascular accident (CVA), stroke.

Cheilosis (Gr *cheilos,* lip) A general symptom of tissue inflammation and breakdown producing swelling and reddening of the lips, a chapped appearance, and fissures at the corners of the mouth; associated with general malnutrition, especially a deficiency of riboflavin.

Cholecalciferol Chemical name for vitamin D in its inactive dietary form (D_3). Formerly measured in terms of International Units (IU), a concept based on the "biologic activity" of a vitamin as measured in rats according to its ability to forestall the development of a disease associated with a deficiency of that specific vitamin. Now, instead, vitamin recommendations are given in direct quantity (mg or μg) needed for health based on current population studies. In the case of vitamin D, 10 μg as cholecalciferol equals 400 IU. When the inactive cholecalciferol is consumed, it is activated first in the liver and then completed in the kidney to its active vitamin D hormone form *calcitriol* (1,25-dihydroxycholecalciferol [$1,25(OH)_2D_3$]). Additional amounts of D_3 are generated by effect of sunlight on 7-dehydrocholesterol in the skin, a precursor cholesterol compound.

Chronic diseases (Gr *chronos,* time) Diseases of aging or long duration.

Chronologic age Age of an individual based on the number of years lived, compared, for example, with *biologic age,* the relative age of a person based on physiologic capacity and measurements.

Chymotrypsin (Gr *chymos,* chyme, creamy gruel-like material produced by gastric digestion of food) One of the protein-splitting and milk-curdling pancreatic enzymes, activated in the intestine from precursor chymotrypsinogen; breaks peptide linkages of the amino acids phenylalanine and tyrosine.

Cineradiographs (Gr *cine-,* kinesis, movement; L *radius,* ray; Gr *graphein,* to write) Fluoroscopic motion film records of internal structures and functions.

Citric acid cycle Final energy production pathway in the cell mitochondria that transforms the ultimate fuel acetyl CoA from carbohydrate and fat, capturing this energy in the cell's metabolic enzyme cycle production of high-energy phosphate bonds of ATP.

Clinical care process An interactive process between health care professional and client of planning personal health care through five phases of assessment and data collection, analysis of findings, planning care according to a written individual care plan, implementing the plan, and evaluating and recording results.

Cobalamin Chemical name for vitamin B_{12}, from its structure as a complex red crystalline compound of high molecular weight, with a single cobalt atom at its core. Its food sources are of animal origin, but the ultimate source is from colonies of synthesizing microorganisms inhabiting the gastrointestinal tract of herbivorous animals.

Coefficient of variation Change or effect produced by the variation in certain factors, or the ratio between two different quantities.

Coenzyme factors A major metabolic role of the micronutrients, vitamins, and minerals as essential partners with cell enzymes in a variety of reactions in both energy and protein metabolism.

Cognitive goal (L *cognito,* to know) Communications goal related to the process of knowing and learning; mental processes of thinking and remembering.

Colostrum (L *colostrum,* bee sting swelling and secretions) Thin, yellowish, milky liquid; mother's initial breast secretion before and immediately after birth of her baby; rich in immune factors and nutrition, especially protein and minerals; foremilk.

Communication Process of giving or interchanging information, thoughts, or feelings by speaking, writing, signing, discussing, listening, responding.

Community care process Program planning to meet defined community health needs through assessment procedures, objectives, program plan, and evaluation.

Complement Series of enzymatic proteins that interact with an antigen-antibody complex to promote phagocyte activity or destroy other cells; component of the body's immune system.

Complementary amino acids Combinations of amino acids from a variety of combined protein foods that complete one another according to their relative amounts of individual amino acids in order to meet growth requirements for the nine essential amino acids that the body does not sufficiently synthesize.

Complete protein A protein food containing all of the essential amino acids; animal food sources are milk, cheese, meat, eggs. Plant proteins alone are incomplete, but complementary combinations may be planned to make a complete protein mix, as a vegetarian would do.

Complex carbohydrates Main dietary carbohydrate; the polysaccharide starch in various foods such as legumes, grains, breads, pasta, cereals, and potatoes.

Condom (L *condus,* a receptacle) A penile sheath serving not only as a barrier method of contraception but also as a means of preventing the spread of sexually transmitted diseases.

Congregate meals Group meals for older adults, served in a social setting in the community and funded by Title III-C of the Older Americans Act.

Constipation (L *constipation,* a crowding together) Infrequent, sometimes difficult, passage of feces; condition is often a source of anxiety to elderly persons and may be perceived more in mental attitude than in physiologic reality; sometimes called "irritable bowel."

Corpus luteum (Gr *corpus,* body; *luteum,* yellow) Mass of estrogen and progesterone secretory cells; produced monthly from the ovarian follicle in the postovulation phase of the female sexual cycle.

Cortical bone (Gr *corticis,* bark, shell) Long bones of the body extremities with heavy outer cortex layer, giving strength to body movements.

Corticosteroid (L *corticis,* bark, shell) Any of the steroids affecting carbohydrate, fat, and protein metabolism, that are produced in the outer region (cortex) of the adrenal glands in response to stimulus of the adrenocorticotropic hormone (ACTH) from the pituitary gland, or any of their synthetic derivatives. These compounds include *glucocorticoids* affecting glucose metabolism, and *mineralocorticoids* affecting electrolyte (Na^+) concentration and hence fluid-electrolyte balance.

Counseling A dynamic process of communication that is client-centered; the role of counselor is to guide the client to identify problems and priorities and to set goals and possible solutions.

Crohn's disease Inflammatory disease first described by New York physician Bernard Crohn (born 1884), involving any part of the gastrointestinal tract, but commonly affecting the lower small intestine and colon.

Cushing's syndrome A condition first described by Boston surgeon Harvey Cushing (1869-1939), due to hypersecretion of adrenocorticotropic hormone (ACTH) or excessive intake of glucocorticoids; characterized by rapidly developing fat deposits of face, neck, and trunk, giving an enlarged and rounded "moon-face" or cushingoid appearance.

Cytoplasm (Gr *kytos,* hollow vessel; *plasma,* anything formed or molded) The protoplasm of the cell outside the nucleus, a continuous gel-like aqueous solution in which the cell organelles are suspended; site of major cell metabolism.

Deamination Process by which the nitrogen radical (NH_2) is split off from amino acids, important in maintaining nitrogen balance.

Decubitus ulcer A bedsore which is caused by prolonged pressure on the skin and tissues covering a bony area; occurs in elderly people who are confined to bed or immobilized.

Dementia (L *de* + *mens,* mind) Progressive organic mental disorder causing changes in personality, disorientation, deterioration in intellectual function, and loss of memory and judgment; dementia caused by drug overdose, electrolyte or fluid imbalance, or insulin shock will be reversed on treatment; dementia caused by injury or degenerative changes in brain tissue is not reversible.

De novo (L *anew,* from the beginning) To make a new product from the beginning with the principal components; akin to "from scratch" as in cooking.

Dental caries (L *caries,* "rottenness") Molecular decay or death of hard tissue; disease of the calcified tissues of the teeth resulting from action of microorganisms on carbohydrate producing acid erosion of the tooth surface; characterized by disintegration of hard outer enamel, followed by breakdown of softer inner dentin material, leaving cavities and exposed soft tissue.

Dentin (L *dens,* tooth) Chief substance of the tooth; surrounds the innermost tooth pulp and is covered by the enamel of the crown and the cementum on the roots.

Depot fat Body fat stored in adipose tissue.

Desquamation (L *de-,* from; *squama,* scale) The shedding of epithelial tissue, mainly from the skin and oral mucosa, in scales or small sheets.

Diagnosis related groups (DRGs) A U.S. government cost-containment management classification scheme for predesignation of Medicare payments based on specific diagnosis categories of disease.

Dietary fiber Nondigestible form of carbohydrate; of nutritional importance in gastrointestinal disease such as diverticulosis, and in management of serum lipid and glucose levels in risk-reduction related to chronic conditions such as heart disease and diabetes.

Dietary guidelines for Americans Diet and health guidelines for planning a healthy diet and reducing disease risks.

Diuresis (Gr *diourein,* to urinate) Increased excretion of urine.

Diuretics (Gr *diouretikos,* promoting urine) Drugs that stimulate urination.

Docosahexaenoic acid (DHA) (Gr *docosa,* 22; *hexa,* 6) Long chain polyunsaturated omega-3 fatty acid, having a 22 carbon chain with 6 double bonds; a metabolic product of omega-3 eicosapentaenoic (*eicosa,* 20; *penta,* 5)—EPA, long-chain fatty acid with 20 carbon atoms and 5 double bonds. Both are found in fatty fish. The body also synthesizes both EPA and DHA from the essential fatty acid linoleic and its product linolenic acid.

Dysgeusia (Gr *dys,* bad; *geusis,* taste) Abnormally perverted sense of taste, or bad taste in the mouth.

Ectoderm (Gr *ektos,* outside; *derma,* skin) The outermost of the three primary cell layers of the embryo.

Edema (Gr *oidema,* swelling) An unusual accumulation of fluid in the intercellular tissue spaces of the body.

Edentulous (L *e-,* without; *dens,* tooth) Absence of natural teeth.

Eicosapentaenoic acid (EPA) (Gr *eicosa,* 20; *penta,* 5) Long-chain polyunsaturated fatty acid composed of a chain of 20 carbon atoms with 5 double (unsaturated) bonds; one of the omega-3 fatty acids found in fatty fish and fish oils.

Electrolyte (Gr *electron,* amber [which emits electricity when rubbed]; *lytos,* soluble) A chemical element or compound that in solution dissociates as ions carrying a positive or negative charge, for example, H^+, Na^+, K^+, Ca^{++}, Mg^{++}, and Cl^-, HCO^-_3, HOP^-_4, SO^-_4. Electrolytes constitute a major force controlling fluid balances within the body through their concentrations and shifts from one place to another to restore and maintain balance—*homeostasis.*

Elemental formula Infant formula produced with elemental, ready to be absorbed components of free amino acids and carbohydrate as simple sugars.

Enamel The very hard white surface substance that covers and protects the soft inner dentin of a tooth.

Endoderm (Gr *endon,* within; *derma,* skin) The innermost of the three primary embryonic cell layers.

Endometrium (Gr *endon,* within; *metra,* uterus) The inner mucous membrane of the uterus.

Endoplasmic reticulum (Gr *endon,* within; *plassein,* to form; L *rete,* net) A protoplasmic network in cells of flattened double membrane sheets; important metabolic cell organelles, some with rough surfaces bearing ribosomes for protein synthesis and other smooth surfaces synthesizing fatty acids.

Energy (Gr *energeia,* energy) The power to overcome resistance, to do work.

Energy balance Physiologic aspect of weight management, based on balance between energy intake in food and energy output in physical activity and internal metabolic work.

Energy intake Energy value of the three energy-yielding macronutrients in food—carbohydrate, fat, and protein, measured in kilocalories; abbreviated kcalories or kcal.

Enmeshed To catch, as in a net, and entangle; intertwined family relationships that capture and diminish individual autonomy or self-regard.

Epidemiology (Gr *epidemios,* prevalent; *-ology,* study) The study of factors determining the frequency, distribution, and strength of diseases in population groups.

Epiglottis (Gr *epi-,* on; *glottis,* vocal apparatus of the larynx) Lid-like cartilaginous structure overhanging the entrance to the larynx and preventing food from entering the larynx and trachea while swallowing.

Epipharynx (Gr *epi-,* on; *pharynx,* throat) Nasopharynx that lies above the level of the soft palate.

Episiotomy (Gr *epision,* pubic region; *tome,* a cutting) Surgical incision into the peritoneum and vagina for obstetrical purposes.

Epithelium (Gr *epi-,* on, upon, over; *thele,* nipple) The covering tissue of internal and external surfaces of the body, including linings of vessels and other small cavities.

Erythrocyte (Gr *erythro-,* red; *cyte,* hollow vessel) Red blood cell.

Erythropoiesis (Gr *erythros,* red; *poiesis,* making) The production of erythrocytes, red blood cells.

Essential amino acid Any one of nine amino acids that the body cannot synthesize at all or in sufficient amounts to meet body needs so it must be supplied by the diet, hence a *dietary* essential for these nine specific amino acids: histidine, isoleucine, leucine, lysine, methionine, phenylalanine, threonine, tryptophan, and valine.

Esterification Chemical process of converting an acid into an *ester,* catalyzed by the enzyme *esterase.* An ester is any compound formed from an alcohol and an acid by removal of water, for example, cholesterol esterification by attaching a fatty acid to the sterol base.

Estrogen Generic group name for the ovarian hormones—beta-estradiol (the most potent), estrone, and estriol, which function to develop and maintain the female sexual organs and to stimulate bone growth.

Ethanol Chemical name for beverage alcohol.

Evaluation Process of determining the value of an educational or clinical program in terms of its initial identified objectives.

Extracellular fluid (ECF) The total body water compartment composed of the collective water outside of cells.

Extracellular water Alternate term for collective body water or fluids outside of cells.

18:2 fatty acid Naming system for fatty acids according to structure: carbon chain length and number of double (unsaturated) bonds. Thus, an 18:2 fatty acid would have a long chain of 18 carbon atoms with 2 double bonds. This is the chemical shorthand for linoleic acid, the essential fatty acid.

Ferrous sulfate Iron fortification compound in infant formulas used as needed to prevent anemia.

Flatulence (L *flatus,* a blowing) Excessive formation and expulsion of gases in the gastrointestinal tract.

Follicle (L *follis,* leather bag) Sac-like secretory cavity encasing an ovum and nourishing its growth.

Food abuse Misuse and excessive eating of food as a reflection of underlying personal needs or problems, rather than in normal amount and nature as an essential part of good health and enjoyment.

Food exchange lists (groups) A meal-planning food guide of six food exchange lists, with indicated portion sizes and equivalent food values for each item in a group, hence items may be exchanged within each group to maintain both variety and food values. The six food groups are bread/cereal, vegetable, fruit, milk, meat, and fat. Easily used for nutrient and energy calculations for management of diabetes and weight.

Food frequency questionnaire (FFQ) A tool for collecting nutrition information about food habits. Consists of a comprehensive list of foods and a scale for checking frequency of use over a period of time.

Food guide A model for planning and evaluating a daily diet.

Food record A 3- to 7-day record of all food consumed, detailed with portion sizes, amounts, and preparation methods or recipes, for nutrition analysis as part of a total nutrition assessment process for planning nutrition care and education, or as an ongoing tool for monitoring nutritional therapy.

Fortified cereal Cereal food products enriched by additions of minerals such as iron and zinc, and vitamins such as thiamin, riboflavin, niacin, folate, B_6, and B_{12}.

Free radical An unstable, high-energy cell molecule with an unpaired electron that causes oxidation reactions in unsaturated fatty acids and may act as a carcinogen.

Frontal bossing (ME *boce,* lump, growth) A rounded protuberance of the forehead. In general terms, a boss is a knob-like rounded protuberance on the body or some body organ.

Functional disability Disability that interferes with activities of daily living, such as bathing, dressing, shopping, preparing meals, eating.

Galactosemia A rare genetic disease in newborns caused by a missing enzyme (galactose-1-phosphate uridyltransferase-G-1-PUT) required for conversion of galactose to glucose for metabolic use in the body. Untreated, galactose (from lactose) accumulates in the blood, causing extensive tissue damage and potential death. Normal growth and development now follows mandatory newborn screening and immediate initiation of a galactose-free diet with a special soy-based formula.

Gastrectomy Surgical removal of all or part of the stomach.

Gastric (Gr *gaster,* stomach) Pertaining to the stomach.

Gastric pH (Gr *gaster,* stomach; *pH,* power of the hydrogen ion—H^+) Chemical symbol relating to H^+ concentration or activity in a solution; expressed numerically as the negative logarithm of H^+ concentration: pH 7.0 is neutral—above it alkalinity increases, and below it acidity increases. The hydrochloric acid (HCl) gastric secretions maintain a gastric pH of about 2.0.

Generativity (L *generatio,* generation) The dynamic psychosocial process of renewing a society's values from one generation to the next.

Gerontology The study of aging including biologic, physiologic, psychologic, and sociologic aspects. Contrast with *geriatrics,* which is the medical specialty dealing with chronic disease, as well as physical health, in older adults.

Gestation (L *gestare,* to bear) Intrauterine fetal growth period (40 weeks) from conception to birth.

Gestational age Period of embryonic-fetal growth and development from ovum fertilization to birth, varying from preterm development of a premature infant to a full-term mature newborn.

Gingivitis (L *gingiva,* "gum of the mouth") Inflammation of the gum tissue surrounding the base of the teeth.

Glomerular filtration rate A measure of the amount of blood filtered by the cup-like glomerulus at the head of each kidney nephron, per unit of time (ml/min).

Gluconeogenesis (Gr *gleukos,* sweetness; *neos,* new; *gennan,* to produce) Production of glucose from keto-acid carbon skeleton from deaminated amino acids and the glycerol portion of fatty acids.

Glucose Simple sugar, basic refined body fuel, circulated in the blood to cells for energy production.

Glycogen A briefly stored form of carbohydrate in the liver and muscle tissues, available for energy fuel during brief fasting periods of sleep; built up in larger storage amounts by high starch meals prior to endurance athletic events for sustained energy.

Glycogen loading Practice among athletes in endurance events of increasing intake of complex carbohydrates in days before the event to increase glycogen storage for energy reserve fuel during the event.

Glycolysis Initial energy production enzyme pathway outside the mitochondria, by which 6-carbon glucose is changed to active 3-carbon fragments of acetyl CoA, the fuel ready for final energy production in the mitochondria to the high-energy phosphate bone compound adenosine triphosphate (ATP).

Goitrogens Natural substances in certain foods such as soybeans that cause hypothyroidism and a compensatory enlargement of the thyroid gland, producing symptoms of iodine-deficiency goiter; effect diminished by adequate heating of the soy meal and adding iodine supplementation.

Golgi apparatus A complex cup-like structure of membranes with associated vesicles, first described by Italian Nobel prize-winning histologist Camillo Golgi (1843-1926); site for synthesis of numerous carbohydrate metabolic products such as lactose, glycoproteins, and mucopolysaccharides.

Granulosa cells Cells surrounding the primitive ovarian follicle and forming its outer layer and the mature ovary.

Grazing Informal descriptive label for food pattern of frequent small snacks throughout the day rather than more formal regular meals. Term taken from animal pattern of constant eating in a pastureland.

Growth acceleration Period of increased speed of growth at different points of childhood development.

Growth channel The progressive regular growth pattern of children, guided along individual genetically controlled channels, influenced by nutritional and health status.

Growth deceleration Period of decreased speed of growth at different points of childhood development.

Growth grid Chart indicating weight-height growth rates of infants and children by percentiles of a representative population, on which an individual child's growth may be plotted for comparison and monitoring over time.

Growth velocity (L *velocitas,* speed) Rapidity of motion or movement; rate of childhood growth over normal periods of development, as compared with a population standard.

Guaiac test A laboratory test for occult (unseen) blood in the stool.

Gynecologic age (Gr *gynaikos,* women) Length of time from onset of menses to present time of conception.

Hematocrit (Gr *haima,* blood; *krinein,* to separate) The volume percentage of red blood cells in whole blood, showing ratio of RBC volume to total blood volume, normally about 35% in women; abbreviated HCT.

Heme iron Dietary iron from animal sources, from heme portion of hemoglobin in red blood cells. More easily absorbed and transported in the body than nonheme iron from plant sources, but supplying the smaller portion of the body's total dietary iron intake.

Hemochromatosis (Gr *haima,* blood; *chroma,* color) Disorder of iron metabolism characterized by excess iron deposits in the tissues, especially the liver and pancreas; results from iron overload from prolonged use of iron supplements or from transfusions.

Hemoglobin (Gr *haima,* blood; L *globus,* a ball) Oxygen-carrying pigment in red blood cells; a conjugated protein containing 4 heme groups combined with iron and 4 long polypeptide chains forming the protein globin, named for its ball-like form; made by the developing RBC in bone marrow.

Hemolytic anemia (Gr *haima,* blood; *lysis,* dissolution) An anemia (reduced number of red blood cells) caused by breakdown of red blood cells and loss of their hemoglobin.

Hemorrhoids (Gr *haima,* blood; *rhoia,* to flow) Enlarged veins in the mucous membranes inside or outside of the rectum; causes pain, itching, discomfort, and bleeding.

Heterozygote (Gr *hetero,* other; *zygotos,* yoked together) An individual possessing different *alleles* (gene forms occupying corresponding chromosome sites) in regard to a given character trait.

Hirsutism (L *hirsutus,* shaggy hair) A condition marked by abundant and excessive hair; abnormal hairiness, especially an adult male pattern of body hair distribution in women.

Homeostasis (Gr *homoios,* like, unchanging; *stasis,* standing, steady) The life-sustaining relative dynamic equilibrium within the body's internal environment; a biochemical and physiologic balance achieved through the constant operation of numerous interrelated homeostatic mechanisms.

Homogenization (Gr *homos,* same; *genos,* kind) Process of forming a permanent emulsion by breaking up fat portion into fine globules and dispersing them equally throughout the milk for uniform quality.

Hydrocephalus (Gr *hydro-,* water; *kephale,* head) A condition characterized by enlargement of the cranium caused by abnormal accumulation of fluid.

Hydrolysis (Gr *hydro-,* water; *lysis,* dissolution) Process by which a chemical compound is split into other simpler compounds by taking up the elements of water, as in the manufacture of infant formulas to produce easier-to-digest derivatives of the main protein casein in the cow's milk base; process occurs naturally in digestion.

Hydroscopic (Gr *hydro-,* water; *skopein,* to measure or examine) Possessing tendency to take up and hold water readily.

Hydroxyapatite The inorganic compound of calcium, phosphate, and hydroxide found in the matrix of bones and teeth, giving rigidity and strength to the structure.

Hypercalcemia Elevated level of calcium in the blood.

Hyperinsulinemia (Gr *hyper* + L *insula,* island) An excessively high level of insulin in the blood.

Hyperlipidemia (Gr *hyper,* above; *lipos,* fat; *haemia,* blood) General term for elevated concentrations of any or all of the lipids in the blood plasma.

Hypernatremic dehydration An abnormally high sodium ion (Na^+) concentration in the extracellular fluid, due to water loss or restriction, drawing cell water to restore osmotic balance, causing dangerous cell dehydration. Compare with *hyponatremia.*

Hyperplasia (Gr *hyper,* above; *plasis,* formation) Enlargement of tissue due to a process of rapidly increasing cell number. Compare with *hypertrophy.*

Hypertrophy (Gr *hyper,* above; *trophe,* nutrition) Enlargement of an organ or part due to the process of increasing cell size.

Hyperventilation (Gr *hyper,* above; L *ventilatio,* ventilation) Increased respiration with larger intake and consequent oxygen-carbon dioxide exchange in the lungs above the normal amount.

Hypogeusia (Gr *hypo-,* under; *geusis,* taste; *aisthesis,* perception) An abnormally diminished acuteness of the sense of taste.

Hyponatremia Abnormally low levels of sodium (Na^+) in the blood; can be easily caused by excess water intake to point of water intoxication, with resulting dilution of the major electrolyte (Na^+) in extracellular circulating fluids.

Hypothalamus (Gr *hypo-,* under; *thalamos,* inner chamber) A small gland adjacent to the pituitary in the midbasal brain area; serves as a collection and dispatching center for information about the internal well-being of the body, using much of this neuroendocrine information to stimulate and control many widespread important pituitary hormones.

Hypovolemia (Gr *hypo-,* under; ME *volume,* volume; Gr *haima,* blood) Low blood volume.

Ideal weight Optimal weight for an individual of a given height, sex, or age in relation to personal health.

Immunoglobulins (L *immunis,* free, exempt; *globulus,* globule, ball) Special components of the body's immune system, proteins synthesized by lymphocytes and plasma cells that have specific antibody activity.

Infant mortality Number of infant deaths during the first year of life (1 month to 1 year) per 1000 live births.

Insensible water loss Daily water loss through the skin and respiration, so named because a person is not aware of it. An additional smaller amount is lost in normal perspiration, the amount varying with the surrounding temperature.

Interpolation (L *interpolare,* to make new) Process of injecting new interpretation or application of data to expand meaning or use, as in deriving data from one age group and applying it to another.

Intracellular water Collective body water or fluids inside of cells; in body composition measures a large portion assigned to total lean body mass, a vital component in cell metabolism.

Intubation Passage of a tube into a body hole, specifically the insertion of a breathing tube through the mouth or nose or into the trachea to ensure a patent airway for the delivery of an anesthetic gas or oxygen.

Involution (L *involutio,* in, into; *volvere,* to roll) A process of rolling or turning inward, shrinking an organ to its normal size, as the uterus after childbirth.

Ions (Gr *ion,* wanderer) Activated form of certain minerals, such as sodium (Na^+), potassium (K^+), and chloride (Cl^-), that carry an electrical charge and perform a variety of essential metabolic tasks.

Iron absorption Degree of iron absorption, relativity small at best, depends upon its acid reduction, either by accompanying food such as orange juice or by the gastric HCl secretions, from the ferric form (Fe^{+++}) in foods to the ferrous form (Fe^{++}) required for absorption. After absorption (about 30% of the total intake) it is oxidized back to the ferric form required for incorporation in body metabolism.

Isomaltase (Gr *isos,* equal; L *maltum,* grain) Enzyme of the intestinal mucosa that splits isomaltose, an *isomer* of maltose (an isomer is a compound like another compound capable of behaving in a similar manner), a digestive product of starch in grains.

Juxtaglomerular apparatus (L *juxta,* near; *glomus,* ball) A complex of special cells located near or adjoining the cup-like glomerulus at the head of each kidney nephron; responsible for sensing the level of sodium in the blood.

Ketones Class of organic compounds, including three keto-acid basis that occur as intermediate products of fat metabolism: acetoacetate, hydroxybutyrate, and acetone; excess production, as in the initial stages of starvation from burning body fat for energy fuel, leads to ketoacidosis, which if continued uncontrolled can bring coma and death.

Kilocalorie (kcalorie, kcal) Unit of measure for energy produced in the body by the energy-yielding macronutrients carbohydrate, fat, and protein.

Kwashiorkor Classic protein-deficiency disease, frequently encountered in children in developing countries, but also seen in developed countries such as the United States in poverty areas and in metabolically stressed and debilitated hospitalized patients.

Kyphosis (Gr *kyphos,* hunchbacked) An abnormal outward curvature of the upper back resulting from age-related bone loss from the vertebrae.

Lactation (L *lactare,* to suckle) The process of milk production and secretion in the mammary glands.

Lactiferous ducts (L *lac,* milk; *ferre,* to bear; *ducere,* to lead or draw) Vessels conducting milk from producing cells to storage and release areas of the breast; tube or passage for secretions.

Lactobacillus bifidus (L *bifidus*) A predominant fermentative lactobacillus in the intestinal flora of breastfed infants.

Lactoferrin (L *lac,* milk; *ferrum,* iron) An iron-binding protein found in human milk.

Lactoperoxidase Enzyme found in human milk that catalyzes the oxidation of organic substrate, including harmful microorganisms, thereby protecting the infant.

Lacunae (L *lacuna,* small pit or hollow cavity) Blood spaces of the placenta in which the fetal villi are found.

Lanolin (L *lana,* wool) Fatty substance extracted from wool, used in ointments and salves.

Larynx (Gr *larynx,* upper part of windpipe) Structure of muscle and cartilage lined with mucous membrane, connected to top part of the trachea and to the pharynx; essential sphincter muscle guarding the entrance to the trachea and functioning secondarily as the organ of the voice.

Laws of thermodynamics (Gr *therme,* heat; *dynamis,* power) Basic three laws of physics relating to heat-energy balance: (1) energy-like matter is neither created nor destroyed, only constantly transformed and recycled, thus conserving energy in any process; (2) there is always an increase in *entropy* (Gr *entrope,* a turning inward), a measure of the part of heat or other energy form in a system that is not available to perform work, thus entropy increases in all natural (spontaneous and irreversible) processes; and (3) absolute zero in energy balance is unattainable.

Lean body mass Collective fat-free mass of body composition; most metabolically active portion of body tissues.

Life expectancy The average remaining years a person of a given age may expect to live, based on statistical population averages.

Lifestyle A person's unique pattern of living which, depending on its form, can be negative or positive in its health result.

Linear growth (L *linearis,* a line) Linear measure of growing body length; height.

Linoleic acid The ultimate essential fatty acid for humans.

Lipase (Gr *lipos,* fat; *-ase,* as, ending indicating an enzyme, attached to a stem that indicates the substrate upon which it works) Group name for enzymes that work on lipids (fats), splitting fatty acids from the glycerol base.

Lipids Chemical group name for fats and fat-related compounds such as cholesterol, lipoproteins, and phospholipids; general group name for organic substances of a fatty nature, including fats, oils, waxes, and related compounds.

Lipolysis (Gr *lipos,* fat; *lysis,* dissolution) The breakdown of fat; fat digestion.

Lobule (L *lobus,* lobe, a well-defined area) A small lobe, one of the primary divisions of a larger lobe; smaller branching vessels or subdivisions that make up a lobe of the mammary gland.

Locus of control (L *locus,* place, site) A person's perceived control center over his life.

Long-term care Medical, personal, or homemaking services provided within an institution or in the community for older adults who are no longer able to care for their own needs.

Longitudinal study Study of persons or populations over a long period of time to measure effects of specific factors on the aging process and incidence and course of disease.

Low birth weight Birth weight less than 2500 g (5.4 lb); very low birth weight, less than 1500 g (3.2 lb).

Lymphoblasts (L *lympha,* water; Gr *blastos,* germ) The immature stage of the mature lymphocyte.

Lymphocytes Mature leukocytes, special lymphoid white blood cells, T cells and B cells, major components of the body's immune system; found in human milk.

Lymphoid tissue (L *lympha,* water) Tissues related to the body system of lymphatic fluids; body tissues giving rise to lymphocytes of the immune system, such as intestinal mucosa and lymph gland.

Lyophilization (Gr *lyein,* to dissolve; *philein,* to love, having an affinity for a stable solution) Process of rapid freezing and dehydration of the frozen product under high vacuum to stabilize or preserve a biologic substance.

Lysozyme (Gr *lysis,* dissolution; *zyme,* leaven) A crystalline basic enzyme in many body fluids such as saliva, tears, and human milk; an antibacterial agent.

Macronutrients (Gr *makros,* large; L *nutriens,* nourishment) Group name for the three large energy-yielding nutrients—carbohydrate, fat, and protein—all organic compounds of large molecular size.

Macrophage (Gr *makros,* large; *phagein,* to eat) Large phagocytes, cells of the immune system that engulf and consume microorganisms, other cells, or foreign particles, and interact with T cells and B cells to produce inflammatory process and antibodies.

Major minerals Minerals that occur in relatively large quantities in the body and hence have greater dietary requirements.

Maltase Enzyme acting on the disaccharide maltose, from starch breakdown, into its two component monosaccharides, two units of glucose.

Mammalian Any vertebrate animal belonging to the class *Mammalia,* or humans, who give birth to live young and nourish them with milk from the female mammary glands.

Mammary glands (Gr *mamme,* mother's milk) Milk-producing glands in females of all mammalian species, humans and animals, who are distinguished from all other life by bearing live young and producing milk to nourish them.

Marsupial (L *marsupium,* a pouch) A member of the animal class of mammals who bear undeveloped young, which they carry in an abdominal pouch and nourish with their milk until development is complete; includes such animals as kangaroos and koala bears.

Mastitis (Gr *mastos,* breast; *-itis,* inflammation) Breast infection; inflammation of the mammary gland.

Maturation (L *maturus,* mature) The process or stage of attaining one's full physical, psychosocial, and mental development. Individual genetic potential guides physical and mental development, which in turn bears the imprint of environmental, psychosocial, and cultural influence.

Mean Mathematical term for the average numerical value of a group of numbers.

Median (L *medianus,* middle) The middle value in a distribution of numbers, with half of the values falling above and half falling below.

Megaloblastic anemia (Gr *mega,* great size; *blastos,* embryo, germ) Anemia due to faulty production of abnormally large immature red blood cells, due to a deficiency of vitamin B_{12} and folate.

Menarche (Gr *men,* month; *arche,* beginning) Onset of menses.

Menopause (Gr *meno-,* month; *pausis,* cessation) Cessation of menses, occurring in North American women at approximately 50 years of age.

Menses Monthly menstrual periods.

Menstruation The monthly discharge of blood and mucosal tissue from the nonpregnant uterus; final phase of the female sexual cycle.

Mesoderm (Gr *mesos,* middle; *derma,* skin) An intermediate layer of embryonic cells developing between the ectoderm (outer layer) and endoderm (inner layer).

Metabolic acidosis Abnormal rise in acid partner of the carbonic acid-base bicarbonate buffer system by excess of organic acids, which displace part of the base bicarbonate in the buffer system and cause the H^+ concentration (acidity) to rise.

Metabolic activity Sum of biochemical actions and reactions in the body that build and maintain tissue, regulate body functions, and require a constant energy source. The most metabolically active tissue is the lean body mass.

Metabolism (Gr *metaballein,* to change) Sum of all the various biochemical and physiologic processes by which the body grows and maintains itself (anabolism) and breaks down and reshapes tissue (catabolism), transforming energy to do its work.

Micelle (L *micella,* small body) A microscopic colloid particle of fat and bile formed in the small intestine for initial stage of fat absorption.

Microcephaly (Gr *mikros,* small; *kephate,* head) Small size of the head in relation to the rest of the body.

Micronutrients (Gr *mikros,* small; L *nutriens,* nourishing) Group name for the nonenergy-yielding nutrients, the vitamins, organic compounds of small molecular size, and minerals, single inert elements; essential coenzyme factors in metabolism and tissue structure.

Microphthalmia (Gr *micro,* small; *ophthalmos,* eye) Abnormal smallness of one or both eyes.

Mid-upper arm muscle circumference (MAMC) Indirect measure of the body's skeletal muscle mass based on mid-arm muscle circumference (MAMC) and triceps skinfold (TSF): MAMC (cm) = MAC (cm) − [0.314 × TSF (mm)].

Milieu (Fr *milieux,* surroundings) Environment, social or physical; an important concept in nutrition, referring to both external sociophysical setting and internal biochemical environments, and interacting balances between them.

Milliosmoles (mOsm/L) Osmole (Gr *osme,* small), standard unit of osmotic pressure; equal to the gram molecular weight of solute divided by the number of particles (ions) into which a substance dissociates in solution. Thus milliosmole would be a much smaller unit of measure of osmotic pressure — $\frac{1}{1000}$ of an osmole, equal to $\frac{1}{1000}$ gram molecular weight of a substance divided by the number

of ions into which a substance dissociates in 1 liter (L) of solution. The term *osmolality* refers to this concentration of solutes per unit of solvent.

Mineral compartment Smallest part of the body composition, found mainly in the skeletal bone mass.

Mitochondria (Gr *mitos,* thread; *chondrion,* granule) Cells' "powerhouse," small elongated organelles located in the cell cytoplasm; principal site of energy generation (ATP synthesis); contains enzymes of the final energy cycle (citric acid cycle) and cell respiration, as well as ribonucleic acid (RNA) and deoxyribonucleic acid (DNA) for some synthesis of protein.

Mortality rate Total number of deaths in a specific category divided by the total number of deaths in the total population.

Morula (L *morus,* mulberry) A solid mass of cells resembling a mulberry, formed by cleavage of a fertilized ovum.

Motivation Forces that affect individual goal-directed behavior toward satisfying needs or achieving personal goals.

Multigravida (L *multus,* many; *gravida,* pregnant) A woman who has had two or more pregnancies.

Multiparous (L *multus,* many, much; *parere,* to bring forth) Women who have had two or more pregnancies resulting in live births.

Myelin (Gr *myelos,* marrow) High lipid-to-protein substance forming sheath to insulate and protect neuron axons and facilitate their neuromuscular impulses.

Myocardial infarction (MI) (Gr *mys,* muscle; L *infarcire,* to stuff it; Gr *kardia*) Death of heart muscle tissue resulting from blockage of blood flow to or through the coronary arteries, usually caused by fatty plaques and blood clot formation from their tissue irritation to the surrounding blood vessel, effectively "stuffing" the vessel at that point and cutting off blood supply to the heart muscle tissue served by the vessel. This event is commonly called a heart attack.

Myocardium (Gr *mys,* muscle; *kardia,* heart) Heart muscle; middle and thickest layer of heart wall.

Myoepithelial cells (Gr *mys,* muscle; *epi-,* on; *thele,* nipple) Tissue composed of contractile epithelial cells surrounding the alveoli and duct system of the lactating breast.

Nanogram (abbreviated ng) (Gr *nano-,* dwarf)

One billionth gram; also called millimicrogram.

Nanomole (abbreviated nmole) (Gr *nanos,* dwarf; *molekul,* molecule) Metric system unit for measuring very small amounts. Prefix *nano-* used in naming very small amounts to indicate one billionth of the unit with which it is combined. *Mole* is chemical term for the molecular weight of a substance expressed in grams — gram molecular weight.

Narcissism Self-love; from Narcissus, a character in Greek mythology who saw his image mirrored in a pool of water and fell in love with his own reflection.

Necrotizing enterocolitis (Gr *nekrosis,* deadness; *enterion,* intestine) An infectious tissue destroying intestinal disease of the small intestine and the colon; acute inflammation of intestinal mucosa.

Negative nitrogen balance Situation in which the amount of nitrogen consumed is less than the amount of nitrogen lost through all excretory routes resulting in a net loss of body nitrogen.

Neonatal (Gr *neos,* new; L *natus,* born) The period surrounding birth; especially the first four weeks after birth when the infant is called a neonate.

Neonatal mortality Number of newborn deaths during the neonatal period (birth to 1 month postpartum) per 1000 live births.

Neonate A newborn infant; term usually refers to the first 4 weeks of life.

Nephron Functional unit of the kidneys, constantly filtering the blood, selectively reabsorbing its components as needed to maintain normal blood values, and excreting the remainder in a concentrated urine. At birth, each kidney has about a million of these minute units, far more than actually needed.

Neuromotor (Gr *neuron,* nerve; L *motorium,* movement center) Movement involving nerve impulses to muscles.

Neurotransmitter (Gr *neuron,* nerve; L *trans,* through, across; *missio,* sending) Large group of some 40 different chemical substances, including compounds as diverse as acetylcholine, various hormones, and several amino acids, which function as essential synaptic transmitters, chemical messengers for sending (or inhibiting) nerve impulses across synapses of connecting nerve endings.

Niacin equivalent (NE) Current international measure for recommended amounts of B vitamin niacin that accounts for both the preformed vitamin and the amino acid precursor tryptophan, from which the vitamin can be synthesized. Thus 1 NE equals 1 g niacin or 60 mg dietary tryptophan.

Nitrogen balance The metabolic balance between nitrogen intake in dietary protein and output in urinary nitrogen compounds such as urea and creatinine. For every 6.25 g dietary protein consumed 1 g nitrogen is excreted.

Nonheme iron The larger portion of dietary iron, including all the plant food sources and 60% of the animal food sources, that lacks the more easily absorbed and bioavailable heme iron in the remaining 40% of the animal food sources that contain hemoglobin residues of iron-containing heme.

Normochromic Normal red blood cell color.

Normocytic Normal cell size.

Nulliparity (L *nullus,* none; *parere,* to bring forth) Reproductive status of a woman who has never borne a viable child.

Nutrient density The protein, vitamin, or mineral content of a food expressed in relation to its energy (caloric) content.

Nutrition assessment (L *nutritio,* nourishment; *assessare,* to assess, to estimate property or income value for purposes of taxation) Process of determining individual or group nutritional status as a basis for identifying needs and goals and planning personal health care or community programs to meet these identified goals.

Nutrition care plan The person-centered care plan, based on nutritional assessment data and evaluation, for individual nutritional care and education to promote health and prevent or treat disease.

Nutrition education The process of helping individuals obtain the knowledge, skills, and motivation needed to make appropriate food choices for positive health throughout life.

Nutrition environment (L *nutritio,* nourishment; Fr *environner,* to surround, encircle) The sum of substances, materials, and processes involved in taking in food and nutrients and assimilating and using them for body health and strength.

Nutrition label Food product label providing nutrition information concerning nutrient and energy values per designated size portion.

Nutritional status (L *status,* condition, situation) Condition of an individual's body tissues and health, especially as related to the nutrients that are essential to the structure, function, and maintenance of body tissues.

Obligatory nitrogen loss The lowest level of nitrogen excretion that can be reached by an individual despite all body conservation mechanisms.

Odd-numbered carbon-chain fatty acids Most fatty acid carbon chains in the human diet are even numbered, broken down by beta oxidation, successively clipping off 2-carbon fragments of *acetyl-CoA* to feed into the final energy production pathway, the citric acid cycle. A few odd-numbered ones do exist, however. When they do occur, they go through the same beta-oxidation process, clipping off 2-carbon fragments until the final 3-carbon residue remains, *proprionyl-CoA,* which is also an intermediate metabolic product of the essential amino acid threonine. These 3-carbon fragments from both sources are converted to *succinyl-CoA,* a 4-carbon compound in the citric acid cycle, so they feed into the final energy production cycle at this point.

Oligosaccharides (Gr *oligos,* little; *saccharide,* sugar) Intermediate products of polysaccharide carbohydrate breakdown, containing a small number (from 4 to 10) of single sugar units of the monosaccharide glucose.

Omega-3 fatty acids Group of long chain polyunsaturated fatty acids having important precursor roles in producing highly active hormone-like substances, the *eicosanoids,* involved in critical metabolic activities such as vascular muscle tone and blood clotting.

Omnivorous (L *omnia,* all; *vorare,* to eat) Eating all kinds of foods, from both animal and plant sources.

Organohalides (Gr *organon,* organ; Chem *halides,* compounds of fluorine, chlorine, bromine, or iodine) Chemical compounds used as pesticides or in industrial processes, for example, DDT and PCBs.

Orofacial muscles (L *os, oris,* mouth) Adjoining muscles of the mouth and face.

Osmolality (Gr *osmos,* impulsion through a membrane) Property of a solution that depends on the concentration of the particles (solutes) in solution per unit of solvent base; measured as milliosmoles per liter (mOsm/L).

Osteoarthritis (Gr *osteon* + *arthron,* joint; *-itis,* inflammation) A form of arthritis in which joints undergo degenerative changes resulting in stiffness, pain, and swelling; arthritis in the hip, knee, or spine can result in some degree of disability.

Osteomalacia (Gr *osteon,* bone; *malakia,* softness) Condition marked by softening of the bones due to impaired mineralization with excess accumulation of osteoid (immature young bone matrix that has not had mineralization to harden it); results from deficiency of vitamin D and calcium.

Osteoporosis (Gr *osteon,* bone; *poros,* passage, pore) Abnormal thinning of bone, producing a porous, fragile, lattice-like bone tissue of enlarged spaces, prone to fracture or deformity.

Ovulation Monthly process in female sexual cycle of secreting a mature ovum for transport through the fallopian tubes to the uterus.

Ovum (L *ovum,* egg) The female reproductive cell (egg) capable of fertilization and development into a new organism.

Oxalic acid A compound in a variety of foods, including green leafy vegetables, corn, soy products such as tofu, and wheat germ, that binds calcium in the food mix and hinders its absorption.

Oxyhemoglobin Hemoglobin with bound oxygen for transport by the red blood cells from the lungs to the body tissue cells for vital metabolic work.

Oxytocin (Gr *oxys,* sharp, sour; *tokos,* birth) Pituitary hormone causing uterine contractions and milk ejection.

Palate (L *palatum,* palate) The partition separating the nasal and oral cavities, with a hard bony front section and a soft fleshy back section.

Palmar grasp Early grasp of the young infant, clasping an object in the palm and wrapping the whole hand around it.

Paraprofessional (Gr *para-,* along side) A nonprofessional person, often from the community being served and thus having valuable insights concerning needs, who is trained to assist the professional community or clinical nutrition specialist in carrying out the nutrition program.

Parenteral nutrition (Gr *para,* beyond, beside; *enteron,* intestine) Nourishment received not through the gastrointestinal tract but rather by an alternate route such as injection into a vein; intravenous feeding of elemental nutrients.

Parietal cells (L *parietes,* wall) Cells lining the stomach that secrete hydrochloric acid; chief cells.

Parity (L *parere,* to bring forth, produce) Number of pregnancies a woman has had producing viable offspring.

Parkinson's disease A neurologic disorder, described by English physician James Parkinson (1755-1824), characterized by tremor, muscular rigidity, and abnormally decreased motor function and ability, affecting mobility.

Parturition (L *parturitio,* to give birth) Act or process of childbirth; maternal labor and delivery.

Pattern for daily food choices Expanded accompaniment to dietary guidelines to apply them to practical meal planning.

Percentile (L *per,* through; *centrum,* a hundred, "by the hundred") Rate or proportion per hundred; statistical term indicating status of a value in relation to 100 equal parts of a series of values in order of their measurable magnitude. For example, a value at the 60th percentile would mean that 60% of all the values in the distribution of the population studies lie at or below the 60th percentile, 40% above it.

Perinatal mortality (Gr *peri-,* around; L *natus,* born) Infant deaths in the perinatal period, shortly before and after birth, approximately from week 20-28 of gestation to 1-4 weeks postpartum, per 1000 live births.

Periodontal disease (Gr *peri,* around + *odove,* tooth) Inflammation and breakdown of the tissues and ligaments that surround the tooth and hold it in place; peridontal disease is often the cause of tooth loss in older people.

Peristalsis (Gr *peri,* around; *stalsia,* contraction) A wave-like progression of alternate contraction and relaxation of the muscle fibers of the gastrointestinal tract.

Pernicious anemia A chronic macrocytic anemia occurring most commonly after age 40; caused by absence of the intrinsic factor normally present in the gastric juices and necessary for the absorption of cobalamin (B_{12}); controlled by intramuscular injections of vitamin B_{12}.

Phagocytosis (Gr *phagein,* to eat; *-cyte,* hollow vessel, anything that contains or covers) The engulfing of microorganisms, other cells, or foreign particles by phagocytes.

pH Power of the hydrogen ion (H^+), a measure indicating degree of acidity or alkalinity of solutions. A pH of 7.0 indicates neutrality, with numbers above it indicating increasing alkalinity and those below increasing acidity.

Pharynx (Gr *pharynx,* throat) The muscular membranous passage between the mouth and the posterior nasal passages and the larynx and esophagus.

Phenylketonuria (PKU) A genetic disease caused by a missing enzyme, phenylalanine hydroxylase, required for the metabolic conversion of the essential amino acid phenylalanine to the amino acid tyrosine. Untreated, profound mental retardation occurs. Normal growth and development now follows current mandatory newborn screening and immediate initiation of a low phenylalanine diet with special "low-phe" formula such as Lofenalac.

Physiologic age Rate of biologic maturation in individual adolescents which varies widely and accounts, far more than does chronologic age, for wide and changing differences in their metabolic rates, nutritional needs, and food requirements.

Phytic acid A compound in certain grains, such as wheat, that binds calcium and hinders its absorption.

Pincer grasp Later digital grasp of the older infant, usually picking up smaller objects with a precise grip between thumb and forefinger.

Pinocytosis (Gr *pinein,* to drink; *kytos,* cell) The uptake of fluid nutrient material by a living cell by means of incupping and invagination of the cell membrane, which closes off and forms free cell vacuoles.

Placebo (L *placere,* to please) An inactive substance or preparation used in controlled drug or nutrient studies to determine the efficacy of an agent under study.

Placenta (L *placentas,* a flat cake) A characteristic organ of mammals during pregnancy joining mother and offspring, providing supportive nourishment and endocrine secretions for embryonic-fetal development and growth.

Polymer (Gr *poly-,* many; *meros,* part) A large compound formed by chains of simpler repeating molecules, for example, the glucose polymer oligosaccharide.

Postpartum (L *post,* after; *partum,* separate part) Period following childbirth or delivery.

Postprandial Following a meal.

Poverty line The minimum income required to provide the basic necessities of food, clothing, and shelter for an individual or family as determined by a U.S. government agency.

Precursor A substance from which another substance is produced.

Preeclampsia (Gr *pre-*, before; *eklampein*, to shine forth) Abnormal condition of late pregnancy marked by rather sudden hypertension and increased edema, usually accompanied by proteinuria; may progress to eclampsia with convulsions and coma; better prevented by good prenatal care and optimal nutrition throughout the pregnancy.

Preterm milk Milk produced by mothers of premature infants.

Preventive approach Positive health care that seeks to identify and reduce risk factors for disease.

Primigravida (L *prima*, first; *gravida*, pregnant) A woman pregnant for the first time.

Primiparous (L *prima*, first; *parere*, to bring forth) State of a woman bearing or having borne only one child.

Primordial follicle Primitive ovarian follicle (*follis*, a leather bag), formed during fetal life; a sac- or pouch-like cavity, a small secretory sac or gland; an ovarian follicle, ovum surrounded by specialized epithelial cells.

Primordial ova (L *primordia*, the beginning; *ovum*, egg) Primitive ova cells produced in large life-supply numbers in the female fetal ovaries before birth.

Progesterone Ovarian hormone that regulates secretory function of the mucosal linings of the uterus and fallopian tubes, and stimulates development of milk-producing structures of the breast.

Prolactin (Gr *pro-*, before; L *lac*, milk) A hormone of the anterior pituitary gland that stimulates and maintains lactation in postpartum mothers.

Prophylactic (Gr *prophylassein*, to keep guard before) Preventive treatment to avoid disease, for example, vitamin K for newborns to prevent the formerly widespread hemorrhagic disease of newborns, since they are born with a sterile gastrointestinal tract and lack the microorganisms that synthesize vitamin K.

Proprietary (L *proprietarius*, owner) Referring to commercial products such as infant formulas and medical items that are designed, manufactured, and sold for profit only by the owner of the patent, formula, brand name, or trademark associated with the product.

Prostaglandins Highly active hormone-like eicosanoid substances produced from essential fatty acid precursors and acting locally in various body tissues with many physiologic effects.

Protein turnover The metabolic process in the body by which proteins are being constantly synthesized, broken down, and the resulting amino acids resynthesized into new proteins.

Proteolytic (Gr *protos*, first, protein; *lysis*, dissolution) Protein-splitting by a series of enzymes through hydrolysis of the peptide bonds into smaller peptides and amino acids.

Prothrombin (Gr *pro-*, before; *thrombos*, clot) Blood-clotting factor (number II), synthesized in the liver from glutamic acid and CO_2, catalyzed by vitamin K.

Protocol (Gr *protokollon*, leaf or tag attached to a rolled papyrus manuscript containing notes as to its contents) A set of governing rules; the plan and procedures for carrying out a scientific study or a person's treatment regimen.

Psychotropic (Gr *psyche* + *trepein*, to turn) To exert an effect on the mind, altering behavior, mental activity, or emotional experience.

Pubertal development The rapid physical growth and sexual development of puberty.

Pyridoxine Chemical name for vitamin B_6, derived from its ring-like structure. In its active form, pyridoxal phosphate, it acts as a coenzyme factor in many types of transamination and decarboxylation reactions in amino acid metabolism.

Radioimmunoassay (L *radius*, ray; *immunis*, free, exempt; *assay*, examine, analyze) Technique using radioactive labeling of the material being studied, for measuring minute quantities of antigen or antibody, hormones, certain drugs, and other substances.

Recommended Dietary Allowances (RDAs) Nutrient and energy standards for healthy population groups in the United States by age and sex, updated every 4-5 years by expert committees of scientists to reflect current research, and issued by the National Research Council of the National Institutes of Health.

Renal solute load Collective number and concentration of solute particles in solution, carried by the blood to the kidney nephrons for excretion in the urine, usually nitrogenous products from protein metabolism, and the electrolytes Na^+, K^+, Cl^-, and HPO_4^{--}.

Requirement The amount of a nutrient that

when fed to a human or animal will prevent the appearance of deficiency symptoms and maintain health.

Resorption (L *resorbere,* to swallow again) The process by which bone is lost; the mineral crystals are dissolved and the protein matrix is broken down and removed.

Resting energy expenditure (REE) Energy expended by a person at rest in a neutral surrounding temperature, neither hot nor cold; similar to other measures of energy needs, such as the classic test of basal metabolic rate (BMR) and the calculated basal energy expenditure (BEE). The three values are often used interchangeably.

Retinol Chemical name for vitamin A derived from its function relating to the retina of the eye and light-dark adaptation. Daily RDA standards are stated in retinol equivalents (RE) to account for sources of the preformed vitamin A and its precursor provitamin A beta-carotene.

Retinol equivalent (RE) Unit of measure for dietary sources of vitamin A, both preformed vitamin, retinol, and the precursor provitamin, beta-carotene. 1 RE = μg retinol or 6 μg beta-carotene.

Reverse peristalsis (Gr *peri-,* around; *stalsis,* contraction) Wave-like contractions of longitudinal and circular muscles of the gastrointestinal tract that normally propel the food mass forward, but may act in reverse in upper GI tract of young infants causing easy spitting up of milk.

Salicylates Compound salts of salicylic acid, found in certain plants and in drugs such as common aspirin (acetylsalicylic acid—ASA).

Senescence (L *senescere,* to grow old) Normal process or condition of growing old.

Senile dementia of the Alzheimer type (SDAT) A type of senile dementia first described by German physician Alois Alzheimer (1864-1915); causes progressive, irreversible degenerative changes in the brain, resulting in loss of neuromuscular function and mental capacity.

Sexual maturity ratings Scale defining stages of sexual maturation during puberty.

Simple carbohydrates The monosaccharides glucose, fructose, and galactose, and the disaccharides sucrose, maltose, and lactose.

Skeletal muscle Muscles attached to skeletal bones for control of body movements; major component of lean body mass.

Sociodemographic Relating to the characteristic social and cultural values, geographic distribution, and physical environments of persons and populations.

Solutes (Gr *solvere,* to dissolve) Particles of a substance in solution; a solution consists of solutes and a dissolving medium (solvent), usually a liquid.

Stereotype An oversimplified and generalized conception or image held by persons and groups that have distorted or unreal meaning, but influences attitudes and behavior of persons holding such views.

Stress Sum of biologic reactions to adverse stimuli, physical, mental, or emotional, internal or external, that disturbs the state of homeostasis and sense of well-being.

Sucrase Intestinal enzyme that splits the disaccharide sucrose into its two component monosaccharides glucose and fructose.

Supine Lying on the back.

Tactile (L *tactio,* to touch) Sense of touching, perception by the touch.

Tannic acid Compound of certain plants such as tea leaves, giving an astringent taste and having astringent properties that promote local tissue healing; an herbal remedy.

Tetany (Gr *teinein,* to stretch) Condition caused by decrease in ionized serum calcium, marked by intermittent spastic muscle contractions and muscular pain; manifest by characteristic carpopedal spasm of the arm muscles causing flexion of the wrist and thumb with extension of the fingers, called *Trousseau's sign.* A so-called "milk tetany" has been reported in young infants fed undiluted cow's milk, due to the greater ratio of phosphorus to calcium in cow's milk than in human milk, and these infants could not clear the phosphate load, which then accumulated in the blood and caused a compensatory decrease in the serum calcium, resulting in the typical muscular spasms of tetany.

Tidal volume The amount of gases, oxygen, and carbon dioxide passing into and out of the lungs in each respiratory cycle.

Title III-C The statute of the Older Americans Act authorizing congregate and home-delivered meals for people age 60 and over.

Tocopherol (Gr *tokos,* childbirth; *pherein,* to carry) Chemical name for vitamin E, so named by early investigators because their initial work with rats indicated a reproductive function, which did not turn out later to be the case with humans, in whom it functions as a strong antioxidant to preserve structural membranes such as cell walls.

Tonsils (L *tonsilla*, tonsil) Small rounded mass of lymphoid tissue in the roof and posterior wall of the nasopharynx.

Trabeculae (L *trabs*, a little beam) Small bones at the ends of long bones at joints such as wrist, vertebrae, and hips.

Trabecular bone General term for small meshwork of bones at ends of long bones forming attached joints, and part of the connecting network between vertebrae.

Trace elements Minerals that occur in small amounts or traces in the body, and hence are required in very small amounts.

Tretinoin A form of retinoic acid, a vitamin A derivative, used as a drug in the medical treatment of chronic acne as a topical keralytic agent (Gr *keras*, horn; *lysis*, dissolution). Keratin is a hard protein; it is the principal constituent of skin, hair, nails, and scar tissue.

Triglyceride Chemical name for fat, indicating structure: attachment of three fatty acids to a glycerol base. A neutral fat, synthesized from carbohydrate, stored in adipose tissue. It releases free fatty acids into the blood when hydrolyzed by enzymes.

Trophoblast (Gr *trophe*, nutrition; *blastos*, embryo, germ) Extraembryonic ectodermal tissue on the surface of the cleaving, fertilized ovum, that is responsible for contact with the maternal circulation and supply of nutrients to the embryo.

Trypsin (Gr *trypein*, to rub; *pepsis*, digestion) A protein-splitting enzyme formed in the intestine by action of enterokinase on the inactive precursor trypsinogen.

Trypsin inhibitor A natural substance in raw soybeans that is responsible for a toxin in the bean. Fortunately this substance is destroyed by heat and rendered inactive.

Ulnar deviation Turning and articulation of the *ulna* (inner and larger bone of the forearm on the side opposite the thumb) with the wrist joint to accomplish coordinated movement of the wrist and hand.

U.S. dietary guidelines A set of seven statements to guide food choices that reflect current health promotion and disease prevention national health objectives.

U.S. RDA A condensed food-labeling version of the regular National Research Council's Recommended Dietary Allowances, not to be confused with the regular NRC standards. This U.S. RDA, set up by the FDA in 1974 to replace the old minimum daily requirements (MDA), was compiled at the time from the 1968 regular RDAs using the highest value within age/sex categories. Cost of label changing prevents updating with revised RDA editions, causing confusion to consumers.

Vascular spaces Spaces within fluid vessels in the body, blood vessels and lymph vessels; contain body fluids in transit, greater amount in blood and remainder in the interconnecting lymphatic system.

Vasodilation (L *vas*, vessel; *dilatare*, to spread out) Expansion or stretching of a blood vessel.

Vasopressin Hormone formed in the hypothalamus and stored in the posterior pituitary gland. Stimulates muscle contraction of capillaries and arterioles to maintain blood pressure and acts on the epithelial cells of the distal tubule of the nephron to cause water reabsorption, producing a concentrated urine and preventing water loss. Thus it is also called the antidiuretic hormone (ADH).

Vegan diet Strict vegetarian diet allowing no animal protein; requires careful food combinations of incomplete plant proteins to complement one another and achieve an overall adequacy of essential amino acids for growth needs.

Venipuncture A technique in which a vein is punctured through the skin by a sharp, rigid stylet or cannula carrying a flexible plastic catheter or by a steel needle attached to a syringe or catheter.

Venous stasis (L *venosus*, vein; Gr *stasis*, standing still) A stoppage, or decreased flow, of blood in the veins draining an organ causing engorgement of the affected vessels and tissues.

Vesicle (L *vesica*, bladder) A small bladder or sac containing liquid; secretory transport sacs that move out into the cell cytoplasm to aid metabolism.

Visceral organs (L *viscus*, large body organ) Large internal organs of the body, located in the chest and abdomen.

Vital capacity Volume of air moved in and out of the lungs with each breath. The residual volume is the amount of air remaining in the lungs after the person has exhaled.

Vitamin A non–energy-yielding micronutrient

required in very small amounts for specific metabolic tasks, but cannot be synthesized by the body so must be supplied in the diet.

Water intoxication An abnormal increase in the amount of water in the body; sodium concentration of body fluids is lowered causing confusion, stupor, seizures, and harmful effects on the central nervous system.

Wellness approach An approach to health care that promotes the planning of a healthy positive lifestyle for maintaining physical and mental well-being.

Whey The thin liquid of milk remaining after the curd, containing the major protein casein, and the cream have been removed; contains other milk proteins lactalbumin and lactoferrin.

Xerostomia (Gr *xeros,* dry; *stoma,* mouth) Dryness of the mouth from lack of normal secretions.

Index

NOTE: Page numbers in italics indicate illustrations; *t* indicates tables.

Median Heights and Weights and Recommended Energy Intake

Category	Age (years) or Condition	Weight (kg)	Weight (lb)	Height (cm)	Height (in)	REE[a] (kcal/day)	Average Energy Allowance (kcal)[b] Multiples of REE	Per kg	Per day[c]
Infants	0.0–0.5	6	13	60	24	320		108	650
	0.5–1.0	9	20	71	28	500		98	850
Children	1–3	13	29	90	35	740		102	1,300
	4–6	20	44	112	44	950		90	1,800
	7–10	28	62	132	52	1,130		70	2,000
Males	11–14	45	99	157	62	1,440	1.70	55	2,500
	15–18	66	145	176	69	1,760	1.67	45	3,000
	19–24	72	160	177	70	1,780	1.67	40	2,900
	25–50	79	174	176	70	1,800	1.60	37	2,900
	51 +	77	170	173	68	1,530	1.50	30	2,300
Females	11–14	46	101	157	62	1,310	1.67	47	2,200
	15–18	55	120	163	64	1,370	1.60	40	2,200
	19–24	58	128	164	65	1,350	1.60	38	2,200
	25–50	63	138	163	64	1,380	1.55	36	2,200
	51 +	65	143	160	63	1,280	1.50	30	1,900
Pregnant	1st Trimester								+ 0
	2nd Trimester								+ 300
	3rd Trimester								+ 300
Lactating	1st 6 months								+ 500
	2nd 6 months								+ 500

[a] Resting energy expenditure (REE); calculation based on FAO equations, then rounded.

[b] In the range of light to moderate activity, the coefficient of variation is ±20%.

[c] Figure is rounded.